STUDENT WORKBOOK FOR USE WITH

MEDICAL ASSISTING

Administrative and Clinical Procedures with Anatomy and Physiology

Kathryn A. Booth, RN-BSN, RMA (AMT), RPT, CPhT, MS
Total Care Programming, Inc.

Leesa G. Whicker, BA, CMA (AAMA)
Central Piedmont Community College

Terri D. Wyman, CPC, CMRS
Wing Memorial Hospital

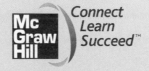

Connect
Learn
Succeed™

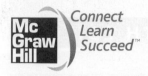

Student Workbook for use with Medical Assisting: Administrative and Clinical Procedures with Anatomy and Physiology, Fifth Edition
Kathryn A. Booth, Leesa G. Whicker, and Terri D. Wyman

Published by McGraw-Hill, a business unit of The McGraw-Hill Companies, Inc., 1221 Avenue of the Americas, New York, NY 10020. Copyright © 2014 by The McGraw-Hill Companies, Inc.

6 7 8 9 0 RMN/RMN 1 0 9 8 7 6 5

ISBN   978-0-07-752588-0
MHID   0-07-752588-4

Cover Image: *bottom 2 hands:* © Violin/ww.fotosearch.com; *Juggling balls:* © Thomas J Peterson, gettyimages.

WARNING NOTICE: The clinical procedures, medicines, dosages, and other matters described in this publication are based upon research of current literature and consultation with knowledgeable persons in the field. The procedures and matters described in this text reflect currently accepted clinical practice. However, this information cannot and should not be relied upon as necessarily applicable to a given individual's case. Accordingly, each person must be separately diagnosed to discern the patient's unique circumstances. Likewise, the manufacturer's package insert for current drug product information should be consulted before administering any drug. Publisher disclaims all liability for any inaccuracies, omissions, misuse, or misunderstanding of the information contained in this publication. Publisher cautions that this publication is not intended as a substitute for the professional judgment of trained medical personnel.

The Internet addresses listed in the text were accurate at the time of publication. The inclusion of a website does not indicate an endorsement by the authors or McGraw-Hill, and McGraw-Hill does not guarantee the accuracy of the information presented at these sites.

www.mhhe.com

Contents

Procedures

INSTRUCTIONS FOR THE PROCEDURE COMPETENCY CHECKLISTS

General Instructions
Review and practice the correct performance of each procedure prior to attempting the procedure. The rationales for all critical steps are given in the performance guidelines within your textbook. Review these steps and rationales carefully before beginning the procedure. As you become more proficient in the procedure, you should perform the procedure without guidance from the textbook or the reviewer. In any procedure, certain steps are considered to be more "important" than others. These steps are referred to as **critical steps**. If any of these steps are missed or performed incorrectly, you should continue to practice the procedure to perfect the technique. Steps with an * are considered critical steps.

Scoring System
The scoring system is based on 100 points so that they are easily converted to 100 percent. Each step has been given a point value based on its importance to completing the procedure. Note that steps with an * are considered **critical steps**. If a critical step is not done correctly, you may be considered unsuccessful in completing the procedure during that attempt.

PROCEDURES LIST

The *Student Workbook* provides you with an opportunity to review and master the concepts and skills introduced in your student textbook, *Medical Assisting: Administrative and Clinical Procedures with Anatomy and Physiology*, Fifth Edition. Chapter by chapter, the workbook provides the following:

Vocabulary Review, which tests your knowledge of key terms introduced in the chapter. Formats for these exercises include Matching, True or False, and Passage Completion.

Content Review, which tests your knowledge of key concepts introduced in the chapter. Formats for these exercises include Multiple Choice, Sentence Completion, and Short Answer (including labeling).

Critical Thinking, which tests your understanding of key concepts introduced in the chapter. These questions require you to use higher-level thinking skills, such as comprehension, analysis, synthesis, and evaluation.

Applications, which provide opportunities to apply the concepts and skills introduced in the chapter. For example, using role play, you will perform such activities as developing a personal career plan and interviewing a medical specialist.

Case Studies, which provide opportunities to apply the concepts introduced in the chapter to lifelike situations you will encounter as a medical assistant. For example, you may be asked to decide how to respond to a patient who calls the doctor's office to say that she is having difficulty breathing or you may be requested to give information about the thyroid gland to a patient who has just been referred for thyroid testing.

Procedure Competency Checklists, which enable you to monitor your mastery of the steps in the procedure(s) introduced in a chapter, such as Preparing a Patient Medical Record/Chart and Performing a Surgical Scrub. Each procedure is correlated with the CAAHEP and ABHES competencies you will need to know to become a medical assistant. Answers to the material in the *Student Workbook* are found in the *Instructor Manual,* on the *Online Learning Center.*

Procedure Work Documentation Forms, for both Administrative and Clinical procedures, are provided in a separate new section. These forms can be used when practicing and testing your skills. Make extra copies because you may use them more than once.

Ask your instructor for permission to check your work against these answers.

Together, your student textbook and the *Student Workbook* form a complete learning package. *Medical Assisting: Administrative and Clinical Procedures with Anatomy and Physiology,* Fifth Edition, will prepare you to enter the medical assisting field with the knowledge and skills necessary to become a useful resource to patients and a valued asset to employers and to the medical assisting profession.

Introduction to Medical Assisting

Name_____ Class_____ Date_____

R E V I E W

Vocabulary Review

Matching

Match the key terms in the right column with the definitions in the left column by placing the letter of each correct answer in the space provided.

_____ 1. Education or training received after a medical assistant is credentialed

_____ 2. The only professional association devoted exclusively to the medical assisting profession

_____ 3. Official authorization or approval of schools or programs that teach medical assisting

_____ 4. The granting of a title or license by a board that gives permission to practice in a profession

_____ 5. Government regulations that help ensure continuity and privacy of healthcare

_____ 6. The credential earned by taking an AAMA-approved course and passing the licensing exam

_____ 7. Skills and knowledge attained for both personal development and career advancement

_____ 8. An organization that accredits both public and private postsecondary institutions that offer medical assisting programs

_____ 9. The credential earned by taking an AMT-approved course and passing the licensing exam

_____ 10. A computer-generated document that summarizes your employment and educational history

_____ 11. An organization that accredits private postsecondary institutions that offer medical assisting programs

_____ 12. A professional organization for medical assistants and other allied healthcare personnel

_____ 13. Confirmation by an organization that an individual is qualified to perform a job to professional standards

_____ 14. Training for other jobs in your department or in other departments, in addition to medical assisting

a. ABHES
b. accreditation
c. AAMA
d. AMT
e. certification
f. CAAHEP
g. CMA
h. continuing education
i. cross-training
j. HIPAA
k. professional development
l. RMA
m. registration
n. résumé

True or False

Decide whether each statement is true or false. In the space at the left, write T for true or F for false. On the lines provided, rewrite the false statements to make them true.

_____ 15. The current trend to hire multiskilled individuals increases the cost of healthcare.

_____

_____ 16. The American Association of Medical Assistants (AAMA) works to raise standards of medical assisting to a professional level.

_____

_____ 17. You do not need to pass the American Medical Technologists certification examination to qualify as a Registered Medical Assistant (RMA).

_____

_____ 18. A Certified Medical Assistant [CMA (AAMA)] credential is automatically renewed.

_____

_____ 19. Accreditation is the process by which programs are officially authorized.

_____

_____ 20. Externships are voluntary in accredited schools.

_____

_____ 21. When a medical assistant is able to perform many duties in the office, the medical assistant is considered to be cross-trained.

_____

_____ 22. The Medical Assistant Occupational Analysis provides the basis for education and evaluation in the medical assistant field.

_____

Content Review

Multiple Choice

In the space provided, write the letter of the choice that best completes each statement or answers each question.

_____ 1. To receive certification or registration as a medical assistant, you must
   a. Graduate from an approved program with a bachelor's degree in medical assisting
   b. Become a member of the AAMA or American Medical Technologists (AMT)
   c. Graduate from an approved medical assistant program and pass the AAMA or AMT examination
   d. Pass the AAMA or AMT examination
   e. Become a multiskilled professional

_____ 2. Formal training programs in medical assisting
   a. Are offered only at 2-year colleges
   b. Can be replaced by on-the-job training
   c. Must be approved by the AAMA
   d. Last 9 months to 2 years and award a certificate, diploma, or associate degree
   e. Result in a bachelor's degree in nursing

_____ 3. Entry-level duties of a clinical medical assistant are *most* likely to include which of the following?

  a. Payroll

  b. Phlebotomy

  c. Insurance processing

  d. Answering telephones

  e. Bookkeeping

_____ 4. The organization that was established in 1989 as an information resource and network for healthcare professionals is the

  a. National Healthcareer Association

  b. National Center for Competency Testing

  c. National Association for Health Professionals

  d. American Medical Technologists

  e. American Association of Medical Assistants

_____ 5. Confirmation by an organization that an individual is qualified to perform a job to professional standards is

  a. Registration

  b. Certification

  c. Accreditation

  d. Professional development

  e. Continuing education

Short Answer

Write the answer to each question on the lines provided.

6. List three administrative duties performed by a medical assistant.

_____

_____

_____

7. List three clinical duties performed by a medical assistant.

_____

_____

_____

8. List three laboratory duties performed by a medical assistant.

_____

_____

_____

9. List three reasons why credentialing is important for a medical assistant's entry and advancement in the medical environment.

_____

_____

_____

10. Why is continuing education important for medical assistants?

_____

_____

_____

Critical Thinking

Write the answer to each question on the lines provided.

1. Explain the importance of making sure the medical assisting program you choose is accredited.

_____

_____

_____

2. Why do accredited medical assisting programs require an externship?

_____

_____

_____

3. What is *scope of practice*, and why is it important to know what your scope of practice includes?

_____

_____

_____

A P P L I C A T I O N

Follow the directions for each application.

1. AAMA Creed

Go to the website for the AAMA (www.aama-ntl.org) and look up the AAMA Medical Assistant Creed. Write each of the eight statements in the Creed as follows. Then choose one statement, circle it, and give an example on the following lines of a situation in which the statement might apply.

Statement 1: _____

Statement 2: _____

Statement 3: _____

Statement 4: _____

Statement 5: _____

Statement 6: _____

Statement 7: _____

Statement 8: _____

_____

_____

_____

_____

2. AAMA Code of Ethics

Go to the website for the AAMA (www.aama-ntl.org) and look up the AAMA Medical Assistant Code of Ethics. What five things do medical assistants pledge to strive to accomplish?

a. _____

b. _____

c. _____

d. _____

e. _____

Choose one of the preceding items and explain how following this guideline can help a medical assistant (1) do a better job and (2) advance his or her career.

_____

_____

_____

_____

C A S E   S T U D I E S

Write your response to each case study on the lines provided.

Case 1

Suppose you work as a medical assistant in a cardiologist's office. In your spare time, you read about new advances in heart medications. Even though only the physician can prescribe these medications, how might this knowledge help you in your job?

_____

_____

_____

Case 2

Your friend Ana started the medical assisting program at the same time you did. Both of you decide to volunteer at a local hospital to learn more about the field. Ana confides to you that she sometimes becomes queasy at the sight of blood or vomit, but she really wants to be a medical assistant. What advice might you give to Ana?

_____

_____

_____

PROCEDURE 1-1 Obtaining Certification/Registration Information through the Internet

Goal
To obtain information from the Internet regarding professional credentialing.

OSHA Guidelines
This procedure does not involve exposure to blood, body fluids, or tissue.

Materials
Computer with Internet access and printer.

Method

Step Number	Procedure	Points Possible	Points Earned
1.	Open an Internet browser and use a search engine to search for a medical assisting credential. If unsure of the credential you would like to pursue, you may just want to search for "Medical Assisting Credentials."	5	
2.	Select the site for the credential you are pursuing. Avoid sponsored links. These links are paid for and typically will not bring you to the site of a credentialing organization.*	10	
3.	Navigate to the home page: • For the CMA (AAMA) credential, enter the site www.aama-ntl.org. • For the RMA (AMT) or CMAS (AMT) credential, enter the site www.amt1.com.	10	
4.	Determine the steps you must take to obtain the selected credential.ˣ • For CMA (AAMA), go to the drop-down menu "CMA (AAMA) Exam" and select the link "How to Become a CMA (AAMA)." • For RMA (AMT), go to the menu on the left, click "Certification," and then select "Medical Assistant" for RMA (AMT). Navigate to the tab "Qualifications."	15	
5.	Print or write down the qualifications you must obtain. RATIONALE: Maintaining a record of needed qualifications will be a reference as you pursue your chosen credential.	10	
6.	Once you have met the qualifications, you will need to apply for the examination or certification. Download the application and the application instructions for the RMA (AMT) or the CMAS (AMT) or the candidate application and handbook for the CMA (AAMA).	5	
7.	To view or print these instructions, you may need to download Adobe Reader. You can click on a link to download Adobe Reader after you click on the "Apply for Certification" link for AMT or the "Apply for the CMA (AAMA) Exam" for AAMA.	5	
8.	Before or after you apply for the examination, you will need to prepare for the examination. Select the link "Prepare for the CMA (AAMA) Exam" on the AAMA site or the "Prepare for Exam" link under the "Medical Assistant" or "Medical Assistant Specialist" drop-down menus on the AMT site.	10	
9.	Prepare for the exam by reviewing the content outline, obtaining additional study resources, or taking a practice exam online.*	10	

(continued)

Copyright © 2014 by The McGraw-Hill Companies, Inc.

Step Number	Procedure	Points Possible	Points Earned
10.	Print or save downloaded information in a file folder on your desktop labeled "Credentials" or something that you can recognize. To print, click on the printer icon found at the bottom of the Web page or click on the printer icon in your browser.	10	
11.	Return to the appropriate site if you have additional questions. For the CMA (AAMA) site, you may want to check the "FAQs on CMA (AAMA) Certification" link. On the AMT site for RMA or CMAS, click on the "Take Exam" link and download the FAQs regarding the testing process.	5	
12.	Any questions you have that are not addressed on the sites can be e-mailed to the organizations. For RMA, send an e-mail to the link rma@amt1.com. On the AAMA site for the CMA credential, click on the "Contact" link on the top right-hand side of the screen.	5	
Total Points		100	

CAAHEP Competencies Achieved

    IX. C (5)   Discuss licensure and certification as it applies to healthcare providers

ABHES Competencies Achieved

    1. (c) Understand medical assistant credentialing requirements and the process to obtain the credential. Comprehend the importance of credentialing

Healthcare and the Healthcare Team

Name_____ Class_____ Date_____

R E V I E W

Vocabulary Review

Matching

Match the key terms in the right column with the definitions in the left column by placing the letter of each correct answer in the space provided.

_____ 1. The channels through which qi flows

_____ 2. Physicians who oversee and coordinate patients' long-term healthcare

_____ 3. Foods that have little or no processing before they are eaten

_____ 4. A life-threatening swelling of the airways or nasal passages

_____ 5. A sampling of cells that could be malignant or cancerous

_____ 6. Assessing the urgency and type of medical condition and immediate medical needs

_____ 7. Examination of the body of a deceased person to determine the cause of death

_____ 8. Screening tests and drugs to prevent disease

_____ 9. Education, exercise, and therapy for patients who have a cardiovascular disease or disorder

_____ 10. Fitness and general good health

_____ 11. A system of hands-on techniques that help relieve pain, restore motion, support the body's natural functions, and influence the body's structure

_____ 12. An electronic form of medical record that allows quick access to all of a patient's data

_____ 13. Physicians who have been educated, licensed, and certified by the American Board of Medical Specialties

a. anaphylactic shock
b. autopsy
c. biopsy
d. board-certified physician
e. cardiac rehabilitation
f. electronic health records
g. meridians
h. osteopathic manipulative medicine
i. preventive care
j. primary care physician
k. triage
l. wellness
m. whole foods

True or False

Decide whether each statement is true or false. In the space at the left, write T for true or F for false. On the lines provided, rewrite the false statements to make them true.

_____ 14. Baby boomers are people who were born between 1946 and 1964.

_____

_____ 15. Outpatient care is also known as ambient care.

_____

_____ **16.** The purpose of long-term care is to provide care for people who have fewer than six months to live.

_____

_____ **17.** Physicians who are generalists and treat all types of illnesses and ages of patients are known as *family practitioners.*

_____

_____ **18.** Endocrinologists stabilize patients who have a medical crisis, such as injury or sudden illness, so that they can then be managed by their PCP or other specialist.

_____

_____ **19.** Another term for a *geriatrician* is *gerontologist.*

_____

_____ **20.** Neurologists study, diagnose, and manage diseases of the kidney.

_____

_____ **21.** A radiographer is a medical doctor with a specialty in radiography.

_____

_____ **22.** A nutritionist has specialized training to assist ill patients with their nutritional needs.

_____

_____ **23.** Compliance officers create policies and procedures to help a facility avoid releasing information incorrectly.

_____

_____ **24.** Part of the job of a medical transcriptionist is to process insurance claims.

_____

_____ **25.** The American Hospital Association is a nonprofit organization that accredits healthcare organizations.

_____

Content Review

Multiple Choice

In the space provided, write the letter of the choice that best completes each statement or answers each question.

_____ **1.** Radiology is the branch of medical science that
  a. Is a subspecialty of neurology
  b. Uses X-rays and radioactive substances to diagnose and treat disease
  c. Provides the scientific foundation for all medical practice
  d. Studies and records the electrical activity of the brain
  e. Determines whether tumors are benign or malignant

_____ **2.** A professional who has studied the chemical and physical qualities of drugs and dispenses prescribed medications to the public is a
  a. Nurse practitioner   **d.** Pharmacist
  b. Physiatrist   **e.** Radiologist
  c. Oncologist

_____ **3.** Which of the following professionals takes health histories, performs physical exams, conducts screening tests, and educates patients and families about disease prevention?
  a. Occupational therapist   **d.** Licensed practical nurse
  b. Associate degree nurse   **e.** Clinical laboratory technician
  c. Independent nurse practitioner

Name_____ Class_____ Date_____

4. A healthcare professional who works under the direction of a physician and manages medical emergencies that occur away from the medical setting is a(n)
a. Emergency medical technician
b. Surgeon's assistant
c. Radiation therapy technologist
d. Physician assistant
e. Pathologist's assistant

5. In which of the following practices are you most likely to encounter patients with a variety of different diseases or conditions, as well as patients having wellness exams?
a. Gynecology
b. Gastroenterology
c. Emergency medicine
d. Cardiology
e. Family practice

6. In which medical specialty do physicians practice a "whole-person" approach to healthcare?
a. Surgery
b. Neurology
c. Nephrology
d. Osteopathy
e. Urology

7. Which specialty treats disorders involving hormones?
a. Gastroenterology
b. Gerontology
c. Endocrinology
d. Emergency medicine
e. Oncology

8. Which medical professional fills prescriptions for glasses and contact lenses?
a. Pharmacist
b. Optician
c. Ophthalmologist
d. Optometrist
e. Otolaryngologist

9. An RN who functions in an expanded nursing role to perform physical exams, conduct screening tests, and educate patients is a(n)
a. Nurse practitioner
b. Associate degree nurse
c. Baccalaureate nurse
d. Physician assistant
e. Licensed practical nurse

10. Which of the following professionals can prescribe medications, when state law permits?
a. Massage therapist
b. Registered nurse
c. Respiratory therapist
d. Physician assistant
e. Medical technologist

Sentence Completion

In the space provided, write the word or phrase that best completes each sentence.

11. Using therapy with electricity, heat, cold, ultrasound, massage, and exercise, a(n) _____ helps restore physical function and relieve pain following disease or injury.

12. A(n) _____ works with emotionally disturbed and mentally challenged patients and assists the psychiatric team.

13. Working under the supervision of a physician and a respiratory therapist, a(n) _____ performs procedures such as artificial ventilation.

14. _____ are allied health professionals trained to draw blood for diagnostic laboratory testing.

15. Working under the supervision of a physician or medical technologist, a(n) _____ performs routine procedures in hematology, serology, blood banking, urinalysis, microbiology, and clinical chemistry.

11. _____
12. _____
13. _____
14. _____
15. _____

Short Answer

Write the answer to each question on the lines provided.

16. When might a family practitioner send a patient to a specialist?

_____

_____

17. What is the difference between a gynecologist and an obstetrician/gynecologist?

_____

_____

18. What is the difference between an ophthalmologist and an optometrist?

_____

_____

19. Discuss the differences in the training and job duties of a licensed practical nurse (LPN) and a medical assistant.

_____

_____

_____

20. Explain the difference between an LPN and a registered nurse (RN).

_____

_____

_____

21. What is osteopathic manipulative medicine?

_____

_____

_____

22. Describe the manual treatments and diagnostic testing that chiropractors use to treat patients.

_____

_____

_____

23. Describe the principles of acupuncture.

_____

_____

_____

24. Describe two conditions that a proctologist would treat.

_____

_____

_____

Critical Thinking

Write the answer to each question on the lines provided.

1. What are the benefits of learning about the medical specialties and subspecialties?

_____

_____

_____

2. What are the differences between medical assistants and physician assistants?

_____

_____

_____

3. Discuss how a medical assistant may interact with other healthcare professionals or specialists.

_____

_____

_____

4. Compare a doctor of osteopathy (DO) to a chiropractor. How are their practices different? How are they similar or the same?

_____

_____

_____

A P P L I C A T I O N

Follow the directions for each application.

1. Specialist Interview

As a follow-up to studying the various specialties, choose a medical specialist to interview and report on your findings.

a. Review the specialty careers described in the textbook. Select one.

b. Check the telephone book or other sources to find specialists in the area you chose. Write down the names and phone numbers of three to five specialists.

c. Call the offices of the specialists until you find a specialist who will grant you a 15- to 30-minute interview. Make an appointment for the interview.

d. Prepare a list of 6 to 10 interview questions. Include questions that address the type and amount of education required, responsibilities and duties, and advantages and disadvantages of the specialty. Also include a question about what personal skills are required. Conclude by asking for advice that the specialist can offer someone interested in pursuing the specialty.

e. Dress professionally for the interview. Take your list of questions and a pen and paper or other recording device to the interview.

f. Conduct the interview, keeping it within the time limit you promised. Thank the specialist for her time.

g. Send a thank-you note to the specialist within a week of the interview.

h. Share your findings with your classmates through a format of your choice: oral presentation, written report, or interview "question and answer" news article.

2. Medical Specialties

Research the Internet for specialties in which a medical assistant may be employed. Research the credentials needed and the experience required for the job. Then find a position within the specialty and research what duties are performed by the position and how you may gain those skills. Report your findings to the class.

C A S E   S T U D I E S

Write your response to each case study on the lines provided.

Case 1

You are currently working for an internist who treats a variety of skin conditions, such as acne, eczema, and hives. A patient presents with a small lesion that has not healed in several months. The physician requests that you submit a referral to a dermatologist. Why would this patient seek medical care from a dermatologist instead of being treated by the internist?

_____

_____

_____

Case 2

You are working in an OB/GYN practice. One of your patients confides in you that her husband is suffering from the sexual dysfunction impotence. She would like her husband to seek medical attention for his condition, but she does not know what type of medical specialty treats this condition. What type of specialist should her husband see?

_____

_____

_____

Professionalism and Success

Name_____ Class_____ Date_____

R E V I E W

Vocabulary Review

Matching
Match the key terms in the right column with the definitions in the left column by placing the letter of each correct answer in the space provided.

_____ 1. Speaking on behalf of a patient's needs and well-being

_____ 2. Values of hard work held by employees

_____ 3. Feedback given to help improve performance

_____ 4. Attributes that enhance an individual's performance and career prospects

_____ 5. Striving for excellence on the job

_____ 6. Judgment based upon analysis

_____ 7. A step-by-step approach to critical thinking

_____ 8. Technical ability

_____ 9. Utilizing time to accomplish desired results

_____ 10. Variety of belief systems and social structures

a. constructive criticism
b. critical thinking
c. cultural diversity
d. hard skills
e. patient advocacy
f. problem solving
g. soft skills
h. time management
i. work ethic
j. work quality

Content Review

Multiple Choice
In the space provided, write the letter of the choice that best completes each statement or answers each question.

_____ 1. When interacting with patients of other cultures or ethnic groups,
   a. Assume that they have the same attitude toward modern medicine that you have
   b. Never involve other family members
   c. Never try to speak their language
   d. Never allow yourself to make value judgments
   e. Assume that modesty is not essential

_____ 2. A medical assistant shows integrity by
   a. Discussing patients with coworkers
   b. Being honest and dependable
   c. Refusing to help patients with insurance forms
   d. Wearing nicely groomed artificial nails
   e. Giving presents to pediatric patients

_____ **3.** Burnout from jobs and other conditions tends to build up stress. To avoid burnout, the medical assistant should

    a. Be realistic about his or her expectations and have balance in his or her life

    b. Feel good by spending more time on what he or she likes

    c. Discuss problems with patients and coworkers

    d. Become aggressive and stand up for himself/herself

    e. Avoid all stress

Short Answer

Write the answer to each question on the lines provided.

4. Place the steps of the problem-solving process in order on the drawing. Use the following steps:

- Analyze the potential solutions
- Evaluate the results
- Identify the effects of the problem
- Identify potential solutions
- Identify the problem
- Implement the best solution
- Identify the objectives or outcome

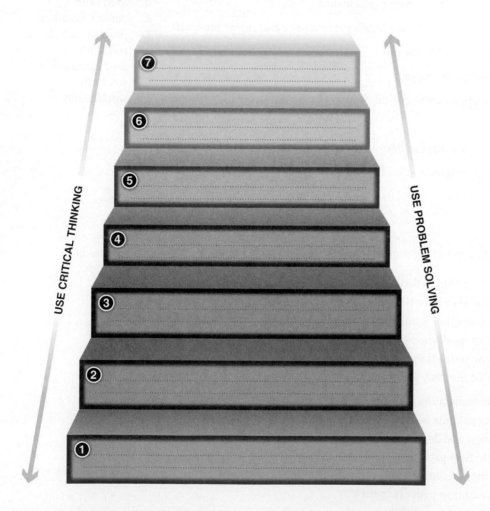

5. List five professional behaviors and then provide an example of how you should display that behavior as a medical assistant.

_____

_____

_____

6. You are getting behind with your classwork and made a failing grade on your last exam. How could you improve yourself or your behavior to be successful?

_____

_____

_____

7. Give five examples of hard skills performed by a medical assistant.

_____

_____

_____

8. Identify one thing that you consider good stress and one thing that you consider bad stress in your life

_____

_____

_____

Critical Thinking

Write the answer to each question on the lines provided.

1. You are sitting in the lounge having lunch with another medical assistant and she begins to gossip about a staff member who is not present. You do not like gossip but don't want to upset your coworker. What should you say?

_____

_____

_____

2. Why do you think the school has a strict policy on punctuality and attendance?

_____

_____

_____

3. Should tardiness be excused if it is not the student's fault?

_____

_____

_____

A P P L I C A T I O N

Follow the directions for each application.

1. **Appropriate Work Dress**

   Work with a partner to collect information on appropriate dress for work in a medical office.

   a. Request and collect uniform catalogs from the Internet. Here are two popular sites: www.Jascouniform.com and www.Allheart.com.

   b. Clip pictures of uniforms that you like and complete the "perfect" medical wardrobe.

   c. Research and find pictures of clothing and accessories that are not suitable for the medical profession.

   d. Make a collage of the two types of clothing—appropriate and inappropriate—and discuss with the class and instructor.

2. **Personal Qualifications of Medical Assistants**

   Make a list of at least 10 personal qualifications of medical assistants and write a sentence or two describing how these qualifications enhance quality patient care and contribute to professional relationships with the allied health team in the medical facility. Facilitate a class discussion about your statements.

3. **Qualities that Portray Confidence**

   Ask five people outside of your medical assisting program what gives them confidence in the staff in their doctor's office. Inform them they are not to include technical skills. Create a list and share it with your class.

4. **Schedule and Goals**

   Create a schedule for yourself for this course. Include your daily, weekly, and course completion goals. Write in detail what you need to do to accomplish each daily goal and include the amount of time to do so.

5. **Burnout Test**

   Unmanaged stress can often lead to job burnout in the profession of medical assisting. Answer the following questions *True* or *False* and check your score at the end to see if you are likely to become a victim of burnout.

   _____ 1. I feel that the people I know who are in authority are no better than I am.

   _____ 2. Once I start a job I have no peace until I finish it.

   _____ 3. I like to tell people exactly what I think.

   _____ 4. Although many people are overly conscious of feelings, I like to deal only with the facts.

   _____ 5. I worry about business and financial matters.

   _____ 6. I often have anxiety about something or someone.

   _____ 7. I sometimes become so preoccupied by a thought that I cannot get it out of my mind.

   _____ 8. I find it difficult to go to bed or to sleep because of the thoughts that bother me.

   _____ 9. I have periods in which I cannot sit or lie down; I need to be doing something.

   _____ 10. My mind is often occupied by thoughts about what I have done wrong or not completed.

   _____ 11. My concentration is not what it used to be.

   _____ 12. My personal appearance is not what it used to be.

   _____ 13. I feel irritated when I see another person's messy desk or cluttered room.

   _____ 14. I am more comfortable in a neat, clean, and orderly room than in a messy one.

   _____ 15. I cannot get through a day or a week without a schedule or a list of jobs to do.

   _____ 16. I believe that the person who works the hardest and longest deserves to get ahead.

   _____ 17. If my job/school/family responsibilities demand more time, I will cut out pleasurable activities to see that they get done.

_____ **18.** My conscience often bothers me about things I have done in the past.

_____ **19.** There are things that I have done that would embarrass me greatly if they become public knowledge.

_____ **20.** I feel uncomfortable unless I get the highest grade.

_____ **21.** It is my view that many people become confused because they do not bother to find out all the facts.

_____ **22.** I frequently feel angry without knowing what or who is bothering me.

_____ **23.** I can't stand to have my checkbook or financial matters out of balance.

_____ **24.** I think that talking about feelings to others is a waste of time.

_____ **25.** There are times when I become preoccupied with washing my hands or keeping things clean.

_____ **26.** I always like to be in control of myself and to know as much as possible about things happening around me.

_____ **27.** I have few or no close friends with whom I share warm feelings openly.

_____ **28.** I feel that the more you can know about future events, the better off you will be.

_____ **29.** There are sins I have committed that I will never live down.

_____ **30.** I always avoid being late to a meeting or an appointment.

_____ **31.** I rarely give up until the job has been completely finished.

_____ **32.** I often expect things from myself that no one else would ask.

_____ **33.** I sometimes worry about whether I was wrong or made a mistake.

_____ **34.** I would like others to see me as not having any faults.

_____ **35.** The groups and organizations I join have strict rules and regulations.

Scoring

Count your number of true statements.

≤ 10 = Relaxed

11 to 20 = Average Stress

≥ 21 = Excess stress, possible workaholic and burnout

C A S E   S T U D I E S

Write your response to each case study on the lines provided.

Case 1

You notice that you have not been feeling well lately, and you suspect that it is job-related stress. What kinds of activities can you take part in to help reduce stress and prevent job burnout?

_____

_____

_____

Case 2

You are sitting in the staff lounge having lunch. Another medical assistant begins to gossip about a staff member who is not present. She is talking about the staff member's son and the problems he has had at school. You prefer not to gossip, but are reluctant to stop your lunch companion since you don't want to upset her. You would like not to be a partner in this discussion but don't want to hurt the relationship with your coworker. What should you do or say? Use the steps in the problem-solving process to help you decide what to do.

_____

_____

_____

Case 3

You are involved in a group interview. The medical assistant that you are interviewing is credentialed and has a lot of good experience. She seems pleasant, but you notice that she has a "Right to Life" tattoo on her forearm, a tongue ring, and facial piercings. How do you think your elderly patients and female patients will perceive her? How might the physician perceive her?

_____

_____

_____

Case 4

You are working with another medical assistant and you notice that she is recording vital statistics in the chart but is not actually taking measurements. What should you do? How does ethical behavior apply here?

_____

_____

_____

PROCEDURE 3-1 Self-Evaluation of Professional Behaviors

WORK // DOC

Goal
To identify necessary professional behaviors and relate them to yourself in order to improve your performance as a medical assistant

OSHA Guidelines
This procedure does not involve exposure to blood, body fluids, or tissue.

Materials
Self-Evaluation of Professional Behaviors Form.

Method

Step Number	Procedure	Points Possible	Points Earned
1.	Read and review each professional behavior.	10	
2.	Rate yourself on each behavior, considering the level at which you exhibit them.*	20	
3.	Identify at least one measure to improve yourself on each behavior, as needed.*	20	
4.	Place the completed form in your portfolio and review it on an ongoing basis.	10	
5.	Reevaluate your professional behavior prior to your applied training experience (practicum).	10	
6.	Compare the two scores and identify any weaknesses.	15	
7.	Obtain feedback about your professional behaviors from your instructor, coworkers, classmates, practicum coordinator, or employer.	15	
Total Points		100	

CAAHEP Competencies Achieved

IV. A (9)   Recognize and protect personal boundaries in communicating with others

X. A (1)   Apply ethical behaviors, including honesty/integrity in performance of medical assisting practice

X. A (2)   Examine the impact personal ethics and morals may have on the individual's practice

ABHES Competencies Achieved

11. b. (1) Exhibiting dependability, punctuality, and a positive work ethic

11. b. (2) Exhibiting a positive attitude and a sense of responsibility

11. b. (4) Being cognizant of ethical boundaries

11. b. (7) Expressing a responsible attitude

Interpersonal Communication

Name_____ Class_____ Date_____

REVIEW

Vocabulary Review

Matching

Match the key terms in the right column with the examples in the left column by placing the letter of each correct answer in the space provided.

_____ 1. "You appear tense today."

_____ 2. "Please, go on."

_____ 3. Allowing the patient time to think without pressure.

_____ 4. "I follow what you said."

_____ 5. "Hi, Mr. Smith. Florida sure agrees with you."

_____ 6. "Can I help you with your shoes, Mrs. Adams?

_____ 7. "Is there something you would like to talk about?"

_____ 8. "So, you are here today because of your swollen ankles and dizziness?"

_____ 9. "Describe your level of pain on a scale from 1 to 5, with 5 being the most severe."

_____ 10. "Tell me when you feel anxious."

_____ 11. "So what you are saying is that you feel the most pressure when you exercise?"

_____ 12. Patient states: "Do you think this is serious enough to discuss with the doctor?" Medical assistant replies: "Do you think it is?"

_____ 13. "Your granddaughter's first birthday sounded wonderful. Now tell me more about your headaches."

_____ 14. "You're visiting the doctor today regarding a cough. How long have you been coughing?"

a. acceptance
b. offering self
c. making observations
d. reflecting
e. clarifying
f. exploring
g. offering general leads
h. giving broad openings
i. mirroring
j. recognizing
k. silence
l. summarizing
m. encouraging communication
n. focusing

True or False

Decide whether each statement is true or false. In the space at the left, write T for true or F for false. On the lines provided, rewrite the false statements to make them true.

_____ 15. Passive listening does not require a response.

_____

_____ 16. Active listening involves two-way communication in which the listener gives feedback or asks questions.

_____

_____ **17.** Empathy is the process of feeling sorry for someone.

_____

_____ **18.** An aggressive person tries to impose his position on others or tries to manipulate them.

_____

_____ **19.** Rapport is a conflictive and argumentative relationship.

_____

_____ **20.** Conflict in the workplace arises when two or more coworkers have the same opinions or ideas.

_____

_____ **21.** An assertive person has low self-esteem.

_____

_____ **22.** Sitting in a chair with your arms crossed is described as having a closed posture.

_____

_____ **23.** Personal space is an area that is approximately 4 feet around a person.

_____

_____ **24.** Feedback is a verbal or nonverbal response from a patient that she understood what has been communicated.

_____

_____ **25.** The manner in which a person interacts with people is referred to as interpersonal skills.

_____

_____ **26.** Patients will see a medical assistant as standoffish and reserved when he has an open posture.

_____

Content Review

Multiple Choice

In the space provided, write the letter of the choice that best completes each statement or answers each question.

_____ **1.** Noise is anything that
- **a.** Helps the patient give feedback
- **b.** Is a part of verbal communication
- **c.** Interferes with the communication process
- **d.** Is part of a communication circle
- **e.** Helps the medical assistant send a message

_____ **2.** Positive communication with patients may involve
- **a.** Getting them to limit their questions to save time
- **b.** Being attentive and encouraging them to ask questions
- **c.** Telling patients who ask questions that their concerns are foolish
- **d.** Allowing patients to act on angry or abusive feelings
- **e.** Explaining that only the physician can answer their questions

_____ 3. Which of the following is an example of negative communication?
   a. Maintaining eye contact
   b. Displaying open posture
   c. Listening carefully
   d. Asking questions
   e. Mumbling

_____ 4. Which of the following is *not* a communication skill?
   a. Active listening
   b. Anxiety
   c. Empathy
   d. Assertiveness
   e. Respect

_____ 5. When interacting with patients of other cultures or ethnic groups,
   a. Assume that they have the same attitude toward modern medicine that you have
   b. Never involve other family members
   c. Do not try to speak their language
   d. Never allow yourself to make value judgments
   e. Assume that modesty is not essential

_____ 6. Which of the following is *not* a deficiency need as defined by Abraham Maslow?
   a. Safety
   b. Love
   c. Esteem
   d. Physiological needs
   e. Empathy

_____ 7. The most effective manner in which to deal with an angry patient is to
   a. Remind the patient that you are an educated medical assistant
   b. Defend the medical facility to the patient
   c. Walk away because a medical assistant should not put up with this behavior
   d. Demonstrate your sincerity and respect by remaining calm
   e. Demand that the patient calm down before you speak to him

_____ 8. According to Erikson, the life stage that exposes children to people other than their immediate family is
   a. Stage I
   b. Stage II
   c. Stage III
   d. Stage IV
   e. Stage V

_____ 9. When a teenager begins to smoke at a young age because his peers are doing it, the child is most likely experiencing
   a. Autonomy
   b. Ego identity
   c. Role confusion
   d. Inferiority
   e. Isolation

Sentence Completion

In the space provided, write the word or phrase that best completes each sentence.

10. A communication circle involves a message, a source, and a(n) _____.

11. Being _____ when communicating with patients shows them that you, the doctors, and other staff members care about them and their feelings.

12. Your _____, which is the way you hold or move parts of your body, can send strong nonverbal messages.

13. If a patient leans back or turns her head away when you lean forward, you may be invading her _____.

14. The _____ syndrome refers to the anxiety that some patients feel in a doctor's office or other healthcare setting.

15. Positive communication with superiors involves keeping them informed, asking questions, minimizing interruptions, and showing _____.

16. Explaining procedures to patients, expediting insurance referral requests, and creating a warm and reassuring environment are all examples of _____ in the physician's office.

17. _____, a well-known behaviorist, developed a human behavior model that states that human beings are motivated by unsatisfied needs.

18. A world-renowned authority on death and dying, _____, developed a model of behavior that an individual will experience on learning of his condition. These behaviors are referred to as *the stages of dying* or *the stages of grief*.

10. _____

11. _____

12. _____

13. _____

14. _____

15. _____

16. _____

17. _____

18. _____

Short Answer

Write the answer to each question on the lines provided.

19. What are three examples of negative communication?

_____

_____

_____

20. List Erik Erikson's life stages and discuss the expected development traits of each.

_____

_____

_____

21. What is the difference between a stereotype and a generalization of different cultures?

_____

_____

_____

22. What are three rules for establishing positive communication with coworkers?

_____

_____

_____

23. List and briefly describe Elisabeth Kübler-Ross's five stages of death and dying.

_____

_____

_____

_____

_____

Critical Thinking

Write the answer to each question on the lines provided.

1. How does a person's nonverbal communication convey his true feelings even when his words say otherwise?

_____

_____

_____

2. Explain why learning developmental life span models can help you communicate with patients.

_____

_____

_____

3. Explain how Elisabeth Kübler-Ross's model of the stages of death and dying can help both the families of terminally ill patients and the patients themselves.

_____

_____

_____

4. From the statements by the medical assistant in each scenario listed as follows, determine which statements are assertive and which are aggressive. Rewrite the aggressive statements to make them assertive.

a. A new patient to your office has begun taking antidepressants. When asking the patient about the new medication, you discover that the patient is only taking the medication when she feels anxious. You respond by saying, "Do you really expect to feel better when you are not following the physician's directions?"

_____

_____

_____

b. A patient has a billing question on a statement that he received recently. You respond, "Let me find the appropriate person to answer the question for you."

_____

_____

_____

c. A coworker uses a profane word by the reception window. You respond by telling her, "You're nasty."

_____

_____

_____

d. Your physician is in her office reviewing lab results when you burst into the room and say, "I have to talk to you now regarding my vacation."

_____

_____

_____

e. You are receiving your annual performance review by your supervisor, and you don't agree on several of the improvement items. You respond by saying, "What do you know? You're not a clinical expert."

_____

_____

_____

f. A patient is yelling at you over the telephone and is using profanity with you. You respond by saying, "Please stop cursing at me, and let's solve this problem together."

_____

_____

_____

A P P L I C A T I O N

Follow the directions for each application.

1. Therapeutic Communication Skills

Make a list of at least 10 therapeutic communication techniques a medical assistant can use. For each technique, explain how the technique improves communication between the medical assistant and the patient.

_____

_____

_____

_____

_____

_____

_____

_____

_____

2. **Maslow's Hierarchy of Human Needs**

List the five levels in Abraham Maslow's hierarchy of human needs. For each level, provide an example of a statement a patient may make that would indicate that these needs are not being met.

_____

_____

_____

_____

_____

C A S E   S T U D I E S

Write your response to each case study on the lines provided.

Case 1

You are having a problem with a coworker. Both of you have the same job title and often work together to interview and prepare patients. This coworker cuts you off when you speak and contradicts you in front of patients. Her actions are affecting the way patients see you as a professional. How should you handle this situation?

_____

_____

_____

Case 2

A male patient is waiting in the exam room to see the physician. He is seeing the physician for sexual dysfunction. You and several medical assistants are outside his room at the nurse's station and burst into laughter about a comment unrelated to the patient. A few minutes later, the patient leaves. What could have happened to cause the patient to leave? How could this have been avoided?

_____

_____

_____

Case 3

A mother brings her 3-year-old into the pediatrician's office. The child is presenting with behavioral issues regarding potty training. The mother states that the child hides behind furniture instead of using the potty or alerting her of her need to use the bathroom. The mother states that she has strict consequences when the child has an accident, such as time-outs when an accident occurs. In addition, the older sibling teases the child about accidents. According to Erikson, what is the life stage level for this child and a possible reason for this behavior?

_____

_____

_____

PROCEDURE 4-1 Communicating with the Anxious Patient

Goal
To use communication and interpersonal skills to calm an anxious patient.

OSHA Guidelines
This procedure does not involve exposure to blood, body fluids, or tissue.

Materials
None.

Method

Step Number	Procedure	Points Possible	Points Earned
1.	Identify signs of anxiety in the patient.*	5	
2.	Acknowledge the patient's anxiety. (Ignoring a patient's anxiety often makes it worse.)	5	
3.	Identify possible sources of anxiety, such as fear of a procedure or test result, along with supportive resources available to the patient, such as family members and friends.	10	
4.	Do what you can to alleviate the patient's physical discomfort. For example, find a calm, quiet place for the patient to wait, a comfortable chair, a drink of water, or access to the bathroom.	10	
5.	Allow ample personal space for conversation. Note: You would normally allow a 1- to 4-ft distance between yourself and the patient. Adjust this space as necessary.	5	
6.	Create a climate of warmth, acceptance, and trust.* **a.** Recognize and control your own anxiety. Your air of calm can decrease the patient's anxiety. **b.** Provide reassurance by demonstrating genuine care, respect, and empathy. **c.** Act confidently and dependably, maintaining truthfulness and confidentiality at all times.	10	
7.	Using the appropriate communication skills, have the patient describe the experience that is causing anxiety, her thoughts about it, and her feelings. Proceeding in this order allows the patient to describe what is causing the anxiety and to clarify her thoughts and feelings about it.* **a.** Maintain an open posture. **b.** Maintain eye contact, if culturally appropriate. **c.** Use active listening skills. **d.** Listen without interrupting.	15	
8.	Do not belittle the patient's thoughts and feelings. This can cause a breakdown in communication, increase anxiety, and make the patient feel isolated.	10	
9.	Be empathic to the patient's concerns.	10	
10.	Help the patient recognize and cope with the anxiety.* **a.** Provide information to the patient. Patients are often fearful of the unknown. **b.** Suggest coping behaviors, such as deep breathing or other relaxation exercises.		
11.	Notify the doctor of the patient's concerns.	10	
Total Points		100	

CAAHEP Competencies Achieved

IV. C (3)   Recognize communication barriers

IV. C (4)   Identify techniques for overcoming communication barriers

IV. C (7)   Identify resources and adaptations that are required based on individual needs, i.e., culture and environment, developmental life stage, language, and physical threats to communication

IV. P (11) Respond to nonverbal communication

IV. A (2)   Apply active listening skills

IV. A (3)   Use appropriate body language and other nonverbal skills in communicating with patients, family, and staff

ABHES Competencies Achieved

5. (a) Define and understand abnormal behavior patterns

5. (b) Identify and respond appropriately when working/caring for patients with special needs

8. (aa) Are attentive, listen, and learn

8. (bb) Are impartial and show empathy when dealing with patients

8. (ee) Communicate on the recipient's level of comprehension

8. (ii) Recognize and respond to verbal and non-verbal communication

8. (kk) Adapt to individualized needs

PROCEDURE 4-2 Communicating with the Angry Patient

Goal
To use communication and interpersonal skills to calm an angry patient.

OSHA Guidelines
This procedure does not involve exposure to blood, body fluids, or tissue.

Materials
None.

Method

Step Number	Procedure	Points Possible	Points Earned
1.	Recognize anger and its causes. Anger is easy to recognize in most people, but it can be subtle in others. Patients who speak in a tense tone, are stubborn, or appear to ignore your attempts at communication may be angry.*	5	
2.	Remain calm and continue to demonstrate genuineness and respect. Communicate that you respect and care about the patient's feelings.	10	
3.	Focus on the patient's physical and medical needs.	10	
4.	Maintain adequate personal space. Place yourself on the same level as the patient. If the patient is standing, encourage him to sit down. Maintain an open posture and eye contact but avoid staring.	10	
5.	Listen attentively and with an open mind to what the patient is saying. Avoid the feeling that you need to defend yourself or to give reasons why the patient should not be angry.*	15	
6.	Encourage patients to be specific in describing the cause of their anger, their thoughts about it, and their feelings. Be empathic and acknowledge the patient's feelings and perceptions. Follow through with any promises you might make concerning correction of a problem, but avoid totally agreeing or disagreeing with the patient. State what you can and cannot do for the patient.	10	
7.	Present your point of view calmly and firmly to help the patient better understand the situation. If patients are receptive to your viewpoint, their perspective may change for the better.	10	
8.	Avoid a breakdown in communication. Allow the patient to voice anger. Trying to outtalk the patient or overexplain will only annoy and irritate him. If needed, suggest that the patient spend a few moments alone to gather his thoughts or to cool off before continuing any type of communication.ˣ	10	
9.	If you feel threatened by a patient's anger or if it looks as if the patient's anger may become violent, leave the room and seek assistance from one of the physicians or other members of the office staff.	10	
10.	Document any actual threats in the patient's chart.	10	
Total Points		100	

CAAHEP Competencies Achieved

IV. C (3)   Recognize communication barriers

IV. C (4)   Identify techniques for overcoming communication barriers

IV. C (7)   Identify resources and adaptations that are required based on individual needs, i.e., culture and environment, developmental life stage, language, and physical threats to communication

IV. A (2)   Apply active listening skills

IV. A (3)   Use appropriate body language and other nonverbal skills in communicating with patients, family, and staff

ABHES Competencies Achieved

5. (a) Define and understand abnormal behavior patterns

5. (b) Identify and respond appropriately when working/caring for patients with special needs

8. (aa) Are attentive, listen, and learn

8. (bb) Are impartial and show empathy when dealing with patients

8. (ee) Communicate on the recipient's level of comprehension

8. (ii) Recognize and respond to verbal and non-verbal communication

8. (kk) Adapt to individualized needs

PROCEDURE 4-3 Communicating with the Assistance of an Interpreter

Goal
To demonstrate techniques to effectively communicate with a non-English-speaking patient through an interpreter.

OSHA Guidelines
This procedure does not involve exposure to blood, body fluids, or tissue.

Materials
Pen, forms, or computer and appropriate pictures and other visual aids if available.

Method

Step Number	Procedure	Points Possible	Points Earned
1.	Identify the patient by name and ask if you pronounced the name correctly. Be sure to smile, even if you are feeling slightly awkward or unsure of yourself.*	10	
2.	Introduce yourself with your title to the patient and the interpreter.	5	
3.	Ask the interpreter to spell his or her full name and provide you with identification, such as his agency's identification or a business card. Retain his business card to file in the patient's medical record. If he or she does not have a business card, obtain contact information, which will also be filed in the patient's medical record.*	15	
4.	Do not take it personally if the patient appears abrupt or even rude; this behavior may be considered appropriate in the patient's culture. For example, in some cultures, male patients may not deal with a female staff member, and that should be respected if possible. Ascertain from the interpreter if there is a problem.	5	
5.	Inquire of the interpreter if the patient speaks or understands any English and if there are any communication traditions or other customs that you should be aware of. For example, traditional Navajo people consider it rude to have direct eye contact.	10	
6.	Provide a quiet comfortable area.	5	
7.	Speak directly to the patient and speak slowly if the patient has any understanding of English.	10	
8.	If forms are to be completed, instruct the interpreter to translate with appropriate intervals and give opportunities for the patient to ask questions to ensure understanding. For example, if providing general consent for treatment, permission to send information and receive payment directly from the insurance company, and privacy decisions, have one area translated at a time. Instruct the interpreter to ask if there are questions at each portion.*	15	
9.	If the patient and interpreter are discussing an issue in depth or appear to be leaving you out of the conversation, ask the translator what is being said.	5	
10.	Provide the same information, services, and courtesies that you would to a native English speaker. If possible, provide written information in the patient's native language.	10	
11.	Document what you would ordinarily document; note on all forms that "translation was done by" and include the name, credential, and agency of the interpreter, as well as the date and time.*	10	
Total Points		100	

CAAHEP Competencies Achieved

IV. C (3)   Recognize communication barriers

IV. C (4)   Identify techniques for overcoming communication barriers

IV. C (7)   Identify resources and adaptations that are required based on individual needs, i.e., culture and environment, developmental life stage, language, and physical threats to communication

IV. A (2)   Apply active listening skills

IV. A (3)   Use appropriate body language and other nonverbal skills in communicating with patients, family, and staff

IV. A (10) Demonstrate respect for individual diversity, incorporating awareness of one's own biases in areas including gender, race, religion, age, and economic status

ABHES Competencies Achieved

5. (a) Define and understand abnormal behavior patterns

5. (b) Identify and respond appropriately when working/caring for patients with special needs

8. (aa) Are attentive, listen, and learn

8. (bb) Are impartial and show empathy when dealing with patients

8. (ee) Communicate on the recipient's level of comprehension

8. (ii) Recognize and respond to verbal and non-verbal communication

8. (kk) Adapt to individualized needs

Legal and Ethical Issues

Name_____ Class_____ Date_____

REVIEW

Vocabulary Review

Passage Completion
Study the key terms in the box. Use your textbook to find definitions of terms you do not understand.

abandonment	consent	libel
arbitration	contract	minors
assault	credentialing	misdemeanor
battery	criminal law	negligence
bioethics	durable power of attorney	slander
breach of contract	ethics	tort
civil law	fraud	

In the space provided, complete the following passage, using some of the terms from the key terms list. You may change the form of a term to fit the meaning of the sentence.

If a healthcare worker does not perform an essential action or performs the action improperly, the patient may bring a charge of 1. _____ against the practice. If a practitioner stops care without providing an equally qualified substitute, a charge of 2. _____ may be filed. Physicians and their patients work under an implied contract. A violation of that contract is a 3. _____. Some charges resulting in lawsuits are brought to trial; others are settled through a mediator in a process known as 4. _____.

Medical assistants may assist patients with completing paperwork known as the 5. _____, which appoints someone to carry out the patient's wishes regarding healthcare decisions should the patient become unable to make these decisions for himself. Some of these decisions include those involving 6. _____ or moral decisions not necessarily related to the law. These decisions for healthcare workers may also include what is known as 7. _____, which frequently revolve around dilemmas resulting from medical advances. 8. _____ consists of crimes against the state. 9. A(n) _____ is included in this type of law, and practicing medicine without a license will result in this charge. A crime against a person is known as a 10. _____, and it comes under the heading of 11. _____ law. The open threat of bodily harm may result in a charge of 12. _____ whereas 13. _____ consists of an action that causes bodily harm.

1. _____
2. _____
3. _____
4. _____
5. _____
6. _____
7. _____
8. _____
9. _____
10. _____
11. _____
12. _____
13. _____

Defamation (of character) damages a person's reputation. When this occurs through speech, it is known as 14. _____, and if it occurs in print, the charge is changed to 15. _____.

14. _____

15. _____

Content Review

Multiple Choice

In the space provided, write the letter of the choice that best completes each statement or answers each question.

_____ 1. The term *res ipsa loquitur* refers to cases in which
   a. The patient has a previously existing condition
   b. The physician abandons the patient
   c. The patient has already filed a lawsuit
   d. The doctor's error was caused by faulty recordkeeping
   e. The doctor's mistake is clear to everyone

_____ 2. If a physician decides to terminate his care of a patient, the physician must
   a. Tell the patient face to face
   b. Leave a message for the patient on the patient's answering machine
   c. Obtain the patient's consent
   d. Inform the patient's family
   e. Send the patient a certified letter

_____ 3. Which of the following is *not* a legal procedure for medical assistants to perform?
   a. Maintaining licenses and accreditation
   b. Recruiting qualified medical assistants for the medical office
   c. Determining needs for documentation and reporting
   d. Diagnosing a condition
   e. Assisting a patient with completing a durable power of attorney

_____ 4. A physician's receptionist asks patients to sign in and list the reason for their visit. This receptionist is violating the patients' right to
   a. Confidentiality
   b. A second opinion
   c. Sue for malpractice
   d. Be seen by the physician in a timely manner
   e. Comprehensive medical care

_____ 5. While practicing within the context of an implied contract with a patient, the physician is obligated to do all of the following *except*
   a. Use due care
   b. Provide complete information and instructions to the patient about diagnoses, options, and methods of treatment
   c. Promise the patient that he or she will recover completely
   d. Stay current regarding all technology and treatments available
   e. Provide appropriate medical coverage when the physician is not available

_____ 6. Crimes such as attempted burglary and disturbing the peace are examples of
   a. Felonies
   b. Misdemeanors
   c. Civil law
   d. Intentional crimes
   e. Social crimes

_____ 7. If a medical assistant gives a patient an injection after the patient has refused the procedure, it could result in a charge of
   a. Assault
   b. Battery
   c. False imprisonment
   d. Not applicable; no charge would result because the physician ordered the procedure
   e. Negligence

_____ 8. Preventing a patient from leaving the medical facility after administration of an allergy injection could be seen as

    a. An invasion of privacy   **d.** Malpractice

    b. False imprisonment   **e.** Battery

    c. An acceptable practice as long as it is documented in the chart

_____ 9. If a patient can prove that she felt "reasonable apprehension of bodily harm," it can result in what type of charge?

    a. Defamation of character   **d.** Negligence

    b. Battery   **e.** Slander

    c. Assault

_____ 10. Documenting in a patient's chart that she is a "whack job" who makes up symptoms because she has "a crush on the doctor" could produce charges of _____ for the practice.

    a. Defamation of character   **d.** Malpractice

    b. Slander   **e.** Libel

    c. Negligence

Sentence Completion

In the space provided, write the word or phrase that best completes each sentence.

11. The four Ds of negligence are duty, dereliction, _____ and damages.

12. The relationship between a doctor and a patient is called a(n) _____.

13. Damaging a person's reputation by making public statements that are both false and malicious is considered _____.

14. Healthcare practitioners who promise patients miracle cures or accept fees from patients while using mystical or spiritual powers to heal are considered _____.

15. A contract that is stated in written or spoken words is considered a(n) _____.

16. Torts that are committed without the intention to cause harm but are committed unreasonably or with a disregard for the consequences are _____.

17. A patient who does not follow medical advice and consistently misses appointments maybe considered in _____ contract.

18. A document that communicates patient rights under HIPAA is called _____.

19. Misfeasance refers to a lawful act that is _____ performed.

20. The _____ lists what patients should expect from their healthcare provider. It was formerly known as the Patient Bill of Rights.

11. _____

12. _____

13. _____

14. _____

15. _____

16. _____

17. _____

18. _____

19. _____

20. _____

Short Answer

Write the answer to each question on the lines provided.

21. What is the difference between malfeasance and nonfeasance?

_____

_____

_____

22. List eight types of personal information that is considered individually identifiable health information under HIPAA.

_____

_____

_____

23. HIPAA allows the provider to share what type of patient healthcare information with outside entities?

_____

_____

_____

24. List and briefly define the four essential elements of a contract.

_____

_____

_____

25. List the five types of medical practice and provide an advantage of each.

_____

_____

_____

26. How can office personnel help prevent lawsuits?

_____

_____

_____

27. Describe the Federal False Claims Act.

_____

_____

_____

28. How can careless use of office equipment compromise privacy of personal health information?

_____

_____

_____

29. Looking at healthcare today, list two bioethical issues that are in today's headlines.

_____

_____

_____

30. List the six principles for preventing improper release of patient information.

_____

_____

_____

A P P L I C A T I O N   `WORK//DOC`

Follow the directions for the application.

Writing a Letter of Withdrawal

Work with two partners. Take turns being a medical assistant, a doctor, and an evaluator. Assume that the doctor has asked the medical assistant to write a letter of withdrawal to a patient.

a. The doctor should explain to the medical assistant what the problem with the patient is and why he has decided to withdraw from the case. The medical assistant should take notes and ask questions as necessary.

b. The medical assistant should then write the letter for the doctor. She should make clear the doctor's reason for withdrawing from the case. She should also include the doctor's recommendation that the patient seek medical care from another doctor as soon as possible. The final copy of the letter should be produced on BWW letterhead.

c. After the foregoing tasks have been completed, the evaluator should critique the letter, keeping in mind the following questions: Does the letter include the doctor's reason for withdrawing from the case? Does the letter include the doctor's recommendation that the patient seek medical care elsewhere? Is the letter free of spelling, punctuation, and grammatical errors? Does it follow a business letter format?

d. The medical assistant and the doctor should discuss the evaluator's comments, noting the strengths and weaknesses of the letter.

e. Exchange roles and repeat the procedure with another student as a doctor who wishes to terminate care of a patient for a different reason.

f. Exchange roles again so that each member of the team has the opportunity to roleplay the medical assistant, the doctor, and the evaluator.

C A S E   S T U D I E S

Write your response to each case study on the lines provided.

Case 1

A patient has a sexually transmitted infection (STI) but does not want you or the doctor to contact any former sex partners. The doctor has asked you to handle this case. How much can you do to make sure these people are notified?

_____

_____

_____

Case 2

A doctor is about to leave on a special family vacation for two months. A new patient comes to the office with a collection of unusual symptoms that do not seem to be serious. The doctor tells the patient to make another appointment after his return from vacation so that he can order some tests. What kind of lawsuit is the doctor risking? What should the doctor do instead?

_____

_____

_____

Case 3

You work in a large medical office with three other medical assistants. One of the other assistants discusses her patients with you during your lunch break together. What, if anything, has the medical assistant done wrong? What should you do about it?

_____

_____

_____

PROCEDURE 5-1 Obtaining Signature for Receipt of Privacy Practices

WORK//DOC

Goal
To follow HIPAA guidelines and obtain the patient's signature that he or she has received and understands the office privacy policies.

OSHA Guidelines
This procedure does not involve exposure to blood, body fluids, or tissues.

Materials
Preprinted receipt of privacy practices information form (see Figure 5-9), pens, copy machine.

Method

Step Number	Procedure	Points Possible	Points Earned
1.	Explain to the patient the office privacy policy regarding protected health information.*	18	
2.	Ask the patient to read the policy carefully and to feel free to ask any questions he or she may have regarding the policy. Answer any questions that may arise.*	18	
3.	When the patient's questions have been answered, witness the patient (or guardian) sign and print his or her name. Note any restrictions that may be placed on the document.*	18	
4.	Print your name and sign the document as witness, including your title.	18	
5.	Date the document when all signatures have been completed.	18	
6.	Make a copy of the document to file in the patient medical record, and give the original to the patient.*	10	
Total Points		100	

CAAHEP Competencies Achieved

IX. P (1)   Respond to issues of confidentiality

ABHES Competencies Achieved

4. (b) Institute federal and state guidelines when releasing medical records or information

4. (f) Comply with federal, state, and local health laws and regulations

11. b. (3) Maintaining confidentiality at all times

PROCEDURE 5-2 Completing a Privacy Violation Complaint Form

WORK // DOC

Goal
To assist the patient in completing a Privacy Violation Complaint form if she feels her PHI has been compromised.

OSHA Guidelines
This procedure does not involve exposure to blood, body fluids, or tissues.

Materials
Privacy Violation Complaint Form (see Figure 5-10), pens, private room to complete form, copy machine.

Method

Step Number	Procedure	Points Possible	Points Earned
1.	Explain to the patient that all formal complaints must be made in writing.ˣ	13	
2.	Ask the patient if she feels assistance will be needed completing the form. If not, the patient may complete the form on her own. Answer any questions she may have regarding completion of the form.	11	
3.	When the patient completes the form, read it carefully, making sure it is complete and legible and the information regarding the breach of privacy is clear.	13	
4.	If the patient requires that any copies be made for documentation backing the claim, make the copies, returning any originals to the patient.	13	
5.	Make sure the patient signs and dates the complaint.*	13	
6.	As the person receiving the complaint, sign the document as indicated and date it.	13	
7.	Explain to the patient that the office will respond to the complaint within 30 days of today's receipt.	13	
8.	Make a copy of the document for the patient, and keep the original for the office files.ˣ	11	
Total Points		100	

CAAHEP Competencies Achieved

IX. P (1)   Respond to issues of confidentiality

ABHES Competencies Achieved

4. (e) Perform risk management procedures

4. (f) Comply with federal, state, and local health laws and regulations

PROCEDURE 5-3 Obtaining Authorization to Release Health Information

WORK//DOC

Goal
To follow HIPAA guidelines when obtaining the patient's protected health information without violating confidentiality regulations.

OSHA Guidelines
This procedure does not involve exposure to blood, body fluids, or tissues.

Materials
Preprinted Authorization to Release Health Information form (see Figure 5-11), pens, copy machine.

Method

Step Number	Procedure	Points Possible	Points Earned
1.	Explain to the patient the need for the requested medical information.*	8	
2.	Obtain the name and address of the practice to which the authorization is to be mailed.	8	
3.	Fill in the patient's name, address, and DOB as required.	8	
4.	Enter the physician's or practitioner's name from your practice who is requesting the PHI.	8	
5.	Enter the information that is being requested.*	10	
6.	Complete the reason for request area, explaining why the patient is requesting the information be sent to your office.*	8	
7.	Enter an expiration date for the authorization, giving a reasonable amount of time for the request to be fulfilled.	8	
8.	Prior to signing the release, go over the information contained within the release with the patient, answering any questions that may arise. Be sure the patient understands the request may be withdrawn (in writing) at any time.	10	
9.	Witness the patient (or guardian) signature and date; if necessary, be sure the guardian relationship area is completed.	8	
10.	Sign and date the document as witness, including your title.	8	
11.	Make a copy of the document to file in the patient medical record and, if requested, give a copy to the patient as well.	8	
12.	Make a notation in the medical record of the document signing and note the date the authorization is mailed.*	8	
Total Points		100	

CAAHEP Competencies Achieved

IX. P (3)   Apply HIPAA rules in regard to privacy/release of information

ABHES Competencies Achieved

4. (b) Institute federal and state guidelines when releasing medical records or information

4. (f) Comply with federal, state, and local health laws and regulations

11. b. (3) Maintaining confidentiality at all times

Basic Safety and Infection Control

Name_____ Class_____ Date_____

REVIEW

Vocabulary Review

Matching

Match the key terms in the right column with the definitions in the left column by placing the letter of each correct answer in the space provided.

_____ 1. An infection caused when an abnormality or malfunction in routine body processes has caused normally beneficial or harmless microorganisms to become pathogenic

_____ 2. A shortened version of the Material Safety Data Sheet

_____ 3. A reservoir of disease who exhibits no symptoms of the disease

_____ 4. An infection caused by introduction of a pathogen from an outside source to the body

_____ 5. An infection acquired by a patient at a medical facility

_____ 6. An inanimate object capable of serving as a reservoir for pathogens

_____ 7. An organism that can carry microorganisms from an infected person to another

_____ 8. An OSHA directive that requires employers to maintain a safe workplace

_____ 9. A microorganism capable of causing disease

_____ 10. The absence or control of pathogens

a. carrier
b. fomite
c. endogenous infection
d. General Duty Clause
e. Healthcare Associated Infection
f. pathogen
g. exogenous infection
h. hazard label
i. asepsis
j. vector

Content Review

Multiple Choice

In the space provided, write the letter of the choice that best completes each statement or answers each question.

_____ 1. Which of the following is the acronym used to illustrate correct use of a fire extinguisher?
a. SWEEP
b. PASS
c. ACT
d. HAI
e. PULL

_____ 2. Where would you find detailed information about a chemical substance you are about to use in the medical office?
a. On the hazard label
b. In the written safety plan
c. On the biohazard label
d. In the MSDS
e. In the hazard communication

Copyright © 2014 by The McGraw-Hill Companies, Inc.

_____ 3. The study of the way people work is known as
    a. Work practice controls
    b. Fomites
    c. Ergonomics
    d. NIOSH
    e. Safety engineering

_____ 4. A reservoir host who is unaware of the presence of a pathogen and therefore spreads disease is called
    a. Transmission
    b. A portal of exit
    c. A portal of entry
    d. A susceptible host
    e. A carrier

_____ 5. Which of the following must an employer make available to employees so as to be in compliance with the OSHA Bloodborne Pathogens Standard?
    a. Polio vaccine
    b. Health insurance
    c. Performance ratings for handling bloodborne pathogens
    d. Hepatitis B vaccine
    e. Clothing allowance

_____ 6. An animal, insect, or human whose body is capable of sustaining the growth of a pathogen is known as
    a. a reservoir host
    b. a susceptible host
    c. a pathogen
    d. flora
    e. an environmental factor

_____ 7. A microorganism's disease-producing power is called
    a. a pathogen
    b. convalescence
    c. immunity
    d. virulence
    e. resistance

_____ 8. An insect that carries microorganisms from one infected person to another is a
    a. fomite
    b. pathogen
    c. host
    d. vector
    e. droplet

_____ 9. An infection in a reservoir host in which an abnormality or malfunction in routine body process has caused normally beneficial or harmless microorganisms to become pathogenic is called a(n)
    a. endogenous infection
    b. subclinical case
    c. exogenous infection
    d. carrier state
    e. Healthcare Associated Infection

_____ 10. The way a pathogen moves from one host to another is what part of the cycle of infection?
    a. Means of exit
    b. Means of entrance
    c. Reservoir host
    d. Transmission
    e. Susceptible host

Short Answer

Write the answer to each question on the lines provided.

11. Label each step in the cycle of infection illustrated in the image below.

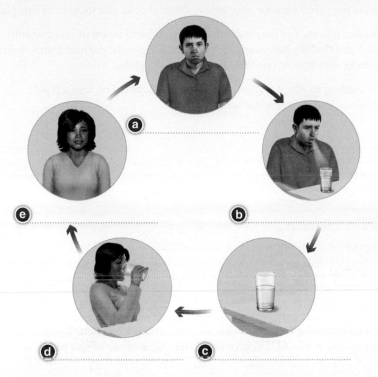

12. On the basis of the labeled figure in the previous exercise, give three examples of each step of the cycle of infection.

a. _____

b. _____

c. _____

d. _____

e. _____

13. If you must use an extension cord in the medical office what steps should you take to ensure that it is used safely?

_____

_____

_____

14. Give five examples of biohazardous waste.

_____

_____

_____

15. Describe a biohazard symbol label.

_____

_____

_____

A P P L I C A T I O N

Follow the directions for each application.

1. You have been asked to write a comprehensive fire safety plan for your office. What should you include in this plan?

2. With a partner, practice removing contaminated gloves. You may want to apply simulated blood or another substance such as strawberry jam to help remind you that the gloves are contaminated. Have the partner watch to make sure that you do not touch your skin or clothing with the contaminated surface of the glove.

3. Label each of the following types of waste according to where it should be properly disposed of. Use a **B** for biohazard waste container, **S** for sharps container, and **R** for regular waste.

    a. Lancet _____

    b. Unsoiled table paper _____

    c. Capillary tube _____

    d. Gloves used during a pelvic exam _____

    e. Wrapper from a bandage _____

    f. Syringe with the safety device activated _____

    g. Alcohol prep pad used to cleanse the skin prior to injection _____

    h. Surgical wound dressing _____

    i. Disposable gown used during a minor surgical procedure _____

    j. Mask used while caring for a patient who has the flu _____

4. Describe the principles of proper hand hygiene including methods of hand disinfection, when your hands should be washed or disinfected, when it is not appropriate to use AHDs, proper nail length, and use of nail polish and nail extensions.

C A S E   S T U D I E S

Write your response to each case study on the lines provided.

Case 1
After taking a shipment of supplies for the clinical and laboratory areas, you notice that one of the boxes is leaking a clear liquid. What action should you take to reduce the risk of exposing yourself and others to a potentially hazardous chemical?

_____

_____

_____

Case 2
As part of your job, you are responsible for maintaining the office's eyewash station. How often should you check the eyewash station? Describe the steps you should take to maintain the eyewash station.

_____

_____

_____

Case 3

You are the clinical supervisor in a pediatric office. You notice that a coworker does not wash her hands after taking a child's temperature. You know the child has chickenpox, a contagious viral disease. After mentioning to the medical assistant that she did not wash her hands, she states, "I will be fine. I had the chickenpox when I was a child." Based on what you have learned about the cycle of infection, why is this statement unacceptable? What should you tell the medical assistant? What part of the cycle of infection does the patient represent? The medical assistant?

_____

_____

_____

Case 4

A patient enters your reception area with a severe laceration on his arm. The blood is dripping from his arm onto the carpet and the front desk area. What actions should you take?

_____

_____

_____

Name_____ Date_____

Evaluated by_____ Score_____

PROCEDURE 6-1 Handling a Fire Emergency

Goal
To ensure safe use of a fire extinguisher during a fire emergency.

OSHA Guidelines
This procedure does not involve exposure to blood, body fluids, or tissue.

Materials
Fully charged fire extinguisher that has been professionally serviced on a yearly basis.

Method

Step Number	Procedure	Points Possible	Points Earned
1.	In the case of an open fire or continuous smoke, pull the fire alarm or call emergency services to alert the local fire authorities.*	15	
2.	Move patients out of the area.*	15	
3.	Remove the fire extinguisher from its stored location.	10	
4.	Assess the fire. If it is too large do not attempt to extinguish the fire. Leave the building immediately and wait for the fire department to arrive.*	15	
If the Fire Cannot Be Easily Contained			
5.	Calmly and quickly ask each employee to follow the established fire plan.	5	
6.	Remove all patients to the outside of the building; ensure patient comfort and safety at all times.*	10	
If the Fire Is Small and Easily Contained			
7.	Hold the fire extinguisher upright.	5	
8.	Pull the safety pin on the fire extinguisher.	5	
9.	Aim at the base of the fire.	5	
10.	Squeeze the trigger.	5	
11.	Sweep side to side until the fire is out.	5	
Once Action Has Been Taken			
12.	Do not reenter the area until the fire department assesses and clears the area.	5	
Total Points		100	

CAAHEP Competencies Achieved

XI. C (2)   Identify safety techniques that can be used to prevent accidents and maintain a safe work environment

XI. C (7)   Describe fundamental principles for evacuation of a healthcare setting

XI. C (8)   Discuss fire safety issues in a healthcare environment

XI. P (5)   Demonstrate proper use of the following equipment:

        b. Fire extinguishers

XI. P (8)   Demonstrate methods of fire prevention in the healthcare setting

ABHES Competencies Achieved

None

PROCEDURE 6-2 Maintaining and Using an Eye Wash Station

WORK // DOC

Goal

To ensure safe use of an eye wash station following a splash or splatter accident.

OSHA Guidelines

Materials

Eye wash station. This may be plumbed or freestanding. Gloves, moisture proof lab coat, and goggles or face mask.

Method

Step Number	Procedure	Points Possible	Points Earned
On a Weekly Basis			
1.	Check that the path to the eye wash station is clear and no more than 10 seconds from the hazard.*	15	
2.	Ensure that the Eyewash sign is easily visible.	10	
3.	Make sure the covers are in place.	10	
4.	Ensure that the unit comes on in 1 second and stays on once it is activated.*	15	
5.	Check the flow of the eye wash to ensure it is of sufficient flow to wash the eye but is not so strong it will damage the eye tissues. Approximately 0.4 gallons per minute is required for an eye wash and 3 gallons per minute is required for an eye/face wash station.*	15	
6.	Check that the temperature of the water is above 60°F and below 100°F.*	15	
7.	Flush the system for one minute.*	15	
8.	Complete the Safety Inspection record attached to the eyewash station.	5	
Total Points		100	
During a Splash or Splatter Emergency			
1.	Assist the victim to the eye wash station.*	20	
2.	Activate the system.*	20	
3.	Have the victim lean in to the eye wash, keeping her eyes continuously open. You may have to don gloves and gown and assist the victim by holding her eye or eyes open.*	20	
4.	Continuously flush the eyes for at least 15 minutes or the length of time recommended on the MSDS if applicable.*	20	
5.	Alert the physician or EMS.*	20	
Total Points		100	

Source: www.nclabor.com/osha/etta/indguide/ig28.pdf.

CAAHEP Competencies Achieved

XI. C (2)   Identify safety techniques that can be used to prevent accidents and maintain a safe work environment

XI. P (5)   Demonstrate proper use of the following equipment

a. Eye wash

ABHES Competencies Achieved

None

PROCEDURE 6-3 Using a Biohazardous Sharps Container

Goal
To ensure safe use of a sharps disposal unit.

OSHA Guidelines

Materials
Approved sharps container and gloves.

Method

Step Number	Procedure	Points Possible	Points Earned
1.	Wash your hands and put on gloves.	5	
2.	Ensure that biohazardous waste containers are close to the place where the waste material is generated.	5	
3.	Hold article by the blunt end.	5	
4.	Drop the object directly into an approved puncture-proof container for sharps Engage safety device If Indicated.*	15	
5.	Place hazardous waste/sharps in appropriate biohazardous waste container immediately or as soon as possible.*	15	
6.	Keep containers closed when not in use. Close them before removing them from the area or use and keep them upright to avoid spills.	5	
7.	Place the container in a secondary container if the outside of the primary container becomes contaminated.	5	
8.	Drop—do not push—intact contaminated needles into the biohazardous waste container for sharps.*	15	
9.	Never break off, recap, reuse, or handle needles after use.*	15	
10.	Do not open, empty, or clean sharps containers.	5	
11.	Discard sharps containers that are two-thirds full in large biohazardous waste containers.	5	
12.	Remove the gloves and wash your hands.	5	
Total Points		100	

CAAHEP Competencies Achieved

XI. C (2)   Identify safety techniques that can be used to prevent accidents and maintain a safe work environment

XI. P (5)   Demonstrate proper use of the following equipment

        c. Sharps disposal containers

ABHES Competencies Achieved

10. (c) Dispose of biohazardous materials

PROCEDURE 6-4 Disposing of Biohazardous Waste

Goal
To correctly dispose of contaminated waste products, including sharps and contaminated cleaning and paper products.

OSHA Guidelines

Materials
Biohazardous waste containers, gloves, waste materials.

Method

Step Number	Procedure	Points Possible	Points Earned
1.	Wash your hands and put on gloves.	15	
2.	Carefully deposit the biohazardous materials in a properly marked biohazardous waste container.*	25	
3.	Never "dump" the contents of one biohazardous waste container into another.	20	
4.	If the container is full, secure the inner liner and place it in the appropriate area for biohazardous waste.*	25	
5.	Remove the gloves and wash your hands.	15	
Total Points		100	

CAAHEP Competencies Achieved

XI. C (2)   Identify safety techniques that can be used to prevent accidents and maintain a safe work environment

ABHES Competencies Achieved

10. (c) Dispose of biohazardous materials

Name_____ Date_____

Evaluated by_____ Score_____

PROCEDURE 6-5 Aseptic Hand Washing

Goal
To remove dirt and microorganisms from under the fingernails and from the surface of the skin, hair follicles, and oil glands of the hands.

OSHA Guidelines
This procedure does not involve exposure to blood, body fluids, or tissues.

Materials
Liquid soap, nailbrush or orange stick, paper towels.

Method

Step Number	Procedure	Points Possible	Points Earned
1.	Remove all jewelry (plain wedding bands may be left on and scrubbed).	5	
2.	Turn on the faucets using a paper towel, and adjust the water temperature to moderately warm. (Sinks with knee-operated faucet controls prevent contact of the surface with the hands.)	10	
3.	Wet your hands and apply liquid soap. Use a clean, dry, paper towel to activate soap pump. Liquid soap, especially when dispensed with a foot pump, is preferable to bar soap.	10	
4.	Work the soap into a lather, making sure that all of both hands are lathered. Rub vigorously in a circular motion for 2 minutes. Keep your hands lower than your forearms so that dirty water flows into the sink instead of back onto your arms. Your fingertips should be pointing down. Interlace your fingers to clean between them, and use the palm of one hand to clean the back of the other. It is important that you wash every surface of your hands.*	40	
5.	Use a single-use nailbrush or plastic, single-use nail cleaner under running water to dislodge dirt around your nails and cuticles.*	15	
6.	Rinse your hands well, keeping the hands lower than your forearms and not touching the sink or faucets.	10	
7.	With the water still running, dry your hands thoroughly with clean, dry paper towels and then turn off the faucets using a clean, dry paper towel. Discard the towels.	10	
Total Points		100	

CAAHEP Competencies Achieved
III. P (4)   Perform hand washing

ABHES Competencies Achieved
4. (c) Apply principles of aseptic techniques and infection control

Name_____ Date_____

Evaluated by_____ Score_____

PROCEDURE 6-6 Using an Alcohol Hand Disinfectant

Goal
To use an alcohol-based hand-cleansing substance to reduce pathogens on the hand surfaces and prevent recontamination.

OSHA Guidelines
This procedure does not involve exposure to blood, body fluids, or tissue.

Materials
60–95% alcohol-based foam, gel, or liquid rub.

Method

Step Number	Procedure	Points Possible	Points Earned
1.	Remove all jewelry (plain wedding bands may be left on).	10	
2.	Pump the recommended amount of AHD onto the palm of the hand.*	25	
3.	Rub the hands together vigorously, ensuring the alcohol comes in contact with all surfaces, including backs of hands, between fingers, and fingernails.*	40	
4.	Continue to rub the solution in a rotary fashion until it is evaporated and the hands are dry.*	25	
Total Points		100	

CAAHEP Competencies Achieved

III. P (4)   Perform hand washing

ABHES Competencies Achieved

4. (c) Apply principles of aseptic techniques and infection control

⬤

PROCEDURE 6-7 Removing Contaminated Gloves

Goal
To remove gloves contaminated with blood, body fluids, or other potentially hazardous substances, avoiding cross contamination of your hands or other surfaces.

OSHA Guidelines
This procedure does not involve exposure to blood, body fluids, or tissue.

Materials
Contaminated gloves, lined trash container or biohazard waste container.

Method

Step Number	Procedure	Points Possible	Points Earned
1.	Using your dominant hand, grasp the palm of the glove of your nondominant hand.	15	
2.	Gently pull the glove off the nondominant hand, turning it inside out and holding it in your dominant hand.	15	
3.	Encase the removed glove completely in the dominant hand.	15	
4.	Place the thumb or two fingers of the ungloved hand under the cuff of the remaining glove, being careful not to touch the outside of the glove with your bare hand.	15	
5.	Pull the glove over your hand, turning it inside out over the other glove and leaving no outside surface exposed.	15	
6.	Throw the gloves away in the appropriate waste container.	10	
7.	Wash your hands.	15	
Total Points		100	

CAAHEP Competencies Achieved

    III. P (2)   Practice Standard Precautions

ABHES Competencies Achieved

    9. (b) Apply principles of aseptic techniques and infection control

    9. (i) Use standard precautions

PROCEDURE 6-8 Removing a Contaminated Gown

Goal
To remove a gown contaminated on the front and sleeves with blood, body fluids, or other potentially hazardous substances, avoiding cross contamination of your hands, body, or other surfaces.

OSHA Guidelines
This procedure does not involve exposure to blood, body fluids, or tissue.

Materials
Contaminated gloves, lined trash container or biohazard waste container.

Method

Step Number	Procedure	Points Possible	Points Earned
1.	Unfasten ties from the neck, then from behind your back.	10	
2.	Peel the gown down and away from neck and shoulders, touching inside of gown only.	25	
3.	Continue pulling the gown down from the neck and shoulders away from your body.	25	
4.	Turn gown inside out making sure you do not touch the outer surface of the gown.	25	
5.	Slowly fold or roll into a bundle and discard in appropriate waste container.	15	
Total Points		100	

CAAHEP Competencies Achieved

III. P (2)   Practice Standard Precautions

ABHES Competencies Achieved

9. (b) Apply principles of aseptic techniques and infection control

9. (i) Use standard precautions

PROCEDURE 6-9 Notifying State and County Agencies about Reportable Diseases

WORK // DOC

Goal
To report cases of infection with reportable disease to the proper state or county health department.

OSHA Guidelines
This procedure does not involve exposure to blood, body fluids, or tissues.

Materials
Communicable disease report form, pen, envelope, stamp.

Method

Step Number	Procedure	Points Possible	Points Earned
1.	Check to be sure you have the correct form.	15	
2.	Fill in all blank areas unless they are shaded (generally for local health department use).	30	
3.	Follow office procedures for submitting the report to a supervisor or physician before sending it out.	25	
4.	Sign and date the form. Address the envelope, put a stamp on it, and place it in the mail.	30	
Total Points		100	

CAAHEP Competencies Achieved

IV. P (2)   Report relevant information to others succinctly and accurately

IX. P (8)   Apply local, state, and federal healthcare legislation and regulation appropriate to the medical-assisting practice setting

ABHES Competencies Achieved

None

Patient Reception

Name_____ Class_____ Date_____

R E V I E W

Vocabulary Review

True or False

Decide whether each statement is true or false. In the space at the left, write T *for true or* F *for false. On the lines provided, rewrite the false statements to make them true.*

_____ 1. The appearance of the reception area helps to create a patient's impression of the practice.

_____

_____ 2. The Americans with Disabilities Act protects people against discrimination because of their mental disability.

_____

_____ 3. A contagious disease can be spread among patients waiting in a reception area.

_____

_____ 4. People from different countries or cultures are considered to have special needs.

_____

_____ 5. A color family is a group of colors that work well together.

_____

_____ 6. Examples of specialty items in a reception area include chairs and sofas.

_____

_____ 7. Patients should have clear, easy access from the parking lot to the medical office door as well as within the office.

_____

_____ 8. A TTY is a device for hearing-impaired patients.

_____

_____ 9. A bulletin board is appropriate in a medical practice.

_____

_____ 10. Health magazines geared toward the general public are a good choice for reading material in a medical office.

_____

_____ 11. It is not necessary to read pamphlets and brochures that are displayed in the reception areas as long as they are published by major publishing companies.

_____

_____ 12. Some states have a relay service for patients with hearing impairments or those with speech disabilities.

_____

_____ 13. No matter how tastefully it is decorated, the reception area will be unappealing if it is not clean.

_____

_____ 14. The primary pastime in the patient reception area is watching television.

_____

_____ 15. Stuffed animals are appropriate for pediatric reception areas because they are soft.

_____

Content Review

Multiple Choice

In the space provided, write the letter of the choice that best answers each question or completes each statement.

_____ 1. The use of videos in a medical practice is
  a. Always inappropriate in the reception area
  b. Becoming a more common activity
  c. Appropriate only for the children's reception area
  d. Appropriate only for adults in the reception area
  e. Appropriate only for adults for teaching purposes

_____ 2. The best toys for children in a reception area are
  a. Toys intended for quiet play
  b. Toys that can be easily cleaned
  c. Toys that can be enjoyed while the child sits
  d. All of the above
  e. None of the above

_____ 3. A double door leading from the medical office to the outside of the building
  a. Helps patients feel safe in the waiting area
  b. Discourages salespeople from entering
  c. Helps patients locate the office
  d. Minimizes drafts in the reception area
  e. All of the above

_____ 4. Which of the following items would be a good addition to a pediatrician's reception area?
  a. DVD player and children's DVDs
  b. Sponge ball and bat
  c. Stuffed animals
  d. Bottle of bubble-blowing liquid
  e. Bag of marbles

_____ 5. Items on a reception bulletin board should be
  a. Written in very large print
  b. Only related to government reports on food and drugs
  c. Changed daily
  d. Never contain information about drugs
  e. Tailored to patients' interests

_____ 6. Older patients may require furniture that is
  a. Plastic
  b. Firm with arms
  c. Brightly colored
  d. Extra soft to accommodate for their loss of muscle tissue
  e. Straight backed without arms

_____ 7. The correct amount of furniture in a reception area
   a. Is enough furniture so that all patients and family members or friends who accompany the patient can sit comfortably, no matter how busy the office schedule is
   b. Is six chairs and one sofa
   c. Is 10 chairs and no sofas
   d. Depends on the size of the room and the number of windows and is usually six to eight chairs
   e. Is specified by OSHA safety regulations

_____ 8. The patient information packet includes
   a. Magazine articles
   b. Billing and insurance processing policies
   c. Drug information
   d. Medical brochures
   e. All of the above

_____ 9. Pediatric reception areas
   a. Are designed to meet the special size and needs of children
   b. Are required under federal law for all family practice offices
   c. Are different from traditional reception areas only in that all the furniture is smaller
   d. Are designed only for sick children
   e. Do not differ in any way from adult reception areas

_____ 10. A cleaning communications notebook is
   a. A means of communication between the office staff and the cleaning staff
   b. A way to list special cleanup needs for the cleaning staff
   c. A way to congratulate and thank the cleaning staff
   d. All of the above
   e. None of the above

_____ 11. A telecommunications machine for the deaf
   a. Is required by federal law in medical practices
   b. Looks just like a regular telephone
   c. Looks like a laptop computer with a cradle for the receiver of a traditional telephone
   d. Is not capable of communicating with another TYY machine
   e. Is required by the Americans with Disabilities Act

_____ 12. The Americans with Disabilities Act
   a. Specifies that bars or rails are attached exactly 30 inches above the floor
   b. Does not address types of discrimination
   c. Maintains the rights of disabled people, including those for employment
   d. Has no impact on the patient reception area of a medical practice
   e. Relates to all of the above

Sentence Completion

In the space provided, write the word or phrase that best completes each sentence.

13. Many elderly patients feel colder because of _____.

14. Music in the reception area should reflect the interests of the _____.

15. The path patients must take to get from the parking area or street to the office and then back again is called the office _____.

16. _____ is waste that can be dangerous to those who handle it or to the environment.

17. In a large medical office, the routine cleaning of the office is performed by _____.

13. _____

14. _____

15. _____

16. _____

17. _____

18. One odor that can be prevented by displaying a sign in a patient reception area is _____.

19. OSHA requires the regular use of _____ as part of a cleaning schedule.

20. To protect patients and staff from being trapped by a fire, medical offices are legally required to install _____.

21. Reading materials in a patient reception area can be organized on tables or in a _____.

22. To protect all patients, but especially those who are immunocompromised, it is best to take _____ patients directly into the exam room.

23. The office _____ can be used to alert patients of local meetings and support groups that may be of interest to them.

24. Coat racks, aquariums, plants, and wall hangings are known as _____ and are used to add a "finishing touch" to the reception area.

25. The reception area creates a significant, visual _____ of the office, as the greeting area for all patients.

18. _____

19. _____

20. _____

21. _____

22. _____

23. _____

24. _____

25. _____

Short Answer

Write the answer to each question on the lines provided.

26. Why are ramps important for a medical practice?

_____

_____

_____

27. What are five daily tasks involved in cleaning a reception area?

_____

_____

_____

_____

28. Why should you take special care in cleaning up after a patient who has vomited or bled on the furniture in the reception area?

_____

_____

_____

29. How much furniture should there be in a patient reception area?

_____

_____

_____

30. How do you best clean a stain?

_____

_____

_____

31. Give two reasons why a medical office should have at least two exits.

_____

_____

_____

32. What are four types of appropriate reading material for the patient reception area?

_____

_____

_____

33. What is the best way to wash artificial flowers?

_____

_____

_____

34. List three ways you could make a reception area more comfortable for elderly patients.

_____

_____

_____

35. List four aspects of a reception area that can make a stay there seem longer than it actually is.

_____

_____

_____

_____

36. How can you best determine the correct temperature for a medical office?

_____

_____

_____

37. List six guidelines for safety in the reception area.

_____

_____

_____

_____

_____

_____

38. List three warm colors.

_____

_____

_____

39. What kind of specialty items would you choose to add to the reception area of a geriatric practice?

_____

_____

_____

40. Why is it important to clean a patient reception area on a daily basis?

_____

_____

_____

A P P L I C A T I O N

Follow the directions for each application.

Creating a Reception Area

Working with a partner, imagine that you have been asked to create a patient reception area for a small medical office. As you plan the area, keep the needs and comfort of the patients foremost in your minds.

a. With your partner, decide on the kind of practice for which you will be creating a reception area, such as a gerontology, orthopedic, or family practice. Then brainstorm a list of the characteristics, needs, and interests of the patients of this practice. Put the kind of practice and your list in writing.

b. Determine the size of the reception area. Base the size on the number of patients who will be using the reception area at one time. Make a diagram or floor plan of the area. If you wish, use graph paper and draw the area to scale. For example, you might decide that one square on the graph paper equals 2 feet in the reception area. Locate all doors and windows. Draw them to scale on the diagram.

c. Discuss the decor. Choose a color family, and select colors for the carpeting, furniture, walls, window treatments, and so on. Keep written notes of your selections.

d. Decide what furniture you will purchase and how it will be arranged. Keep in mind the needs of the kinds of patients who will use the reception area. Locate each piece of furniture on your diagram of the area, drawing each to scale.

e. Choose music, specific magazines and books, and special items for the reception area. Write down your choices.

f. Along with other pairs of students, share your diagram and written notes with the class. Join in a class discussion of the various reception area plans and how each area will meet the specific needs of the medical practice and its patients.

C A S E   S T U D I E S

Write your response to each case study on the lines provided.

Case 1

The physician is especially fond of tropical fish and wants to add a tropical fish aquarium to the office. You don't know how to correctly care for an aquarium of fish and fear it might be a hazard to young patients. What should you do?

_____

_____

_____

Case 2

One patient visits the medical office where you work at least once a week and brings her two preschoolers. At first, she asked you to keep an eye on them while she was in the exam room. Now she just leaves the children in the reception area, expecting you to babysit without being asked. You cannot stay in the reception area and watch her children. How can you handle this problem?

_____

_____

_____

Case 3

You are working in a large medical office along with two other medical assistants. You notice that you are the only one who routinely picks up and cleans the patient reception area. You feel others should be helping maintain this important area. What should you do?

_____

_____

_____

PROCEDURE 7-1 Creating a Pediatric Reception Area

Goal
To create an appropriate environment for children in the patient reception area of a medical (pediatric) practice.

OSHA Guidelines
This procedure does not involve exposure to blood, body fluids, or tissues.

Materials
Children's books and magazines, games, toys, nontoxic crayons and coloring books, television and DVD player, children's DVDs, child- and adult-size chairs, child-size table, bookshelf, boxes or shelves, decorative wall hangings or educational posters (optional).

Method

Step Number	Procedure	Points Possible	Points Earned
1.	Place all adult-size chairs against the wall. Position some of the child-size chairs along the wall with the adult chairs.	14	
2.	Place the remainder of the child-size chairs in small groupings throughout the room. In addition, put several chairs with the child-size table.	14	
3.	Put the books, magazines, crayons, and coloring books on the bookshelf in one corner of the room near a grouping of chairs.	14	
4.	Choose toys and games carefully. Avoid toys that encourage active play, such as balls or toys that require a large area. Make sure that all toys meet safety guidelines. Watch for loose or small (smaller than a golf ball) parts. Toys should also be easy to clean.*	14	
5.	Place the activities for older children near one grouping of chairs and the games and toys for younger children near another grouping. Keep the toys and games in a toy box or on shelves designated for them. Consider labeling or color-coding boxes and shelves and the games and toys that belong there to encourage children to return the games and toys to the appropriate storage area.	14	
6.	Place the television and DVD player on a high shelf, if possible, or attach them to the wall near the ceiling. Keep children's DVDs behind the reception desk, and periodically change the video in the DVD player.*	16	
7.	To make the room more cheerful, decorate it with wall hangings or posters.	14	
Total Points		100	

CAAHEP Competencies Achieved

None

ABHES Competencies Achieved

8. (x) Maintain medical facility.

PROCEDURE 7-2 Creating a Reception Area Accessible to Patients with Special Needs

Goal
To arrange elements in the reception area to accommodate patients with special needs.

OSHA Guidelines
This procedure does not involve exposure to blood, body fluids, or tissues.

Materials
Ramps (if needed), doorway floor coverings, chairs, bars or rails, adjustable-height tables, magazine rack, television/DVD player, large-type and Braille magazines.

Method

Step Number	Procedure	Points Possible	Points Earned
1.	Arrange chairs to create gaps that allow substantial space along walls and near other chair groupings for wheelchairs. Keep the arrangement flexible so that chairs can be removed to allow room for additional wheelchairs if needed.*	10	
2.	Remove any obstacles that may interfere with the space needed for a wheelchair to swivel around completely. Also, remove scatter rugs or any carpeting that is not attached to the floor. Such carpeting can cause patients to trip and create difficulties for wheelchair traffic.*	10	
3.	Position coffee tables at a height and location that is accessible to people in wheelchairs.	10	
4.	Place office reading materials, like magazines, at a height that is accessible to people in wheelchairs (for example, on tables or in racks attached midway up the wall).	10	
5.	Locate the television and DVD within full view of patients sitting on chairs and in wheelchairs so that they do not have to strain their necks to watch.	10	
6.	For patients who have a vision impairment, include large-type and Braille reading materials.	10	
7.	For patients who have difficulty walking, make sure bars or rails are attached securely to walls 34 to 38 inches above the floor, to accommodate requirements set forth in the Americans with Disabilities Act. Make sure the bars are sturdy enough to provide balance for patients who may need it. Bars are most important in entrances and hallways, as well as in the bathroom. Consider placing a bar near the receptionist's window for added support as patients check in.*	10	
8.	Eliminate sills of metal or wood along the floor in doorways. Otherwise, create a smoother travel surface for wheelchairs and pedestrians with a thin rubber covering to provide a graduated slope. Be sure that the covering is attached properly and meets safety standards.*	10	
9.	Make sure the office has ramp access.*	10	
10.	Solicit feedback from patients with physical disabilities about the accessibility of the patient reception area. Encourage ideas for improvements. Address any additional needs.*	10	
Total Points		100	

CAAHEP Competencies Achieved

IX. C (11)   Identify how the Americans with Disabilities Act (ADA) applies to the medical assisting profession

ABHES Competencies Achieved

5. (b) Identify and respond appropriately when working/caring for patients with special needs

8. (x) Maintain medical facility

PROCEDURE 7-3 Opening and Closing the Medical Office

WORK // DOC

Goal
To ensure readiness and to receive and care for patients in an efficient, organized, and safe manner.

OSHA Guidelines
This procedure does not involve exposure to blood, body fluids, or tissues.

Materials
Checklist for opening and closing the office (Tables 7-2 and 7-3 may be used as samples), pen, telephone, pad of paper.

Method

Step Number	Procedure	Points Possible	Points Earned
1.	Using Table 7-2, Daily Checklist for Opening the Office, as a guide, simulate the functions of opening the office. Enter the week ending date.*	5	
	a. Begin by disarming the security system.	15	
	b. Telephone the answering service to pick up messages or do the same using the office answering machine or voicemail system. Document any messages and notify the appropriate person of the call.	15	
	c. Conduct each task on the form, placing your initials in the column for the correct day of the week.*	15	
2.	Using Table 7-3, Daily Checklist for Closing the Office, as a guide, simulate the functions of closing the office. Enter the week ending date.*	5	
	a. Begin with logging out and turning off the computers.	15	
	b. Use the telephone to turn on the answering machine/voicemail or notify the answering service that the office is closing.	15	
	c. Conduct each task on the form, placing your initials in the column for the correct day of the week.*	15	
Total Points		100	

CAAHEP Competencies Achieved

None

ABHES Competencies Achieved

8. (d) Apply concepts for office procedures

Office Equipment and Supplies

Name_____ Class_____ Date_____

R E V I E W

Vocabulary Review

Matching

Match the key term in the right column with the definitions in the left column by placing the letter of each correct answer in the space provided.

_____ 1. The physical components of a computer system

_____ 2. A blinking line on the computer screen showing where the next character that is keyed will appear

_____ 3. Instructions a computer needs to function

_____ 4. A device that scans printed information, translating it into electronic impulses over telephone lines, which when received is translated back into an exact replica of the original document

_____ 5. A computer's temporary, programmable memory

_____ 6. A computer disk similar to an audio compact disc that stores huge amounts of data

_____ 7. Software that uses more than one medium—such as graphics, sound, and text—to convey information

_____ 8. A printout of information from a computer

_____ 9. A type of machine that forms characters using a series of dots created by tiny drops of ink

_____ 10. A system that allows users to run two or more software programs simultaneously

_____ 11. A collection of records created and stored on a computer

_____ 12. A method of sending and receiving messages through a network

_____ 13. A global network of computers

_____ 14. A software package that automatically changes the computer monitor at short intervals or shows moving images to prevent burn-in

_____ 15. A device that scans documents for transmission

_____ 16. A machine that consists of a meter and a mailing machine

_____ 17. Transforming the spoken word into writing

_____ 18. A feature of many copiers

_____ 19. Equipment used to assist with protecting confidentiality

a. CD-ROM
b. cursor
c. database
d. electronic mail
e. hard copy
f. hardware
g. ink-jet printer
h. Internet
i. operating systems
j. multimedia
k. multitasking
l. random-access memory (RAM)
m. scanner
n. screen saver
o. postage meter
p. paper shredder
q. collating
r. warranty
s. transcription
t. backup system
u. inventory
v. fax machine
w. unit price
x. MSDS
y. purchase order

_____ **20.** A contract guaranteeing free service and replacement parts for a specific time frame

_____ **21.** A guarantee that information will be available if there is a system failure

_____ **22.** A listing of supplies used in the office

_____ **23.** A document used to order supplies from a vendor

_____ **24.** The price per item

_____ **25.** A description of the chemical breakdown of products as well as use and safety precautions

Content Review

Multiple Choice

In the space provided, write the letter of the choice that best completes each statement or answers each question.

_____ **1.** Another name for a laptop is a

    a. Minicomputer   **d.** Microcomputer

    b. Mainframe   **e.** PDA

    c. Notebook

_____ **2.** The keyboard is the most common input device. Other input devices include

    a. A mouse   **d.** Speakers

    b. Earphones   **e.** File folders

    c. Software

_____ **3.** Which statement about ROM is *true*?

    a. It is permanent memory   **d.** You can make changes to ROM

    b. It is the same as RAM   **e.** None of the statements are true

    c. It is programmable

_____ **4.** A "multitasking" system means

    a. Many different types of expenses are involved

    b. The system has multiple uses

    c. Users can run two or more software programs simultaneously

    d. All of the above

    e. None of the above

_____ **5.** The first step in selecting new computer equipment is

    a. To set up a trial run of a new system for 30 days

    b. To research the needs of the office and the capabilities of the equipment

    c. To remove the old system

    d. To convert back to a manual system

    e. To set up a search committee

_____ **6.** A computer password

    a. Backs up computer files

    b. Can be shared by more than one employee performing the same functions

    c. Stores information

    d. Helps protect confidential information

    e. All of the above

_____ **7.** Which of the following is considered the most important piece of hardware in a computer system?

    a. RAM   **d.** The instruction set

    b. ROM   **e.** The CPU

    c. The USB port

____ 8. Which group of items is considered general supplies?
    a. Lancets, tongue depressors, and sutures
    b. Lubricating jelly, alcohol swabs, and needles
    c. Paper cups, toilet paper, and liquid soap
    d. Copy paper, stamps, and pens
    e. File folders, insurance manuals, and forms

____ 9. You should order by "rush order"
    a. Only as absolutely required
    b. On Fridays to avoid the weekend
    c. Routinely
    d. On Mondays to compensate for the weekend
    e. Never

____ 10. The Federal Trade Commission (FTC) requires supply companies to provide merchandise within how many days or to give you the option of canceling with a full refund?
    a. 90
    b. 60
    c. 180
    d. 30
    e. 14

____ 11. A purchase requisition is
    a. A form that can be used only when faxing an order
    b. Another name for an invoice
    c. Another name for an MSDS sheet
    d. Used only when purchasing through a buying pool
    e. A formal request from a staff member or doctor

____ 12. The best place to store the office holiday decorations is
    a. In a storage area away from heat and water
    b. As close to the ceiling as possible because this item is used only once a year
    c. By the furnace
    d. Near the water heater
    e. In the patient bathroom

____ 13. When the physician determines that a chart can be discarded, you should
    a. Throw it in the trash
    b. Shred it
    c. Burn it
    d. Keep it for 7 years
    e. Store it in a confidential location

____ 14. The postage meter
    a. Is a convenient and cost-efficient way to apply postage to office correspondence and packages
    b. Functions only when there is money in the postal account
    c. Automatically senses the weight of a letter or package
    d. A and B only
    e. None of the above

____ 15. A leasing agreement for large office equipment is
    a. Always preferable to buying
    b. Advantageous when you do not have enough money to buy the equipment but you need the service it provides
    c. Always less expensive over the long term
    d. Always more expensive over the long term
    e. Never price negotiable

Sentence Completion

In the space provided, write the word or phrase that best completes each sentence.

16. Word processing, database, and accounting software are examples of software that is written for a specific purpose, or _____.

17. _____ are high-resolution printers that use a technology similar to that of photocopiers.

18. Requiring a(n) _____ limits the computer users who can access files.

19. A(n) _____ operates over telephone lines but uses a different frequency than the telephone frequency.

20. A(n) _____ is a type of pointing device and is common on laptop and notebook computers.

21. Photocopiers can be configured with a(n) _____ that can transmit the images of documents to computers.

22. A(n) _____ is a modem that operates over cable television lines to provide fast Internet access.

23. OSHA stands for _____.

24. New calendars and appointment books are examples of _____ supplies.

25. _____ must be stored out of site and in a locked cabinet.

26. The rules of good housekeeping and _____ apply to storage areas for clinical supplies.

27. _____ are groups of physicians who order supplies together to obtain a quantity discount.

28. A(n) _____ is a machine that applies postage to an envelope or package.

29. Medical assistants may be asked to _____ tape-recorded words into written text.

30. A(n) _____ imprints a check with the date, payee's name, and payment amount.

31. If the price of the equipment or terms of the sale are not firm, there is room for _____, or for bargaining for additional savings or more flexible terms.

32. A(n) _____ tells how a piece of equipment works, what its special features are, and how to troubleshoot problems.

33. Periodically, it will be necessary to conduct an equipment _____, which is a list of a business's equipment.

34. Most software packages offer _____ if you are unable to troubleshoot a software problem successfully.

35. A(n) _____ is an option for renting office equipment instead of purchasing equipment outright.

16. _____
17. _____
18. _____
19. _____
20. _____
21. _____
22. _____
23. _____
24. _____
25. _____
26. _____
27. _____
28. _____
29. _____
30. _____
31. _____
32. _____
33. _____
34. _____
35. _____

Short Answer

Write the answer to each question on the lines provided.

36. Compare a mouse and a trackball.

_____

_____

37. Patient records are stored on the hard disk drive of a computer. What are three ways that you could give a copy of those records to a consulting physician?

_____

_____

38. What are three sources of information you might turn to if you are having problems using a software program?

_____

_____

_____

39. How does a surge protector help maintain a computer system?

_____

_____

40. Why might it be a good idea to take a computer course at an adult school or community college every few years?

_____

_____

_____

41. Describe how to establish an online account for ordering supplies.

_____

_____

_____

42. What tasks are likely to be included in the medical assistant's responsibilities for maintaining supplies?

_____

_____

_____

43. List items that are important to include on an inventory card.

_____

_____

_____

44. Explain how inventory cards and colored adhesive flags can be used to track supplies that must be reordered.

_____

_____

_____

45. Explain how to calculate a unit price.

_____

_____

_____

46. What procedure should you follow when receiving a supply shipment?

_____

_____

_____

47. You notice that some items are always running out. What might you do to handle this situation?

_____

_____

_____

48. What are the benefits of faxing a document?

_____

_____

_____

49. Why is using a check writer safer than handwriting a check?

_____

_____

_____

50. List three steps in troubleshooting a problem with a piece of equipment.

_____

_____

_____

A P P L I C A T I O N

Follow the directions for each application.

1. You have been asked to research whether the office should purchase a new copier/fax/scanner combination or continue with the separate units that many in the office feel are adequate. Where will you start?

2. You are setting up an inventory system for the office. Your first task is to design inventory pages to place in a binder. What information should you include for each item? List each category of needed information on the lines provided. Use a sheet of paper to design the inventory page.

3. You are ordering 2-liter plastic bottles of saline solution for the office. Apex Medical Supply sells a 10-bottle package for $12.50. Acme Medical Supply sells the same brand and size in an 8-bottle package for $11.20. Which package is the better buy?

4. Work with two partners. One should take the role of a medical assistant who has worked in a medical practice for a while and knows how to operate all the office equipment. The second partner should take the role of a new medical assistant who is not familiar with the equipment. The third person should serve as an observer and evaluator.

   a. The observer should choose a piece of office equipment, such as the photocopier. The experienced medical assistant should then give step-by-step directions on how to use the equipment. The new medical assistant should ask questions to clarify the directions.

   b. The evaluator should observe the training session while checking the directions given against those presented in the text.

   c. When the training session is complete, the evaluator should provide feedback by citing any omissions or errors in the instructions. All three partners should discuss the effectiveness of the session.

   d. Now exchange roles. The new evaluator should choose another piece of equipment to describe in another round of training.

   e. Exchange roles again so that each member of the team plays each role at least once. Repeat the activity until all partners achieve confidence in using each piece of equipment.

5. Design a cover sheet to accompany a confidential faxed transmittal from a medical practice.

   a. Decide on the type of medical practice. Create the names of the physicians and the address and phone number of the practice.

   b. On an 8½- by 11-inch sheet of paper, decide what information to include. Then design your cover sheet.

   c. Type the finished cover sheet. Check spelling, grammar, and punctuation.

   d. Compare your cover sheet with those of other students. Decide whether you have provided all necessary information. Discuss whether cover sheets should be typed or handwritten and why.

CASE STUDIES

Write your response to each case study on the lines provided.

Case 1
The medical office where you work has just begun converting to a computer system. The doctors are concerned about the confidentiality of the files. What will you recommend?

_____

_____

_____

Case 2
As the person at your office in charge of ordering supplies, you take a call from an unknown vendor. He tells you that he has an overstock of your brand of photocopier toner. He wants to get rid of it, so he will let you have it for half the regular price. He instructs you to send a check to a box number he gives you; then he will ship the toner to you. What should you do? Why?

_____

_____

_____

Case 3

You receive a letter from a vendor threatening collection if an invoice that is now 6 months old is not paid immediately. You know that the invoice has been paid. How can you support your claim that your office has paid its bill?

_____

_____

_____

Case 4

The office manager leaves you a note asking you to fax a document. You place the document in the sending tray of the machine and key in the phone number, but nothing happens. What do you do?

_____

_____

_____

PROCEDURE 8-1 Using a Facsimile (Fax) Machine [WORK // DOC]

Goal
To correctly prepare and send a fax document while following all HIPAA guidelines to guard patient confidentiality.

OSHA Guidelines
This procedure does not involve exposure to blood, body fluids, or tissues.

Materials
Fax machine, fax line, cover sheet with statement of disclaimer, area code and phone number of fax recipient, document to be faxed, telephone line, and telephone.

Method

Step Number	Procedure	Points Possible	Points Earned
1.	Prepare a cover sheet, which provides information about the transmission. Cover sheets can vary in appearance but usually include the name, telephone number, and fax number of the sender and the receiver; the number of pages being transmitted; and the date of the transmission. Preprinted cover sheets can be used. (See Figure 8-10 in the text.)*	10	
2.	All cover sheets must carry a statement of disclaimer to guard the privacy of the patient. A disclaimer is a statement of denial of legal liability. (A sample cover sheet is shown in Figure 8-10 in the text.)*	10	
3.	Place all pages of the document, including the cover sheet, either face down or face up in the fax machine's sending tray, depending on the directions stamped on the sending tray.	10	
4.	If the documents are placed face down, write the area code and fax number on the back of the last page.	5	
5.	Dial the telephone number of the receiving fax machine, using either the telephone attached to the fax machine or the numbers on the fax keyboard. Include the area code for long-distance calls.	10	
6.	When using a fax telephone, listen for a high-pitched tone. Then press the "Send" or "Start" button, and hang up the telephone. This step completes the call circuit in older-model fax machines. Your fax is now being sent. Newer fax machines do not require this step.*	10	
7.	If you use the fax keyboard, press the "Send" or "Start" button after dialing the telephone number. This button will start the call.	10	
8.	Watch for the fax machine to make a connection. Often a green light appears as the document feeds through the machine.	10	
9.	If the fax machine is not able to make a connection, as when the receiving fax line is busy, it may have a feature that automatically redials the number every few minutes for a specified number of attempts.	5	
10.	When a fax has been successfully sent, most fax machines print a confirmation message. When a fax has not been sent, the machine either prints an error message or indicates on the screen that the transmission was unsuccessful.*	5	
11.	Attach the confirmation or error message to the documents faxed. File appropriately.*	10	

(continued)

Name_____ Date_____

Evaluated by_____ Score_____

Step Number	Procedure	Points Possible	Points Earned
12.	If required by office policy, the sender should call the recipient to confirm the fax was received.	5	
Total Points		100	

CAAHEP Competencies Achieved

V. P (6)   Use office hardware and software to maintain office systems

ABHES Competencies Achieved

8. (d) Apply concepts for office procedures

8. (ll) Apply electronic technology

Name_____ Date_____

Evaluated by_____ Score_____

PROCEDURE 8-2 Using a Photocopier Machine

Goal
To produce copies of documents.

OSHA Guidelines
This procedure does not involve exposure to blood, body fluids, or tissues.

Materials
Copier machine, copy paper, documents to be copied.

Method

Step Number	Procedure	Points Possible	Points Earned
1.	Make sure the machine is turned on and warmed up. It will display a signal when it is ready for copying.	15	
2.	Assemble and prepare your materials, removing paper clips, staples, and self-adhesive flags.*	15	
3.	Place the document to be copied in the automatic feeder tray as directed, or upside down directly on the glass. The feeder tray can accommodate many pages; you may place only one page at a time on the glass. Automatic feeding is a faster process, and you should use it when you wish to collate or staple packets. Page-by-page copying is best if you need to copy a single sheet or to enlarge or reduce the image. To use any special features, such as making double-sided copies or stapling the copies, press a designated button on the machine.	15	
4.	Set the machine for the desired paper size.*	15	
5.	Key in the number of copies you want to make, and press the "Start" button. The copies are made automatically.	15	
6.	Press the "Clear" or "Reset" button when your job is finished.*	10	
7.	If the copier becomes jammed, follow the directions on the machine to locate the problem (for example, there may be multiple pieces of paper stuck inside the printer), and dislodge the jammed paper. Most copy machines will show a diagram of the printer and the location of the problem.*	15	
Total Points		100	

CAAHEP Competencies Achieved

V. P (6)   Use office hardware and software to maintain office systems

ABHES Competencies Achieved

8. (d) Apply concepts for office procedures

8. (ll) Apply electronic technology

Name_____ Date_____

Evaluated by_____ Score_____

PROCEDURE 8-3 Using a Postage Meter

Goal
To correctly apply postage to an envelope or package for mailing, according to U.S. Postal Service guidelines.

OSHA Guidelines
This procedure does not involve exposure to blood, body fluids, or tissues.

Materials
Postage meter, addressed envelope or package, postal scale.

Method

Step Number	Procedure	Points Possible	Points Earned
1.	Check that there is postage available in the postage meter.*	10	
2.	Verify the day's date.*	10	
3.	Check that the postage meter is plugged in and switched on before you proceed.	10	
4.	Locate the area where the meter registers the date. Many machines have a lid that can be flipped up, with rows of numbers underneath. Months are represented numerically, with the number "1" indicating the month of January, "2" indicating February, and so on. Check that the date is correct. If it is incorrect, change the numbers to the correct date.	10	
5.	Make sure that all materials have been included in the envelope or package. Weigh the envelope or package on a postal scale. Standard business envelopes weighing up to 1 oz require the minimum postage (the equivalent of one first class stamp). Oversize envelopes and packages require additional postage. A postal scale will indicate the amount of postage required.	10	
6.	Key in the postage amount on the meter, and press the button that enters the amount. For amounts over $1, press the "$" sign or the "Enter" button twice.*	10	
7.	Check that the amount you typed is the correct amount. Envelopes and packages with too little postage will be returned by the U.S. Postal Service. Sending an envelope or package with too much postage is wasteful to the practice.	10	
8.	While applying postage to an envelope, hold it flat and right side up (so that you can read the address). Seal the envelope (unless the meter seals it for you). Locate the plate or area where the envelope slides through. This feature is usually near the bottom of the meter. Place the envelope on the left side, and give it a gentle push toward the right. Some models hold the envelope in a stationary position. (If the meter seals the envelope for you, it is especially important that you insert it correctly to allow for sealing.) The meter will grab the envelope and pull it through quickly.	10	
9.	For packages, create a postage label to affix to the package. Follow the same procedure for a label as for an envelope. Affix the postmarked label on the package in the upper-right corner.	10	
10.	Check that the printed postmark has the correct date and amount and that everything written or stamped on the envelope or package is legible.	10	
Total Points		100	

CAAHEP Competencies Achieved

V. P (6)   Use office hardware and software to maintain office systems

ABHES Competencies Achieved

8. (d) Apply concepts for office procedures

8. (ll) Apply electronic technology

PROCEDURE 8-4 Using a Check-Writing Machine

Goal
To produce a check using a check-writing machine.

OSHA Guidelines
This procedure does not involve exposure to blood, body fluids, or tissues.

Materials
Check-writing machine, blank checks, office checkbook or accounting system.

Method

Step Number	Procedure	Points Possible	Points Earned
1.	Assemble all equipment.	15	
2.	Turn on the check-writing machine.	10	
3.	Place a blank check or a sheet of blank checks into the machine.	15	
4.	Key in the date, the payee's name, and the payment amount. The check-writing machine imprints the check with this information, perforating it with the payee's name. The perforations are actual little holes in the paper, that prevent anyone from changing the name on the check.	15	
5.	Turn off the check-writing machine.	15	
6.	A doctor or another authorized person then signs the check.*	15	
7.	To complete the process, record the check in the office checkbook or accounting system.*	15	
Total Points		100	

CAAHEP Competencies Achieved

V. P (6)   Use office hardware and software to maintain office systems

ABHES Competencies Achieved

8. (d) Apply concepts for office procedures

8. (ll) Apply electronic technology

PROCEDURE 8-5 Step-by-Step Overview of Inventory Procedures

Goal

To set up an effective inventory program for a medical office.

OSHA Guidelines

This procedure does not involve exposure to blood, body fluids, or tissues.

Materials

Pen, paper, file folders, vendor catalogs, index cards or loose-leaf binder and blank pages, reorder reminder cards, vendor order forms.

Method

Step Number	Procedure	Points Possible	Points Earned
1.	Discuss and define with your physician/employer the extent of your responsibility in managing supplies. Know whether the physician's approval or supervision is required for certain procedures, whether any systems have already been established, and if the physician has any preference for a particular vendor or trade-name item. If your medical practice is large, determine which medical assistant is responsible for each aspect of supply management.	8	
2.	Know what administrative and clinical supplies should be stocked in your office. Create a formal supply list of vital, incidental, and periodic items, and keep a copy in the office's procedures manual.*	8	
3.	Start a file containing a list of current vendors with copies of their catalogs.	5	
4.	Create a wish list of brands or products the office does not currently use but might like to try. Inform other staff members of the list so that they can make entries.	5	
5.	Make a file for supply invoices and completed order forms. (Keep these documents on file for at least 3 years.)*	8	
6.	Devise an inventory system of index cards, loose-leaf pages, or a computer spreadsheet for each item. List the following data for each item on its card: • Date and quantity of each order • Name and contact information for the vendor and sales representative • Date each shipment was received • Total cost and unit cost, or price per piece for the item • Payment method used • Results of periodic counts of the item • Quantity expected to cover the office for a given period of time • Reorder quantity (the quantity remaining on the shelf that indicates when reorder should be made)	9	
7.	Have a system for flagging items that need to be ordered and those that are already on order. For example, mark their cards or pages with a self-adhesive tab or note. Make or buy reorder reminder cards to put into the stock of each item at the reorder quantity level.*	5	
8.	Establish with the physician a regular schedule for taking inventory. Every 1 to 2 weeks is usually sufficient. As a backup system for remembering to check stock and reorder, estimate the times for these activities. Mark them on your calendar, or create a tickler file on your computer.*	5	

(continued)

Step Number	Procedure	Points Possible	Points Earned
9.	Order at the same times each week or month, after inventory is taken. However, if there is an unexpected shortage of an item, and more than a week or so remains before the regular ordering time, place the order immediately.	5	
10.	Fill in the vendor's order form (or type a letter of request). Order by telephone, fax, e-mail, or online. Online ordering will expedite the order. Follow procedures that have been approved by the physician or office manager. When placing an order, have all the necessary information at hand, including the correct name of the item and the order and account numbers. Record the order information in the inventory file for that item. Be sure to obtain from the vendor an estimated arrival time for the order, and mark that date and order number on your calendar.*	5	
11.	When ordering online, save the website to "Favorites" for easy, one-click future access. Select the website and establish an account with the company. To establish an account, you will need to give information about your office practice, including the name of the practice, contact name, the address, the phone number, an e-mail address, and a payment source. Ask about adding the practice to any special contact lists for promotional materials and discounts.	5	
12.	When you receive the shipment, record the date and the amount received on the item's inventory card or record page. Check the shipment against the original order and the packing slip inside the package to ensure that the right items, sizes, styles, packaging, and amounts have arrived. Initial each item on the packing slip as a record that the correct item and amount was received. If there is any error, immediately call or e-mail the vendor, with the catalog page and the inventory card or record page at hand.*	8	
13.	Check the invoice carefully against the original order and the packing slip, making sure that the amount of the bill matches the items listed on the invoice and the packing list, and ensure that the bill has not already been paid. Sign or stamp the invoice to show that the order was received.	8	
14.	Write a check to the vendor to be signed by the physician. (Check writing procedures are described in the *Financial Management* chapter.) Be sure to show the physician the original order, packing slip, and invoice. Record the check number, date, and amount of payment on the invoice, and initial it or have the physician do so. Write the invoice number on the front of the check.*	8	
15.	Mail the check and the vendor's copy of the invoice to the vendor within 30 days, and file the office copy of the invoice with the original order and packing slip.	8	
Total Points		100	

CAAHEP Competencies Achieved

   V. P (10)   Perform an office inventory

ABHES Competencies Achieved

   8. (z) Maintain inventory equipment and supplies

9

Examination and Treatment Areas

Name_____ Class_____ Date_____

REVIEW

Vocabulary Review

Matching

Match the key terms in the right column with the definitions in the left column by placing the letter of each correct answer in the space provided.

_____ 1. An exam performed to confirm a patient's health or diagnose a medical problem

_____ 2. Complete destruction of all living organisms

_____ 3. The ease with which people can move in and out of a space

_____ 4. Instrument used to enlarge the opening of the nose to permit viewing

_____ 5. Thick-walled, reproductive bodies capable of resisting harsh conditions

_____ 6. A process that destroys most organisms, except for spores and some viruses

_____ 7. Instrument used for inspecting the ear

_____ 8. Blood that is not visible to the naked eye

_____ 9. Water-soluble gel used during a physical exam of the rectum or vagina

_____ 10. Description of items that are used up or emptied during an exam

_____ 11. Chemical spray used to preserve a specimen obtained from the body for pathologic exam

_____ 12. Sending sound waves through a cleaning solution to clean delicate instruments

_____ 13. Instrument used to examine the interior of the eye

_____ 14. Scrubbing with special brushes and detergent to remove blood, mucus, and other contaminants or media where pathogens can grow

_____ 15. Instrument used to establish an artificial airway

a. accessibility
b. consumable
c. disinfection
d. endotracheal tubes
e. fixative
f. general physical exam
g. lubricant
h. nasal speculum
i. occult blood
j. ophthalmoscope
k. otoscope
l. sanitation
m. spores
n. sterilization
o. ultrasonic cleaning

True or False

Decide whether each statement is true or false. In the space at the left, write T for true or F for false. On the lines provided, rewrite the false statements to make them true.

_____ 16. Putting the exam room in order is the physician's responsibility.

_____

_____ 17. The three methods of infection control are sanitization, disinfection, and sterilization.

_____ 18. Sanitization is a scrubbing process used to remove the microorganisms that cause disease.

_____ 19. Bleach is an effective means of sterilization.

_____ 20. The thermostat in an exam room should be set at 55°F to discourage the growth of bacteria.

_____ 21. A glass slide is an example of a consumable supply.

_____ 22. After washing your hands, you should use a clean paper towel to handle doorknobs.

_____ 23. ADA accessibility guidelines require doorways to be trimmed in metal casing.

_____ 24. An instrument used to examine the external ear canal and tympanic membrane is a tuning fork.

_____ 25. Sanitization involves raising the number of microorganisms on an object or surface to a fairly safe level.

Content Review

Multiple Choice

In the space provided, write the letter of the choice that best completes each statement or answers each question.

_____ 1. Ideally, how many exam rooms should a doctor have reserved for exclusive use?

a. 0　　　　　　　　　　　　　d. 3

b. 1　　　　　　　　　　　　　e. 4

c. 2

_____ 2. A common disinfectant used in exam areas and on surfaces is

a. Ammonia　　　　　　　　　d. Window cleaner

b. Dish detergent　　　　　　　e. A 10% bleach solution

c. A 5% vinegar solution

_____ 3. The ADA requires that doorways be at least

a. 22 inches wide　　　　　　　d. 60 inches tall

b. 30 inches wide　　　　　　　e. 96 inches tall

c. 36 inches wide

_____ 4. An instrument used to check pupil response in the eye is a(n)

a. Otoscope　　　　　　　　　d. Penlight

b. Exam light　　　　　　　　　e. Laryngoscope

c. Stethoscope

_____ 5. If a medical assistant accidentally brings a patient into a room before it is cleaned, which of the following would be the most appropriate action to take?

   a. Have the patient wait in the room while it is cleaned

   b. Put a clean sheet on the examining table and ignore the rest of it

   c. Ignore the whole situation

   d. Clean the table, have the patient sit on the table, and then remove the waste

   e. Ask the patient to wait outside just for a moment while it is cleaned

_____ 6. An instrument used to measure size or development of a body part is a

   a. Thermometer

   b. Tuning fork

   c. Tape measure

   d. Speculum

   e. Penlight

_____ 7. An instrument used to measure blood pressure is a(n)

   a. Stethoscope

   b. Anoscope

   c. Ophthalmoscope

   d. Tuning fork

   e. Sphygmomanometer

_____ 8. The first step in preventing infection transmission in the exam room is

   a. Disinfecting work surfaces

   b. Handwashing

   c. Arranging supplies

   d. Keeping the examining table clean

   e. Maintaining proper room temperature

_____ 9. A chemical agent that leaves an instrument clean but not sterile is a(n)

   a. Lubricant

   b. Antiseptic

   c. Detergent

   d. Disinfectant

   e. Antibiotic

_____ 10. The use of alcohol is an effective means of

   a. Sterilization

   b. Immunization

   c. Disinfection

   d. Sanitization

   e. Decontamination

Short Answer

Write the answer to each question on the lines provided.

11. What are three medical instruments you can sanitize and reuse without further disinfection or sterilization?

_____

_____

_____

12. List three factors that can have an impact on the effectiveness of a disinfectant.

_____

_____

_____

13. What are the disadvantages of using acid products to disinfect instruments and equipment?

_____

_____

_____

14. Describe the process you would use to sanitize surgical instruments.

_____

_____

_____

15. Where in the exam room should the examining table be placed?

_____

_____

_____

16. Why is it important to maintain proper ventilation in an exam room?

_____

_____

_____

17. List four general cleaning tasks a janitorial service might perform in a medical office.

_____

_____

_____

18. When must you disinfect surfaces in the exam room?

_____

_____

_____

19. Good lighting serves many purposes in an exam room. Name three.

_____

_____

_____

20. The illustrations show a variety of instruments used during a general physical exam. On the lines provided, write the name of each instrument and briefly explain its use.

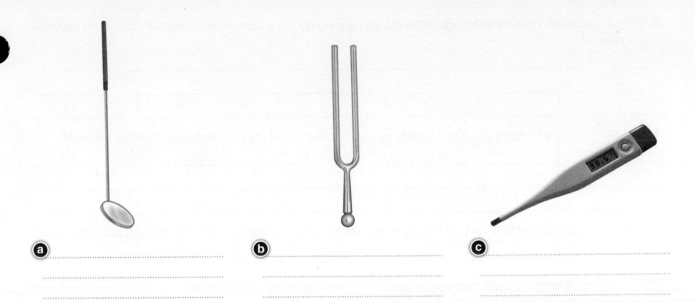

a ....
....
....

b ....
....
....

c ....
....
....

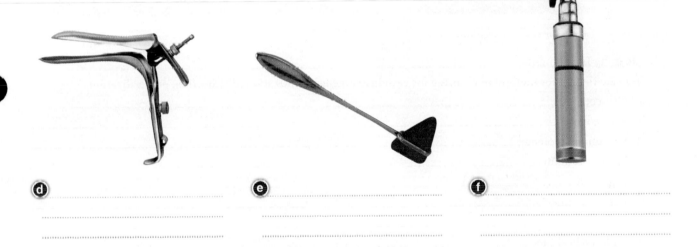

d ....
....
....

e ....
....
....

f ....
....
....

21. What tasks are involved in maintaining the instruments and supplies needed in the exam room?

_____

_____

_____

Critical Thinking

Write the answer to each question on the lines provided.

1. What tasks in the preparation of the exam and treatment area can influence a patient's perception of a medical practice?

_____

_____

_____

2. Why do you think OSHA regulations prohibit applying cosmetics in a room where potentially infectious materials are present?

_____

_____

_____

3. What tasks in preparing the exam and treatment areas are done to aid the physician in performing his work?

_____

_____

_____

4. Why is it important to maintain proper temperature in the laboratory refrigerator? How will you accomplish this?

_____

_____

_____

A P P L I C A T I O N

Follow the directions for each application.

1. **Cleaning Instruments**

   Indicate the proper method of cleaning for each instrument—sanitization, disinfection, or sterilization.

   a. Otoscope _____

   b. Anoscope _____

   c. Sphygmomanometer _____

   d. Nasal speculum _____

   e. Glassware _____

   f. Reflex hammer _____

   g. Stethoscope _____

   h. Endotracheal tube _____

2. **Sanitizing Instruments and Equipment**

   Work with one partner and sanitize a group of instruments. One person should sanitize the instruments and equipment. The second should act as an evaluator and should refer to the detailed description provided in the text while observing the procedure. Assume that a surgical procedure has just been completed.

   a. Collect all the instruments from the procedure.

   b. Put on utility gloves and separate the sharp instruments from all other equipment.

   c. Rinse each piece of equipment in hot running water. Scrub the instruments and equipment with hot, soapy water and a plastic scrub brush. Use a neutral-pH detergent. Then rinse and dry them properly.

   d. When the sanitizing process is complete, the observer should present a critique of the procedure, pointing out any errors in the procedure and offering suggestions for improved technique.

   e. Exchange roles so that each of you has the opportunity to practice the procedure while the other observes and offers comments and suggestions.

3. Inspecting the Medical Office

Suppose you are a health and safety inspector for your state. Describe the things you would look for, in each area listed as follows, when inspecting a medical office.

a. Compliance with the Americans with Disabilities Act

_____

_____

_____

_____

b. Infection control

_____

_____

_____

_____

C A S E   S T U D I E S

Write your responses to each case study on the lines provided.

Case 1

While reviewing the patient list for the next day, you notice that the patient for Dr. Tejada's 10:00 a.m. appointment is in a wheelchair. What "reasonable accommodations" have already been made for this patient?

_____

_____

_____

Case 2

You have been asked to train Sam, a newly hired medical assistant. Sam's main responsibility will be to keep the exam rooms in proper order. What information will you give Sam?

_____

_____

_____

Case 3

At a weekly staff meeting, a coworker announces her intention of cutting overhead costs by turning thermostats down to 65°F and using only under-cabinet lights rather than overhead lights. She then asks the group for feedback on these ideas. What would you say?

_____

_____

_____

PROCEDURE 9-1 Performing Sanitization with an Ultrasonic Cleaner

Goal
To decontaminate items safely and effectively using an ultrasonic cleaner.

OSHA Guidelines

Materials
Ultrasonic cleaner, contaminated items and instruments, ultrasonic cleaning fluid, manufacturer's directions.

Method

Step Number	Procedure	Points Possible	Points Earned
1.	Review the manufacturer's directions.	5	
2.	Fill the container of the ultrasonic cleaner with water.	5	
3.	Add the directed amount of ultrasonic cleaning fluid. Check the directions carefully.	5	
4.	Plug in and turn on the ultrasonic cleaner. Allow a warm-up period if needed. Check the instructions.	5	
5.	Separate instruments and equipment made of different metals.*	15	
6.	Separate instruments with sharp points.*	15	
7.	Open hinges on instruments and equipment.*	10	
8.	Place instruments and equipment in the ultrasonic cleaner, but do not overfill.	5	
9.	Close the lid, turn on the machine or timer, and wait for the cycle to be completed.	5	
10.	Rinse each instrument or piece of equipment in cool running water and then distilled or demineralized water as policy dictates.*	10	
11.	Dry each instrument or piece of equipment.	5	
12.	Prepare each item for storage or further disinfection or sterilization.	5	
13.	Replace ultrasonic cleaning solution according to office policy and manufacturers' guidelines.*	10	
Total Points		100	

CAAHEP Competencies Achieved

III. C (3)   Discuss infection control procedures

III. C (6)   Compare different methods of controlling the growth of microorganisms

ABHES Competencies Achieved

9. (b) Apply principles of aseptic techniques and infection control

9. (k) Prepare and maintain examination and treatment area

PROCEDURE 9-2 Guidelines for Disinfecting Exam Room Surfaces

Goal
To reduce the risk of exposure to potentially infectious microorganisms in the exam room.

OSHA Guidelines

Materials
Utility gloves, disinfectant (10% bleach solution or EPA-approved disinfecting product), paper towels, dustpan and brush, tongs, forceps, clean sponge or heavy rag.

Method

Step Number	Procedure	Points Possible	Points Earned
1.	Wash your hands and put on utility gloves.*	15	
2.	Remove any visible soil from exam room surfaces with disposable paper towels or a rag.	10	
3.	Thoroughly wipe all surfaces with the disinfectant.		
4.	Use tongs, a dustpan and brush, or forceps to pick up shattered glass, which may be contaminated.*	20	
5.	Remove and replace protective coverings, such as plastic wrap or aluminum foil, on equipment if the equipment or the coverings have become contaminated. After removing the coverings, disinfect the equipment and allow it to air dry. (Follow office procedures for the routine changing of protective coverings.)	10	
6.	When you finish cleaning, dispose of the paper towels or rags in a biohazardous-waste receptacle.*	20	
7.	Remove the gloves and wash your hands.*	15	
8.	If you keep a container of 10% bleach solution on hand for disinfection purposes, replace the solution daily to ensure its disinfecting potency.	10	
Total Points		100	

CAAHEP Competencies Achieved

III. C (3)   Discuss infection control procedures

III. C (6)   Compare different methods of controlling the growth of microorganisms

Name_____ Date_____

Evaluated by_____ Score_____

ABHES Competencies Achieved

9. (b) Apply principles of aseptic techniques and infection control

9. (k) Prepare and maintain examination and treatment area

10. (c) Dispose of biohazardous materials

Written and Electronic Documents

Name_____ Class_____ Date_____

Vocabulary Review

Passage Completion
Study the key terms in the box. Use your textbook to find definitions of terms you do not understand.

annotating	full-block letter style	salutation
body	inside address	signature block
clarity	letterhead	simplified letter style
complimentary closing	modified-block letter style	subject line
concise	optical character reader (OCR)	template
editing	proofreading	

In the space provided, complete the following passage, using some of the terms from the box. You may change the form of a term to fit the meaning of the sentence.

Most business letters are written on (1)_____ paper, which identifies the business. The (2)_____, which is placed about two lines below the dateline, states the name and address of the person receiving the letter. The (3)_____ acts as the greeting for the letter and a (4)_____ may be included so that the recipient immediately has a clue as to the contents of the (5)_____ or main section of the letter. In the (6)_____ letter style, all lines are flush left, but in the (7)_____ style, the dateline and (8)_____ begin slightly to the right of the center of the page. The (9)_____ style omits the salutation and the complimentary closing altogether. When a letter is received, your physician may ask you to highlight or make notes on a letter, pointing out important sections, in a process known as (10)_____.

1. _____
2. _____
3. _____
4. _____
5. _____
6. _____
7. _____
8. _____
9. _____
10. _____

True or False
Decide whether each statement is true or false. In the space at the left, write T for true or F for false. On the lines provided, rewrite the false statements to make them true.

_____ **11.** Tan Kraft envelopes are also called clasp envelopes.

_____

_____ **12.** You need to capitalize all the words in the complimentary close of a business letter.

_____

_____ 13. The USPS abbreviation PA stands for Pennsylvania.

_____ 14. Office letterhead should be used for every page of a business letter.

_____ 15. Using standardized templates can simplify making mailing labels.

_____ 16. The term clarity means your letter should be brief and to the point.

_____ 17. The signature block is always placed in or slightly to the right of the horizontal center of the letter.

_____ 18. The modified-block style includes indented paragraphs.

_____ 19. A separate signed consent regarding e-mail is not required as long as the patient provides an e-mail address on the office registration form.

_____ 20. The terms editing and proofreading may be used interchangeably.

Content Review

Multiple Choice

In the space provided, write the letter of the choice that best completes each statement or answers each question.

_____ 1. What attribute should come through in business correspondence?
   a. Compassion
   b. Concern
   c. Professionalism
   d. Efficiency
   e. Clarity

_____ 2. Which of the following tells you that paper is of high quality?
   a. Bond
   b. Letterhead
   c. Color
   d. Watermark
   e. Price

_____ 3. Which of the following is NOT considered part of effective writing?
   a. Clarity
   b. Active voice
   c. Passive voice
   d. Conciseness
   e. Politeness

_____ 4. Which of the following demonstrates an INCORRECT courtesy title?

    a. Dr. Gerald Ward, M.D.

    b. Dr. Gerald Ward

    c. Gerald Ward, M.D.

    d. Mr. Gerald Ward

    e. All of the above are correct

_____ 5. What form of communication is affecting the USPS?

    a. Business communication

    b. Personal, written communication

    c. Package shipping

    d. Face-to-face communication

    e. Electronic communication (e-mail)

_____ 6. How is proofreading/editing best accomplished?

    a. As soon as possible after the document is written

    b. By someone other than the writer of the document

    c. Several hours after the document has been written

    d. b and c are the best combination

    e. a and b are the best combination

_____ 7. Which proofreading/editing tool provides synonyms to avoid repetitive wording within a document?

    a. Medical dictionary

    b. English dictionary

    c. Thesaurus

    d. PDR

    e. Grammar/usage manual

_____ 8. Which word is spelled correctly?

    a. Arrhythmia

    b. Antiflexion

    c. Psoriasus

    d. Paliative

    e. Pshychiatry

_____ 9. Which of the following procedures for preparing mail may be automated in some offices?

    a. Signature

    b. Preparing the envelope

    c. Folding/inserting

    d. Calculating postage

    e. Applying postage

_____ 10. Which of the following is the first step in processing incoming mail?

    a. Distributing

    b. Annotating

    c. Recording

    d. Opening

    e. Sorting

Sentence Completion

In the space provided, write the word or phrase that best completes each statement.

11. The _____ is similar to full block but it differs in that the dateline, complimentary closing, signature block, and notations are aligned and begin at the center of the page or slightly to the right.

12. Two different styles of punctuation used in correspondence are _____ and _____.

13. The USPS abbreviation for Kansas is _____.

14. _____ include information such as the number of enclosures that are included with the letter and the names of other people who will be receiving copies of the letter.

15. _____ means thoroughly checking a document for errors.

16. The USPS uses electronic _____ to help speed mail processing.

17. The Web address for the USPS Web page is _____.

18. The USPS abbreviation for center is _____.

19. Most correspondence generated in a medical office, such as letters, postcards, and invoices, is sent by _____.

20. _____ is also called parcel post.

21. The first step in processing mail is to _____ it.

22. To _____ means to underline or highlight key points of the letter or to write reminders, comments, or suggested actions in the margins or on self-adhesive notes.

23. Business letters written with the modified-block letter style with indented paragraphs are identical to the modified block style except that the paragraphs are _____.

24. When writing a business letter, it is proper to include at least _____ in each paragraph.

25. *Enc* in a business letter means _____.

26. The space around the edges of a form or letter that is left blank is called the _____.

27. The letter _____ must be appropriate for the reader so that the contents may be easily understood.

28. Mistyped monetary figures are an example of a(n) _____ error.

29. When a business letter is folded for mailing, it is folded into horizontal _____ for easy insertion into the envelope.

30. To obtain notification of delivery of a letter, utilize _____ mail offered by the USPS.

31. The _____ of a letter consists of single-spaced lines that are the content of a business letter.

32. _____ is the action the post office will take when a piece of mail does not reach its destination.

33. _____ written on the outside of a letter or package means that the letter or package should not be opened by anyone but the addressee.

34. _____ is the process that ensures that a document is accurate, clear, and complete; free of grammatical errors; organized logically; and written in an appropriate style.

35. Formatting, data, and mechanical errors may all be detected by carefully _____ documents.

11. _____

12. _____

13. _____

14. _____

15. _____

16. _____

17. _____

18. _____

19. _____

20. _____

21. _____

22. _____

23. _____

24. _____

25. _____

26. _____

27. _____

28. _____

29. _____

30. _____

31. _____

32. _____

33. _____

34. _____

35. _____

Short Answer

Write the answer to each question on the lines provided.

36. List three types of envelopes commonly used in a medical office, and briefly describe their uses.

_____

_____

_____

37. What is the difference between a modified-block letter style and a simplified letter style?

_____

_____

_____

38. Describe the voice of the following sentence. Then rewrite the sentence, changing the voice to make it more direct and concise.

The patient's blood sample was sent to you by our office on November 4, 20xx.

_____

_____

_____

39. Why is an envelope with a typed address likely to be delivered more quickly than one with a handwritten address?

_____

_____

_____

40. Describe the difference between certified and registered mail.

_____

_____

_____

Labeling

1. Label the parts of the letter illustrated in the following figure.

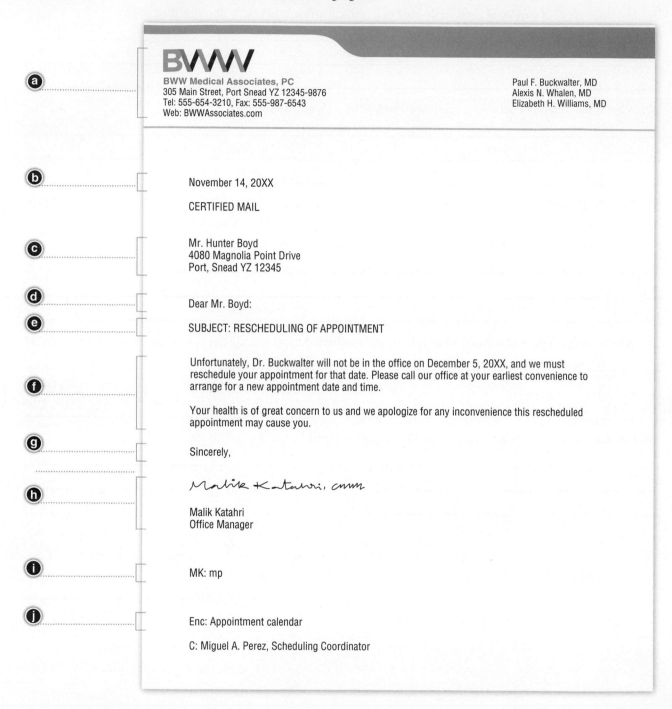

(a)

BWW

BWW Medical Associates, PC
305 Main Street, Port Snead YZ 12345-9876
Tel: 555-654-3210, Fax: 555-987-6543
Web: BWWAssociates.com

Paul F. Buckwalter, MD
Alexis N. Whalen, MD
Elizabeth H. Williams, MD

(b)

November 14, 20XX

CERTIFIED MAIL

(c)

Mr. Hunter Boyd
4080 Magnolia Point Drive
Port, Snead YZ 12345

(d)

Dear Mr. Boyd:

(e)

SUBJECT: RESCHEDULING OF APPOINTMENT

(f)

Unfortunately, Dr. Buckwalter will not be in the office on December 5, 20XX, and we must reschedule your appointment for that date. Please call our office at your earliest convenience to arrange for a new appointment date and time.

Your health is of great concern to us and we apologize for any inconvenience this rescheduled appointment may cause you.

(g)

Sincerely,

(h)

Malik Katahri, CMM

Malik Katahri
Office Manager

(i)

MK: mp

(j)

Enc: Appointment calendar

C: Miguel A. Perez, Scheduling Coordinator

A P P L I C A T I O N

WORK // DOC

Follow the directions for each application.

1. Applying Basic Rules of Effective Writing

Read each of the following sentences looking for errors in spelling, word division, and capitalization, as well as errors in the use of plurals, possessives, and numbers. If a sentence is incorrect, rewrite it correctly on the lines provided. Compare your corrections with those of a partner. Did you find the same errors? Did you miss any? Are there any writing rules that you need to study further?

a. The Patients left oricle showed evidence of a recent infarktion.

_____

b. The abcess developed during the patients' recent trip to see his aunt.

_____

c. The patient was given a perscription for a 10-day supply of ilosone, a form of erythromycin.

_____

d. This 6-year-old patient reports falling from a slide at Ridge Street school this past tuesday.

_____

e. X-rays indicate hare-line fraktures of two cervical vertebra.

_____

2. Handling Incoming Mail

You are a medical assistant whose duties include processing incoming mail. Some of the procedures that you follow are described as follows. For procedures that are correct, write *correct* on the lines provided. For procedures that are incorrect, write the correct procedures on the lines provided.

a. Collect everything from the office mailbox and process it a few items at a time throughout the day.

_____

b. In the top-priority pile, place letters and packages sent by overnight mail delivery, special delivery, registered mail, or certified mail. To this pile, also add any newspapers or magazines.

_____

c. After sorting the mail, open all the envelopes at once—except for those marked "personal" or "confidential"—and remove their contents, making sure to take everything out of each envelope.

_____

d. Throw away the envelopes as soon as you have removed their contents.

_____

e. Compare enclosure notations on each letter with the actual enclosures to make sure all items were included. Then make notes about missing items so that senders can be contacted.

_____

f. Staple each letter to its enclosures so they cannot become separated.

_____

g. Stamp any bills or statements with the date they are received.

_____

3. Preparing a Business Letter

Read the following case study: You are a medical assistant working at the BWW medical office. Dr. Buckwalter says to you, "Please prepare a letter to go to Mr. Ford. He is the attorney for Mrs. Smith. Just check her chart to get his address. Tell him that Mrs. Smith has not been coming to her scheduled appointments. Tell him that I can't help if she doesn't want my help!"

Instructions:

a. What questions might you have before you prepare this letter—use the following lines.

_____

_____

_____

_____

b. Type the letter, using the BWW Letterhead provided after you prepare the letter; use block style format. The phone number for the office may be found on the letterhead, but you should include it within the body of the letter in case the attorney has any questions.

You found the attorney's address within the patient's chart. It is, William Ford, Esq/Ford, Wilkins Law Offices/ 135 Cinceros Ave./Ste. 3200/Plainfield, XY 55555

4. Commonly Misspelled Words

Correct the spelling of the following words.

a. abcess _____

b. laynx _____

c. chancrer _____

d. nocomial _____

e. defibillator _____

f. parentral _____

g. sphymomanometer _____

h. Febuary _____

i. comittee _____

j. occassion _____

k. truely _____

C A S E   S T U D I E S

Write your response to each case study on the lines provided.

Case 1

A new coworker asks you to proofread a business letter that he wrote. You notice that the letter contains numerous formatting and mechanical errors. You also suspect that there may be data errors in the letter. What should you do?

_____

_____

_____

Case 2

While opening the office mail, you discover that a patient has enclosed a check for more than she owes. Should you take a moment from processing the mail to call the patient? Why or why not?

_____

_____

_____

Case 3

You have just finished preparing several letters for signing by Dr. Morris, a physician in your office. Most of the letters need to be sent out today, but he will be extremely busy with patients for the rest of the day. Dr. Fuchs, another physician in your office, has authorized you to sign her letters. Should you sign Dr. Morris's letters and send them out right away? Explain your answer.

_____

_____

_____

PROCEDURE 10-1 Creating a Professional Letter   WORK // DOC

Goal
To follow standard procedure for constructing a business letter.

OSHA Guidelines
This procedure does not involve exposure to blood, body fluids, or tissue.

Materials
Word processor or personal computer, letterhead paper, dictionaries or other professional tools.

Method

Step Number	Procedure	Points Possible	Points Earned
1.	Format the letter according to the standard office procedure. Use the same punctuation and style throughout.*	15	
2.	Start the dateline three lines below the last line of the printed letterhead. (Note: Depending on the length of the letter, it is acceptable to start between two and six lines below the letterhead.)*	5	
3.	Two lines below the dateline, type in any special mailing instructions (such as REGISTERED MAIL, CERTIFIED MAIL, and so on).	5	
4.	Three lines below any special instructions, begin the inside address. Type the addressee's courtesy title (Mr., Mrs., Ms.) and full name on the first line. If a professional title is given (M.D., RN, Ph.D.), type this title after the addressee's name instead of using a courtesy title.	5	
5.	Type the addressee's business title, if applicable, on the second line. Type the company name on the third line. Type the street address on the fourth line, including the apartment or suite number. Type the city, state, and zip code on the fifth line. Use the standard two-letter abbreviation for the state, followed by one space and the zip code.	5	
6.	Two lines below the inside address, type the salutation, using the appropriate courtesy title (Mr., Mrs., Ms., Dr.) prior to typing the addressee's last name.*	5	
7.	Two lines below the salutation, type the subject line, if applicable.	5	
8.	Two lines below the subject line, begin the body of the letter. Single-space between lines. Double-space between paragraphs.	5	
9.	Two lines below the body of the letter, type the complimentary closing.	5	
10.	Leave three blank lines (return four times), and begin the signature block. (Enough space must be left to allow for the signature.) Type the sender's name on the first line. Type the sender's title on the second line.*	5	
11.	Two lines below the sender's title, type the identification line. Type the sender's initials in all capitals and your initials in lowercase letters, separating the two sets of initials with a colon or a forward slash.	5	
12.	One or two lines below the identification line, type the enclosure notation, if applicable.	5	
13.	Two lines below the enclosure notation, type the copy notation, if applicable.	5	
14.	Edit the letter.	10	
15.	Proofread and spell-check the letter.*	15	
Total Points		100	

CAAHEP Competencies Achieved

    IV. P (10)   Compose professional/business letters

ABHES Competencies Achieved

    7. a. Perform basic keyboarding skills, including

          (1) Locating the keys on a keyboard

          (2) Typing medical correspondence and basic reports

PROCEDURE 10-2 Writing an Interoffice Memo

Goal
To follow standard procedure for writing an interoffice memo.

OSHA Guidelines
This procedure does not involve exposure to blood, body fluids, or tissue.

Materials
Word processor or personal computer, plain paper, dictionaries or other professional references as needed.

Method

Step Number	Procedure	Points Possible	Points Earned
1.	Gather all necessary materials and documents needed to compose the memo.	10	
2.	Decide whether the memo will be created "freehand" or by using an existing template.	18	
3.	If using a template, fill in the headings as listed with the appropriate information. If the memo is being created freehand, use the headings, DATE:, TO:, FROM:, and RE: or SUBJECT:. Fill in each heading with the appropriate information.*	18	
4.	Double or triple space after the memo headings or, if using a template, move to the body area of the memo and begin typing the information to be included in the memo.	18	
5.	Single space the information within the memo and double space between paragraphs. Use either the block or indented paragraph format, depending on office policy.	18	
6.	Spell-check and proofread the document carefully, correcting errors as necessary.*	18	
Total Points		100	

CAAHEP Competencies Achieved

IV. C (8)　　Recognize elements of fundamental writing skills

IV. P (10)　　Compose professional/business letters

ABHES Competencies Achieved

7. a. Perform basic keyboarding skills, including

(1) Locating the keys on a keyboard

(2) Typing medical correspondence and basic reports

7. b. Identify and properly utilize office machines, computerized systems, and medical software such as

(1) Efficiently maintain and understand different types of medical correspondence and medical reports

PROCEDURE 10-3 Composing a Professional E-mail Message

Goal
To follow standard procedure for writing a professional e-mail message.

OSHA Guidelines
This procedure does not involve exposure to blood, body fluids, or tissue.

Materials
Computer with e-mail (Internet) capabilities, dictionary or other professional references as needed.

Method

Step Number	Procedure	Points Possible	Points Earned
1.	Verify that the patient's medical record contains a signed "Consent to Use E-mail" form, allowing communication by this method.*	10	
2.	Use a classic easy-to-read font such as Times New Roman at 12–14 pt. Use black ink only.	8	
3.	If responding to a patient e-mail, open the e-mail and choose "Reply." If composing a new message, choose "New" to open a new e-mail document. Carefully enter the patient's e-mail address.	8	
4.	Add the e-mail address to the office address book for easy reference, if it is not saved in the office EHR program.	8	
5.	If answering a patient e-mail, you may keep the subject line from the original message. If you are writing a new e-mail, enter a descriptive subject line.	8	
6.	Insert a salutation, using the patient's surname as you would with an ordinary letter.	8	
7.	Compose the body of the message, aligning the information with the left margin.	8	
8.	Double space at the end of the message and enter your name, including a signature line with the practice information, and a phone number.	8	
9.	Spell-check and proofread the message carefully for any errors.*	10	
10.	Click "Send" and wait for the message informing you the message has been sent.	8	
11.	If the message is returned as undeliverable, verify the e-mail address was entered correctly. If necessary, correct the address and attempt delivery again.	8	
12.	If the message is returned a second time as undeliverable, contact the patient by phone or an alternate communication method to be sure that he or she receives the required information.	8	
Total Points		100	

CAAHEP Competencies Achieved

IV. C (8)   Recognize elements of fundamental writing skills

IV. P (10)   Compose professional/business letters

ABHES Competencies Achieved

7. a. Perform basic keyboarding skills, including

   (2) Typing medical correspondence and basic reports

7. b. Identify and properly utilize office machines, computerized systems, and medical software such as

   (1) Efficiently maintain and understand different types of medical correspondence and medical reports

   (2) Apply computer application skills using a variety of different electronic programs including both practice management software and EMR software

8. (jj) Perform fundamental writing skills including correct grammar, spelling, and formatting techniques when writing prescriptions, documenting medical records, etc.

PROCEDURE 10-4 Composing an Electronic Patient Letter

Goal
To create and send an electronic letter to a patient.

OSHA Guidelines
This procedure does not involve exposure to blood, body fluids, or tissue.

Materials
EHR software program with letter templates, information necessary to compose the letter, dictionary or other professional references as needed.

Method

Step Number	Procedure	Points Possible	Points Earned
1.	After verifying that there is a signed "Consent to Use E-mail" in the patient's record, access the *New* menu in the appropriate screen of the software program. Choose *New Letter Template*.	12	
2.	In the *RE:* window, key the subject line such as "Welcome to BWW Medical Associates, PC."	12	
3.	In the *Text* box, key the body of the letter. Begin the letter with an introductory statement, such as "Welcome to BWW Medical Associates, and thank you for choosing us for your healthcare needs. We look forward to working with you." Enter all pertinent information required for the letter. If continuing a "welcome to the practice" letter, be sure to include the practice name, address, phone numbers, and website information, as well as the names of the medical staff and office personnel. Don't forget the usual office hours as well.	12	
4.	When you complete the letter, give the template an easily identifiable name, such as *Welcome New Patient Letter.**	12	
5.	Open the EHR software and enter the appropriate patient's medical record. Select the *New* menu and choose the letter template you just created. Because you are in the patient's medical record, most software programs will automatically enter the patient's address in the inside address section of the letter. The standard greeting and closure should also be inserted from the medical record. Check to be sure the information listed is correct.	14	
6.	Add a signature to the signature block of the letter by using the "Sign" icon within the EHR program. Choose the correct provider/staff member from the drop-down list and verify that the correct signature is inserted.	12	
7.	If the signed "Consent to Use E-mail" is in the patient's chart, the letter may be sent by clicking "Send." If the consent is not signed, print the letter and send it to the patient via USPS.*	12	
8.	Be sure to click "Save" or "Done" depending on the EHR software used, so that the template is saved for future use.	14	
Total Points		100	

CAAHEP Competencies Achieved

    IV. C (8)   Recognize elements of fundamental writing skills

    IV. P (10)   Compose professional/business letters

ABHES Competencies Achieved

    7. a. Perform basic keyboarding skills, including

        (2) Typing medical correspondence and basic reports

    7. b. Identify and properly utilize office machines, computerized systems, and medical software such as

        (1) Efficiently maintain and understand different types of medical correspondence and medical reports

        (2) Apply computer application skills using a variety of different electronic programs including both practice management software and EMR software

    8. (jj) Perform fundamental writing skills including correct grammar, spelling, and formatting techniques when writing prescriptions, documenting medical records, etc.

PROCEDURE 10-5 Sorting and Opening Mail

Goal
To follow a standard procedure for sorting, opening, and processing incoming office mail.

OSHA Guidelines
This procedure does not involve exposure to blood, body fluids, or tissue.

Materials
Letter opener, date and time stamp (manual or automatic), stapler, paper clips, adhesive notes.

Method

Step Number	Procedure	Points Possible	Points Earned
1.	Check the address on each letter or package to be sure that it has been delivered to the correct location.	7	
2.	Sort the mail into piles according to priority and type of mail. Your system may include the following: • Top priority. This pile will contain any items that were sent by overnight mail delivery in addition to items sent by registered mail, certified mail, or special delivery. (Faxes and e-mail messages are also top priority.) • Second priority. This pile will include personal or confidential mail. • Third priority. This pile will contain all first-class mail, airmail, and Priority Mail items. These items should be divided into payments received, insurance forms, reports, and other correspondence. • Fourth priority. This pile will consist of packages. • Fifth priority. This pile will contain magazines and newspapers. • Sixth priority. This last pile will include advertisements and catalogs.	7	
3.	Set aside all letters labeled "Personal" or "Confidential." Unless you have permission to open these letters, only the addressee should open them.	7	
4.	Arrange all the envelopes with the flaps facing up and away from you.	7	
5.	Tap the lower edge of the envelope to shift the contents to the bottom. This step helps to prevent cutting any of the contents when you open the envelope. *	7	
6.	Open all the envelopes.	7	
7.	Remove and unfold the contents, making sure that nothing remains in the envelope.	7	
8.	Review each document, and check the sender's name and address. • If the letter has no return address, save the envelope, or cut the address off the envelope, and tape it to the letter. • Check to see if the address matches the one on the envelope. If there is a difference, staple the envelope to the letter, and make a note to verify the correct address with the sender.	7	
9.	Compare the enclosure notation on the letter with the actual enclosures to make sure that all items are included. Make a note to contact the sender if anything is missing.	7	
10.	Clip together each letter and its enclosures.*	9	
11.	Check the date of the letter. If there is a significant delay between the date of the letter and the postmark, keep the envelope.	7	

(continued)

Step Number	Procedure	Points Possible	Points Earned
12.	If all contents appear to be in order, you can discard the envelope.	7	
13.	Review all bills and statements. • Make sure the amount enclosed is the same as the amount listed on the statement. • Make a note of any discrepancies.	7	
14.	Stamp each piece of correspondence with the date (and sometimes the time) to record its receipt. If possible, stamp each item in the same location—such as the upper-right corner.*	7	
Total Points		100	

CAAHEP Competencies Achieved

None

ABHES Competencies Achieved

7. b. Identify and properly utilize office machines, computerized systems, and medical software such as

(1) Efficiently maintaining and understanding different types of medical correspondence and medical reports

8. (a) Perform basic clerical functions

8. (hh) Receive, organize, prioritize, and transmit information expediently

Medical Records and Documentation

Name_____ Class_____ Date_____

REVIEW

Vocabulary Review

Matching

Match the key terms in the right column with the definitions in the left column by placing the letter of each correct answer in the space provided.

_____ 1. Documentation of patient medical history

_____ 2. Charting method based on symptoms, diagnosis, and treatment

_____ 3. Adding notes to the patient chart

_____ 4. Objective, external factors

_____ 5. Turning words into written format

_____ 6. Oral review of patient's body systems by physician

_____ 7. Charting method beginning with CC; ending with return visit or referral information

_____ 8. Base information for each patient

_____ 9. Medical record filing system using each document's source

_____ 10. Subjective internal conditions felt by the patient

_____ 11. Chart documentation sorted by the patient problem list

_____ 12. Patient who does not follow prescribed treatment plan

_____ 13. Examination and review medical records for accuracy

_____ 14. Physician findings

_____ 15. The patient's symptoms

a. audit
b. CHEDDAR
c. demographics
d. documentation
e. noncompliant
f. objective
g. patient record
h. POMR
i. ROS
j. sign
k. SOAP
l. SOMR
m. subjective
n. symptom
o. transcription

True or False

Decide whether each statement is true or false. In the space at the left, write T for true or F for false. On the lines provided, rewrite the false statements to make them true.

_____ 16. It is not necessary to document in the medical record when a patient is noncompliant.

_____

_____ 17. Patient records may be used to evaluate the quality of treatment a facility or physician's office provides.

_____

_____ 18. Informed consent forms state that a patient has agreed to treatment.

_____

_____ 19. All written correspondence from the patient, doctor's office, laboratory, hospital or independent healthcare agency should be kept in the patient's chart.

_____ 20. When creating the patient medical record, the first document to be placed in the chart is the registration form.

_____ 21. Transcription is the transforming of written notes into accurate spoken form.

_____ 22. Problem-oriented medical records are a way to overcome the disadvantages of SOMR medical charting.

_____ 23. Subjective data comes from the physician as well as from exams and test results.

_____ 24. External record audits are done on a periodic basis by the medical office staff.

_____ 25. If a life insurance company calls asking for patient medical records, they may be released to the company.

Content Review

Multiple Choice

In the space provided, write the letter of the choice that best completes each statement or answers each question.

_____ 1. When you are in doubt regarding who is authorized to sign a release of records form for a minor,
   a. Always ask the oldest person
   b. Always ask the minor who is authorized
   c. Do not allow anyone to sign
   d. You must ask a lawyer for guidance
   e. You must always ask your superior

_____ 2. When children reach this age, most states consider them adults with the right to privacy regarding all of their medical information.
   a. 16
   b. 18
   c. 20
   d. 21
   e. 22

_____ 3. Test results received from sources outside the practice are best organized in sections within what part of the medical chart?
   a. Laboratory and other test results
   b. A special section in the chart especially for outside source material
   c. The very front of the chart
   d. The very back of the chart
   e. a or b depending on where the material comes from

_____ 4. Which of the following elements of SOAP charting describes the data that comes directly from the patient?

    a. S

    b. O

    c. A

    d. P

    e. S or A

_____ 5. Which of the following elements of SOAP charting describes the course of treatment to be followed?

    a. S

    b. O

    c. A

    d. P

    e. A or P

_____ 6. What does the abbreviation PT mean?

    a. Partial

    b. Physical therapy

    c. Patient

    d. Preoperative

    e. Professional tone

_____ 7. The six Cs of charting include

    a. Conformity, clarity, cleanliness, conciseness, chronological order, and confidentiality

    b. Conformity, clarity, completeness, conciseness, chronological order, and creativity

    c. Client's words, clarity, completeness, conciseness, chronological order, and confidentiality

    d. Client's words, conformity, cleanliness, conciseness, chronological order, and confidentiality

    e. Client's words, clarity, conciseness, conformity, chronological order, and confidentiality

_____ 8. Conventional records are

    a. Also called SOMR

    b. Also called POMR

    c. Organized by problems of the patient

    d. Especially easy for tracking a specific ailment in a patient

    e. Also called CHEDDAR

_____ 9. The P in SOAP documentation stands for

    a. Purpose

    b. Procedures

    c. Physical

    d. Plan

    e. Prescription

_____ 10. As a general rule, if information is not documented,

    a. It is not important

    b. It is not useful

    c. No one can prove that an event or procedure took place

    d. It is illegal

    e. Malpractice will result

_____ **11.** The S in SOAP documentation stands for

    a. Subjective

    b. Serious

    c. Sensitive

    d. Statistics

    e. Secret

_____ **12.** Original documentation

    a. Is always selected instead of a copy to be given to the patient on request

    b. Cannot be faxed

    c. Legally belongs to the patient

    d. Legally belongs to the physician and belongs in the patient's medical chart

    e. Belongs in the medical chart but is the property of the patient

_____ **13.** Completeness in charting means

    a. Using the patient's exact words

    b. Dating all entries into a chart

    c. Not leaving any blank lines when charting

    d. Using precise descriptions and accepted medical terminology

    e. Not leaving out information

_____ **14.** The first form used in initiating a patient financial record is the

    a. Informed consent form

    b. Doctor's diagnosis form

    c. Patient medical history form

    d. Patient registration form

    e. Patient physical examination form

_____ **15.** The term noncompliant means that the patient

    a. Does not understand

    b. Does not hear well

    c. Is not literate

    d. Does not follow medical advice and direction

    e. a, b, and c

_____ **16.** If a physician who is dictating speaks with an accent and you find it difficult to understand the dictation, you should

    a. State you don't understand and stop

    b. Ask others in the office if they understand the physician and ask them to take dictation

    c. Record the dictation

    d. Do the best you can

    e. Ask the physician to speak more slowly than normal

Sentence Completion

In the space provided, write the word or phrase that best completes each sentence.

17. The patient's past medical history, family medical history, and social and occupational history are included in a part of the chart called the _____.

18. It is important to date and _____ every entry you put in the patient chart so that it is easy to tell which items the medical assistant enters and which items other people enter.

19. When filling out patient charts, it is important to record patients' _____, not your interpretation of them.

20. To make chart data more concise, medical workers use standard medical abbreviations, such as "patient got _____" instead of "patient got out of bed."

21. All information in a patient's chart is _____ to protect the patient's privacy.

22. In a conventional, or source-oriented medical record, all the patient's problems and treatments are recorded in the record in _____ order.

23. In problem-oriented medical recordkeeping, each _____ is listed separately, making it easier for the physician to track a patient's progress.

24. When documenting problems, you must be careful to distinguish between signs, which are external factors that can be seen and measured, and symptoms, which are _____ that can be felt only by the patient.

25. Because documentation is useless if it is not _____, make sure your handwriting is clear when documenting by hand in a medical record.

26. The doctor's transcribed notes for the patient's chart should be initialed by the _____.

27. If information is not entered in the medical record in a _____ fashion, a patient's health may be in jeopardy because of missing or incomplete information.

28. The _____ method of charting describes a patient's condition by the use of four letters. The letters describe what the patient says, what the medical personnel see, an evaluation of the problem, and a directive for care.

29. _____ in medical records are not uncommon but must be changed immediately in the proper manner.

30. The "C" in CHEDDAR stands for _____.

31. Age _____ is the age at which most states consider an individual to be an adult.

32. To maintain patient _____, never discuss a patient's records, forward them to another office, fax them, or show them to anyone but the physician unless you have the patient's written permission to do so.

33. A _____ contains a record of the patient's history; information from the initial interview with the patient; all findings and results from physical exams; and any tests, x-rays, and other procedures.

34. In the _____, patient information is arranged according to who supplied the data—the patient, the doctor, a specialist, or someone else.

35. _____ means to be brief and to the point.

17. _____
18. _____
19. _____
20. _____
21. _____
22. _____
23. _____
24. _____
25. _____
26. _____
27. _____
28. _____
29. _____
30. _____
31. _____
32. _____
33. _____
34. _____
35. _____

Short Answer
Write the answer to each question on the lines provided.

36. Explain the difference between patient signs and symptoms. List three examples of each.

_____

_____

_____

37. Describe why it is so important to use care when making corrections to medical charts.

_____

_____

_____

38. List four additions that a physician might want to make to a patient's chart.

_____

_____

_____

_____

39. Describe the SOAP approach to medical record documentation.

_____

_____

_____

40. Explain the 6 Cs of charting

_____

_____

_____

_____

_____

_____

A P P L I C A T I O N

WORK // DOC

Follow the directions for each application.

1. Initiating a Patient Record

Work with two partners. Each of you should take turns being a medical assistant, a patient, and an observer/evaluator. Assume that this is the patient's first visit to the medical office.

a. Working together, create a model for a patient record. It must contain all the standard chart information, including Patient Registration Form, Patient Medical History Form, and Patient Physical Examination Form. (You may use the forms shown in Figures 11-1 and 11-3 of the textbook as a guide.)

b. Have one partner play the role of the medical assistant and another partner play the role of a patient complaining of headaches. The third partner should act as the observer and evaluator. Have the medical assistant help the patient complete the Patient Registration Form. Then have the medical assistant interview the patient and record the medical history, using standard abbreviations where appropriate, ending with a description of the patient's reason for the visit. The medical assistant should document any signs, symptoms, or other information the patient wishes to share.

c. Have the evaluator critique the interview and the documentation in the patient chart. The critique should take into account the accuracy of the documentation, the order in which the medical history was taken, and the history's completeness. The evaluator also should note the medical assistant's ability to follow the 6 Cs of charting, including the correct use of medical abbreviations.

d. The medical assistant, the patient, and the observer should discuss the observer's comments, noting the strengths and weaknesses of the interview and the quality of the documentation.

e. Exchange roles and repeat the exercise with a new patient. Allow the student playing the patient to choose a different medical problem.

f. Exchange roles again so that each member of the team has an opportunity to play the interviewer, the patient, and the observer once.

2. **Correcting a Patient Record**

a. Using the same patient information as in the model for a patient record created in Application 1, make a correction to three different parts of the record. Pay special attention to Procedure 11-2. Each team member should take turns making three corrections each.

b. Ask your instructor to review each correction and comment on your work. There should be no blacking out or the use of white correction fluid. All corrections should be clear and neat. All corrections should be dated and initialed. Make sure you indicate the reason you made the correction.

C A S E   S T U D I E S

Write your response to each case study on the lines provided.

Case 1

You accidentally throw out a sheet of a patient's medical chart. The trash has already been taken away, so there is no chance for you to get it back. You are new in the office, and you are afraid of losing your job if you tell the doctor what you have done. You remember the information that was on the sheet. You think you can easily rewrite it. What should you do?

_____

_____

_____

Case 2

A former patient of the doctor you work for calls and asks you to send her medical records to her new physician. She says it is important that the records get to her new doctor by this afternoon and asks you to fax them. Would you have a problem with this request? Why or why not?

_____

_____

_____

Case 3

Dr. Buckwalter receives laboratory results from a test performed on Willie Jones. He calls Mr. Jones at home on Monday, July 6, at 10:00 a.m. He gets no answer, but he leaves a message on Mr. Jones's answering machine asking him to call the office. By 10:00 a.m. the next morning, Dr. Buckwalter has received no response from Mr. Jones. He calls again and reaches Mrs. Jones and asks her to have her husband call the office. Mr. Jones calls the doctor's office at 2:30 that afternoon. Dr. Smith discusses the test results with Mr. Jones and asks him to make an appointment for the following week. Mr. Jones is connected with the receptionist. He makes an appointment for 11:00 a.m. on July 12. As a medical assistant, how would you record this series of events in Mr. Jones's chart?

_____

_____

_____

PROCEDURE 11-1 Preparing a New Patient Paper Medical Record

⬚ **WORK // DOC**

Goal
To assemble a new patient paper medical record.

OSHA Guidelines
This procedure does not involve exposure to blood, body fluids, or tissue.

Materials
File folder, labels as appropriate (alphabet, numbers, dates, insurance, allergies, etc.), forms (patient registration, medical history, advance directives, physician progress notes, laboratory forms), hole punch.

Method

Step Number	Procedure	Points Possible	Points Earned
1.	Carefully create a chart label according to practice policy. This label may include the patient's last name followed by the first name, or it may be a medical record number for those offices that utilize numeric or alphanumeric filing.*	17	
2.	Place the chart label on the right edge of the folder, extending the label the length of the tab on the folder.	17	
3.	Place the date label on the top edge of the folder, updating the date according to practice policy. (The date is usually updated annually, if the patient has come into the office within the last year.)	17	
4.	If alpha or numeric filing labels are utilized, place a patient name label on the chart according to practice policy.	17	
5.	Punch holes in the appropriate forms for placement within the patient's medical record.	15	
6.	Place all the forms in appropriate sections of the patient's medical record.*	17	
Total Points		100	

CAAHEP Competencies Achieved
V. P (3) Organize a patient's medical record

ABHES Competencies Achieved
8. (b) Prepare and maintain medical records

PROCEDURE 11-2 Correcting Paper Medical Records

Goal
To follow standard procedures for correcting a paper medical record.

OSHA Guidelines
This procedure does not involve exposure to blood, body fluids, or tissue.

Materials
Patient file, other pertinent documents that contain the information to be used in making corrections (for example, transcribed notes, telephone notes, physician's comments, correspondence), good ballpoint pen.

Method

Step Number	Procedure	Points Possible	Points Earned
1.	Corrections and additions should be made so that the original information remains readable, so that there can be no suggestion of intent to conceal information. Draw a single line through the information to be replaced.*	20	
2.	Write or type in the correct information above or below the original line or in the margin. The location in the chart for the new information should be clear. If a separate sheet of paper or another document is required for the correction or addition, clearly note in the record, "See attached document A" or use similar wording to indicate where the corrected information can be found.	20	
3.	Place a note near the correction or addition, stating why it was made (for example, "error, wrong date; error, interrupted by phone call"). Make sure you initial and date the correction. This indication can be a brief note in the margin or an attachment to the record. Do not make any changes or additions in a record without noting the reason for them.*	20	
4.	Enter the date and time, and initial the correction or addition.*	20	
5.	If possible, have another staff member or the physician witness and initial the correction to the record when you make it.	20	
Total Points		100	

CAAHEP Competencies Achieved
   IX. C (14)   Describe the process to follow if an error is made in patient care

ABHES Competencies Achieved
   8. (b) Prepare and maintain medical records

PROCEDURE 11-3 Entering (Adding) Information into a Paper Medical Record

Goal

To document continuity of care by creating a complete, accurate, timely record of the medical care provided to a patient in your medical facility.

OSHA Guidelines

This procedure does not involve exposure to blood, body fluids, or tissue.

Materials

Patient medical record, pertinent documents (test results, X-ray results, telephone notes, correspondence, etc.), blue ballpoint pen, notebook, keyboard, transcription equipment.

Method

Step Number	Procedure	Points Possible	Points Earned
1.	Verify that you have the correct chart for the documents to be filed. Carefully check the patient's name, DOB, and medical record number (if available) as verification.*	10	
2.	Transcribe any dictated notes as soon as possible and enter them into the patient record. If notes are handwritten, be sure they are filed in the correct location within the medical record.	9	
3.	Spell out the names of disorders, diseases, medications, and other terms the first time you enter them into the patient record, followed by the appropriate abbreviation. For example: "congestive heart failure (CHF)." Thereafter, you may use the abbreviation alone.	9	
4.	Enter only what the doctor has dictated. Do *not* add your own comments, observations, or evaluations. Use self-adhesive flags or other means to call the doctor's attention to something you have noticed that may be helpful to the patient's case. Date and initial each entry.	9	
5.	Follow office procedure to record routine or special laboratory, X-ray, or other test results. These results may be posted in a particular section of the file or on a separate test summary form. If you use the summary form, make a note in the file that the results were received and recorded. Place the original report in the patient's file if required to do so by office policy. Date and initial each entry. File all correspondence and hospital records in the appropriate area of each chart, using reverse chronological order so that the most recent record is on top. Be sure that each document is initialed or stamped by the physician as having been seen, prior to filing it within the patient's chart.	10	
6.	Make a note in the record of all telephone calls to and from the patient. Date and initial the entries. These entries also may include the doctor's comments, observations, changes in the patient's medication, new instructions to the patient, and so on. If calls are recorded in a separate telephone log, note in the patient's record the time and date of the call and refer to the log. It is particularly important to record such calls when the patient resists or refuses treatment, skips appointments, or has not made follow-up appointments.	9	
7.	Make notations in the medical record of any immunizations and vaccines that have been given to the patient. Notations should be posted in the patient's immunization record inside the medical chart. Input them into your state's public health database as well. Immunization records are kept indefinitely as a permanent part of the patient's medical history.	9	

(continued)

Step Number	Procedure	Points Possible	Points Earned
8.	Read over the entries for omissions or mistakes. Ask the doctor to answer any questions you may have.*	9	
9.	Make sure that you have dated and initialed each entry.*	9	
10.	Be sure that all documents are included in the file and within the appropriate location so they may be located easily when needed.	9	
11.	Return the patient's medical record to its appropriate location in the filing system as soon as possible.*	8	
Total Points		100	

CAAHEP Competencies Achieved

IX. P (7)   Document accurately in the patient record

ABHES Competencies Achieved

4. (a) Document accurately

8. (b) Prepare and maintain medical records

8 (gg) Use pertinent medical terminology

Electronic Health Records

Name_____ Class_____ Date_____

R E V I E W

Vocabulary Review

Matching

Match the key terms in the right column with the definitions in the left column by placing the letter of each correct answer in the space provided.

_____ 1. Adding omitted information or making corrections in the medical record

_____ 2. Ordering labs & x-ray and receiving their results via an EHR program

_____ 3. Electronic patient record program used within one office

_____ 4. Records housed in a computer system

_____ 5. A program created specifically to fit a need or requirement

_____ 6. Health record of one patient created and maintained by the patient

_____ 7. Electronic records to be shared outside the individual practice

_____ 8. An electronic appointment book

_____ 9. A "reminder" calendar

_____ 10. Sending prescriptions by email

_____ 11. Confidential patient information

_____ 12. Passwords and access codes

a. EHR
b. EMR
c. PHR
d. customized
e. PHI
f. e-prescribing
g. computerized records
h. addendum
i. EHR security
j. tickler file
k. scheduler
l. order integration

True/False

Decide whether each statement is true or false. In the space at the left, write T for true or F for false. On the lines provided, rewrite the false statements to make them true.

_____ 13. EHR systems allow medical information to be shared only within a single practice.

_____

_____ 14. Communication problems are the leading cause of medical errors.

_____

_____ 15. The overall goal of EHR is to reduce medical errors.

_____

_____ **16.** EMR systems are created to allow information to be shared by more than one healthcare system.

_____

_____ **17.** PHRs are created and used by an individual patient.

_____

_____ **18.** "Meaningful use" includes three steps for Medicare/Medicaid providers implementing an EHR program in order to receive financial incentives.

_____

_____ **19.** EP stands for electronically connected provider.

_____

_____ **20.** If a physician is qualified for both the Medicare and Medicaid EHR incentive programs, he may participate in both.

_____

_____ **21.** There are more filing issues with EMR/EHR programs than with paper records.

_____

_____ **22.** EHR/EMR programs may be customized for specialty practices.

_____

Content Review

Multiple Choice

In the space provided, write the letter of the choice that best completes each statement or answers each question.

_____ **1.** Medical errors are the _____ leading cause of patient death in the United States.
  a. 2nd
  b. 4th
  c. 6th
  d. 8th
  e. 10th

_____ **2.** In what year did President George W. Bush envision most Americans having access to EHR?
  a. 2012
  b. 2013
  c. 2014
  d. 2015
  e. 2016

_____ **3.** The _____ is quickly becoming a physician's most important business and legal tool.
  a. PHI
  b. Computer
  c. Medical assistant
  d. Legal counsel
  e. Electronic record

_____ 4. Which of the following would result from an EHR's increased access to patient information?
  a. Increased continuity of care
  b. Decreased medical errors
  c. Decreased healthcare costs
  d. a and b
  e. a, b, and c

_____ 5. Which of the following is not a legal document?
  a. EMR
  b. EHR
  c. PHR
  d. Patient financial record
  e. Consent for treatment

_____ 6. Which of the following providers are considered "EPs" for the Medicare EHR incentive program?
  a. Physicians
  b. Dentists
  c. Optometrists and chiropractors
  d. Podiatrists
  e. All of the above

_____ 7. Which of the following providers are considered "EPs" for the Medicaid EHR incentive program?
  a. Physicians
  b. Dentists
  c. NPs/PAs
  d. Nurse midwives
  e. All of the above

_____ 8. What is the number 1 issue for providers regarding EHR implementation?
  a. Financial concerns
  b. Staff training issues
  c. The need for an F/T or P/T IT professional
  d. Possible damage to existing computer systems
  e. The need for hardware/software upgrades

_____ 9. Passcodes and access codes increase what functionality for electronic records?
  a. Access
  b. Availability
  c. Security
  d. Safety
  e. Healthcare alerts

_____ 10. Which additional functions of EHR will be helpful to the billing and coding staff?
  a. Tickler file
  b. Scheduler
  c. Insurance verification
  d. Coding program
  e. c and d

Sentence Completion

In the space provided, write the word or phrase that best completes each sentence.

11. _____ are the 8th leading cause of patient death in the United States.

12. Decreasing medical errors will help _____ healthcare costs.

13. Electronic medical information created, compiled, and managed within one healthcare facility is known as _____.

14. _____ describes the same information if it can be shared outside the healthcare facility where it originated.

15. A(n) _____ is not a legal record but is an electronic file created, used, and maintained by a patient concerning his or her personal health.

16. To be eligible for Medicare and Medicaid EHR incentive programs, _____ must be demonstrated by the provider.

17. _____ are qualified providers for the Medicaid EHR program but not for the Medicare EHR program.

18. All EHR/EMR templates contain _____, which must be completed for each patient.

19. All entries in an electronic system must be checked carefully before clicking _____ as entries cannot be changed once this occurs.

20. _____ is maintained with the EHR program through the use of passwords and access codes.

11._____

12._____

13._____

14._____

15._____

16._____

17._____

18._____

19._____

20._____

Short Answer

Write the answer to each question on the lines provided.

21. As a medical assistant, what five items should be kept in mind when working with EHR?

_____

_____

_____

22. Explain how customized templates may be helpful to specialty practices when creating an EHR program.

_____

_____

_____

23. Aside from making appointments electronically, what other functions may be included with an electronic scheduling program?

_____

_____

_____

A P P L I C A T I O N

Follow the directions for each application.

1. Using the directions that follow, create a new patient face sheet for yourself using the SpringCharts™ EHR program.

SpringCharts Tip

Shortcut:

Open a Patient's Chart
The third speed icon from the right on the Toolbar of the main *Practice View* screen enables the user to quickly open a patient's chart and by-pass the *Actions* menu.

| ∇ Hamilton, Byron R, 05/05/53 |
| File Edit Windows Actions New ▶ |

Show Chart/Face Sheet icon

SpringCharts Tip

Remember that you only need to type the first few letters of the word to conduct a search. The more letters you type, the more likely you are to make a mistake, and the system will not be able to locate the term.

SpringCharts Tip

If you don't see the list of items you added under the *Social Hx* section of the *Category Preferences* window in Exercise 5.1, you may need to close SpringCharts and restart the program.

SpringCharts Tip

Place your cursor after the *Preferences* category item you selected and then click on the pop-up text item. The placement of the cursor determines where the pop-up text is inserted.

Building a New Patient's Face Sheet

If your SpringCharts program was not shut down and reopened after completing your previous exercise, you may do so now. This will refresh the program to include the new items added in any previous exercise.

1. Open your own chart by selecting the *Open a Patient's Chart* icon (shown in margin) on the main menu. Type the first few letters of your last name in the search field of the *Choose Patient* window and click on the *Search* icon.
2. Select your name, and your chart will open. It will be empty except for your demographic information.
3. Within your chart, click on the *Show Chart/Face Sheet* icon, located at the far right of the menu bar, to open the *Edit Face Sheet* window.

Allergies

4. The window opens to the *Allergies* section.
5. In the *Allergy* field on the right side, type "peni" and press the *Search* icon.
6. Select *Penicillins* from the list. The program adds this drug to your allergy list on the left side.
7. Repeat these steps to add the drug *Codeine* and the allergen *Peanut Containing Prod.*
8. In the *Other Sensitivities* field, in the lower part of the window, type the medication *Erythromycin*. Then select *causes nausea* from the *Allergy Notes* pop-up text (to the right).

Social History

9. Click on the (Social Hx) button to open the *Social History* window.
10. In the *Preferences* list in the lower right, select the *Alcohol Use*: category.
11. Select the appropriate item from the *Social Hx* pop-up text field in the upper window, for example, *Alcohol Use: Non Drinker*.
12. Repeat these steps to add information in the *Caffeine Use* and *Living Arrangements* preference categories, using the pop-up text of your choice.

Past Medical History

13. Click on the [PMHX] navigation button to open the *Past Medical History* window.
14. Select several items of your choice from the *Preferences* list to build your past medical history.
15. Add a medical condition that is not in the *Preferences* list by searching for a diagnosis in the *Dx* field in the upper right. Type *HTN* for hypertension, click the *Search* icon, and select the diagnosis.

Family Medical History

16. Click on the [FMHX] navigation button to open the *Family Medical History* window.
17. Select several medical conditions of your choice from the *Preferences* list to build your family medical history.
18. Select Father. Died At Age: and Cause of Death: from the *Preferences* list. Place your cursor at the end of the *Died at Age*: phrase in the *Other FMHX* field and then type a fictitious age. Hit the [Enter] key.
19. Place your cursor at the end of the *Cause of Death*: phrase and select a medical condition from the list.
20. In the *Parents Information* section in the lower left, check the box to indicate the father is deceased. Select the date from the calender icon 6/9/1969.

Chart Note

21. Click on the [Chart Note] navigation button to open the *Chart Note* section.
22. Select *Prefers Hospital* in the pop-up text on the right side. Then select *St. Judes* from the right side.
23. Click in the *Chart Note* field on the left side of the window. Hit the [Enter] key to move your cursor to a new line.
24. Select *Religion* in the pop-up text on the right side. Place your cursor at the end of this word and type a specific religion (can be fictitious).

Routine Medications

25. Click on the [Routine Meds] navigation button to open the *Routine Medications* window.
26. In the upper right quadrant, search for and select each of the following medications: *Diovan, Glucophage,* and *Lipitor*. You can select the strength of your choice. All three medications should now appear on the left side of the window.
27. In the *Notes and OTC Meds* field, select several OTC (over-the-counter) items from the *Routine Meds* pop-up text in the lower-right quadrant.

(continued)

Problem List

28. Click on the [Problem List] navigation button to open the *Problem List* window.
29. In the *Dx* field in the upper right, type in htn (*for hypertension*) and conduct a search. Select *HTN 401.9 for hypertension.*
30. In the same field, type the code *250* and conduct a search. Select *Diabetes.*
31. In the *Dx* field, type *hypercholest* and conduct a search. Select *Hypercholesterolemia 272.0.*
32. Search for and select *Allergic Rhinitis—Pollen 477.0.*

Chart Alert

33. Click on the [Chart Alert] navigation button (shown in margin) to open the *Chart Alert* window.
34. Click on the *Edit PopUp text* icon on the far right. Place your [Caps Lock] key on and type *SPANISH-ENGLISH IS SECOND LANGUAGE* on the next empty line in the *Edit Pop-up Text* window. Click the [Done] button.
35. Select *SPANISH-ENGLISH IS SECOND LANGUAGE* from the available pop-up text.

| Chart Alert | ▾ | ✎ |

Edit PopUp Text icon

Printing the Face Sheet

36. Click the [Print FS] button in the lower left corner of the *Edit Face Sheet* window.
37. Click the [Print] button in the *Document Printing Options* window. Select the printer and print your documents.
38. Click on the [Back] button in the *Edit Face Sheet* window. All the data selected is now positioned in the various face sheet categories within your chart.
39. Close your patient's chart.
40. Collect your printed face sheet document and turn it in to your instructor.

Source: Byron R. Hamilton, *Electronic Health Records*, 3rd ed., pp. 18–20, Exercise 5.2.

2. Using the instructions that follow, edit your medical records in the SpringCharts™ EHR program to add an insurance to your medical record.

Adding the Patient's Primary Insurance

1. Open your chart by clicking on the *Open a Patient's Chart* icon on the main *Practice View* screen toolbar, entering your last name in the *Choose Patient* field, conducting a search, and selecting your name.
2. Right-click in the *Insurance* section of your face sheet and select the *Edit* option.
3. In the *Edit Patient Insurance* window, enter the following information:
   • Group Name: *Springfield School System*
   • Group No.: *SSS24589*
   • Policy No.: *4578954*
   • Details: *Deductible for procedures and tests—$250.00*
   • Co-pay: *$25.00*
   • Insured (Guarantor): Click in the *Pt is the guarantor* check box
   • Insurance Company: *Principal Financial Group*
4. Save the primary insurance information by clicking the [Save] button.

Note: The primary insurance information will not appear on your face sheet until the chart has been closed and reopened.

5. Close the chart.
6. Click on the *Recent Charts* menu in the *Practice View* window. Select your name. The primary insurance information will appear on your face sheet. Close your chart.

Source: Byron R. Hamilton, *Electronic Health Records*, 3rd ed., p. 24, Exercise 5.3.

3. Follow the instructions given below and, using the SpringCharts™ EHR software program, complete the following tasks:

   a. Add an Existing Patient to the schedule

   b. Block out Time on the schedule

   c. Add a New Patient to the schedule

   d. Add a Note to the schedule

   e. Add Additional Patients to the schedule

Adding an Existing Patient to the Schedule

1. Log on to SpringCharts. Close the Tutorial window.
2. Click on an OPEN icon on the appointment schedule.
3. When the Edit Appointment window displays, click on the [Choose Patient] button.
4. With the Choose Patient window open, type the first few letters of your last name, and then press the Search button.
5. Select your name from the list.
6. Enter a fictitious reason for your visit in the Note field of the Edit Appointment window.
7. Add your initials after the note.

Blocking Out Time on the Schedule

2. Click on the OPEN time slot for the beginning of the last hour of the work day, where you will block out time on the schedule for a staff meeting.
3. Type "Staff Meeting" in the Note field of the Edit Appointment window.
4. Click on the [Block This Time] button.
5. Repeat this exercise for each 10-minute increment until the entire hour is blocked. (You do not need to repeat "Staff Meeting" for subsequent time slots.).

Adding a New Patient to the Schedule

2. Click on an OPEN time slot on the appointment schedule.
3. When the Edit Appointment window displays, type Jeremie Hill in the Patient field.
4. Type in Physical for the visit reason in the Note field.
5. Add your initials after the note.
6. Click the [Done] button.

Adding a Note to the Schedule

1. Add two established patients, Sally Dalton and Robert Underhagen, to the appointment schedule. Note: Refer back to Exercise 4.2 if you need help adding existing patients to the schedule.
2. Add the reason note "UTI" (urinary tract infection) to Sally's appointment and the reason note "Lab" to Robert.

Adding Additional Patients to the Schedule

1. Add two new patients to the appointment schedule, along with appropriate reason notes. You may make up the names of your patients and the reasons for their visits.

Note: Remember, these are 'new' patients, so you will not search for them in the data base.

Source: Byron R. Hamilton, *Electronic Health Records*, 3rd ed., pp. 8–9, Exercises 4.2–4.6.

C A S E S T U D I E S

Write your response to each case study on the lines provided.

Case 1

The former boyfriend of one of the administrative medical assistants comes into the office for treatment—he did not know she works in the office. He is concerned she will be able to access his medical record because "she is on the computer all the time, and I know you have electronic records here." What can you tell him to ease his fears?

_____

_____

Case 2

The ED at the local hospital calls. Mr. Sanderson has just been in a car accident. The hospital needs his medical history quickly. The new EHR program in the office is compatible with that of the ED. What can you do to help?

_____

_____

_____

Case 3

BWW Medical Associates, PC has just finished installing the new EHR program in your office. Some of the patients are concerned that now "everyone will have access to my medical file." What can you tell these concerned patients?

_____

_____

_____

Name_____ Date_____

Evaluated by_____ Score_____

PROCEDURE 12-1 Creating a New Patient Record Using EHR Software

Goal
To create a new patient record using EHR Software.

OSHA Guidelines
This procedure does not involve exposure to blood, body fluids, or tissue.

Materials
Initial patient forms (patient information, advance directives, physician notes, referrals, laboratory orders).

Method

Step Number	Procedure	Points Possible	Points Earned
1.	Open the New Patient window of the EHR program as directed by the software vendor.	14	
2.	Enter the patient's full name as directed, being careful to enter the name in the correct order.*	15	
3.	If the patient has a family member who also comes to the practice, you may be able to use a shortcut to copy the patient's address from the existing patient information; otherwise, carefully enter the patient's demographic information, including address, phone number, birth date, etc.	14	
4.	Follow the software directions for completing each screen, including the patient's insurance, guarantor, and employer information.	15	
5.	Depending on office policy, you may also enter the patient's medical history information. Open the software program's medical history screen and carefully key in the information required for each screen.	14	
6.	Carefully inspect all information for accuracy, and save the new patient record as directed by the software program instructions.*	15	
7.	Depending on office policy, information from a hard copy medical record may be scanned into the EHR or a manual file created to maintain it. Follow your office procedure for filing this information.	13	
Total Points		100	

CAAHEP Competencies Achieved

V. P (5) Execute data management using electronic healthcare records such as the EMR

ABHES Competencies Achieved

7. b (2) Apply computer application skills using variety of different electronic programs including both practice management software and EMR software

8. (ll) Apply electronic technology

Name_____ Date_____

Evaluated by_____ Score_____

PROCEDURE 12-2 Making an Addition or Addendum (Correction) to an Electronic Health Record

Goal
To follow standard procedures for correcting or making an addendum to an electronic health record.

OSHA Guidelines
This procedure does not involve exposure to blood, body fluids, or tissue.

Materials
Access to the patient's EHR, other pertinent documents containing the information to be used in making corrections (for example, handwritten notes, telephone notes, physician comments, correspondence, or test results).

Method

Step Number	Procedure	Points Possible	Points Earned
1.	Open the patient record requiring the correction or addendum, following the software program instructions.	25	
2.	Following the software program instructions, obtain the *Edit* feature of the software program for this health record.*	25	
3.	When the pop-up window appears stating the record is *not editable* but asking if an addendum (or change) is required, answer *Yes*.	25	
4.	The program will now automatically date and time stamp the new entry with the current date and time, as well as initial stamp the entry with the current user's initials when the save feature is used.	25	
Total Points		100	

CAAHEP Competencies Achieved

V. P (5)   Execute data management using electronic healthcare records such as the EMR

IX. C (14)   Describe the process to follow if an error is made in patient care

IX. P (7)   Document accurately in the patient record

ABHES Competencies Achieved

7. b (2) Apply computer application skills using variety of different electronic programs including both practice management software and EMR software

8. (b) Prepare and maintain medical records

8. (ll) Apply electronic technology

Name_____ Date_____

Evaluated by_____ Score_____

PROCEDURE 12-3 Creating an Appointment Matrix for an Electronic Scheduling System

Goal
Using an electronic scheduling system, indicate the days and times when the office is not scheduling appointments.

OSHA Guidelines
This procedure does not involve exposure to blood, body fluids, or tissue.

Materials
Electronic scheduling program, physician schedule of meetings, conferences, vacations, and other times of unavailability, including staff meetings and hours when patients are not seen.

Method

Step Number	Procedure	Points Possible	Points Earned
1.	Using the physician schedule of availability as the base for the matrix, confer with the physician or office manager to assure that no additional schedule changes are planned.	10	
2.	Open the office appointment scheduler per the program format.	15	
3.	Block the dates and times when the general office or physician will not be available for patient appointments, using the physician and office schedules as guides.*	15	
4.	Choose the appropriate option if the time frame is repeatedly unavailable.	15	
5.	Enter a reason that the time is not available for future reference. The office program may use color coding to assist with this process.	15	
6.	If cluster scheduling is used for the office, most schedulers allow you to specify what types of appointments may be entered; again, the scheduler may use color coding to outline specific types of appointments.	15	
7.	Many programs will allow you to specify specific time frames necessary for different types of appointments, and these may be set up now also. For instance, physical exams for new patients may require 45 minutes, and visits for a BP check or a typical sick visit may be set up for 15 minutes. If the program allows, set up these matrixes now, too.*	15	
Total Points		100	

CAAHEP Competencies Achieved

V. P (1)   Manage appointment schedule, using established priorities

V. P (6)   Use office hardware and software to maintain office systems

ABHES Competencies Achieved

8. (c) Schedule and manage appointments

8. (d) Apply concepts for office procedures

8. (ll) Apply electronic technology

PROCEDURE 12-4 Scheduling a Patient Appointment Using an Electronic Scheduler

Goal
Utilizing the previously created matrix, book patient appointments, applying the correct amount of time for each appointment.

OSHA Guidelines
This procedure does not involve exposure to blood, body fluids, or tissue.

Materials
Electronic scheduler, template outlining time frames for patient appointment types.

Method

Step Number	Procedure	Points Possible	Points Earned
1.	Establish the type of appointment required by the patients, particularly noting if the appointment is for a new patient or an established patient.	20	
2.	If needed, consult the office template for the amount of time required for the patient appointment. Keep in mind the reason for the appointment, as that may affect timing.	20	
3.	When possible, schedule appointments earlier in the day first, and then move to later time frames. Do ask if the patient has a preferred time frame and, if possible, honor the request.	20	
4.	Following the electronic scheduler instructions, use the search option to find the next available appointment for the time frame required for the patient's appointment. Once the patient agrees to the appointment offered, enter the patient name, phone number, and reason for the appointment. Save the appointment per software instructions.	20	
5.	Repeat the appointment information to the patient, giving any necessary instructions regarding preparation for the appointment.*	20	
Total Points		100	

CAAHEP Competencies Achieved

V. P (1)   Manage appointment schedule, using established priorities

V. P (6)   Use office hardware and software to maintain office systems

ABHES Competencies Achieved

8. (c) Schedule and manage appointments

8. (d) Apply concepts for office procedures

8. (ll) Apply electronic technology

Telephone Techniques

Name_____ Class_____ Date_____

REVIEW

Vocabulary Review

Matching
Match the key terms in the right column with the definitions in the left column by placing the letter of each correct answer in the space provided.

_____ 1. Document listing the types of calls each staff member is responsible for handling

_____ 2. How words are said

_____ 3. Automated telephone answering system

_____ 4. Deciding the necessary action to take

_____ 5. Categorizing calls

_____ 6. Transferring calls to the correct person

_____ 7. Saying words clearly and distinctly

_____ 8. The level of your voice

_____ 9. Telephone device allowing you to speak with patients who are deaf

_____ 10. Handling calls politely and professionally

a. automated voice response unit
b. enunciation
c. etiquette
d. pitch
e. pronunciation
f. routing
g. routing list
h. screening
i. TDD
j. telephone triage

Content Review

Multiple Choice
In the space provided, write the letter of the choice that best completes each statement or answers each question.

_____ 1. When checking for understanding during a call,
   a. Watch for visual signals
   b. Ask the caller if there are any questions
   c. Repeat everything at least twice
   d. Ask the caller to explain the information to a third person
   e. Talk more loudly than normal

_____ 2. The correct use of a telephone log includes
   a. Keeping three copies of each phone message
   b. Keeping two copies of each phone message
   c. Using only a spiral-bound book
   d. Using only a message pad
   e. Giving the original message to the appropriate person and retaining a copy

_____ 3. If a caller refuses to discuss his symptoms with anyone but the physician,
   a. Schedule an appointment immediately
   b. Try to talk the patient into talking with you
   c. Have the doctor return the call
   d. Call the patient the next day to see whether he has changed his mind
   e. Route the call to the office manager

_____ 4. When reaching a patient's voice mail system
   a. Hang up immediately
   b. Leave a message if you have written permission from the patient to leave such messages on voice mail
   c. Leave the office name and phone number
   d. Leave a detailed message asking the patient to call you back
   e. Leave the office phone number only, with no other information

_____ 5. An automated telecommunications system
   a. Is inappropriate for use in a medical practice
   b. Is used in many hospitals and ambulatory care settings
   c. Is more expensive than using a phone operator
   d. Requires that the caller know exactly who he wants to speak to
   e. Is preferred by most patients calling physician offices

_____ 6. When using an answering system during the day, the best time to check for messages is
   a. At the beginning and end of the day
   b. At the end of the day so you are not interrupted by patient phone calls
   c. At lunch time
   d. Whenever it is convenient
   e. At preset times throughout the day

_____ 7. Prescription refills are commonly called in by this member of the office staff.
   a. Medical assistant   d. RN or LPN
   b. Office manager   e. Physician
   c. Receptionist

_____ 8. After identifying the office, an automated voice response unit should then provide this piece of information.
   a. How to reach an operator
   b. How to obtain an alphabetical listing of employees
   c. What to do if the call pertains to an emergency
   d. How to reach the covering physician after hours
   e. How to leave prescription refill information

_____ 9. What is the most important reason cell phone use should be avoided in the medical office?
   a. It is impolite to patients and coworkers
   b. They are a distraction
   c. Discussions may center around PHI, which should not be heard by others
   d. Patients busy texting may not hear important information
   e. Cell phones may interfere with office equipment

_____ 10. Which of the following is not part of telephone etiquette?
   a. Smiling   d. Enunciation
   b. Pronunciation   e. Pitch
   c. Other facial expressions

_____ **11.** A patient calls and tells you he is having severe vomiting. What should you do?

   a. Make an appointment for the next day

   b. Immediately put the call through to a doctor or handle the call according to the established office procedures for patients that need immediate medical help

   c. Make an appointment for the patient within the next 3 days

   d. Make an appointment for an annual physical exam

   e. Ask the patient to hold and ask for help evaluating the situation

_____ **12.** If you are in doubt about whether a situation is a medical emergency,

   a. You should treat it like an emergency

   b. You can ignore the situation if the patient tells you he does not want to see the doctor

   c. You should ask the patient to sit down so he can be observed

   d. You should rely on your intuition to do the right thing

   e. Use "Google" or another search engine to research the situation

_____ **13.** Pronunciation is

   a. The high or low level of speech

   b. The pitch of the voice

   c. The tone of the voice

   d. Saying words correctly

   e. Speaking without any accent

_____ **14.** The best way to hold a telephone when you are using it is

   a. With one hand

   b. With a telephone rest

   c. Propped on your shoulder so you have both hands free

   d. Propped on your shoulder, making sure you change shoulders every 3 minutes to avoid fatigue

   e. Both a and b

_____ **15.** How should a medical assistant respond to patient complaints?

   a. Listen carefully but never admit mistakes

   b. Defend the doctor and the policies of the practice

   c. Be careful to raise your voice only when the patient raises his voice

   d. Acknowledge the patient's anger

   e. Do not allow the patient to talk down to you

Sentence Completion

In the space provided, write the word or phrase that best completes each sentence.

16. The medical assistant handles calls that deal with _____ issues.

16. _____

17. _____ is a medical emergency in which there is a drop in body temperature during prolonged exposure to cold.

17. _____

18. If you will be discussing clinical matters over the telephone, it is a good idea to shut the _____ between the reception area and the administrative area.

18. _____

19. _____

19. Never release any patient information to an outside caller unless the _____ asks you to do so.

20. _____

20. The medical assistant may be responsible for making routine _____ to verify that patients are following treatment instructions.

21. _____ is clear and distinct speaking.

22. Before ending a telephone call, it is good professional behavior to always _____ the important points of the conversation.

23. Keeping a _____ on the desk allows you to easily find frequently used telephone numbers.

24. When taking a telephone message, always record the date and _____ of the call.

25. _____ is a medical emergency in which the patient experiences paleness; feeling faint; and a weak, rapid pulse.

21. _____

22. _____

23. _____

24. _____

25. _____

Short Answer

Write the answer to each question on the lines provided.

26. List the features of good communication skills.

_____

_____

_____

27. List three types of calls that a medical assistant would handle.

_____

_____

_____

28. List the steps to screen calls appropriately in the office.

_____

_____

_____

29. List three types of incoming calls.

_____

_____

_____

30. List at least eight symptoms or conditions that would qualify as a medical emergency.

_____

_____

_____

31. What are five ways you can make your telephone voice effective?

_____

_____

_____

32. What is the typical procedure for putting a call on hold?

_____

_____

_____

33. How is telephone triage conducted?

_____

_____

_____

34. The physician requests that you contact a patient and ask him to come in for an appointment, but the patient refuses to come in. What do you do?

_____

_____

_____

35. Discuss guidelines for dealing with an angry caller.

_____

_____

_____

A P P L I C A T I O N

Follow the directions for each application.

1. **Handling a Patient Call**

   Work with two partners. Have one partner play the role of an angry patient calling to complain about being billed for a procedure that never took place. Have the second partner act as a medical assistant handling the call. Have the third partner act as an observer and evaluator.

   a. Role-play the telephone call. The medical assistant should listen carefully to the caller, taking notes about the details of the problem. The medical assistant also should be sure to ask all necessary questions.

   b. The medical assistant should respond to the caller's complaint in a professional manner and explain the specific action that will be taken to address the issue.

   c. Have the observer provide a critique of the medical assistant's handling of the call. The critique should evaluate the use of proper telephone etiquette, the proper routing of the call, and the assistant's telephone notes. Comments should include both positive feedback and suggestions for improvement.

   d. Exchange roles and repeat the exercise. Allow the student playing the caller to choose another reason for the call.

   e. Exchange roles again so that each member of the group has an opportunity to play the role of the medical assistant.

   f. Discuss the strengths and weaknesses of each group member's telephone etiquette.

2. **Taking Telephone Messages**

   Work with a partner to design the best possible telephone message pad or telephone log for a medical office.

   a. Consider the various types of incoming calls that the medical practice receives. Review the different types of information that a person taking a message might need to obtain. Make a list of the types of calls and types of information. Think about the order in which the information is obtained. Decide how much space is needed for each entry.

b. Choose which you will design—a telephone message pad or a telephone log. As you work with your partner to design it, consider these questions: What is the best size for the pad or log? How many messages will fit on one page? How will copies be made? What color will the pad or log be? Pay attention to the information that must be included, the space available for each message, and the layout of the page.

c. Test your telephone message pad or log. Have your partner role-play a patient calling a medical office. Use your message pad or log to take the message.

d. Then trade roles and repeat the role playing. Discuss the strengths and weaknesses of your message pad or log. Revise your design as needed.

e. Share your message pad or log with other pairs of students. Critique each other's designs. Discuss how the designs are different and how they are similar. Assess the strengths and weaknesses of each design. Offer suggestions for revisions.

f. Make final adjustments to the design of your telephone message pad or telephone log on the basis of your classmates' feedback.

C A S E   S T U D I E S

Write your response to each case study on the lines provided.

Case 1
You overhear another medical assistant speaking rudely to a patient. What should you do?

_____

_____

_____

Case 2
In a single morning, you receive calls from a patient with an emergency, an attorney, a physician from another medical office, and a salesperson. Describe how you would route each of these calls.

_____

_____

_____

Case 3
A patient calls and says that he thinks he is having a heart attack. What do you do?

_____

_____

_____

Case 4
A physician calls and asks to speak to the physician in your practice. The physician is with a patient. What do you do?

_____

_____

_____

PROCEDURE 13-1 Using a Telecommunications Device for the Deaf (TDD)

Goal
To properly communicate with the hearing-impaired patient using a TDD.

OSHA Guidelines
This procedure does not involve exposure to blood, body fluids, or tissue.

Materials
Telephone, TDD (if available), patient chart for documentation, pen.

Method

Step Number	Procedure	Points Possible	Points Earned
Answering a Call with TDD			
1.	Answer the phone as usual. If you hear a rapid clicking sound, you know you have a TDD call. You may hear no sound at all; do not hang up, it may still be a TDD call.	7	
2.	If you know (or believe) this is a TDD call, place your phone receiver on the TDD as directed.*	7	
3.	Type your normal office greeting: "BWW Medical Associates, this is Miguel. How may I help you?"	8	
4.	When you complete your message, type "GA," which stands for "Go Ahead." This tells the patient you have completed your message and it is his turn to respond.*	7	
5.	Give the patient time to type his response. When you see "GA" at the end of his message, it is your turn to respond.	7	
6.	When the patient receives all of the information required, he will type "Bye, SK," which stands for Good-Bye, Stop Keying.	7	
7.	If you agree the call is completed, you may also reply "Bye, SK." This will give the patient the opportunity to be the one to end the call.	7	
8.	When you receive a response of SKSK (Stop Keying, Stop Keying), the conversation is complete and you may hang up and turn off the TDD.*	7	
Making a Call with a TDD			
1.	Turn on the TDD.	7	
2.	Dial the patient's phone number on your standard telephone and listen for the phone to ring.	7	
3.	When you hear the TDD sound, place the phone receiver on the TDD as directed.*	7	
4.	After the patient types a greeting and "GA" appears on the TDD display, identify yourself and proceed with the conversation.	8	
5.	Remember to type "GA" when you complete your message so that the patient knows it is his turn to respond.	7	
6.	Even though you were the one to initiate the call, you should still allow the patient to make the decision that the call is completed by keying "SKSK."*	7	
Total Points		100	

CAAHEP Competencies Achieved

IV. P (7)   Demonstrate telephone techniques

VII. A (2)   Demonstrate sensitivity in communicating with both providers and patients

ABHES Competencies Achieved

8. (ee) Use proper telephone techniques

8. (hh) Receive, organize, prioritize, and transmit information expediently

PROCEDURE 13-2 Renewing a Prescription by Telephone

WORK // DOC

Goal
To ensure that a complete and accurate prescription is received by the patient.

OSHA Guidelines
This procedure does not involve exposure to blood, body fluids, or tissue.

Materials
Telephone, appropriate phone numbers, message pad or prescription refill request form, pen and patient chart with prescription order.

Method

Step Number	Procedure	Points Possible	Points Earned
1.	Take the message from the call or the message system. For the prescription to be complete, you must obtain the patient's name, date of birth, phone number, pharmacy name and/or phone number, medication, and dosage.	8	
2.	Follow your facility policy regarding prescription renewals. Typically, the prescription is usually called into the pharmacy the day it is requested. An example policy may be posted at the facility and may state, "Nonemergency prescriptions refill requests must be made during regular business hours. Please allow 24 hours for processing."	7	
3.	Communicate the policy to the patient. You should know the policy and the time when the refills will be reviewed. For example, you might state, "Dr. Williams will review the prescription between patients and it will be telephoned within one hour to the pharmacy. I will call you back if there is a problem."	8	
4.	Obtain the patient's chart or reference the electronic chart to verify you have the correct patient and that the patient is currently taking the medication. Check the patient's list of medications, which are usually part of the chart.	8	
5.	Give the prescription refill request and the chart to the physician or prescriber. Do not give a prescription refill request to the physician without the chart or chart access information. Wait for an authorization from the physician before you proceed.	7	
6.	Once the physician authorizes the prescription, prepare to call the pharmacy with the renewal information. You cannot call in Schedule II or III medications. Be certain to have the physician order, the patient's chart, and the refill request in front of you when you make the call. The request should include the name of the drug, the drug dosage, the frequency and mode of administration, the number of refills authorized, and the pharmacy's name and phone number.*	8	
7.	Telephone the pharmacy. Identify yourself by name, the practice name, and the doctor's name.	7	
8.	State the purpose of the call. (Example: "This is Miguel Perez from BWW Medical Associates. I am calling to request a prescription refill for a patient.")	8	
9.	Identify the patient. Include the patient's name, date of birth, address, and phone number.*	8	
10.	Identify the drug (spelling the name when necessary), the dosage, the frequency and mode of administration, and any other special instructions or changes for administration (such as "take at bedtime").*	8	

(continued)

Step Number	Procedure	Points Possible	Points Earned
11.	State the number of refills authorized.*	8	
12.	If leaving a message on a pharmacy voicemail system set up for physicians, state your name, the name of the doctor you represent, and your phone number before you hang up.	7	
13.	Document the prescription renewal in the chart after the medication has been called into the pharmacy. Include the date, the time, the name of pharmacy, and the person taking your call. Also include the medication, dose, amount, directions, and number of refills. Sign your first initial, last name, and title.*	8	
Total Points		100	

CAAHEP Competencies Achieved

IV. P (7)   Demonstrate telephone techniques

IX. P (7)   Document accurately in the patient record

ABHES Competencies Achieved

8. (dd) Serve as liaison between physician and others

8. (ee) Use proper telephone techniques

8. (hh) Receive, organize, prioritize, and transmit information expediently

8. (jj) Perform fundamental writing skills including correct grammar, spelling and formatting techniques when writing prescriptions, documenting medical records, etc.

Name_____ Date_____

Evaluated by_____ Score_____

PROCEDURE 13-3 Screening and Routing Telephone Calls

Goal
To properly screen incoming telephone calls.

OSHA Guidelines
This procedure does not involve exposure to blood, body fluids, or tissue.

Materials
Telephone, telephone pad, pen or pencil, appointment book or computerized scheduling software (computer), office routing list.

Method

Step Number	Procedure	Points Possible	Points Earned
1.	Make sure all of the materials are within reach of the telephone equipment.	10	
2.	Answer the telephone promptly within two to three rings	15	
3.	Identify the medical office and identify yourself. Make sure you know office procedure for answering the phone in your facility even if a telephone answering system is employed to route calls to you. For example: "BWW Medical Associates, this is Malik, how may I help you?"	15	
4.	If the caller does not identify himself, ask him to do so and the number he is calling from, and write down this information. Find out the reason for the call. Is it an emergency? (Refer to Table 13–2.) If so, follow office policy.	15	
5.	If you can handle the call, take care of the query. Listen carefully to what the caller has to say, paying particular attention to tone and feeling.*	15	
6.	If this is a call that needs to be transferred to someone (per the routing list), tell the caller to whom and to what number you will be transferring the call. Make sure you write down the caller's name and phone number in case the call is accidentally dropped. If the other staff member does not answer promptly or is on another line, ask the caller if he would like to be transferred to the staff member's voicemail (if available) or would like to leave a message.	15	
7.	If you need to take a message, make sure you repeat the information that is given to you, especially the name of the person and his phone number. Take a complete message.*	15	
Total Points		100	

CAAHEP Competencies Achieved
IV. P (7) Demonstrate telephone techniques

VII. A (2) Demonstrate sensitivity in communicating with both providers and patients

ABHES Competencies Achieved
8. (dd) Serve as liaison between physician and others

8. (ee) Use proper telephone techniques

8. (hh) Receive, organize, prioritize, and transmit information expediently

Copyright © 2014 by The McGraw-Hill Companies, Inc.

Chapter 13: Telephone Techniques **177**

PROCEDURE 13-4 Handling Emergency Calls

Goal
To determine whether a telephone call involves a medical emergency and to learn the steps to take if it is an emergency call.

OSHA Guidelines
This procedure does not involve exposure to blood, body fluids, or tissue.

Materials
Office guidelines for handling emergency calls; list of symptoms and conditions requiring immediate medical attention; telephone numbers of area emergency rooms, poison control centers, and ambulance transport services; telephone message forms or telephone message log.

Method

Step Number	Procedure	Points Possible	Points Earned
1.	When someone calls the office regarding a potential emergency, remain calm.	15	
2.	Obtain the following information, taking accurate notes:*	20	
	a. The caller's name.	(4)	
	b. The caller's telephone number and the address from which the call is being made.	(2)	
	c. The caller's relationship to the patient (if it is not the patient who is calling).	(2)	
	d. The patient's name (if the patient is not the caller).	(2)	
	e. The patient's age.	(2)	
	f. A complete description of the patient's symptoms.	(2)	
	g. If the call is about an accident, a description of how the accident or injury occurred and any other pertinent information.	(2)	
	h. A description of how the patient is reacting to the situation.	(2)	
	i. Treatment that has been administered.	(2)	
3.	Read back the details of the medical problem to verify them.	10	
4.	If necessary, refer to the list of symptoms and conditions that require immediate medical attention to determine if the situation is indeed a medical emergency.	10	
If the Situation Is a Medical Emergency			
1.	Put the call through to the doctor immediately, or handle the situation according to the established office procedures.	10	
2.	If the doctor is not in the office, follow established office procedures. These may involve one or more of the following:	10	
	a. Transferring the call to the nurse practitioner or other medical personnel, as appropriate;	(2)	
	b. Instructing the caller (if not the patient) to hang up and dial 911 to request an ambulance for the patient;	(2)	
	c. Instructing the patient to be driven to the nearest emergency room;	(2)	
	d. Instructing the caller to telephone the nearest poison control center for advice and supplying the caller with its telephone number; and/or	(2)	
	e. Paging the doctor.	(2)	

(continued)

Step Number	Procedure	Points Possible	Points Earned
If the Situation Is Not a Medical Emergency			
1.	Handle the call according to established office procedures.	15	
2.	If you are in doubt about whether the situation is a medical emergency, treat it like an emergency. You must always alert the doctor immediately about an emergency call, even if the patient declines to speak with the doctor.	10	
Total Points		100	

CAAHEP Competencies Achieved

IV. P (7)   Demonstrate telephone techniques

VII. A (2)   Demonstrate sensitivity in communicating with both providers and patients

ABHES Competencies Achieved

8. (dd) Serve as liaison between physician and others

8. (ee) Use proper telephone techniques

8. (hh) Receive, organize, prioritize, and transmit information expediently

PROCEDURE 13-5 Retrieving Messages from an Answering Service or System

WORK // DOC

Goal
To follow standard procedures for retrieving messages from an answering service or system.

OSHA Guidelines
This procedure does not involve exposure to blood, body fluids, or tissue.

Materials
Telephone message pad, manual telephone log, or electronic telephone log.

Method

Step Number	Procedure	Points Possible	Points Earned
1.	Set a regular schedule for calling the answering service (system) to retrieve messages.	12	
2.	Call at the regularly scheduled time(s) to see if there are any messages.	12	
3.	If calling a service, identify yourself and state that you are calling to obtain messages for the practice.	13	
4.	If calling an answering system, when the call is answered, you will enter the passcode for the office.	13	
5.	For each message, write down all pertinent information on the telephone message pad or telephone log, or key it into the electronic telephone log. Be sure to include the caller's name and telephone number, time of call, message or description of the problem, and action taken, if any.*	12	
6.	If calling an answering service, repeat the information, confirming that you have the correct spelling of all names and the complete, correct information.	13	
7.	If calling an answering system, be sure you listen carefully and replay messages if necessary to get complete information given within each message.	12	
8.	When you have retrieved all messages, route them according to the office policy.	13	
Total Points		100	

CAAHEP Competencies Achieved

IV. P (7)   Demonstrate telephone techniques

ABHES Competencies Achieved

8. (ee) Use proper telephone techniques

8. (hh) Receive, organize, prioritize, and transmit information expediently

Patient Education

Name_____ Class_____ Date_____

Vocabulary Review

Matching

Match the key terms in the right column with the definitions in the left column by placing the letter of each correct answer in the space provided.

_____ 1. Teaching targeted to the cognitive domain

_____ 2. Education that is geared, in both content and language, toward the average person

_____ 3. The learning domain that deals with motivation, sensory perception, and behaviors

_____ 4. The repetition by a patient of a demonstration after the medical assistant has demonstrated a skill

_____ 5. The demonstration by a medical assistant of a technique while the patient observes; then the patient repeats the technique

_____ 6. Cognitive, affective, and psychomotor areas of learning

_____ 7. The learning domain that deals with the physical skills necessary to perform a task

_____ 8. Diagnostic testing of a patient who is typically free of symptoms

_____ 9. Teaching targeted to the affective domain

_____ 10. The learning domain that deals with facts and knowledge

_____ 11. The system of values and principles a medical office has adopted in its everyday practices

_____ 12. Teaching targeted to the psychomotor domain

a. affective domain
b. cognitive domain
c. consumer education
d. domains of learning
e. factual teaching
f. modeling
g. participatory teaching
h. philosophy
i. psychomotor domain
j. return demonstration
k. screening
l. sensory teaching

Content Review

Multiple Choice

In the space provided, write the letter of the choice that best completes each statement or answers each question.

_____ 1. Which of the following terms is used to describe an office's set of values and principles?
   a. Screening technique
   b. Benefits
   c. Confidentiality
   d. Philosophy
   e. Privacy rules

_____ 2. Which of the following topics would an educational newsletter most likely contain?
   a. Healthcare tips
   b. A physician's credentials
   c. The payment policies of a medical office
   d. A community resource directory
   e. A list of the office's staff

_____ 3. The process of screening
   a. Prevents an early diagnosis
   b. Teaches patients how to perform healthcare tasks
   c. Differs according to patient age
   d. Is advisable only when symptoms are present
   e. Cannot be done in a medical practice

_____ 4. Some practices create simplified, pictorial versions of their patient information packet for patients
   a. With hearing impairments
   b. With visual impairments
   c. Who do not understand English
   d. Who will undergo surgical procedures
   e. Who are under the age of 10

_____ 5. It is recommended that the water in a water heater be set at what temperature to prevent injury?
   a. 100° F   d. 140° F
   b. 120° F   e. 160° F
   c. 130° F

_____ 6. When developing a patient education plan, the first thing you must do is
   a. Develop the plan
   b. Discuss the idea with the physician
   c. Perform the instruction
   d. Identify how intelligent the patient is
   e. Identify the patient's needs

_____ 7. Which of these is the best definition of patient education?
   a. The use of visual material to educate a patient
   b. The demonstration of a technique to a patient
   c. The use of verbal instruction to educate a patient
   d. The use of verbal and written instruction to educate a patient
   e. The use of verbal, written, or demonstrative instructions to educate a patient

_____ 8. Which statement about patient education is true?
   a. Patient education is always performed according to a well-defined plan
   b. Patient education is only appropriate for intelligent people
   c. Patient education takes many forms and includes a variety of techniques
   d. Medical assistants are not generally involved in patient education
   e. The physician is responsible for providing all patient education

_____ 9. Many accidents happen because people fail to see potential risks. *Potential risks* means
   a. Side effects
   b. Situations or things that can cause harm
   c. Preventive measures
   d. Situations or things that always cause harm
   e. Safety measures

_____ 10. The patient information packet should include
    a. The first bill or invoice
    b. Names of medical practices not associated with the medical office for which you are working
    c. Technical medical brochures describing disease processes
    d. A description of the practice and an introduction to the office
    e. Referrals to other physicians

_____ 11. The patient confidentiality statement
    a. Supplies a place for the patient to sign before any other practice information is released
    b. Is not commonly used in a pediatric practice
    c. States that no patient information will be released without signed authorization from the patient
    d. Is not usually part of the information packet
    e. Requires the patient not to release any information about the practice to others

_____ 12. The guidelines for healthful habits include adequate rest, which is defined as how many hours of sleep each night?
    a. 7 to 8 hours
    b. 8 to 9 hours
    c. 5 to 6 hours
    d. 3 to 5 hours
    e. 10 or more hours

Sentence Completion

In the space provided, write the word or phrase that best completes each sentence.

13. Many accidents happen because people fail to see _____ and do not develop plans of action.

14. A patient information packet should identify office staff members according to their duties and _____.

15. Elderly patients who have problems with memory should receive detailed _____ instructions.

16. Patients who will undergo a surgical procedure must first sign a(n) _____ form.

17. When you provide preoperative education, be aware that the fear and _____ of patients who are about to undergo a surgical procedure can adversely affect the learning process.

18. Instruction to patients before they undergo surgery, also called _____ education, can increase their overall satisfaction with their care.

13. _____

14. _____

15. _____

16. _____

17. _____

18. _____

Short Answer

Write the answer to each question on the lines provided.

19. List at least two benefits of patient education before surgery.

_____

_____

_____

20. List three ways to achieve good health.

_____

_____

_____

21. What are three ways in which a patient information packet can be helpful to patients?

_____

_____

_____

22. What are three ways in which a patient information packet can be helpful to the medical office?

_____

_____

_____

23. List five types of information that should appear in a patient information packet.

_____

_____

_____

24. Identify and describe the three types of patient teaching.

_____

_____

_____

25. List three ways you can relieve a patient's anxiety.

_____

_____

_____

26. List five tips for preventing injury in the workplace.

_____

_____

_____

27. List the seven steps to developing an education plan for a patient.

_____

_____

_____

28. Why is it important for a surgical patient to have someone drive him/her home after surgery?

_____

_____

_____

Critical Thinking
Write the answer to each question on the lines provided.

1. What are the advantages of developing a formal written education plan for a patient?

_____

_____

2. How might your approach to educating children about healthful habits differ from your approach to teaching adult patients?

_____

_____

3. What type of preoperative education plan do you think might be best for a patient who is blind?

_____

_____

4. Of the healthy habits listed in this chapter, which three do you consider the most important? Why?

_____

_____

5. What do you think is the most important tip for preventing injury in the workplace? Why?

_____

_____

A P P L I C A T I O N

Follow the directions for each application.

1. **Preparing an Education Brochure**
   a. Use the Internet to choose a medical topic such as *leukemia* or *sickle cell anemia*.
   b. Write at least two or three paragraphs about this medical topic and prepare the information in a brochure format.
   c. Insert pictures to help explain the information.
   d. Use word processing software to create the brochure. You may be able to locate a specific template for brochures.

C A S E   S T U D I E S

Write your response to each case study on the lines provided.

Case 1

During a physical exam, a teenage patient admits to you that he lives "mainly on hamburgers and French fries," that he rarely exercises, and that he often gets fewer than 6 hours of sleep at night, except on weekends. "I'll worry about my health when I'm older," he tells you. What can you say to the patient to encourage him to adopt healthful habits now?

_____

_____

_____

Case 2

The physician you work for wants you to develop patient information that will fit on two sides of a 4-by-6-inch index card. There will be room for only the most important information. What should appear on the card?

_____

_____

_____

Case 3

The third level of disease prevention involves the rehabilitation and management of an existing illness. What might you say to a patient who thinks that rehabilitation is just a waste of time and money?

_____

_____

_____

Case 4

A patient calls with questions about her upcoming surgery. Her patient record reflects that the physician has already discussed the nature of the surgery with her. As a medical assistant, what are your responsibilities for ensuring that the patient is fully prepared for the surgery?

_____

_____

_____

PROCEDURE 14-1 Creating Electronic Patient Instructions

Goal
To create and administer patient instructions electronically.

OSHA Guidelines
This procedure does not involve exposure to blood, body fluids, or tissue.

Materials
An electronic health records software program (such as SpringCharts™) that includes a patient instructions feature.

Method

Step Number	Procedure	Points Possible	Points Earned
1.	Search the EHR to find the button or icon to create patient instructions. (Check the Help button or review the training manual.)	15	
2.	Determine if you will need to write your own or can select from a previously created list of patient instructions. Select the correct button to proceed.	10	
3.	Create new instructions by either of the following methods:* a. Type your patient instructions directly in the open window or a word processing program. This will depend on the EHR you are using. b. Open the web browser and navigate to a credible Internet site for patient instruction. Highlight the information you want to use from the website. Right-click on any highlighted area and choose Copy. Click in the patient instruction window or in the word processing program and press the [Ctrl] and [V] keys. Close the web page and return to the EHR.	20	
4.	Import instructions by opening a previously created document saved as an .RTF or other word processing file type. Import the document according to the manufacturer's instructions.*	20	
5.	Use existing instructions by selecting them from a list within the EHR or a file folder on your computer. Check the specific directions for the EHR program you are using.	15	
6.	Record in the EHR the instructions that you provided to the patient. In most programs this occurs when you generate the instructions and becomes a permanent record in the patient's chart.*	20	
Total Points		100	

CAAHEP Competencies Achieved

V. P (5) Execute data management using electronic healthcare records such as the EMR

V. P (7) Use internet to access information related to the medical office

ABHES Competencies Achieved

8. (ll) Apply electronic technology

Name_____ Date_____

Evaluated by_____ Score_____

PROCEDURE 14-2 Identifying Community Resources

Goal
To create a list of useful community resources for patient referrals.

OSHA Guidelines
This procedure does not involve exposure to blood, body fluids, or tissue.

Materials
Computer with Internet access, phone directory, printer.

Method

Step Number	Procedure	Points Possible	Points Earned
1.	Determine the needs of your medical office and formulate a list of community resources. The specific needs of your patients will help you formulate your list. Being able to help patients find outside assistance when necessary is the goal.*	20	
2.	Use the Internet to research the names, addresses, web addresses, and phone numbers of local resources such as state and federal agencies, home healthcare agencies, long-term nursing facilities, mental health agencies, and local charities. Use the phone directory to assist in locating local agencies such as Meals on Wheels; Alcoholics Anonymous; shelters for abused individuals; hospice care; Easter Seals; Women, Infants, and Children (WIC); and support groups for grief, obesity, and various diseases.*	20	
3.	Contact each resource and request information such as business cards and brochures. Some agencies may send a representative to meet with you regarding their services. If patients can access information easily, they are more likely to take advantage of the services available to them.	10	
4.	Compile a list of community resources with the proper name, address, phone number, e-mail address, and contact name. Include any information that may be helpful to the office.	10	
5.	Update and add to the information often because outdated information will only frustrate you and your patients, creating even more anxiety.*	20	
6.	Post the information in a location where it is readily available. Maintain an electronic record for easy reference.*	20	
Total Points		100	

CAAHEP Competencies Achieved

IV. P (12)   Develop and maintain a current list of community resources related to patients' healthcare needs

ABHES Competencies Achieved

8. (e) Locate resources and information for patients and employers

8. (ll) Apply electronic technology

PROCEDURE 14-3 Locating Credible Patient Education Information on the Internet

Goal
To determine the credibility of patient education information on the Internet.

OSHA Guidelines
This procedure does not involve exposure to blood, body fluids, or tissue.

Materials
Computer with Internet access.

Method

Step Number	Procedure	Points Possible	Points Earned
1.	Open your Internet browser and locate a search engine. Search engines vary in the way they search so you may want to use more than one search engine for different results.	10	
2.	Search the topic. Be specific when entering the search term. For example, if you want to know about the proper diet for high cholesterol, you should type, "high cholesterol diet." For different or more medical sites, try using different terms; instead of high cholesterol try "hyperlipidemia."	10	
3.	Select a site from the list of results and evaluate the source.* a. Click the "about us" link to find out who developed the site. Sites should have an active link available to contact the webmaster and verify the source. b. Sites developed by professional organizations, educational institutions, or a branch of the federal government are generally better than those developed by an individual or a commercial company.	15	
4.	Review the "about us" page to determine the quality of the information.* a. Review the mission statement or other detailed information about the developer. b. Look for information about the writers or authors of the site. Make sure they are medical professionals.	15	
5.	Check the content of the site.* a. Avoid sites that have sensational writing or make claims that are too good to be true. b. Make sure the language of the information is at a level that you can understand. Avoid sites that use lots of technical jargon for patient instruction.	15	
6.	Make sure the information is current by checking the copyright or by checking the contact information on the site. Medical information changes frequently, so check the date and avoid information over 5 years old.*	15	
7.	Avoid websites that are potentially biased. For example, if the site is written by a pharmaceutical company, the site will present only information about the medication manufactured by that company. There may be alternative medications. Sites written by individuals are interesting but may be biased as well.*	10	
8.	Protect your privacy. If the sites require you to register, review their Privacy Policy. They may be able to share your or your patient's information with other companies.	5	

(continued)

Step Number	Procedure	Points Possible	Points Earned
9.	Once you have evaluated the site and decide to use it, you may want to have your supervisor or licensed practitioner review and approve the information you will be providing to the patient.	5	
Total Points		100	

CAAHEP Competencies Achieved

V. P (7)   Use internet to access information related to the medical office

ABHES Competencies Achieved

8. (e) Locate resources and information for patients and employers

8. (ll) Apply electronic technology

PROCEDURE 14-4 Developing a Patient Education Plan

Goal
To create and implement a patient teaching plan.

OSHA Guidelines
This procedure does not involve exposure to blood, body fluids, or tissue.

Materials
Pen, paper, various educational aids (such as instructional pamphlets and brochures), and/or visual aids (such as posters, videotapes, or DVDs).

Method

Step Number	Procedure	Points Possible	Points Earned
1.	Identify the patient's educational needs in order to provide instruction at the patient's point of need. Consider the following:* a. The patient's current knowledge b. Any misconceptions the patient may have c. Any obstacles to learning (loss of hearing or vision, limitations of mobility, language barriers, and so on) d. The patient's willingness and readiness to learn (motivation) e. How the patient will use the information	20	
2.	Using the various educational aids available, develop and outline a plan that addresses all the patient's needs. Include the following areas in the outline:* a. What you want to accomplish (your goal) b. How you plan to accomplish it c. How you will determine if the teaching was successful	20	
3.	Write the plan. Try to make the information interesting for the patient.	10	
4.	Before carrying out the plan, share it with the physician to get approval and suggestions for improvement.	10	
5.	Perform the instruction. Be sure to use more than one teaching method. For instance, if written material is being given, be sure to explain or demonstrate the material instead of simply telling the patient to read the educational materials.	10	
6.	Document the teaching in the patient's chart for continuity of care and to maintain a legal record.*	20	
7.	Revise your plan as necessary to make it even more effective. To be an effective teacher, you must evaluate the methods you use.	10	
Total Points		100	

CAAHEP Competencies Achieved

IV. P (9)   Document patient education

V. P (7)   Use internet to access information related to the medical office

ABHES Competencies Achieved

8. (e) Locate resources and information for patients and employers

8. (ll) Apply electronic technology

9. (r) Teach patients methods of health promotion and disease prevention

PROCEDURE 14-5 Outpatient Surgery Teaching [WORK//DOC]

Goal
To inform a preoperative patient of the necessary guidelines to follow prior to surgery.

OSHA Guidelines
This procedure does not involve exposure to blood, body fluids, or tissue.

Materials
Patient chart, Surgical Guidelines Sample.

Method

Step Number	Procedure	Points Possible	Points Earned
1.	Review the patient's chart to determine the type of surgery to be performed and then ask the patient what procedure is being performed.*	10	
2.	Tell the patient that you will be providing both verbal and written instructions that should be followed prior to surgery.	5	
3.	Inform the patient about policies regarding makeup, jewelry, contact lenses, wigs, dentures, and so on.	5	
4.	Tell the patient to leave money and valuables at home.	5	
5.	If applicable, suggest appropriate clothing for the patient to wear for postoperative ease and comfort.	5	
6.	Explain the need for someone to drive the patient home following an outpatient surgical procedure.*	10	
7.	Tell the patient the correct time to arrive at the office, surgery center, or hospital for the procedure.	5	
8.	Inform the patient of dietary restrictions. Be sure to use specific, clear instructions about what may or may not be ingested and at what time the patient must abstain from eating or drinking. Also explain these points: a. The reasons for the dietary restrictions b. The possible consequences of not following the dietary restrictions*	10	
9.	Ask patients who smoke to refrain from or reduce cigarette smoking during at least the 8 hours prior to the procedure. Explain to the patient that reducing smoking improves the level of oxygen in the blood during surgery.	5	
10.	Suggest that the patient shower or bathe the morning of the procedure or the evening before.	5	
11.	Instruct the patient about medications to take or avoid before surgery. For example, patients may need to stop taking a daily aspirin or vitamin E before surgery to reduce the risk of bleeding.*	10	
12.	If necessary, clarify any information about which the patient is unclear.	5	
13.	Provide written surgical guidelines, and suggest that the patient call the office if additional questions arise.*	10	
14.	Document the instructions in the patient's chart for continuity of care and as a legal record.*	10	
Total Points		100	

CAAHEP Competencies Achieved

IV. P (5)   Instruct patients according to their needs to promote health maintenance and disease prevention

IV. P (9)   Document patient education

ABHES Competencies Achieved

9. (q) Instruct patients with special needs

9. (r) Teach patients methods of health promotion and disease prevention

Managing Medical Records

Name_____ Class_____ Date_____

Vocabulary Review

Matching
Match the key terms in the right column with the definitions in the left column by placing the letter of each correct answer in the space provided.

_____ 1. Separates the contents in a file drawer

_____ 2. File cabinet that is taller than it is wide

_____ 3. File that is used frequently

_____ 4. Each part of a name or numerical sequence

_____ 5. Traditional filing method

_____ 6. Reminder file

_____ 7. File of patient who has moved away

_____ 8. Often the first unit for numerical filing

_____ 9. Storage units that stack together when not in use

_____ 10. Logical alpha, numerical or date order

_____ 11. Quan Tragh Chu See Chu, Quan Tragh

_____ 12. How long records are kept or destroyed

_____ 13. Files that are used infrequently

_____ 14. How records are created, filed, and maintained

_____ 15. Sequencing records

_____ 16. Placeholder for removed medical records

_____ 17. The sequencing guidelines for alphabetic filing

_____ 18. Filing system using numbers

_____ 19. File cabinet that has wide drawers

_____ 20. System using the center numbered unit as start point

a. active file
b. alphabetic filing
c. closed file
d. compactible file
e. cross-referenced
f. file guide
g. inactive file
h. indexing
i. indexing rules
j. lateral file
k. middle digit
l. numeric filing
m. out guide
n. records management system
o. retention schedule
p. sequential order
q. terminal digit
r. tickler file
s. unit
t. vertical file

True or False
Decide whether each statement is true or false. In the space at the left, write T for true or F for false. On the lines provided, rewrite the false statements to make them true.

_____ 21. If storage space is limited, there are a number of paperless options for storing files.

_____

_____ **22.** No matter where you store files, you must consider the issue of safety as well as security.

_____ **23.** The rules of indexing state that all hyphenated names are always considered to be one unit.

_____ **24.** OSHA states that there must be a "reasonable safeguard" to protect health information from any disclosure, whether intentional or unintentional.

_____ **25.** Wm St. Mary will be filed before William St. Mary.

_____ **26.** In terminal digital filing, numbered units are read from right to left.

_____ **27.** Horizontal file cabinets are also called lateral file cabinets.

_____ **28.** A records management system refers to the way patient records are created, filed, and maintained.

_____ **29.** Commercial records centers manage stored documents for medical practices.

_____ **30.** When inserting documents into folders already in place in the drawer, lift the folders up and out of the drawer.

_____ **31.** You should write the name of a patient on the tab of a file folder to identify the contents.

_____ **32.** It is not important to use an out guide as a placeholder to indicate that a file has been taken out of the filing system.

_____ **33.** File 111-283-091 is filed before 111-283-090 and 111-283-092 in terminal digit filing.

_____ **34.** In an alphabetic filing system, files are placed in alphabetical order according to the patients' last names.

_____ **35.** When counting years in a retention schedule, you should count the year in which the document was produced.

_____ **36.** A file that has been cross-referenced has been placed in more than one location.

_____ **37.** Mother Theresa would be indexed as Theresa, Mother.

_____ **38.** Coding is another term for naming a file.

_____ 39. The best filing plan is to file once or twice a week.

_____

_____ 40. The first indexing unit for Janine Smith-Jackson is Smith.

_____

Content Review

Multiple Choice

In the space provided, write the letter of the choice that best completes each statement or answers each question.

_____ 1. If you are unsure whether to cross-reference a file, the best policy is
   a. To not do it
   b. To do it
   c. To let someone else make the decision
   d. To not put the file away. Set the file on your desk
   e. To place the unlabeled file into the file cabinet or filing system

_____ 2. A numeric filing system
   a. Is not used when patient confidentiality is especially important
   b. Organizes records in a numerical sequence
   c. May include numbers that indicate where in the filing system a file can be found
   d. Is the only practical system for a large practice
   e. b and c

_____ 3. Use color-coding for files
   a. Only when using a numeric filing system
   b. Only to identify files belonging to specific categories of patients
   c. Only when you are using no other filing system
   d. To reduce the risk of misplacing files
   e. To make the file room more colorful to work in

_____ 4. For tickler files to work effectively, they must be
   a. Kept in file folders
   b. Kept in a file box
   c. Listed on a calendar
   d. Placed in the computer
   e. Checked frequently

_____ 5. The *first* step in locating a misplaced file is to
   a. Look for the color of the misfiled chart
   b. Discuss it with the person in charge of the office
   c. Check the doctor's office to see if it is on her desk
   d. Check with the other employees
   e. Determine the last time you knew the file's location

_____ 6. The medical records for patients who have died should be placed in which type of file?
   a. Active
   b. Inactive
   c. Closed
   d. Reserved
   e. Expired

_____ 7. When files are organized in a variety of filing systems that place patient records one after the other in a pattern or an order, it is referred to as a
   a. Sequential order
   b. Labeled order
   c. Tabbed order
   d. Standard order
   e. Chronological order

_____ 8. Which group of names is sequenced correctly?
  a. Johnson, Janice; Johnson, James; Johnsen, Janet; Jonson, Janinie
  b. Johnson, James; Johnsen, Janet; Jonson, Janine; Johnson, Janice
  c. Johnsen, Janet; Jonson, Janine; Johnson, Janice; Johnson James
  d. Jonson, Janine; Johnson, Janice; Johnson, James; Johnsen, Janet
  e. Johnsen, Janet; Johnson, James; Johnson, Janice; Jonson, Janine

_____ 9. To make the best use of a color filing system, you must
  a. Use only bright colors
  b. Use no more than four colors
  c. Always color code a file based on the age of the patient
  d. First identify the classifications that are important in your office
  e. Never combine a color-coding system with any other filing system

_____ 10. Using the terminal digit filing system, which sequence of numbers is correct?
  a. 234 526 318   234 522 318   324 522 316   234 522 613
  b. 234 522 318   324 522 316   234 522 613   234 526 318
  c. 324 522 316   234 522 613   234 526 318   234 522 318
  d. 234 522 613   234 526 318   234 522 318   324 522 316
  e. 324 522 316   234 522 318   234 526 318   234 522 613

_____ 11. Filing guidelines
  a. Help you file more efficiently
  b. Help you select a filing system
  c. Identify who is responsible for all filing
  d. Help you set up a tickler system
  e. Help you organize individual files, readying them for filing

_____ 12. When selecting a commercial records center to assist with patient records, it is important to
  a. Assess the monthly fee
  b. Assess the location
  c. Assess the system for retrieval and delivery of files
  d. All of the above
  e. None of the above

_____ 13. Who can take an original patient medical record out of the medical office?
  a. The office manager   d. No one
  b. The medical assistant   e. The patient
  c. The nurse

_____ 14. The proper order for the steps of filing is
  a. Sort, inspect, code, index, and store
  b. Store, inspect, index, code, and sort
  c. Inspect, index, code, sort, and store
  d. Index, inspect, code, sort, and store
  e. The order does not matter as long as they are all completed

_____ 15. Rotary circular files
  a. Take up a lot of room and should be used only in a spacious office
  b. Can only be operated manually
  c. Are a good option when space is limited
  d. Can only be operated electronically
  e. Can be stored stacked on top of one another

Sentence Completion

In the space provided, write the word or phrase that best completes each sentence.

16. Vertical files have a metal frame from which _____ are hung.

17. _____ can be skipped when filing patient records that have been previously filed.

18. To protect the confidentiality of patient records, always keep them in a(n) _____ area.

19. _____ are large accordion-style folders with tabs in which files can be stored temporarily.

20. When a record can be filed in two or more places, it should be _____.

21. If you need to keep some patient-related materials separate from the patient's medical record, you should create a(n) _____ file.

22. _____ is another term for naming a file.

23. When you put an identifying mark or phrase on a document to ensure that it is properly filed, you are _____ it.

24. Infrequently used files are filed as _____ records.

25. A(n) _____ specifies how long to keep different types of patient records in the office after files have become inactive or closed.

16. _____

17. _____

18. _____

19. _____

20. _____

21. _____

22. _____

23. _____

24. _____

25. _____

Short Answer

Write the answer to each question on the lines provided.

26. Why is it important to completely remove a file from the drawer in order to file correctly?

_____

_____

_____

27. What are two safety concerns when using filing equipment?

_____

_____

_____

28. What is the purpose of the tabs on file folders, and why are they positioned in different places on the folders?

_____

_____

_____

29. What is the purpose of the pockets on some out guides?

_____

_____

_____

30. Name the five steps in the filing process.

_____

_____

_____

_____

_____

31. List four formats in which inactive and closed files can be stored.

_____

_____

_____

32. Describe how supplemental files are different from primary medical records.

_____

_____

_____

33. Describe the "indexing" step in filing. What is included?

_____

_____

_____

34. Describe the steps to follow if a file is misplaced.

_____

_____

_____

Critical Thinking

Write the answer to each question on the lines provided.

1. Why is it important not to misplace patient files?

_____

_____

_____

2. What are some of the things that could possibly occur as a result of a medical file being lost?

_____

_____

_____

3. What filing system would you choose for a practice that has many patients who are celebrities? Explain.

_____

_____

_____

A P P L I C A T I O N

Follow the directions for each application.

1. **Creating a Patient Filing System**

   Work in groups of four students. Within your group, choose partners to work together.

   a. With your partner, prepare a list of 15 hypothetical patients—complete with full names, ages, and primary ailments. Exchange patient lists with the other pair of students in your group.

   b. With your partner, analyze the patient list you have been given. Determine what kind of filing system, alphabetic or numeric, is appropriate.

   c. Organize the patients' names as you would for the filing system you have chosen. If you have chosen the alphabetic system, write each name on a different index card and organize the cards. If you have chosen the numeric system, create a master list that shows the numbers and the corresponding patient names.

   d. Assume that your patient list is part of a much larger filing system that contains a similar mix of patients. Colorcode your filing system. With your partner, decide what categories of information you need to identify through color-coding. Then assign colors to your patient list as appropriate.

   e. After you have completed your filing system, meet with the other pair of students in your group and compare filing systems. How are they different? How are they alike? Each pair should evaluate the other pair's filing system for appropriateness and accuracy. Pairs should be able to justify their choices.

   f. Form different groups of four students. Exchange your original patient list with a different pair of students and repeat steps b through e.

Using the names listed as follows, take 20 index cards and write one patient's name on the front of each index card. On the back of the card, index the name properly. Once indexing has been completed, sort the cards in alphabetical order. Have a classmate check your work, critiquing both the indexing and the final filing results. You do the same for your classmate.

Alexis Nevach Wyman-Gagnon

Dylan Moyer

Brenda Lee Lane

Terri D. Ward, CMA (AAMA)

Bentley Rian Beals

Mari Lou Whalen

Dale Michael Wyman

Mrs. Charles (Bethanie) Lane-Lytle

Eliza Gagnon

Aaron Michael Wyman

Katelyn Moyer

Msg James W. Lane

Jazmyn Beals

Mrs. Eleanor M. Ward

Brendan M. Whalen

Kevin Mathew Wyman

Jennifer Lane

Lexus Beals

Christopher Keith Wyman

Matthew David Whalen

PROCEDURE 15-1 Creating a Filing System for Paper Medical Records

Goal
To create a filing system that keeps related materials together in a logical order and enables office staff to store and retrieve medical records efficiently.

OSHA Guidelines
This procedure does not involve exposure to blood, body fluids, or tissue.

Materials
Vertical or horizontal filing cabinets with locks, tabbed file folders, labels, file guides, out guides, filing sorters.

Method

Step Number	Procedure	Points Possible	Points Earned
1.	Evaluate which filing system is best for your office—alphabetic or numeric. Make sure the doctor approves the system you choose.*	12	
2.	Establish a style for labeling files, and make sure that all file labels are prepared in this manner.	12	
3.	Avoid writing labels by hand. Use a keyboard, label maker, or preprinted adhesive labels.	12	
4.	Set up a color-coding system to distinguish the files (for example, use blue for the letter A, red for B, yellow for C, and so on). Create a chart, suitable to be hung in a professional file room that uses the color-coding system	13	
5.	Use file guides to divide files into sections	12	
6.	Use out guides as placeholders to indicate which files have been taken out of the system. Include a charge-out form to be signed and dated by the person who is taking the file.	13	
7.	To keep files in order and to prevent them from being misplaced, use a file sorter to hold those patient records that will be returned to the files during the day or at the end of the day.	13	
8.	Develop a manual that explains the filing system to new staff members. Include guidelines on how to keep the system in good order.*	13	
Total Points		100	

CAAHEP Competencies Achieved

V. C (5)   Identify systems for organizing medical records

V. A (1)   Consider staff needs and limitations in establishment of a filing system

V. P (4)   File medical records

V. P (8)   Maintain organization by filing

V. C (7)   Discuss pros and cons of various filing methods

V. C (8)   Identify both equipment and supplies needed for filing medical records

ABHES Competencies Achieved

    8. (b) Prepare and maintain medical records

    8. (d) Apply concepts for office procedures

Name_____ Date_____

Evaluated by_____ Score_____

PROCEDURE 15-2 Setting Up an Office Tickler File

Goal
To create a comprehensive office tickler file designed for year-round use.

OSHA Guidelines
This procedure does not involve exposure to blood, body fluids, or tissue.

Materials
12 manila file folders or 3-ring binder with 12 separators, 12 file labels, pen or typewriter, paper.

Method

Step Number	Procedure	Points Possible	Points Earned
1.	Write or type 12 file labels, 1 for each month of the year. Abbreviations are acceptable. Do *not* include the current calendar year, just the month.	10	
2.	Affix one label to the tab of each file folder.	10	
3.	Arrange the folders so that the current month is on the top of the pile. Months should follow in chronological order.	10	
4.	Write or type a list of upcoming responsibilities and activities. Next to each activity, indicate the date by which the activity should be completed. Leave a column after this date to indicate when the activity has been completed. Use a separate sheet of paper for each month.	10	
5.	File the notes by month in the appropriate folders	10	
6.	Place the folders in order, with the current month on top, in a prominent place in the office, such as in a plastic box mounted on the wall near the receptionist's desk.	10	
7.	Check the tickler file at least once a week on a specific day, like every Monday. Assign a backup person to check it in case you happen to be out of the office.*	10	
8.	Complete the tickler activities on the designated days, if possible. Keep notes concerning activities in progress. Be sure to note when activities are completed and by whom.	10	
9.	At the end of the month, place that month's file folder at the bottom of the tickler file. If notes are remaining in that month's folder, move them to the current month's folder.	10	
10.	Continue to add new notes to the appropriate tickler files.	10	
Total Points		100	

CAAHEP Competencies Achieved

V. P (8)   Maintain organization by filing

ABHES Competencies Achieved

8. (d) Apply concepts for office procedures

PROCEDURE 15-3 Developing a Records Retention Program

Goal
To establish a records retention program for patient medical records that meets office needs, as well as legal and government guidelines.

OSHA Guidelines
This procedure does not involve exposure to blood, body fluids, or tissue.

Materials
Updated guide for record retention as described by federal and state law (go to the HIPAA Advisory website), file folders, index cards, index box, paper, pen or typewriter.

Method

Step Number	Procedure	Points Possible	Points Earned
1.	List the types of information contained in a typical patient medical record in your office. For example, a file for an adult patient may include the patient's case history, records of hospital stays, and insurance information.	5	
2.	Research the state and federal requirements for keeping documents. Contact your appropriate state office (such as the office of the insurance commissioner) for specific state requirements, like rules for keeping records of insurance payments and the statute of limitations for initiating lawsuits. If your office does business in more than one state, be sure to research all applicable regulations. Consult with the attorney who represents your practice.*	10	
3.	Compile your research results in a chart. At the top of the chart, list the different kinds of information your office keeps in patient records. Down the left side of the chart, list the headings "Federal," "State," and "Other." Then, in each box, record the corresponding information.	10	
4.	Compare all the legal and government requirements. Indicate which one is for the longest period of time.*	5	
5.	Meet with the physician (or office manager) to review the information. Working together, prepare a retention schedule. Determine how long different types of patient records should be kept in the office after a patient leaves the practice and how long records should be kept in storage. Although retention periods can vary based on the type of information kept in a file, it is often easiest to choose a retention period that covers all records. Determine how files will be destroyed when they have exceeded the retention requirements. Usually, records are destroyed by paper shredding. Purchase the appropriate equipment, or contract with a shredding company as necessary.	10	
6.	Put the retention schedule in writing, and post it prominently near the files. In addition, keep a copy of the schedule in a safe place in the office. Review it with the office staff.*	10	
7.	Develop a system for easily identifying files under the retention system. For example, for each file deemed inactive or closed, prepare an index card or create a master list containing the following information:	15	
	• Patient name and Social Security number	(2)	
	• Contents of the file	(2)	
	• Date the file was deemed inactive or closed and by whom	(2)	

(continued)

Step Number	Procedure	Points Possible	Points Earned
	• Date the file should be sent to inactive or closed file storage (the actual date will be filled in later; if more than one storage location is used, indicate the exact location to which the file was sent)	(2)	
	• Date the file should be destroyed (the actual date will be filled in later)	(2)	
	Have the card signed by the physician (or office manager) and by the person responsible for the files. Keep the card in an index box or another safe place. This is your authorization to destroy the file at the appropriate time.*	(5)	
8.	Use color-coding to help identify inactive and closed files. For example, all records that become inactive in 2013 could be placed in green file folders or have a green sticker with "13" placed on them and moved to a supplemental file. Then, in January 2015, all of these files could be pulled and sent to storage.	10	
9.	One person should be responsible for checking the index cards once a month to determine which stored files should be destroyed. Before retrieving these files from storage, circulate a notice to the office staff stating which records will be destroyed. Indicate that the staff must let you know by a specific date if any of the files should be saved. You may want to keep a separate file with these notices.	5	
10.	After the deadline has passed, retrieve the files from storage. Review each file before it is destroyed. Make sure the staff members who will destroy the files are trained to use the equipment properly. Develop a sheet of instructions for destroying files. Post it prominently with the retention schedule, near the machinery used to destroy the files.	10	
11.	Update the index card, giving the date the file was destroyed and by whom.	5	
12.	Periodically review the retention schedule. Update it with the most current legal and governmental requirements. With the staff, evaluate whether the current schedule is meeting the needs of your office or whether files are being kept too long or destroyed prematurely. With the physician's approval, change the schedule as necessary. *	5	
Total Points		100	

CAAHEP Competencies Achieved

V. C (10)   Discuss filing procedures

ABHES Competencies Achieved

8. (d) Apply concepts for office procedures

Schedule Management

Name_____ Class_____ Date_____

R E V I E W

Vocabulary Review

Matching

Match the key terms in the right column with the definitions in the left column by placing the letter of each correct answer in the space provided.

_____ 1. The scheduling of similar appointments together at a certain time of the day or week

_____ 2. A report of what happened and what was discussed and decided at a meeting

_____ 3. A system of scheduling in which patients arrive at the doctor's office at their convenience and are seen on a first-come, first-served basis

_____ 4. A patient who arrives without an appointment

_____ 5. A substitute physician hired to see patients while the regular physician is away from the office

_____ 6. A system of scheduling where patients arrive at regular, specified intervals, assuring the practice a steady stream of patients throughout the day

_____ 7. A system of scheduling in which two or more patients are booked for the same appointment slot, with the assumption that both patients will be seen by the physician within the scheduled period

_____ 8. Booking an appointment several weeks or even months in advance

_____ 9. A patient who does not call to cancel and does not come to an appointment

_____ 10. A system of scheduling in which the number of patients seen each hour is determined by dividing the hour by the length of the average visit and then giving that number of patients all appointments at the beginning of each hour

_____ 11. The basic format of an appointment book, established by blocking off times on the schedule during which the physician is able to see patients

_____ 12. Leaving large, unused gaps in the doctor's schedule, an approach that does not make the best use of the physician (or staff) time

_____ 13. Scheduling appointments for more patients than can reasonably be seen in the time allowed

_____ 14. A scheduling system similar to the wave system, with patients arriving at planned intervals during the hour, allowing time to catch up before the next hour begins

_____ 15. A detailed travel plan listing dates and times for specific transportation arrangements and events, the location of meetings and lodgings, and phone numbers

a. advance scheduling
b. cluster scheduling
c. double-booking system
d. itinerary
e. locum tenens
f. matrix
g. minutes
h. modified-wave scheduling
i. no-show
j. open-hours scheduling
k. overbooking
l. time-specified scheduling
m. underbooking
n. walk-in
o. wave scheduling

True or False

Decide whether each statement is true or false. In the space at the left, write T for true or F for false. On the lines provided, rewrite the false statements to make them true.

_____ 16. The appointment book is a legal record that should be kept for at least 3 years.

_____

_____ 17. Double-booking assumes that two patients will be seen at least 30 minutes apart.

_____

_____ 18. Cluster scheduling is used to schedule patients with similar appointment needs.

_____

_____ 19. Most minor medical problems, such as sore throats, earaches, or blood pressure (BP) follow-ups, usually require only 10–15 minutes.

_____

_____ 20. Medical offices are not allowed to schedule patients beyond 6 months.

_____

_____ 21. Emergency patients should always be referred to the local emergency room for treatment.

_____

_____ 22. Patients referred by another physician should be scheduled after all the regular patients since they are not regular patients and will probably never return.

_____

_____ 23. You should avoid scheduling a diabetic patient in the late morning before lunch.

_____

_____ 24. Patients who have a habit of arriving late for appointments should be scheduled toward the end of the day.

_____

_____ 25. The abbreviation used to designate a patient who is returning to see the physician for a chronic condition is "cons."

_____

Content Review

Multiple Choice

In the space provided, write the letter of the choice that best completes each statement or answers each question.

_____ 1. When a patient has never been seen at the medical office for an appointment, the following abbreviation should be placed next to the patient's name.
   a. US
   b. RS
   c. PT
   d. NS
   e. NP

_____ **2.** The typical appointment length for a complete physical examination is

    a. 10-15 minutes   **d.** 30-60 minutes

    b. 15-20 minutes   **e.** 60-90 minutes

    c. 20-30 minutes

_____ **3.** Which of the following statements is *false* with regard to the physical appointment book?

    a. The appointment book is considered a legal record

    b. Corrections should be made using an eraser or correction fluid

    c. All entries must be clear and easy to read

    d. The schedule should be written in blue or black ink

    e. The appointment book may be used as evidence in legal proceedings

_____ **4.** When a patient cannot come in for his original scheduled appointment, the abbreviation used next to the patient's name in that time slot is

    a. Sig

    b. Ref

    c. Can

    d. Cons

    e. Resch

_____ **5.** When patients are seen on a first-come, first-served basis, it is called

    a. Open-hours scheduling

    b. Wave scheduling

    c. Double booking

    d. Cluster scheduling

    e. Advance scheduling

_____ **6.** Which of the following represents wave scheduling?

    a. Patient A 10:00 a.m., Patient B 10:15 a.m.

    b. Patient A 10:00 a.m., Patient B 10:30 a.m.

    c. Patient A 10:00 a.m., Patient B 10:00 a.m.

    d. Patient A 10:00 a.m., Patient B 11:00 a.m.

    e. Patient A 10:00 a.m., Patient B 11:30 a.m.

_____ **7.** Time-specified scheduling is also referred to as

    a. Open-hours scheduling

    b. Physician preference scheduling

    c. Stream scheduling

    d. Cluster scheduling

    e. Advance scheduling

_____ **8.** Which of the following is an example of a new patient in the medical office?

    a. A patient who had a medication refilled 6 months ago

    b. A patient who comes into the office for an annual physical examination

    c. A child who needs a school sports physical

    d. A person who saw the physician 4 years ago for a physical

    e. A patient who changed insurance companies after the first of the year

_____ 9. When an office sends reminder cards to patients with their appointment time and date, prior to mailing these cards, they are stored in _____ by the office.
  a. A patient file
  b. A tickler file
  c. A reminder file
  d. A memory file
  e. None of the above

_____ 10. What is the best way to handle no-show patients?
  a. Do not schedule future appointments for these patients
  b. Ask the physician to abandon these patients
  c. Refuse to give these patients the appointment when they want it
  d. Call these patients before their appointments to remind them of the day and time of the appointment
  e. Have the patient's employer remind the employee of the appointment

_____ 11. A patient who needs to be fasting for blood work before seeing the physician should be scheduled
  a. At the beginning of the day
  b. During the noon hour
  c. After lunch
  d. Before the end of the day
  e. In the middle of the morning

_____ 12. Which of the following is appropriate for a patient that habitually arrives late for his/her appointments?
  a. The physician should send the patient a letter stating that if he/she arrives late for his appointments, then he/she will need to find another physician to care for him
  b. Tell the patient to come in 1 hour prior to his/her actual appointment
  c. Document each late arrival in the patient's chart
  d. Try booking the patient later in the day where his/her tardiness will cause less of a disruption
  e. c and d

_____ 13. To schedule an emergency appointment, the medical assistant should
  a. Determine if the patient can wait until the next day and give medical advice about what the patient should do until he/she can be seen
  b. Ask the nature of the emergency and ask how soon before the patient can arrive at the office
  c. Tell the patient that the physician does not have any time left in his/her schedule for the day so the patient should go to the emergency room
  d. Cancel all the patients for the remainder of the day to accommodate the emergency
  e. Determine if the person is a patient of the practice and if his/her insurance covers emergency care in the private office

_____ 14. What is the best way to handle a cancellation?
  a. Reschedule the appointment while the patient is still on the phone
  b. Call the patient the next day to see what time works best for a rescheduled appointment
  c. Contact the patient's family to confirm that the patient needed to cancel the appointment
  d. Notify the patient that the office policy allows for only two cancellations unless he/she can provide a note documenting the reason for the cancellation
  e. None of the above

_____ **15.** Scheduling outside appointments for patients includes the following events *except*
   a. Prescription refills
   b. Laboratory work
   c. X-rays
   d. Hospital stays
   e. Surgery

_____ **16.** A type of scheduling that does not make the best use of the physician's time is
   a. Wave scheduling
   b. Time-specific scheduling
   c. Underbooking
   d. Advance booking
   e. Modified scheduling

_____ **17.** The term *locum tenens* refers to
   a. A subpoena for the physician to go to court
   b. A multiple-physician practice
   c. The abandoning of a patient
   d. A substitute physician
   e. A lawsuit for negligence

_____ **18.** When the medical assistant is planning a meeting for the physician, it is important to know
   a. When the meeting will be held
   b. How many will be attending the meeting
   c. How long the meeting will last
   d. The purpose of the meeting
   e. All of the above

_____ **19.** The double-booking system of scheduling means
   a. One patient will be scheduled every 15 minutes
   b. A patient will be scheduled for two follow-up appointments
   c. The physician can see two patients at the same time
   d. Two or more patients are scheduled for the same appointment slot
   e. None of the above

_____ **20.** A patient booked 2 months prior to an annual gynecological examination is a good example of the use of
   a. Wave scheduling
   b. Open-hours scheduling
   c. Advance scheduling
   d. Time-specified scheduling
   e. Open-ended scheduling

_____ **21.** When scheduling a new patient, it is important to
   a. Obtain the patient's home address and daytime telephone number
   b. Ask the patient about insurance coverage
   c. Ask the patient the reason for the appointment
   d. Ask the patient to arrive 15 minutes ahead of the appointment time
   e. Do all of the above

_____ **22.** When making a return appointment, it is best to
   a. Make the appointment while the patient is still in the office
   b. Have the patient go home and check his/her schedule to ensure there are no conflicts before setting the appointment time
   c. Have the patient call back at the end of the week after he/she has checked his agenda
   d. Call the patient in a day or two to set the return appointment
   e. Ask the physician if the patient can wait until he/she is feeling better

_____ **23.** When scheduling patients for multiple return visits it is best to
  a. Schedule the patient every other day, alternating morning and afternoon time slots
  b. Schedule the patient for the same time and day each week in order to keep a routine
  c. Ask the patient to come in at least once a week when he/she is available
  d. Have the patient call each Monday to set a new appointment for the week
  e. Schedule the patient only if he/she calls and needs to see the physician

_____ **24.** If a patient comes in unexpectedly with an emergency condition, it is vital that
  a. The nearest hospital be notified immediately
  b. The patient be treated as quickly as the schedule will allow
  c. A physician see that patient ahead of patients who may already be waiting
  d. Patients who have appointments at that time be given the chance to reschedule
  e. The patient wait his/her turn

_____ **25.** Most minor medical problems, such as a sore throat, earache, or blood sugar check, usually require an appointment time of
  a. 5 minutes   **d.** 20 to 30 minutes
  b. 10 to 15 minutes   **e.** 30 to 45 minutes
  c. 15 to 20 minutes

Sentence Completion

In the space provided, write the word or phrase that best completes each sentence.

26. The abbreviation NP stands for _____.   **26.** _____

27. To save time when entering information in the appointment book, you could use the standard abbreviation CPE to stand for _____.   **27.** _____

                                                              28. _____

28. _____ scheduling systems can be programmed to lock out selected appointment slots, which can be saved for emergencies.   **29.** _____

                                                              30. _____

29. It is important to document a patient who is a no-show in the appointment book and in the _____.   **31.** _____

                                                              32. _____

30. To see a referral on relatively short notice is a matter of _____ to the referring physician.   **33.** _____

                                                              34. _____

31. The open-hours scheduling system is still used by _____ practices, _____ departments, and _____ care centers.   **35.** _____

32. Online scheduling is relatively new. The patients schedule themselves via the _____ and _____.

33. When a pharmaceutical representative who is unknown to you comes into the office, ask for a _____ and check with the physician before scheduling an appointment.

34. Wave scheduling works effectively in larger medical facilities that have enough _____ and _____ to provide services to _____ patients at the same time.

35. To reduce the chance of error when using an appointment card, enter the appointment in the _____ first, then fill out the card.

Short Answer

Write the answer to each question on the lines provided.

36. Why is it important not to throw away an old appointment book?

_____

_____

_____

37. How can having a list of standard procedures and the time required for each procedure help you be an efficient scheduler?

_____

_____

_____

38. What three pieces of information must you obtain to properly schedule a patient appointment?

_____

_____

_____

39. Give three examples of special scheduling situations that would require you to adjust the patient needs.

_____

_____

_____

40. Which takes more time and why: an established patient visit or a new patient visit?

_____

_____

_____

41. Why is it beneficial to involve the patient in scheduling his/her outside appointments?

_____

_____

_____

42. Why is it important to document a no-show in the appointment book or scheduler as well as in the patient medical record?

_____

_____

_____

A P P L I C A T I O N

Follow the directions for each application.

1. **Setting Up an Appointment Matrix**

   Using the information and figures found in Chapter 16 of the textbook, set up an appointment matrix using the scenarios given.

   a. Tuesday November 12: Office Hours from 9 a.m. to 6 p.m.
   Lunch from 12:30–1:00
   Physician hospital rounds from 11:30–1:00

   b. Wednesday November 13: Office hours from 8 a.m.–4:30 p.m.
   Lunch 12:30–1:00
   School physicals from 2 p.m.–4 p.m.

2. **Scheduling Patient Appointments**

   Book the following appointments in the order given using the appointment matrix you just created. Use Table 16-2 in the textbook as a guide for the time needed for each appointment, if time is not given.

   a. Ken Washington 30 minute F/U with ECG on Tuesday after 3 p.m.

   b. Syliva Gonzales CDE on Wednesday early a.m. (fasting for labs)

   c. Shenya Jones F/U appointment facial swelling, resolving Tuesday 12–1 p.m.

   d. Valarie Ramirez 30 minutes 2–3 p.m. either day

   e. John Miller BP check and weight check only both days between 9–10 a.m.

   f. Mohammad Nassar school physical either day at 2:30 (30 min)

   g. Raja Latau pap and pelvic 3 p.m. or later either day

   h. Cindy Chen F/U appt and CBC 1–2 p.m.

   i. Peter Smith ED calls Wednesday at 8:30 a.m. Cut hand washing dishes, thinks sutures are needed. Can be there in 20 minutes.

   j. Nancy Evans's husband calls at 3:30 Wednesday. She is having N/V ×2 days. He wants to bring her right in.

APPOINTMENT RECORD

Dr. Whalen		DOCTOR	Dr. Whalen	
		AM		
		8:00		
		8:15		
		8:30		
		8:45		
		9:00		
		9:15		
		9:30		
		9:45		
		10:00		
		10:15		
		10:30		
		10:45		
		11:00		
		11:15		
		11:30		
		11:45		
		12.00		
		12:15		
		12:30		
		12:45		
		PM		
		1:00		
		1:15		
		1:30		
		1:45		
		2:00		
		2:15		
		2:30		
		2:45		
		3:00		
		3:15		
		3:30		
		3:45		
		4:00		
		4:15		
		4:30		
		4:45		
		5:00		
		5:15		
		5:30		
		5:45		

REMARKS & NOTES _____

12 November Tuesday

13 November Wednesday

3. Developing a Travel Itinerary

Dr. Williams in your practice is attending the American Medical Association's annual conference, to be held at the Hyatt Regency Hotel in Chicago. Develop a travel itinerary, using the sample itinerary found in Figure 16-10 in the textbook as a guide. You will give a copy to Dr. Williams and also keep a copy in the office for reference.

a. Determine the dates of the conference and the dates of the physician's departure and return. Choose the airline that the physician will fly and note the flight times.

b. Record the itinerary in chronological order. Include telephone numbers and addresses of each location where the physician can be reached as well as the dates and times that the physician can be reached there.

c. Evaluate your itinerary. Are you able to contact the physician at every point during the trip? If not, is there additional information you can list on the itinerary?

d. Examine itineraries developed by your classmates. Is there something they included in their itineraries that you can add to yours?

e. With your classmates, discuss the value of having an itinerary.

CASE STUDIES

Write your response to each case study on the lines provided.

Case 1

The office has just opened for the day, and, on reviewing the appointments for the day, you see the schedule is completely full. There are two new referral patients and four follow-up post-op exams. Also, a patient just called with severe abdominal pain and was directed to come to the office immediately to be seen as soon as the physician arrives. The doctor just called, stating that he has a family emergency and will not be in the office until after lunch.

a. How should the scheduled appointments be handled?

_____

_____

_____

b. What will you do about the patient with abdominal pain?

_____

_____

_____

Case 2

A patient who has been under the physician's care for over 10 years has developed a chronic condition over the past year requiring monthly appointments to regulate medications. In the past 6 months, he has missed four appointments and has been late for the other two. You have a good rapport with the patient, and the physician has asked you to speak with him. How will you handle this situation?

_____

_____

_____

Case 3

You are new to this office. As part of your orientation, you are observing the office scheduling assistant. Today, you notice she appears to be telling patients that she cannot book them today but she can book them for tomorrow or later in the week. When you look at the schedule, there appear to be several openings at the end of the day. When you ask the scheduler why she is not using these appointments, she explains that she has plans for the evening and she does not want to be working late. "Besides," she says, "none of these calls have been emergencies, so it is fine to schedule them on another day."

a. Is this attitude a problem?

_____

_____

_____

b. How will you handle this situation, particularly as a new employee?

_____

_____

_____

PROCEDURE 16-1 Creating an Appointment Matrix   WORK//DOC

Goal
To create an appointment matrix to indicate the days and the hours the physician is not scheduling patients.

OSHA Guidelines
This procedure does not involve exposure to blood, body fluids, or tissue.

Materials
Appointment book; pencil or pen; physician schedule of meetings, conferences, vacations, staff meetings, and other times of unavailability when patients are not seen.

Method

Step Number	Procedure	Possible Points	Points Earned
1.	Using the physician schedule of availability as the base for the matrix, confer with the physician or office manager to ensure that no additional schedule changes are planned.	35	
2.	Indicate within each area the reason why the time is being closed to appointments, such as lunch, hospital rounds, AAMA meeting, etc.*	35	
3.	If the office utilizes cluster scheduling for certain appointments such as physical exams, blood sugar testing, etc., these time frames must also be set apart. Following office policy, such as using brackets, note the appropriate appointment type to be scheduled during this time frame.	30	
Total Points		100	

CAAHEP Competencies Achieved
V. C (2)   Describe scheduling guidelines

V. P (1)   Manage appointment schedule, using established priorities

ABHES Competencies Achieved
8. (dd) Serve as liaison between physician and others

Name_____ Date_____

Evaluated by_____ Score_____

PROCEDURE 16-2 Creating an Appointment Matrix for an Electronic Scheduling System

Goal
Using an electronic scheduling system, indicate the days and times when the office is not scheduling patients.

OSHA Guidelines
This procedure does not involve exposure to blood, body fluids, or tissue.

Materials
Appointment book; pencil or pen; physician schedule of meetings, conferences, vacations, staff meetings, and other times of unavailability when patients are not seen.

Method

Step Number	Procedure	Possible Points	Points Earned
1.	Using the physician schedule of availability as the base for the matrix, confer with the physician or office manager to ensure that no additional schedule changes are planned.	14	
2.	Open the office appointment scheduler per the program format.	14	
3.	Block the dates and times when the general office or physician will not be available for patient appointments, using the physician and office schedules as guides.*	14	
4.	Choose the appropriate option if the time frame is repeatedly unavailable.	14	
5.	Enter a reason that the time is not available for future reference. The office program may use color coding to assist with this process.*	14	
6.	If cluster scheduling is used for the office, most schedulers allow you to specify what types of appointments may be entered; again, color coding may be used by the scheduler to outline specific types of appointments.	14	
7.	Many programs will allow you to specify time frames necessary for different types of appointments, and these may be set up now also. For instance, physical exams for new patients may require 45 minutes, and visits for BP typical sick visits are set up for 15 minutes. If the program allows, set up these matrixes now also.	16	
Total Points		100	

CAAHEP Competencies Achieved

V. C (2)   Describe scheduling guidelines

V. P (1)   Manage appointment schedule, using established priorities

V. P (6)   Use office hardware and software to maintain office systems

ABHES Competencies Achieved

8. (dd) Serve as liaison between physician and others

8. (ll) Apply electronic technology

PROCEDURE 16-3 Scheduling Appointments

WORK//DOC

Goal
Utilizing the previously created matrix, book patient appointments applying the correct amount of time for each appointment.

OSHA Guidelines
This procedure does not involve exposure to blood, body fluids, or tissue.

Materials
Appointment book and pen or pencil, or electronic scheduler (with appropriate matrix), template outlining time frames for patient appointment types.

Method

Step Number	Procedure	Possible Points	Points Earned
1.	Establish the type of appointment required by the patient, particularly if this is a new patient or a returning patient.*	17	
2.	If necessary, consult the template for the amount of time required for the patient appointment. Keep in mind the reason for the appointment when scheduling (i.e., is the patient required to be fasting).	15	
3.	When possible, schedule appointments earlier in the day first and then move to later time frames. Do ask the patient if he/she has a preferred time frame in mind and, if at all possible, accommodate the request.	17	
4.	When using an appointment book, enter the patient name, phone number, and reason for the appointment in the appropriate space, blocking out additional blocks of time if necessary to accommodate a longer appointment time.*	17	
5.	If an electronic scheduler is used, use the search option to find the next available appointment for the time frame required for the appointment. Enter the patient name, phone number, and reason for the appointment.	17	
6.	Repeat the appointment information to the patient, giving any necessary instructions regarding preparation for the appointment, such as early arrival for blood tests, completion of paperwork, etc. Also, this is a good time to remind patients about any copayments that will be due at the time of the appointment.	17	
Total Points		100	

CAAHEP Competencies Achieved

V. P (1)   Manage appointment schedule, using established priorities

V. P (6)   Use office hardware and software to maintain office systems

ABHES Competencies Achieved

8. (c) Schedule and manage appointments

8. (dd) Serve as liaison between physician and others

8. (ll) Apply electronic technology

PROCEDURE 16-4 Completing the Patient Appointment Card

WORK // DOC

Goal
To accurately complete a patient appointment card for the patient's next visit.

OSHA Guidelines
This procedure does not involve exposure to blood, body fluids, or tissue.

Materials
Appointment book or electronic scheduler, pen, and appointment card

Method

Step Number	Procedure	Possible Points	Points Earned
1.	After entering the patient's appointment in the appointment book or electronic scheduler, repeat the appointment date and time to the patient to verify accuracy.	35	
2.	Complete the patient appointment card, entering the appointment date and time on the card. If the practice has multiple providers, there may also be a place for the appropriate physician name to be entered, and you should do so.*	35	
3.	Repeat appointment information to patient one more time when giving the card to him/her, again verifying the information.	30	
Total Points		100	

CAAHEP Competencies Achieved

V. P (1)   Manage appointment schedule, using established priorities

ABHES Competencies Achieved

8. (c) Schedule and manage appointments

8. (dd) Serve as liaison between physician and others

Name_____ Date_____

Evaluated by_____ Score_____

PROCEDURE 16-5 Placing Appointment Confirmation Calls

Goal

To decrease the number of "no-show" patients by making appointment confirmation calls 24–48 hours prior to the scheduled appointment.

OSHA Guidelines

This procedure does not involve exposure to blood, body fluids, or tissue.

Materials

Office appointment book, electronic scheduler, or listing of patients scheduled to be seen tomorrow or the next day with their home phone numbers.

Method

Step Number	Procedure	Possible Points	Points Earned
1.	Starting with the first appointment of the day, call the patient listed.	14	
2.	If the phone is answered, ask for the patient. If you reach the patient, give your name and the name of the practice and state that you are confirming the patient's appointment for the applicable date and time.*	14	
3.	Remind the patient of any special instructions regarding the appointment, such as fasting, bringing in medical record or registration information, and copayments due.*	16	
4.	If the patient is not available, leave your name and phone number, asking that the patient return your call.	14	
5.	If a voice mail or answering machine system is reached, follow the practice confidentiality rules of leaving only your name and phone number, asking the patient to call you back, unless you have permission from the patient to leave more explicit information on voice mail.*	14	
6.	Thank the patient for his/her time, stating you will see them at the stated date and time.	14	
7.	Allow the patient to hang up first, so if there are questions, you may answer them.	14	
Total Points		100	

CAAHEP Competencies Achieved

V. P (1)   Manage appointment schedule, using established priorities

ABHES Competencies Achieved

8. (c) Schedule and manage appointments

8. (dd) Serve as liaison between physician and others

8. (ee) Use proper telephone techniques

PROCEDURE 16-6 Scheduling Outpatient Surgical Appointments

WORK//DOC

Goal
To schedule an outpatient surgical procedure.

OSHA Guidelines
This procedure does not involve exposure to blood, body fluids, or tissue.

Materials
Patient medical record, scheduling form, calendar, telephone, pen.

Method

Step Number	Procedure	Possible Points	Points Earned
1.	Obtain detailed information regarding the procedure to be performed from the physician and patient medical record. Information should include the name of procedure to be performed, the amount of the time the outpatient surgical suite will be needed, and the reason (diagnosis) for the procedure.*	10	
2.	From the patient's medical record, you will need the patient's full name, DOB, allergies, current medications, address, phone number, and insurance information.	10	
3.	Place a call to the appropriate surgery center or outpatient surgical unit at the requested facility. Have the name of the surgeon, assistant, or PA (if they will be used) available, as well as the patient's and physician's preferred dates for the procedure.	10	
4.	When the appointment scheduler answers the phone, identify yourself, the practice, and the procedure you need to schedule, as well as the preferred dates.	10	
5.	When a date for the procedure is agreed upon by the patient, give the scheduler the patient's name, address, phone number, DOB, gender, and insurance information, including the prior authorization number if needed. Also give the patient's diagnosis as required for medical necessity.*	10	
6.	Inquire as to any pre-procedure testing that may need to be done as well as any patient preparation required prior to the procedure, including patient arrival time.*	10	
7.	Confirm the appointment date and time prior to hanging up. If necessary, book any pre-procedure testing for the patient and document these appointments in the patient instructions and appropriate office form(s) such as the surgical check-off sheet and/or within the patient's medical record.*	10	
8.	Provide the patient with written instructions from the physician as well as all information obtained while booking the appointment. The patient should also be informed that he should arrange for someone to drive him to and from this appointment.	10	
9.	Go over the written dates and instructions with the patient, asking the patient if there are any questions, answering them if possible, and, if not, asking a clinical member of the team to do so.	10	
10.	Give a copy of instructions and information to the patient and keep a copy in the patient record. Remind the patient to feel free to call the office at any time with any questions or concerns.	10	
Total Points		100	

CAAHEP Competencies Achieved

V. P (1)   Manage appointment schedule, using established priorities

V. P (2)   Schedule patient admissions and/or procedures

ABHES Competencies Achieved

8. (c) Schedule and manage appointments

8. (f) Schedule inpatient and outpatient admissions

8. (dd) Serve as liaison between physician and others

PROCEDURE 16-7 Scheduling Inpatient Surgical Appointments

WORK // DOC

Goal
To schedule an inpatient surgical procedure.

OSHA Guidelines
This procedure does not involve exposure to blood, body fluids, or tissue.

Materials
Patient medical record, scheduling form, calendar, telephone, pen.

Method

Step Number	Procedure	Possible Points	Points Earned
1.	Obtain detailed information regarding the procedure to be performed from the physician and patient medical record. Information should include the name of procedure to be performed, the amount of the time the outpatient surgical suite will be needed, and the reason (diagnosis) for the procedure.*	10	
2.	From the patient's medical record, you will need the patient's full name, DOB, allergies, current medications, address, phone number, and insurance information.	10	
3.	Place a call to the appropriate surgical unit at the requested hospital. Have the name of the surgeon, assistant, or PA (if they will be used) available, as well as the patient's and physician's preferred dates for the procedure.	10	
4.	When the appointment scheduler answers the phone, identify yourself, the practice, and the procedure you need to schedule, as well as the preferred date.	10	
5.	When a date for the procedure is agreed upon by the patient, give the scheduler the patient's name, address, phone number, DOB, gender, and insurance information, including the prior authorization number if needed. Also give the patient's diagnosis as required for medical necessity.*	10	
6.	Inquire as to any pre-procedure testing that may need to be done as well as any patient preparation required prior to the procedure, including patient arrival time.*	10	
7.	Confirm the appointment date and time prior to hanging up. If necessary, book any pre-procedure testing for the patient and document these appointments in the patient instructions and appropriate office form(s) such as the surgical check-off sheet and/or within the patient's medical record.*	10	
8.	Provide the patient with written instructions from the physician as well as all information obtained while booking the appointment. The patient should also be informed that he should arrange for someone to drive him to and from the hospital.	10	
9.	Go over the written dates and instructions with the patient, asking the patient if there are any questions, answering them if possible, and, if not, asking a clinical member of the team to do so.	10	
10.	Give a copy of instructions and information to the patient and keep a copy in the patient record. Remind the patient to feel free to call the office at any time with any questions or concerns.	10	
Total Points		100	

CAAHEP Competencies Achieved

V. P (1)   Manage appointment schedule, using established priorities

V. P (2)   Schedule patient admissions and/or procedures

ABHES Competencies Achieved

8. (c) Schedule and manage appointments

8. (f) Schedule inpatient and outpatient admissions

8. (dd) Serve as liaison between physician and others

17

Insurance and Billing

Name_____ Class_____ Date_____

REVIEW

Vocabulary Review

Matching

Match the key terms in the right column with the definitions in the left column by placing the letter or each correct answer in the space provided.

_____ 1. The rule stating that the primary insurance plan for all dependents will be that of the policyholder whose birthday comes first in the year

_____ 2. Document explaining the total amount of the claim, the amount allowed and disallowed, subscriber liability, the amount paid, and any notations regarding noncovered services

_____ 3. The legal clause limiting the total payments from all insurance carriers to 100% of the covered charges

_____ 4. The traditional health plan that reimburses policyholders for the costs of healthcare

_____ 5. Billing the patient for the difference between the usual fee charged and the lower allowed charge of the insurance plan

_____ 6. The company that takes nonstandard medical billing software formats and translates them into the standard EDI format

_____ 7. The process by which the provider contacts the insurance carrier to see if the proposed procedure is covered by a specific patient's insurance policy

_____ 8. A procedure or treatment not covered by the patient's insurance policy

_____ 9. Monthly payment received by the physician for each patient covered by an HMO, regardless of how many times a patient is seen in that month

_____ 10. The payment system used by Medicare to calculate acceptable fees

_____ 11. The highest amount a payer will pay any provider for a service or procedure

_____ 12. Another name for the authorization from a physician allowing a patient to seek treatment from another practice (for insurance purposes)

_____ 13. The electronic claim transaction that is the equivalent of the HIPAA paper claim

_____ 14. A listing of the common services and procedures for the practice, including the charge for each

_____ 15. The congressional agency overseeing Medicare and Medicaid

a. allowed charge
b. balance billing
c. benefits
d. birthday rule
e. capitation
f. CMS
g. clearinghouse
h. coinsurance
i. coordination of benefits
j. deductible
k. exclusion
l. EOB/EOP
m. fee-for-service
n. fee schedule
o. participating physician
p. preauthorization
q. premium
r. referral
s. RA
t. RBRVS
u. third party payer
v. X12 837 Healthcare Claim

_____ 16. The other name for insurance payment for medical service

_____ 17. The fixed percentage of covered charges paid by the patient, after the insurer covers its share.

_____ 18. The base or yearly cost for healthcare insurance

_____ 19. The yearly dollar amount that must be paid by the insured before any claims are considered by the insurance carrier

_____ 20. The other abbreviation for EOB or EOP

_____ 21. Physicians who enroll with a managed care plan and abide by their rules and regulations

_____ 22. Insurance plan that accepts the risk of covering the cost of medical services provided to a patient

Sentence Completion

In the space provided, complete the following sentences using the insurance plans discussed in this chapter.

23. _____ is the national health insurance program for Americans aged 65 and older.

24. _____ is the insurance program covering expenses of dependents of veterans with total, permanent, service-related disabilities and also those of dependents of veterans who died in the line of duty due to their service-connected disabilities.

25. Private insurance plans that can be purchased to supplement Medicare to decrease the patient out-of-pocket expense are known as _____ plans.

26. A managed care organization that establishes a network of providers who care for their patients is called a(n) _____.

27. _____ is the program that provides healthcare benefits for dependents of active duty and retired military personnel.

28. PPOs, HMOs, fee-for-service plans, and MSAs are all choices for Medicare beneficiaries in a program known as _____.

29. A(n) _____ is a managed care organization that provides specific services to their members, and the physicians enrolled in the program agree to provide these services in exchange for a capitation payment and/or negotiated fee-for-service rate.

30. _____ is the federally funded, state-run healthcare assistance program for low-income patients, the disabled, and families receiving aid for dependent children.

23. _____

24. _____

25. _____

26. _____

27. _____

28. _____

29. _____

30. _____

Content Review

Multiple Choice

In the space provided, write the letter of the choice that best completes each statement or answers each question.

_____ 1. Which of the following is a Medicare plan that charges a monthly premium and a small copayment for each office visit but no deductible?

    a. Medicare managed care plan

    b. Medicare preferred provider organization plan

    c. Medicare private fee-for-service plan

    d. Original Medicare plan

    e. Medigap plan

_____ 2. At the time of service, if required by the managed care plan, medical assistants collect

    a. Deductibles

    b. Copayments

    c. Premiums

    d. Coinsurance

    e. All of the above

_____ 3. The nationally uniform relative value of a procedure is based on which of the following 3 things?

    a. The physician's specialty, the cost of living, and insurance rates

    b. The age of the patient, the diagnosis of the patient, and the geographic area of the practice

    c. The amount billed by the physician, the cost of the procedure, and the copayment of the patient

    d. The physician's work, the practice's overhead, and the cost of malpractice insurance

    e. The fee schedule of the physician, the geographic area of the practice, and the diagnosis of the patient

_____ 4. Under the concept of the resource-based relative value scale (RBRVS) used by Medicare, the fee for a procedure is based on

    a. A formula based on using the relative value unit, the geographic adjustment factor, and a conversion factor

    b. The generally accepted fee that a physician charges for difficult or complicated services

    c. The average fee that a physician charges for a service or procedure

    d. The 90th percentile of fees charged for a procedure by similar physicians in the same area

    e. A formula based on the relative value usage, the geographic adjustment factor, and a conversion factor

_____ 5. Billing a patient for the difference between a higher usual fee and a lower allowed charge is called _____ and is not allowed by participating physicians.

    a. Capitation

    b. Assignment of benefits

    c. Coordination of benefits

    d. Third-party paying

    e. Balance billing

_____ 6. Under Medicare Part B, patients are required to pay an annual
   a. Deductible
   b. Copayment
   c. Coinsurance
   d. Claim submission charge for reimbursement
   e. Annual premium

_____ 7. Medicare Part A does not pay for
   a. Inpatient expenses up to 90 days for each benefit period
   b. Medical care at home
   c. Outpatient medical services
   d. Psychiatric hospitalization
   e. Respite care

_____ 8. Patients enrolled in the Original Medicare Plan may purchase additional coverage under a
   a. Medicare Part A plan
   b. Coinsurance plan
   c. Medigap plan
   d. Medicare Advantage plan
   e. Fee-for-service

_____ 9. TRICARE has three choices of healthcare benefits, including
   a. Prime, Extra, Basic
   b. Prime, Extra, Standard
   c. Extra, Basic, Civilian
   d. Standard, Basic, Prime
   e. Basic, Standard, Civilian

_____ 10. The primary purpose of the coordination of benefits is to
   a. Ensure that the insured person's medical bills are paid in full
   b. Allow physicians to charge differently based on the patient's insurance
   c. Determine the patient's eligibility for medical services
   d. Prevent duplication of payment
   e. Require insurance companies to pay the bill in full

_____ 11. The explanation of benefits or explanation of payment received from the insurance company is often referred to or called the
   a. Disclosure statement
   b. Remittance advice
   c. Formulary
   d. Coordination of benefits
   e. Receivable statement

_____ 12. The major types of health plans are
   a. Fee-for-service and workers' compensation
   b. Workers' compensation and managed care
   c. Managed care and fee-for-service
   d. Disability and private plan
   e. a and c

_____ 13. Which of the following statements accurately relates to Medicare benefits?
  a. The Medicare part of a hospital plan begins after the patient has been in the hospital 3 days
  b. To be eligible for Medicare Part A the beneficiary is required to be at least 65 years old and no longer employed
  c. Once a person is enrolled in Medicare Part A, she is automatically enrolled in Part B
  d. Medicare Part A covers only 190 days of psychiatric care
  e. The original Medicare plan requires the beneficiary to pay 50% of disallowed charges

_____ 14. Which of the following is true of workers' compensation insurance?
  a. Medical costs arising from an auto accident while on the way to work are covered under worker's compensation
  b. Death benefits are allowed if the death occurred in a work-related setting
  c. Rehabilitation costs are covered if required because of a work-related injury
  d. Payment is made to a patient for a temporary disability due to a work-related illness
  e. b and d

_____ 15. Which of the following is *true* concerning disability insurance?
  a. Disability insurance may be offered by the employer at the employee's expense
  b. Disability insurance is not health insurance
  c. Disability insurance does not cover medical expenses
  d. Disability insurance can be either short-term or long-term
  e. All of the above

True or False

Decide whether each statement is true or false. In the space to the left, write T for true or F for false. On the lines provided, rewrite the false statements to make them true.

_____ 16. CHAMPVA covers the expenses of the dependents of veterans with total, permanent, service-connected disabilities.

_____

_____ 17. TRICARE is a Medicaid program.

_____

_____ 18. A managed care organization (MCO) sets up agreements with physicians as well as with enrolled members.

_____

_____ 19. Copayments are made to insurance companies.

_____

_____ 20. The RBRVS system is the basis for the Medicare payment system.

_____

_____ 21. Preferred provider organizations (PPOs) never allow members to receive care from physicians outside the network.

_____

_____ 22. Exclusions are expenses covered by an insurance company.

_____

_____ **23.** A deductible is a fixed-dollar amount that must be met in full on the first visit each year to a physician.

_____ **24.** The 1500 professional claim form is often referred to as the 1505 because of its 2005 revision date.

_____ **25.** Under a MCO contract, most specialists are compensated for caring for patients under a capitation plan.

Short Answer

Write the answer to each question on the lines provided.

26. List the three major methods used to transmit claims electronically.

_____

_____

_____

27. Explain the purpose of the coordination of benefits clause in insurance policies.

_____

_____

_____

28. What does an eligible person need to do in order to receive Medicare Part B benefits?

_____

_____

_____

29. Explain the purpose of the alpha suffix attached to the Medicare ID number.

_____

_____

_____

30. List the five sections of data elements on the X12 837 Health Care Claim.

_____

_____

_____

_____

A P P L I C A T I O N

WORK // DOC

Follow the directions for each application.

1. Using the figure that follows, answer the questions on the next page about the CMS 1500 claim form.

A completed CMS 1500 Health Insurance Claim Form showing the following details:

1500 HEALTH INSURANCE CLAIM FORM
APPROVED BY NATIONAL UNIFORM CLAIM COMMITTEE 08/05

- 1. MEDICARE: X (Medicare #)
- 1a. INSURED'S I.D. NUMBER: 000 11 2345 A
- 2. PATIENT'S NAME: WARD ELEANOR M
- 3. PATIENT'S BIRTH DATE: 02 02 1929, SEX: F X
- 5. PATIENT'S ADDRESS: 305 MAIN STREET
- CITY: FUNTON, STATE: XY
- ZIP CODE: 12345-6789, TELEPHONE: (521) 628 3270
- 8. PATIENT STATUS: Other X
- 9. OTHER INSURED'S NAME: WARD ELEANOR M
- a. OTHER INSURED'S POLICY OR GROUP NUMBER: 625743289
- b. OTHER INSURED'S DATE OF BIRTH: 02 02 1929, SEX: F X
- d. INSURANCE PLAN NAME OR PROGRAM NAME: MEDEX
- 10. IS PATIENT'S CONDITION RELATED TO: a. EMPLOYMENT? NO X; b. AUTO ACCIDENT? NO X; c. OTHER ACCIDENT? NO X
- 11. INSURED'S POLICY GROUP OR FECA NUMBER: NONE
- d. IS THERE ANOTHER HEALTH BENEFIT PLAN? YES X
- 12. PATIENT'S OR AUTHORIZED PERSON'S SIGNATURE: SIGNATURE ON FILE
- 13. INSURED'S OR AUTHORIZED PERSON'S SIGNATURE: SIGNATURE ON FILE
- 17. NAME OF REFERRING PROVIDER OR OTHER SOURCE: WHALEN MARI LOU; 17a. ZZ 201400000X; 17b. NPI 423 543 6543
- 20. OUTSIDE LAB? NO X
- 21. DIAGNOSIS OR NATURE OF ILLNESS OR INJURY: 1. 482 . 9; 2. 496

24. A. DATE(S) OF SERVICE From MM DD YY	To MM DD YY	B. PLACE OF SERVICE	C. EMG	D. PROCEDURES, SERVICES, OR SUPPLIES CPT/HCPCS	MODIFIER	E. DIAGNOSIS POINTER	F. $ CHARGES	G. DAYS OR UNITS	H. EPSDT Family Plan	I. ID. QUAL.	J. RENDERING PROVIDER ID. #
1	05 10 20xx	05 10 20xx	11		99213	25	1	80 00	1		NPI	9876543210
2	05 10 20xx	05 10 20xx	11		71020		1	120 00	1		NPI	9876543210
3	05 10 20xx	05 10 20xx	11		82805		2	65 00	1		NPI	9876543210
4	05 10 20xx	05 10 20xx	11		85025		1	40 00	1		NPI	9876543210
5											NPI	
6											NPI	

- 25. FEDERAL TAX I.D. NUMBER: 222518600, EIN X
- 27. ACCEPT ASSIGNMENT? YES X
- 28. TOTAL CHARGE: $ 305 00
- 31. SIGNATURE OF PHYSICIAN OR SUPPLIER: Alexis N. Whalen, MD; DATE 15/12/xx
- 33. BILLING PROVIDER INFO & PH #: 555-654-3210; BWW Medical Associates, 305 Main Street, Port Snead YZ 12345-6789; a. 1002003001

NUCC Instruction Manual available at: www.nucc.org

APPROVED OMB-0938-0999 FORM CMS-1500 (08/05)

Source: From Helen Houser and Terri Wyman, ADMINISTRATIVE MEDICAL ASSISTING: A WORKFORCE READINESS APPROACH, 1/e. © 2012 McGraw Hill Companies, Inc. Reprinted with permission.

    a. What insurance does the patient have? What is the policy number?

    b. Which block contains the patient's diagnosis codes?

    c. Which block demonstrates medical necessity for the procedures performed?

    d. What is the NPI for BWW Medical Associates, PC?

    e. Which physician treated the patient?

    f. Does the patient have a secondary insurance plan? If so, what is it?

    g. Does the physician participate in the insurance plan? How do you know?

    h. What is the total charge listed on this claim?

    i. Who referred the patient to BWW Medical Associates?

    j. What is the patient's employment status?

2. Verifying Workers' Compensation Coverage

Use this scenario to assist in performing Procedure 17-1.

    Patient's Information: George Rafael, 102 Stagecoach Drive, Port Snead, XY 12345

    Phone: 555-987-2152. DOB: 8/25/xx. Spouse: Lynda Rafael

    Employer: HangRite Gutter. Phone: 555-781-2461

    Employer Contact: Lynn Santaniello, owner

    Date of Injury: 7/8/xx. First Report of Injury Filed 7/8/xx

    W/C Insurance Carrier: Wausau. Policy Number: 876543 Phone 555-987-6758

    Wausau Contact: James Wrigley

    Claim # 000-12987

3. Use the following scenario to assist in performing Procedure 17-2, obtaining prior authorization:

    Patient: Mari Lou Whalen, 11 Willard Street, Port Snead, XY 12345

    Insurance: Aetna. Policy Number 987654321

    Procedure: Total Thyroidectomy with parathyroidectomy

    Diagnosis: Thyroid/parathyroid lesions causing hyperparathyroidism

    Date of Surgery: 9/2/xx

    Authorization Number: 0902987765432

4. Create a clean 1500 claim form following the outline provided in Procedure 17-3, and using the scenario information that follows to complete the claim. Any information not given means the referenced block on the claim should be left blank. Use the figure from Application #1 to complete the provider information in blocks 25–27 and 31–33.

Patient Information:	Guarantor's Information:
Jazmyn Grover	Kim Carlson (Mom)
210 Archer Way	210 Archer Way
Port Snead, XY 12345-6789	Port Snead, XY 12345-6789
DOB: 5/01/xx	DOB: 7/30/xx
Sex F/Status FT Student	Sex F
Condition not related to employment or accident	Phone: 555-123-4567
Insurance Information:	**Claim Information:**
Carrier: Blue Cross/Blue Shield	Referring MD: Joseph Wright, MD
Policy #: 75621483	Referring MD NPI: 1023459876
Group #: 987456	Outside Lab: No
Insured: Kim Carlson	DOS: 8-22-xx
Procedures: 99212 (office visit) $65.00	POS: 11 (office)
87081 (throat culture) $25.00	Provider: Alexis Whalen, MD
85025 (CBC) $40.00	Provider NPI: 9876543210
Diagnosis: 034.0 (strep throat)	

5. Using the Remittance Advice (EOB/EOP) that follows, answer the questions on the next page about this RA.

PATIENT	INSURANCE CLAIM CONTROL NO.	1 PROCEDURE CODE	NO. SVCS.	2 WHEN (MO DAY YR)	SERVICE CODE	PC1 IMP	3 AMOUNT BILLED	4 AMOUNT APPROVED	5 AMOUNT APPLIED TO DEDUCTIBLE	6 CO-INSURANCE	7 MEDICARE PAYS 80% OF THIS AMOUNT	8 SERVICES PAID IN FULL	9 WITHHELD FOR OFFSET	10 MEDICARE PAID PATIENT	11 MEDICARE PAID PROVIDER	12 MEDICARE DOES NOT PAY FOR THESE SERVICES
MARY DOE 123-45-6789A	11311101414-00	99214	001	0909 09	0911	1	55.57	55.57								
		81000	001	0909 09	611	5	4.37	4.37								
		78730	001	0909 09	611	4	76.80	76.80								
		CLAIMS TOTALS					136.74	136.74	0.00	26.47	132.37	4.37	0.00	0.00	110.27	
JANE JONES 555-44-321-A	11311101415-00	99244	001	0905 09	611	3	131.03	131.03								
		31000	001	0905 09	611	5	4.37	4.37								
		32000	001	0905 09	611	5	150.68	150.68								
		78730	001	0905 09	611	4	76.80	76.80								
		CLAIMS TOTALS					362.88	362.88	0.00	71.71	358.51	4.37	0.00	0.00	291.17	
JACK SMITH 987-65-4321A	11311101436-00	99214	001	0912 09	611	1	55.57	55.57								
		81000	001	0912 09	611	5	4.37	4.37								
		78730	001	0912 09	611	4	76.80	76.80								
		CLAIMS TOTALS					136.74	136.74	0.00	26.47	132.37	4.37	0.00	0.00	110.27	

PAYMENT FOR THE LABORATORY TEST IS BASED ON A FEE SCHEDULE. A COPY OF THIS CLAIM DETERMINATION WILL BE FORWARDED TO THE BENEFICIARY'S SUPPLEMENTAL INSURER WITHIN THE NEXT 30 DAYS. QUESTIONS REGARDING PAYMENT OF SUPPLEMENTAL BENEFITS SHOULD BE DIRECTED TO THAT INSURER. PAYMENT FOR THIS SERVICE IS BASED ON THE MEDICARE FEE SCHEDULE.

	NUMBER OF CLAIMS	AMOUNT BILLED	AMOUNT APPROVED	AMOUNT APPLIED TO DEDUCTIBLE	COINSURANCE	MEDICARE PAYS 80% OF THIS AMOUNT	SERVICES PAID IN FULL	WITHHELD FOR OFFSET	MEDICARE PAID PATIENT	MEDICARE PAID PROVIDER
TOTAL	3	636.26	636.35	0.00	124.65	498.60	13.11	0.00	0.00	511.71
PAGE-										
CHECK-										

PROVIDER NUMBER: 000412000
WEEK ENDING: 10/11/12
CHECK NUMBER: 04750780 6
DATE PAID: 10/15/12

Elizabeth Williams, MD
305 Main Street,
Fort Snead, YZ 12345-9876

SUMMARY ►

Source: From Helen Houser and Terri Wyman, ADMINISTRATIVE MEDICAL ASSISTING: A WORKFORCE READINESS APPROACH, 1/e. © 2012 McGraw Hill Companies, Inc. Reprinted with permission.

   a. What is Jane Jones' ID number?

   b. What is the total amount billed for Mary Doe?

   c. What is the physician's provider number?

   d. What is the check number for this EOB?

   e. What is Jack Smith's coinsurance amount?

   f. What is the total amount of the check received?

   g. What is the procedure code for Jane Jones with a billed amount of $150.68?

   h. How much was paid on Jack Smith's account?

   i. What is the approved (allowed) charge for CPT coder 81000 for Mary Doe?

   j. What is the total amount paid for Jane Jones' visit?

C A S E   S T U D I E S

Write your response to each case study on the lines provided.

Case 1

A new patient is completing your office's patient registration form. The patient tells you that she has insurance but does not have her card with her and does not know the effective date of coverage, the group plan number, or the identification number. Explain one or more ways to obtain the insurance information right away.

_____

_____

_____

Case 2

Mr. Lewis, a new patient, arrives at the office for his first appointment. His neighbor is a patient in the office and referred Mr. Lewis to your office. As you are checking him in, you discover that he is enrolled in a PPO insurance plan and your office is not an in-network provider. You explain to Mr. Lewis that he can still be seen, but he will be responsible for a higher coinsurance and may be subject to a deductible. Mr. Lewis is upset and angry that he was not informed of this fact when he made the appointment.

   a. How could this incident have been avoided?

_____

_____

_____

   b. Is there anything you can do today to assist Mr. Lewis?

_____

_____

_____

Case 3

Your medical office receives a payment and a remittance advice (RA) from an insurer in response to a claim you filed for a patient. The RA notes that one of the services on the claim is not covered in the patient's plan. What steps will you take regarding the rejected portion of the claim?

_____

_____

_____

PROCEDURE 17-1 Verifying Workers' Compensation Coverage

Goal
To verify workers' compensation coverage before accepting a patient.

OSHA Guidelines
This procedure does not involve exposure to blood, body fluids, or tissue.

Materials
Telephone, paper, and a pen.

Method

Step Number	Procedure	Points Possible	Points Earned
1.	Call the patient's employer and verify that the accident or illness occurred on the employer's premises or at an employment-related work site.	17	
2.	Obtain the employer's approval to provide treatment. Be sure to write down the name and title of the person giving approval, as well as his phone number.*	17	
3.	Ask the employer for the name of its workers' compensation insurance company. (Employers are required by law to carry such insurance. It is a good policy to notify your state labor department about any employer you encounter that does not have workers' compensation insurance, although you are not required to do so.) If the employer has not done so, remind them to report the incident to the W/C carrier, using the First Report of Injury or Illness, and to the state labor department within 24 hours of the incident.*	17	
4.	Contact the insurance company and verify that the employer does indeed have an active policy in good standing with the company.	17	
5.	Obtain the claim number assigned to the case from the insurance company. This claim number is placed on all claims and submitted paperwork.*	17	
6.	When the patient begins treatment, create a patient record. If the patient is already an active patient with the practice, create separate medical and financial records for the workers' compensation-related treatment.	15	
Total Points		100	

CAAHEP Competencies Achieved

    IV. P (7)   Demonstrate telephone techniques

    VII. P (1)   Apply both managed care policies and procedures

    VII. P (5)   Obtain preauthorization, including documentation

    VII. P (6)   Verify eligibility for managed care services

ABHES Competencies Achieved

    8. (r) Apply third-party guidelines

    8. (s) Obtain managed care referrals and pre-certification

PROCEDURE 17-2 Submitting a Request for Prior Authorization

WORK // DOC

Goal
To submit a request for prior authorization.

OSHA Guidelines
This procedure does not involve exposure to blood, body fluids, or tissue.

Materials
Patient medical chart with planned procedure and CPT code, diagnosis and ICD code for proof of medical necessity, Standard Prior Authorization Request Form, and patient financial record or the following information: patient name, address, DOB, subscriber name and relationship to patient if not the same, insurance policy group, and ID numbers.

Method

Step Number	Procedure	Points Possible	Points Earned
1.	Place a call to the insurance carrier or access the website if available.	20	
2.	When you reach the nurse manager for the patient's policy, explain that you would like to obtain prior authorization for the requested procedure. She will ask a series of questions regarding the patient, procedure, and diagnosis. Answer these questions using the assembled materials from the patient's medical and financial records.*	20	
3.	If obtaining authorization via the insurance carrier's website, access the website utilizing your user ID and password. Enter the prior authorization area of the website, and enter the required information using the assembled materials from the patient's medical and financial records.*	20	
4.	When prior authorization is obtained, carefully record the authorization number and the name and extension number of the person issuing the authorization (if obtained over the phone). If the authorization is obtained via a website, print out the authorization documentation.	20	
5.	Place the authorization number and/or documentation in the patient medical and financial record for further reference, as it will be required when submitting the patient's health insurance claim.*	20	
Total Points		100	

CAAHEP Competencies Achieved

IV. P (7)   Demonstrate telephone techniques

VII. P (1)   Apply both managed care policies and procedures

VII. P (5)   Obtain preauthorization, including documentation

VII. P (6)   Verify eligibility for managed care services

ABHES Competencies Achieved

8. (r) Apply third-party guidelines

8. (s) Obtain managed care referrals and precertification

PROCEDURE 17-3 Completing the CMS-1500 Claim Form

WORK // DOC

Goal
To complete the CMS-1500 claim form correctly.

OSHA Guidelines
This procedure does not involve exposure to blood, body fluids, or tissue.

Materials
Patient record, CMS-1500 form, typewriter, computer or pen, and patient ledger card or charge slip.

Method
Note: The numbers below correspond to the numbered fields on the CMS-1500.

Step Number	Procedure	Points Possible	Points Earned
Patient Information Section			
1.	Place an X in the appropriate insurance box.	1	
	a. Enter the insured's insurance identification number as it appears on the insurance card.*	2	
2.	Enter the patient's name in this order: last name, first name, middle initial (if any).	2	
3.	a. Enter the patient's birth date using an 8-digit format. b. Indicate the patient's sex: male or female.	2	
4.	If the insured and the patient are the same person, enter SAME. If not, enter the policyholder's name.	2	
5.	Enter the patient's mailing address, city, state, and zip code.	2	
6.	Enter the patient's relationship to the insured. If they are the same, enter SELF.	2	
7.	Enter the insured's mailing address, city, state, zip code, and telephone number. If this address is the same as the patient's, enter SAME. For Medicare, leave blank.*	2	
8.	Indicate the patient's marital, employment, and student status by placing an X in the appropriate boxes.	1	
9.	Enter the last name, first name, and middle initial of any other insured person whose policy might cover the patient. If the claim is for Medicare and the patient has a Medigap policy, enter the patient's name again.	2	
	a. Enter the policy or group number for the other insured person.	2	
	b. Enter the date of birth and sex of the other insured person (listed in field 9).	2	
	c. Enter the other insured's employer or school name.	2	
	d. Enter the other insured's insurance plan or program name. If the plan is Medigap and CMS has assigned it a nine-digit number called PAYERID, enter that number here.	2	
10.	Place Xs in the appropriate YES or NO boxes in a, b, and c to indicate whether the patient's place of employment, an auto accident, or other type of accident precipitated the patient's condition. If an auto accident is responsible, for PLACE, enter the two-letter state postal abbreviation for the location of the accident.*	1	

(continued)

Step Number	Procedure	Points Possible	Points Earned
11.	Enter the insured's policy group number. For Medicare claims, fill out this section only if there is other insurance primary to Medicare; otherwise, enter NONE and leave fields a–d blank.	2	
	a. Enter the insured's date of birth and sex as in field 3, if the insured is not the patient.	2	
	b. Enter the employer's name or school name here. This information will determine if Medicare is the primary payer.	2	
	c. Enter the insurance plan or program name.	2	
	d. Place an X to indicate YES or NO related to another health benefit plan.	2	
12.	The patient or an authorized representative signs and dates the form here. If a representative signs, have the representative indicate the relationship to the patient. If signatures are on file, this may be noted by inserting "Signature on File."*	2	
13.	Have the insured (the patient or another individual) sign here. If signatures are on file, this may be noted by inserting "Signature on File."*	2	
Physician Information Section			
14.	Enter the date of the current illness, injury, or pregnancy using eight digits, if not the same as the date of service.	1	
15.	Enter the date the patient was first seen for illness or injury. Leave it blank for Medicare.	1	
16.	Enter the dates the patient is or was unable to work. This information could signal a workers' compensation claim.	1	
17.	Enter the name of the referring physician, clinical laboratory, or other referring source.	2	
	a. Depending on insurance carrier instructions, enter an approved 2-digit qualifier (refer to Table 17–1) in the small space and the appropriate referring provider identifier next to it. If the carrier requires only the NPI, leave this box blank.	2	
	b. Enter the referring provider NPI number.*	2	
18.	If the patient was hospitalized during this encounter, enter the dates here.	1	
19.	Use the payer's current instructions for this field. In many cases, it may be left blank.	1	
20.	Place an X in the YES box if a laboratory test was performed outside the physician's office, and enter the test price if you are billing for these tests. Place an X in the NO box if the test was done in the physician's office that is billing the insurance company.	1	
21.	Enter the ICD code number for each diagnosis or nature of injury. Enter up to four codes in order of importance.*	2	
22.	Enter the Medicaid resubmission code and original reference number if applicable.	1	
23.	Enter the prior authorization number if required by the payer.	2	
24.	The six service lines in block 24 are divided horizontally to accommodate NPI and other proprietary identifiers per insurance carrier instructions. Otherwise, use the nonshaded areas only if the payer requires just the NPI for claims submission.	2	
	a. Enter the date of each service, procedure, or supply provided. Add the number of days for each and enter them, in chronological order, in field 24g.	2	
	b. Enter the two-digit place-of-service code (see Table 17-5).	2	
	c. EMG stands for emergency care. Check with the insurer to see if this information is needed. If it is required and emergency care was provided, enter Y; if it is not required or care was not on an emergency basis, leave this field blank.	2	

Step Number	Procedure	Points Possible	Points Earned
	d. Enter the CPT/HCPCS codes with modifiers for the procedures, services, or supplies provided.*	2	
	e. Enter the diagnosis code (or its reference number—1, 2, 3, or 4—depending on carrier regulations) that applies to that procedure, as listed in field 21.*	2	
	f. Enter the dollar amount of the fee charged.	2	
	g. Enter the days or units for the number of times the service was performed.	2	
	h. This field is Medicaid-specific for early periodic screening diagnosis and treatment programs. For all other payers, leave this field blank.	1	
	i. (shaded area). If required by the insurance carrier, enter the appropriate non-NPI identifier here. If not required, leave this area blank.	2	
	j. If the carrier requires a non-NPI number, enter the PIN identified in 24i in the shaded area. Use the nonshaded area below this to enter the provider's NPI in 24j.	2	
25.	Enter the physician's or care provider's federal tax identification number or Social Security number and enter an X in the box identifying which number is listed.	2	
26.	Enter the patient's account number assigned by your office, if applicable.	2	
27.	Place an X in the YES box to indicate the physician will accept Medicare or TRICARE assignment of benefits.*	1	
28.	Enter the total charge for the service.	2	
29.	Enter the amount already paid by any primary insurance company or the patient, if it pertains to his deductible.	1	
30.	Enter the balance due to your office. For primary Medicare claims, leave this field blank.	2	
31.	Have the physician or service supplier sign and date the form here. In most cases, because claims are filed electronically, the signature is on file and the typed name of the provider is acceptable in this block.	2	
32.	Enter the name and address of the organization or individual who performed the services. If service was provided in the provider's office or the patient's home, leave this field blank.	1	
	a. If block 32 is completed, enter the NPI for the service facility.	1	
	b. If block 32 is completed and if required by the insurance carrier, enter the appropriate two-digit qualifier immediately followed by the identification number being used. Do not place any spaces or punctuation between the qualifier and the identification number.	1	
33.	List the billing physician's or supplier's name, address, zip code, and phone number.	2	
	a. Enter the billing provider's NPI.	2	
	b. If required by the insurance carrier, enter the non-NPI qualifier in field 33b, immediately followed by the identification number being used. Do not place any spaces or punctuation between the qualifier and the identification number.	2	
Total Points		100	

CAAHEP Competencies Achieved

VII. P (3)   Complete insurance claim forms

ABHES Competencies Achieved

8. (u) Prepare and submit insurance claims

PROCEDURE 17-4 Tracking Insurance Claims Submissions

WORK // DOC

Goal
To create and use a spreadsheet to track insurance claims submissions.

OSHA Guidelines
This procedure does not involve exposure to blood, body fluids, or tissue.

Materials
CMS-1500 claims prepared for submission or record of CMS-1500 claims submitted electronically; spreadsheet or grid for handwritten record with pen or computer with software program such as MS Excel, allowing for the creation of a spreadsheet.

Method

Step Number	Procedure	Points Possible	Points Earned
1.	Using Figure 17-10 as a guide, create columns with the following (or similar) headings: Patient Name (and/or account number); Insurance Company; Date of Submission and Amount of the Claim; Insurance Response and Date of Response; Date of Resubmission; Date of Payment; Payment Amount; Patient Balance; and Date of Patient Billing.	15	
2.	Using the list of claims submitted, complete the blanks for patient name, insurance company, date of submission, and amount of the claim.*	17	
3.	When the RA (EOB) is received, complete the date and response columns, including whether the claim is paid, rejected, denied, or a request was made for more information.*	17	
4.	If resubmission is required, enter the date of resubmission.	17	
5.	If payment is received, enter the date of receipt and the amount of the payment.	17	
6.	Record patient balance (if any) and the date the patient is billed.*	17	
Total Points		100	

CAAHEP Competencies Achieved

VII. P (3)   Complete insurance claim forms

ABHES Competencies Achieved

8. (u) Prepare and submit insurance claims

18

Diagnostic Coding

Name_____ Class_____ Date_____

R E V I E W

Vocabulary Review

Matching

Match the key terms in the right column with the definitions in the left column by placing the letter of each correct answer in the space provided.

_____ 1. The notation within ICD using directions *See* or *See also* after the main terms in the index; notes that another term may be appropriate when coding the referenced diagnosis

_____ 2. Code set based on a system maintained by WHO whose use is mandated by HIPAA for reporting diseases, conditions, signs, and symptoms

_____ 3. The patient's primary reason for seeking care

_____ 4. The alphanumeric designation used to communicate the diagnosis to third-party payers on the healthcare claim form

_____ 5. One of two ways diagnoses are listed in ICD; diagnoses appear in alpha order with their corresponding diagnosis code(s)

_____ 6. Type of ICD-9 code that identifies external causes of injuries and illnesses

_____ 7. One of two ways diagnoses are listed in ICD; diagnoses codes are listed in numeric order with additional instructions regarding the use of the code for each diagnosis

_____ 8. The first diagnosis listed for outpatient claims as the *primary* reason for the patient's visit

_____ 9. Analysis of the connection between diagnostic and procedural information in order to evaluate the medical necessity of the reported charges

_____ 10. Another term for the physician's *assessment* of the patient's condition

_____ 11. The first diagnosis listed for inpatient claims as the *principal* reason found, after study, for the patient's hospitalization

_____ 12. An ICD-9 code used to identify healthcare encounters for reasons other than illness or injury, such as annual exams and immunizations (a Z code in ICD-10)

_____ 13. The list of abbreviations, punctuations, symbols, typefaces, and instructional notes providing guidelines for using the ICD code set

_____ 14. Causes and severity of illness

_____ 15. Subdivisions of the alpha Index for ICD-10 chapters containing clinical descriptions of the code range and guidelines for coding

_____ 16. The cause of a disease or condition

a. Alphabetic Index
b. categories
c. chapters
d. chief complaint
e. code linkage
f. conventions
g. cross-reference
h. diagnosis
i. diagnosis code
j. E code
k. etiology
l. International Classification of Diseases
m. morbidity
n. mortality
o. primary diagnosis
p. principal diagnosis
q. subcategories
r. Tabular List
s. V code
t. WHO

_____ 17. The 3-digit code subdivisions in ICD-10

_____ 18. The organization that maintains and updates ICD

_____ 19. Divisions of ICD-10 named for a body system or a specific disease type

_____ 20. Causes of death

Content Review

Multiple Choice

In the space provided, write the letter of the choice that best completes each statement or answers each question.

_____ 1. An example of a condition requiring a V code in ICD-9 or Z code in ICD-10 is
   a. Chronic bronchitis
   b. A fractured tibia
   c. Influenza
   d. An annual checkup
   e. An acute back sprain

_____ 2. One of the reasons the ICD-9-CM was originally created was to classify statistics of patient "morbidity," which means
   a. Death
   b. Surgeries
   c. Wellness
   d. Sickness
   e. None of the above

_____ 3. When a condition or disease cannot be described more specifically, the abbreviation that may be used is
   a. NOS
   b. SPN
   c. NOT
   d. SNO
   e. NEC

_____ 4. Which of the following descriptions accurately reflects the difference between acute and chronic?
   a. A chronic condition is more serious than an acute condition
   b. Chronic conditions may worsen from time to time and become acute
   c. The onset of an acute illness is slow and lasts a long time
   d. If a patient has an acute and chronic illness, the acute code is listed first, followed by the chronic code
   e. b and d

_____ 5. An E code is used to
   a. Describe chronic illness
   b. Explain how an injury happened
   c. Describe the treatment the patient received
   d. Assign the benefits the patient will receive
   e. c and d

_____ 6. Codes are updated and new ICD manuals are available
   a. Every 6 months
   b. Every year
   c. As needed when new codes are developed
   d. Every 2 years
   e. Every 10 years

_____ 7. When choosing an ICD code, you need to have
   a. A ledger card
   b. An encounter form
   c. A chart note
   d. A superbill
   e. b, c, or d

_____ 8. NOS, NEC, brackets, and parentheses are examples of
   a. Abbreviations
   b. Exclusions
   c. Conventions
   d. Encounter terms
   e. None of the above

_____ 9. The main term for gastroesophageal reflux disease is
   a. GERD
   b. Gastro
   c. Reflux
   d. Disease
   e. Esophagus

_____ 10. When coding malignant neoplasms, the primary site is
   a. The location where the cancer originated
   b. The area where the cancer has spread
   c. The place where chemotherapy drugs are injected
   d. The metastatic location of the cancer
   e. None of the above

_____ 11. The abbreviation NEC is used when
   a. There is more than one diagnosis
   b. The physician does not have a final diagnosis
   c. A patient has a serious illness
   d. There is not a code that is specific enough to match the physician's description
   e. The physician is a specialist

_____ 12. When the word *Excludes* is found in the ICD-9, it means that
   a. It is a supplementary code
   b. It is the primary code
   c. The entry is not classified as part of the preceding code
   d. It is a nonessential code
   e. The code is incomplete without another digit

_____ 13. When the phrase *code first underlying disease* appears beneath a coded condition, you will
   a. Not use this code as the first code
   b. Use the primary diagnosis code first
   c. Use this code as the first code
   d. Place the primary code after this code
   e. a and b

_____ 14. The first step in locating the appropriate code in the ICD is to
   a. Identify the expanded diagnosis phrase
   b. Identify the main term in the Alphabetic Index

    c. Locate the main term in the Tabular List

    d. Determine if there is a secondary diagnosis

    e. None of the above

_____ 15. Which of the following statements is true concerning the x character used in the ICD-10 coding?

    a. The x means that a shorter code must be used

    b. The x is used as a placeholder for future expansion of the subcategory

    c. The x is used for a nonexistent digit when a sixth or seventh digit is required for code specificity.

    d. The x is always used in the fifth digit place

    e. b and c

_____ 16. In the Alphabetic Index, brackets within a code are used

    a. To indicate manifestation (secondary) codes

    b. To enclose supplementary words

    c. To enclose modifiers

    d. If an exclusion exists

    e. None of the above

_____ 17. *Excludes1* is a note that indicates

    a. Codes that are always attached together

    b. Codes that cannot appear together

    c. The patient's condition must be congenital

    d. The patient's condition is an acquired one

    e. The patient's condition is neither acquired nor congenital

_____ 18. Which of the following statements is true about ICD-10?

    a. V codes are still included in the ICD-10

    b. The ICD-10 includes fewer than 68,000 codes

    c. The format of the ICD-10 codes includes 3–7 characters

    d. E codes will be used in the ICD-10 version the same as in the ICD-9

    e. None of the above

_____ 19. When you apply the ICD-10 guidelines for laterality codes, right and left would be coded using

    a. R = right and L = left

    b. 0 = right and 1 = left

    c. 1 = right and 2 = left

    d. D = right (dextro-) and S = left (sinistro-)

    e. b or d

_____ 20. Which of the following code range of ICD-10 represents the "V codes" of ICD-9?

    a. A00–B99

    b. F00–F99

    c. P00–P96

    d. R00–R99

    e. Z00–Z99

_____ 21. In Chapter 19 of the ICD-10, the letters A, D, and S are referred to as

    a. Extensions

    b. Subcategories

    c. Categories

    d. Etiologies

    e. Diagnoses

_____ 22. When you are coding from ICD-10, a patient who sustained an injury from being burned with battery acid would have codes from code range

    a. V01–Y98

    b. S00–T98

    c. M00–M99

    d. H60–H95

    e. E00–E90

_____ 23. The code T36 from ICD-10 is used to code

    a. Diabetes mellitus due to underlying condition with hyperosmolarity

    b. Influenza due to H1N1 influenza virus

    c. Age-related osteoporosis with current pathological fracture

    d. Influenza due to identified avian influenza virus with other manifestations

    e. Poisoning by, adverse effect of, and underdosing of systemic antibiotics

_____ 24. The note *Excludes2* in ICD-10, indicates that

    a. The condition is excluded as not part of the condition represented by the code

    b. One code is used for more than one condition

    c. A separate code is used for all related conditions

    d. Codes cannot appear together

    e. If the patient has more than two conditions, additional codes are not necessary

_____ 25. Burns are classified by the extent of the burn based on the

    a. Agent that caused the burn

    b. Treatment required

    c. Location of the burn on the body

    d. Rule of nines

    e. Code of burns

True or False

Decide whether each statement is true or false. In the space at the left, write T *for true or* F *for false. On the lines provided, rewrite the false statements to make them true.*

_____ 26. The Alphabetic Index is organized by the condition, not by the body part in which the condition occurs.

_____

_____ 27. One of the purposes of the ICD-9-CM is to study healthcare costs.

_____

_____ 28. When coding neoplasms, the secondary site is the area where the cancer originated.

_____

_____ 29. The statement *Excludes1* in ICD-10 means that you should always use the code listed above the Excludes1 note.

_____

_____ 30. One purpose for the ICD-10 is to provide decreased specificity of diagnostic codes.

_____

_____ 31. Parentheses are used to enclose supplemental or nonessential information that will not affect the code selection.

_____

_____ 32. A patient who has an elevated blood pressure should always have a diagnosis code for hypertension.

_____

Short Answer

Write the answer to each question on the lines provided.

33. Why is there a mandate to transition from the ICD-9-CM coding system to ICD-10-CM?

_____

_____

34. List six reasons that ICD codes are used today.

_____

_____

_____

_____

_____

35. What is the difference between an acute and chronic condition?

_____

_____

_____

36. What is a combination code and when is it used?

_____

_____

_____

37. One of the changes in ICD-10 is the use of *laterality* codes. What are they, and when are they used?

_____

_____

_____

38. What is the purpose of the placeholder *x* in ICD-10?

_____

_____

_____

39. Explain the purpose of code linkage.

_____

_____

_____

40. ICD-10 uses the terms *category* and *subcategory.* Explain the (specific) difference(s) between these two coding terms.

_____

_____

_____

A P P L I C A T I O N

Follow the directions for each application.

Diagnosis Coding Exercises

   a. Using an ICD-9 coding manual, locate the appropriate diagnosis codes for the following diseases or conditions, and insert your answers in the middle column.

   b. Using an ICD-10 coding manual, locate the appropriate diagnosis codes for the following diseases or conditions, inserting your answers in the right column.

Diagnosis/Condition	ICD-9 Code	ICD-10 Code
Diabetes with diabetic neuropathy		
Nondisplaced fracture of tibial shaft (left)		
Burn, first degree, (right) forearm		
Corneal abrasion not due to contact lenses (left), initial encounter		
Cellulitis of the right knee		
Postherpetic trigeminal neuralgia		
Uncomplicated senile dementia		
Acute vein thrombosis of the calf		
Mild dysplasia of the cervix		
Genital herpes, unspecified (male)		
Frostbite of the foot (without necrosis)		
Sprain of elbow at the radiohumeral joint (left)		
First-degree sunburn		
Acute cholecystitis with gallstones in ducts, but no obstruction		
Acute, benign pericarditis, idiopathic		
Bell's palsy		
Poisoning (hypersensitivity) by penicillin		
Breech delivery; obstructed labor due to buttocks presentation (single fetus)		
Group B Streptococcus pneumonia		
Cancer of bronchus, metastatic to bone and brain		

Coding Scenarios

   1. Henry Warner is an established patient with Dr. Buckwalter. He has a longtime history of COPD and asthma. The physician has been treating Henry with bronchodilator therapy, oxygen, and steroids when weather changes cause Henry's breathing to worsen. Today Henry has an appointment to see the doctor because of weakness, a nonproductive cough, and an elevated temperature. Upon examination, the physician determines that Henry has an upper respiratory infection exacerbating the asthma and COPD. He orders a complete blood count (CBC), chest x-ray, and pulse oximetry. The examinations and laboratory tests are performed in the clinic.

What conditions should be coded for this patient? List the conditions or diagnoses that should be coded for this patient, giving both the ICD-9 and ICD-10 codes for each.

Diagnosis			
ICD-9			
ICD-10			

2. Kim Beals brings her 4-year-old daughter Jazmyn in for her yearly well-child exam. In addition to her physical exam for preschool, Jazmyn also receives her DPTaP (DPT and polio) immunization and her varicella immunization. Dr. Whalen also completes the required paperwork for the preschool.

What diagnosis codes will be used to code this encounter for Jazmyn?

Diagnosis			
ICD-9			
ICD-10			

3. Emmie Ward was a passenger on a motorcycle that spun out after hitting sand on the roadway when the driver attempted to avoid a car pulling into an intersection. Emmie is complaining of pain and numbness of her left elbow and arm, which is at an "odd" angle. Other than scrapes and abrasions on her left hand and arm, she complains of no other injuries. Examination and x-ray confirm a displaced fracture of the radius and closed fracture of the proximal ulnar head (Monteggia's fracture). The fracture was set and referral to orthopedics made.

What diagnosis codes will be used for Emmie's medical record?

Diagnosis	Monteggia's fracture		
ICD-9			
ICD-10			

PROCEDURE 18-1 Locating an ICD-9-CM Code

Procedure Goal
To analyze diagnoses and locate the correct ICD code.

OSHA Guidelines
This procedure does not involve exposure to blood, body fluids, or tissue.

Materials
Patient record, charge slip or superbill, and ICD-9-CM manual.

Method
Procedure steps.

Step Number	Procedure	Points Possible	Points Earned
1.	Locate the patient's diagnosis on the superbill (encounter form) or elsewhere in the patient's chart. If it is found on the superbill, verify documentation in the medical chart.	17	
2.	Find the diagnosis in the ICD-9's Alphabetic Index. Look for the condition first, then locate the indented subterms that make the condition more specific. Read all cross-references to check all the possibilities for a term, including its synonyms and any eponyms.*	17	
3.	Locate the code from the Alphabetic Index in the ICD-9's Tabular List.	17	
4.	Read all information to find the code that corresponds to the patient's specific disease or condition. Study the list of codes and descriptions. Be sure to pick the most specific code available. Check for the symbol that shows that fourth (and) fifth digits may be required.*	17	
5.	Be sure that all necessary codes are chosen to completely describe each diagnosis. Check for instructions stating an additional code is needed. If more than one code is needed, be sure instructions are followed and the codes are listed in the correct order.	17	
6.	Carefully record the diagnosis code(s) on the insurance claim and proofread the numbers.	15	
Total Points		100	

CAAHEP Competencies Achieved

VIII. C (3)   Describe how to use the most current diagnostic coding classification system

VIII. P (2)   Perform diagnostic coding

ABHES Competencies Achieved

3. Medical Terminology

   (d) Recognize and identify acceptable medical abbreviations

8. Medical Office Business Procedures Management

   (t) Perform diagnostic and procedural coding

PROCEDURE 18-2 Locating a V Code

Procedure Goal
To analyze the patient record (or encounter form) and decide whether a V code is an appropriate diagnosis code.

OSHA Guidelines
This procedure does not involve exposure to blood, body fluids, or tissue.

Materials
Patient record, charge slip or superbill, and ICD-9-CM manual.

Method
Procedure steps.

Step Number	Procedure	Points Possible	Points Earned
1.	Locate the patient's diagnosis. This information may be found on the superbill (encounter form) or elsewhere in the patient's chart. If it is on the superbill, verify documentation in the medical chart.*	15	
2.	If the reason for the patient encounter relates to a physical exam, immunization, well-child visit, or other visit where there is no diagnosis or condition of illness found, a V code will be used to code the reason for the visit (diagnosis).	15	
3.	Find the diagnosis in the ICD-9's Alphabetic Index. Look for the condition first and then locate any indented subterms that make the condition more specific. Read all cross-references.*	15	
4.	Locate the code from the Alphabetic Index in the V code area of the ICD-9's Tabular List.	15	
5.	Read all descriptive information to find the code that corresponds to the patient's specific reason for today's visit. Be sure to pick the most specific code available. Check for the symbol that shows that a fourth and (possibly) a fifth digit is required.*	15	
6.	Be sure that that no other codes are required to describe the patient's reason for the visit. Check for instructions stating an additional code is needed. If more than one code is needed, be sure instructions are followed and the codes are listed in the correct order.	15	
7.	Carefully record the diagnosis code(s) on the insurance claim and proofread the numbers.	10	
Total Points		100	

CAAHEP Competencies Achieved

VIII. C (3) Describe how to use the most current diagnostic coding classification system

VIII. P (2) Perform diagnostic coding

ABHES Competencies Achieved

3. Medical Terminology

(d) Recognize and identify acceptable medical abbreviations

8. Medical Office Business Procedures Management

(t) Perform diagnostic and procedural coding

PROCEDURE 18-3 Locating an E Code

Procedure Goal
To analyze the patient record (or encounter form) and decide whether an E code is required to completely code the encounter.

OSHA Guidelines
This procedure does not involve exposure to blood, body fluids, or tissue.

Materials
Patient record, charge slip or superbill, and ICD-9-CM manual.

Method
Procedure steps.

Step Number	Procedure	Points Possible	Points Earned
1.	Locate the patient's diagnosis. This Information may be found on the superbill (encounter form) or elsewhere in the patient's chart. If it is on the superbill, verify documentation in the medical chart.*	15	
2.	If the patient's diagnosis begs the question "How did that happen?" an E code is required to give the insurance carrier as much information as possible.	15	
3.	After coding the diagnosis of the condition requiring treatment, open the ICD-9 manual to the External Cause Alphabetic Index or, if necessary, use the Table of Drugs and Chemicals. Find the appropriate description in the ICD-9's Alphabetic Index, looking for the condition first, and then locate any indented subterms that make the condition more specific. Read all cross-references.*	15	
4.	Locate the code from the Alphabetic Index in the E code area of the ICD-9's Tabular List.	15	
5.	Read all descriptive information to find the code that corresponds to how the patient's current condition came about. Choose the most specific code available. Check for the symbol that shows that a fourth and (possibly) a fifth digit are required; many E codes require these.*	15	
6.	Carefully record the diagnosis code(s) on the insurance claim and proofread the numbers.	15	
7.	E codes are always secondary, so be sure that that the primary diagnosis code is listed first. Check for instructions stating an additional code(s) is needed. If more than one code is needed, be sure instructions are followed and the codes are listed in the correct order.*	10	
Total Points		100	

CAAHEP Competencies Achieved

VIII. C (3) Describe how to use the most current diagnostic coding classification system

VIII. P (2) Perform diagnostic coding

ABHES Competencies Achieved

3. Medical Terminology

(d) Recognize and identify acceptable medical abbreviations

8. Medical Office Business Procedures Management

(t) Perform diagnostic and procedural coding

PROCEDURE 18-4 Locating an ICD-10-CM Code

Procedure Goal
To analyze diagnoses and locate the correct ICD code.

OSHA Guidelines
This procedure does not involve exposure to blood, body fluids, or tissue.

Materials
Patient record, charge slip or superbill, and access to ICD-10-CM codes on the CMS website: www.cms.hhs.gov/ICD10/01_Overview.asp, or access to a draft copy of the 2010 ICD-10-CM manual.

Method
Procedure steps.

Step Number	Procedure	Points Possible	Points Earned
1.	Locate the patient's diagnosis. This information may be found on the superbill (encounter form) or elsewhere in the patient's chart. If it is on the superbill, verify documentation in the medical chart.	17	
2.	Find the diagnosis in the ICD-10 Alpha Index. Look for the condition first, then locate the indented subterms that make the condition more specific. Read all cross-references to check all the possibilities for a term, including its synonyms and any eponyms.*	17	
3.	Following the directions in the Alpha Index, locate the code or code range from the Alpha Index in the ICD's Tabular List.	17	
4.	Read all information and instructions carefully to find the code that exactly corresponds to the patient's specific disease or condition. Carefully study the list of codes and descriptions. Be sure to pick the most specific code available.*	17	
5.	Watch for instructions advising of the need for additional codes as well as instructions regarding coding sequence and need for 6th and 7th digits or placeholders.*	17	
6.	Document the chosen codes carefully, remembering sequencing instructions.	15	
Total Points		100	

CAAHEP Competencies Achieved

VIII. C (3) Describe how to use the most current diagnostic coding classification system

VIII. P (2) Perform diagnostic coding

ABHES Competencies Achieved

3. Medical Terminology

(d) Recognize and identify acceptable medical abbreviations

8. Medical Office Business Procedures Management

(t) Perform diagnostic and procedural coding

19

Procedure Coding

Name_____ Class_____ Date_____

REVIEW

Vocabulary Review

Matching
Match the key terms in the right column with the definitions in the left column by placing the letter of each correct answer in the space provided.

_____ **1.** Similar care being provided by more than one physician

_____ **2.** A reference with the most commonly used system of codes

_____ **3.** The period of time after many procedures for follow-up care that is considered included in the payment for that procedure

_____ **4.** One or more two-digit alphanumeric codes assigned in addition to the CPT code to show that some special circumstance applies to the service or procedure

_____ **5.** Any CPT code that includes more than one procedure in its description

_____ **6.** Codes that represent medical procedures, diagnostic tests, and examinations to evaluate a patient's condition

_____ **7.** Codes used when discussing questions or concerns regarding test results, prognosis, risks, options, treatment instructions, importance of compliance, risk factor reduction, and patient/family education

_____ **8.** Lab tests frequently ordered together that are organ- or disease-oriented

_____ **9.** Codes used to describe the wide range of time, effort, skill, and locations used by physicians for different patients to diagnose conditions and plan treatments

_____ **10.** Codes that cover many supplies and DME; also referred to as national codes; services and procedures may not be found in CPT

_____ **11.** CPT code that is only reported in addition to the primary code

_____ **12.** The act of separately listing services or procedures instead of using available code that includes all services provided

_____ **13.** Care provided to unstable, critically ill patients; constant bedside attention is needed with explicit information as to time spent

_____ **14.** Purposely choosing a code of a higher level than that of the service provided

_____ **15.** Patient who has not received professional services from the physician within the last 3 years

_____ **16.** Analysis of the connection between diagnostic and procedural information in order to evaluate medical necessity

_____ **17.** Term used when the insurance carrier bases reimbursement on a code level lower than the one submitted by the provider

a. add-on code
b. bundled code
c. code linkage
d. concurrent care
e. consultation
f. counseling
g. critical care
h. CPT
i. downcoding
j. E/M code
k. established patient
l. global period
m. HCPCS Level II codes
n. modifier
o. new patient
p. panel
q. procedure code
r. unbundling
s. upcoding

_____ **18.** Care provided at the request of another healthcare provider

_____ **19.** Patient who has been seen by the physician within the last 3 years

True or False

Decide whether each statement is true or false. In the space at the left, write T for true or F for false. On the lines provided, rewrite the false statements to make them true.

_____ **20.** The CPT manual is updated every 6 months in January and June.

_____

_____ **21.** E/M codes are often considered the most important of all CPT codes because they can be used by all physicians in any medical specialty.

_____

_____ **22.** The period of time that is covered for follow-up care is called the entire service period.

_____

_____ **23.** To code a laboratory testing panel correctly, the physician must order each test listed within the panel, and there must be a need for each of them.

_____

_____ **24.** Claims fraud occurs when physicians or others falsely represent their services or charges to payers.

_____

_____ **25.** Modifier 55 means that the surgeon did not provide the pre- or post-op care.

_____

_____ **26.** The blue triangle symbol tells the user that this is a new code not used in previous editions of the CPT manual.

_____

_____ **27.** Concurrent care is a term used to describe a situation where a patient is being cared for by one physician who is a specialist.

_____

_____ **28.** The expanded problem-focused level of service includes a review of the past family and/or social history of the patient.

_____

_____ **29.** The most difficult aspect of E/M code to document is the MDM or medical decision making.

_____

_____ **30.** You must know if the patient has been at the hospital emergency department (ED) before in order to choose the correct ED E/M Code.

_____

Content Review

Multiple Choice

In the space provided, write the letter of the choice that best completes each statement or answers each question.

_____ **1.** The organization that publishes the CPT reference manual is
- **a.** HIPAA
- **b.** AMA
- **c.** AAMA
- **d.** WHO
- **e.** CMS

_____ 2. The maximum composition of a CPT code is five digits plus
a. One 2-digit modifier
b. Two 2-digit modifiers
c. Three 2-digit modifiers
d. Two 3-digit modifiers
e. Three 3-digit modifiers

_____ 3. When a medical facility uses published superbills or encounter forms with the CPT codes already on them for procedures, it is important to update the forms with the new codes when they are available in
a. January
b. March
c. June
d. September
e. December

_____ 4. HCPCS Level II codes are also called
a. Modifiers
b. National codes
c. Professional codes
d. AMA codes
e. DME codes

_____ 5. HCPCS Level I codes are also known as
a. E/M codes
b. National codes
c. AMA codes
d. Modifiers
e. CPT codes

_____ 6. Healthcare claims must comply with rules imposed by
a. Federal law
b. State law
c. Payer requirements
d. Insurance carrier requirements
e. All of the above

_____ 7. Which of the following would be the possible result of an inaccurately coded claim?
a. Denied claim
b. Reduced payment
c. Downcoding by the payer
d. All of the above
e. None of the above

_____ 8. To decrease the risk of fraud charges, medical offices should have
a. An encounter form
b. A software program for electronic billing
c. A compliance plan
d. A certified medical assistant
e. a and b

_____ 9. When a surgeon provides and administers general anesthesia, the modifier used with the surgical procedure is
a. 22
b. 23
c. 32
d. 47
e. 50

_____ 10. A red dot next to a CPT code in the manual denotes that this code is
a. A new code for this edition
b. Revised from a previous edition
c. Used when coding vaccines pending approval
d. Used when moderate sedation was used with the procedure
e. Being removed this year

_____ 11. Which of the following statements describes the function or result of unbundling?
   a. Codes are broken down into more than one code
   b. It is used to create higher reimbursement
   c. It is not allowed as an acceptable practice
   d. It is used to consolidate more than one coded procedure
   e. a, b, and c

_____ 12. The range of codes used to code radiology procedures is
   a. 00100–01999
   b. 10021–69990
   c. 80048–89356
   d. 70010–79999
   e. 99500–99602

_____ 13. A patient recovering from a surgical procedure is now seen by the physician for an unrelated problem. The unrelated problem is billed
   a. Bundled with the code for the surgical procedure if it is still within the global period
   b. Separately using a modifier
   c. At the end of the global period for the surgical procedure
   d. a and c
   e. b and c

_____ 14. When you submit a claim for immunizations
   a. Two codes are required, one for the injection and one for the vaccine or toxoid given
   b. One code is used for both the injection and the vaccine or toxoid given
   c. An E/M code is required for all submissions
   d. The vaccine is the only item coded and submitted
   e. b and c

_____ 15. Insurance fraud includes practices such as billing
   a. Only once for a service
   b. For procedures that are related to the patient's condition
   c. Separately for services that are bundled in a single procedure code
   d. For medically necessary procedures
   e. For a service that was performed

_____ 16. When a service such as a consult is required by the insurance carrier or a governmental or regulatory agency, the CPT modifier used is called
   a. Unrelated Services
   b. Mandated Services
   c. Technical Component
   d. Professional Component
   e. Increased Procedural Services

_____ 17. The subheading area of the CPT coding manual provides the
   a. General section name, such as Surgery
   b. General body system
   c. Procedures performed
   d. Body area for the body system
   e. Detailed body system

_____ **18.** The # sign is used to

    a. Note that codes are out of numeric sequence

    b. Denote that the code is new for the new edition of the CPT manual

    c. Tell the user that the code has been revised

    d. Separate codes in a section

    e. Designate codes that are pending approval

_____ **19.** When a physician meets with a patient and the family to discuss questions or concerns regarding the patient's prognosis, it is coded as

    a. Concurrent care

    b. Critical care

    c. A consultation

    d. An evaluation

    e. Counseling

_____ **20.** The term *code creep* is also known as

    a. Unbundling   **d.** Upcoding

    b. Downcoding   **e.** Bundling

    c. Underbilling

_____ **21.** The range of codes for the evaluation and management section of the CPT manual is

    a. 99201–99499   **d.** 99500–99602

    b. 90281–99199   **e.** 99602–99800

    c. 99100–99140

_____ **22.** Which of the following is a component used to determine the level of E/M code that is used?

    a. The age of the patient

    b. The specific insurance carrier the patient uses

    c. The extent of the examination that the physician conducted

    d. The level of medication the physician prescribes for the patient

    e. The geographic location of the medical practice

_____ **23.** Which of the following would not be coded using the HCPCS Level II codes?

    a. Durable medical equipment

    b. Procedures performed by the physician

    c. Emergency transport services

    d. Drugs and injections

    e. Routine venipuncture and Pap smear

_____ **24.** Which of the following is not a subcategory title used as a type of E/M code?

    a. Hospital Inpatient Services

    b. Consultations

    c. Office/Other Outpatient Services

    d. OB/GYN Services

    e. Critical Care Services

_____ **25.** Which of the following elements are included when coding using the problem-focused level of service regarding the patient's history?

    a. CC and HPI   **d.** ROS and HPI

    b. CC and ROS   **e.** CC and PFSH

    c. HPI and PFSH

Sentence Completion

In the space provided, write the word or phrase that best completes each sentence.

26. To make coding processes more efficient, medical offices often list frequently used procedures and their applicable CPT codes on _____.

27. HCPCS was developed by the CMS, which stands for _____.

28. When performing a code review or coding audit, the processor needs to ensure that there is a clear and correct link between each _____ and _____.

29. CPT symbols include triangles pointing toward each other, which indicates _____ or _____ text information.

30. The levels for coding a patient history (or examination) include _____, _____, _____, and _____.

31. Using multiple codes to describe a service that can be appropriately described by using one code is called _____.

32. The complexity levels of medical decision making (MDM) include _____, _____, _____ and _____.

33. To use the CPT manual correctly, first look up the description in the _____ and then verify the information in the _____.

34. Indented code information replaces the information following the _____ in the primary code.

35. Modifier 51 exempt codes are denoted with a _____.

36. _____ are used to denote special circumstances surrounding the code being submitted for payment.

37. Modifier 57 would be added to an E/M code in this circumstance: _____.

38. Category III HCPCS codes are (temporary) codes used for _____.

39. In order to use critical care codes, the _____ spent at the bedside must be documented.

40. The _____ is the time frame surrounding a procedure where all related services are considered part of the payment for that procedure.

26. _____
27. _____
28. _____
_____
29. _____
_____
30. _____
_____
_____
_____
_____
31. _____
32. _____
_____
_____
_____
33. _____
_____
34. _____
35. _____
36. _____
37. _____
38. _____
39. _____
40. _____

Short Answer

Write the answer to each question on the lines provided.

41. Cite seven possible consequences of inaccurate coding and incorrect billing.

_____

_____

_____

_____

_____

_____

42. List the six main sections found in the CPT coding manual, in the sequence they are found from the beginning of the manual to the end, including the code ranges found in each.

_____

_____

_____

_____

_____

43. List the common symbols found in CPT and their descriptions. Give an example of each **not** found in the textbook.

_____

_____

_____

_____

_____

44. What materials are needed to properly code with the CPT manual?

_____

_____

45. What are the key components to be checked when performing a coding audit?

_____

_____

_____

A P P L I C A T I O N

Using the scenarios given, code each procedure using the CPT manual.

1. Anesthesia code for a diagnostic arthroscopy _____

2. Destruction of 3.2 cm malignant lesion _____

3. Total hip replacement _____

4. Incision and drainage of foot bursa _____

5. Flexible bronchoscopy with laser destruction of tumor _____

6. Coronary artery bypass graft (CABG) single venous graft _____

7. Repair lacerated diaphragm _____

8. Partial splenectomy for ruptured spleen _____

9. Bone marrow biopsy _____

10. Laparoscopic cholecystectomy _____

11. Appendectomy for ruptured appendix _____

12. Incisional prostate biopsy _____

13. D&C for postpartum hemorrhage _____

14. Total abdominal hysterectomy with bilateral salpingo-oophorectomy _____

15. Hysterotomy with tubal ligation _____

16. Parathyroidectomy _____

17. Removal of foreign body imbedded in eyelid _____

18. AP and lateral chest x-ray _____

19. Complete CBC (automated) _____

20. Sodium (Na), potassium (K), chloride (CI) and carbon dioxide (CO_2) _____

These short scenarios are all related to E/M codes (Hint: one needs a modifier and one requires a procedure code in addition to the E/M—is a modifier needed here too?)

1. Patient admitted to Observation for stomach pain. Detailed history and exam were performed, and MDM is low. _____.

2. This 42-year-old (established) patient comes to the office for a BP check only. _____.

3. Ms. Ward, a new patient, complains of sinus pain. Expanded problem focused history and exam are completed, and sinus x-rays are ordered. Antibiotics are prescribed. _____.

4. The W/C insurance is requiring a confirmatory consult for this patient. A comprehensive history and exam are performed, and MDM is moderately complex. _____.

5. Mr. Sanchez is seen in the ED after an MVA. Comprehensive physical and history are performed, and MDM is of high complexity. _____.

6. Dr. Williams spent 60 minutes at the bedside stabilizing a patient status post myocardial infarction. _____.

7. Dr. Buckwalter performed a housecall for Mrs. Fussy, a longstanding patient. He performed a problem-focused history and exam and considered her MDM straightforward, diagnosing a UTI. _____.

8. A subsequent visit to the SNF (nursing home) was provided for Mr. Bedding who is improving daily S/P CVA (stroke). He hopes to return home soon. _____.

9. Felix Gatto is a new patient who arrives complaining of a furuncle on his neck. Dr. Whalen performed a brief exam and, after straightforward MDM, because she had time, also performed an I&D of the skin boil. _____.

10. Dr. Williams was called to the hospital to consult on a 5- y/o child, who 1 day after surgery, has spiked a fever and suffered a seizure. History and exam are comprehensive, and MDM is complex. _____.

Code Linkage

In each of the coded scenarios, using the midsection given from the CMS 1500 claim form, enter each listed CPT code on the form in block 24D and choose at least one diagnosis code from the one listed, entering number 1, 2, 3, 4 as required to "link" each procedure to its diagnosis to prove medical necessity.

Below is an example:

Ex: Nancy Evans comes in for an office visit (99213) in follow up for her Alzheimer's disease (294.11) and also a CBC (85025) to check on her anemia (280.1).

1. Raja Lautu had her yearly physical 2 weeks ago. As part of the physical, Dr. Williams ordered a screening (turned diagnostic) mammogram (77057-GH). This revealed a small density in the right breast (611.72). Ultrasound of the mass was performed (76645-RT), revealing a solid mass (611.72). Stereotactic breast biopsy (19102-RT) is performed, revealing grade II infiltrating ductal carcinoma (174.9).

2. Sylvia Gonzales returns to the office for follow up (99212) of her Type 2 diabetes (250.00) and hyperlipidemia (272.2). A GTT was performed (82951) as well as a lipid panel (80061)

21. DIAGNOSIS OR NATURE OF ILLNESS OR INJURY (Relate Items 1, 2, 3 or 4 to Item 24E by Line)									22. MEDICAID RESUBMISSION CODE / ORIGINAL REF. NO.				
1. L___ . ___ 3. L___ . ___ 2. L___ . ___ 4. L___ . ___									23. PRIOR AUTHORIZATION NUMBER				
24. A. DATE(S) OF SERVICE			B. PLACE OF SERVICE	C. EMG	D. PROCEDURES, SERVICES, OR SUPPLIES (Explain Unusual Circumstances)		E. DIAGNOSIS POINTER	F. $ CHARGES	G. DAYS OR UNITS	H. EPSDT Family Plan	I. ID. QUAL.	J. RENDERING PROVIDER ID. #
From MM DD YY	To MM DD YY				CPT/HCPCS	MODIFIER						
1											NPI	
2											NPI	
3											NPI	
4											NPI	
5											NPI	
6											NPI	

3. Ken Washington returns for follow up (99214) status post CVA with residual left arm weakness (729.89). He complains today that he has had headaches and dizziness (780.4), possibly related to his hypertension (401.9). His BP today is elevated at 168/92. Dr. Buckwalter is also concerned about Ken's hypothyroidism (244.9) and orders a free T4 (84439), total T4 (84436), and TSH (84443). EKG is also performed (93000) due to the elevated BP.

21. DIAGNOSIS OR NATURE OF ILLNESS OR INJURY (Relate Items 1, 2, 3 or 4 to Item 24E by Line)									22. MEDICAID RESUBMISSION CODE / ORIGINAL REF. NO.				
1. L___ . ___ 3. L___ . ___ 2. L___ . ___ 4. L___ . ___									23. PRIOR AUTHORIZATION NUMBER				
24. A. DATE(S) OF SERVICE			B. PLACE OF SERVICE	C. EMG	D. PROCEDURES, SERVICES, OR SUPPLIES (Explain Unusual Circumstances)		E. DIAGNOSIS POINTER	F. $ CHARGES	G. DAYS OR UNITS	H. EPSDT Family Plan	I. ID. QUAL.	J. RENDERING PROVIDER ID. #
From MM DD YY	To MM DD YY				CPT/HCPCS	MODIFIER						
1											NPI	
2											NPI	
3											NPI	
4											NPI	
5											NPI	
6											NPI	

Source for CMS 1500 forms: From Helen Houser and Terri Wyman, ADMINISTRATIVE MEDICAL ASSISTING: A WORKFORCE READINESS APPROACH, 1/e. © 2012 McGraw Hill Companies, Inc. Reprinted with permission.

C A S E   S T U D I E S

Write your response to each case study on the lines provided.

Case 1

Alice Gagnon is here for her yearly physical exam (she is 25) and also to receive a tetanus booster. How will you code this visit?

_____

_____

_____

Case 2

Kevin Wyman was rushed to the hospital with acute RLQ pain. Dr. Buckwalter examined him in the ED. After a complete history and exam and U/S of his abdomen, it was found that his appendix had ruptured. An emergency appendectomy was performed. Code the ED visit, the abdominal ultrasound (complete), and the appendectomy.

_____

_____

_____

Case 3

The new medical assistant in the office insists on using the "vague" supply code of 99070 because she has never used the HCPCS manual. What can you tell her so that she understands the importance of the HCPCS manual? Why is it important in this case that the HCPCS manual be used instead of the CPT code of 99070?

_____

_____

_____

PROCEDURE 19-1 Locating a CPT Code

Goal
To locate correct CPT codes using the CPT manual.

OSHA Guidelines
This procedure does not involve exposure to blood, body fluids, or tissue.

Materials
Patient record, superbill or charge slip containing procedure(s) performed, CPT manual.

Method

Step Number	Procedure	Points Possible	Points Earned
1.	Find the services listed on the superbill (if used) and in the patient's record.	10	
	a. Check the patient's record to see which services were documented. For E/M procedures, note whether the patient is a new or established patient and then look for clues as to the location of the service, extent of history, examination, and medical decision making that were involved.*	15	
2.	Look up the procedure code(s) in the Alphabetic Index of the CPT manual.	10	
	a. Verify the code number in the numeric index, reading all notes and guidelines for that section.*	10	
	b. If a code range is noted, look up each code in the range and choose the correct code given in the Tabular Index. If the correct description is not found, start the process again. Use the same process if multiple codes are given, looking each one up in the numeric index until you find the correct code description.	15	
3.	Determine appropriate modifiers.	10	
	a. Check section guidelines and Appendix A to choose a modifier if needed to explain a situation involving the procedure being coded, such as bilateral procedure, surgical team, or a discontinued procedure.	5	
4.	Carefully record the procedure code(s) on the healthcare claim, or, if the office is computerized, enter the codes into the office billing system for placement on an electronic health claim form. Usually the primary procedure, the one that is the primary reason for the encounter or visit, is listed first.	10	
5.	Match each procedure with its corresponding diagnosis. The primary procedure is often (but not always) matched with the primary diagnosis.*	15	
Total Points		100	

CAAHEP Competencies Achieved
   VIII. P (1)   Perform procedural coding

ABHES Competencies Achieved
   8. (t) Perform diagnostic and procedural coding

Name_____ Date_____

Evaluated by_____ Score_____

PROCEDURE 19-2 Locating a HCPCS Code

Goal
To locate correct HCPCS codes using the HCPCS manual.

OSHA Guidelines
This procedure does not involve exposure to blood, body fluids, or tissue.

Materials
Patient record, superbill or charge slip containing procedure(s) performed, HCPCS manual.

Method

Step Number	Procedure	Points Possible	Points Earned
1.	Locate the service, supplies, and equipment requiring a HCPCS code from the encounter form from the patient's record. If an encounter form is used, verify procedure completion in the medical record.	15	
2.	Use the Alphabetic Index in the beginning of the manual to locate the section in which the category of codes is found.	20	
3.	Find the code or code range listed, reading descriptions carefully. Do not code from the Alphabetic Index.*	15	
4.	Look up the code or each code in the code range listed in the Tabular Index. Read descriptions carefully.*	20	
5.	Make sure the code is valid for the type of insurance the patient carries.	15	
6.	Enter the correct code(s) on the superbill or encounter form (if necessary) and, if the office uses a computerized billing program, in the patient's computerized record so that it can be used for billing purposes. Otherwise, place the HCPCS code in block 24d of the 1500 claim form for submission to the insurance carrier. Match each HCPCS code with the appropriate diagnosis code to demonstrate medical necessity.	15	
Total Points		100	

CAAHEP Competencies Achieved
VIII. P (1) Perform procedural coding

ABHES Competencies Achieved
8. (t) Perform diagnostic and procedural coding

PROCEDURE 19-3 Entering CPT/HCPCS and ICD Codes into an EHR Program

Goal
To enter procedure and diagnosis codes into the SpringCharts™ EHR /Billing Program.

OSHA Guidelines
This procedure does not involve exposure to blood, body fluids, or tissue.

Materials
Paper or Electronic Superbill, patient's medical record and computer with SpringCharts™ EHR program loaded.

Method

Step Number	Procedure	Points Possible	Points Earned
1.	Open the appropriate patient's record in the EHR Program.	8	
2.	Click **Assessment**.	6	
3.	Click **Add Diagnosis** and then **Search**.	6	
4.	Key in the first few words of the diagnosis, such as **Type II Diabetes**.	6	
5.	Based on the information on the superbill or in the medical record, choose the correct diagnosis for the patient's visit.	8	
6.	When the diagnosis is chosen, click **OK**.	6	
7.	Click **Plan** and then **Search**.	6	
8.	Click **Search for Code**	6	
9.	Locate the correct description/code for the procedure performed in the **Procedure Code Search** field.	8	
10.	Strike the **tab** key to confirm your entry.	6	
11.	Click **Search** and choose the procedure you just found.	8	
12.	Click ***Category**.	6	
13.	Choose the correct service category for the procedure performed.	6	
14.	Click **OK**.	6	
15.	Confirm the entries are correct and saved in the **Orders** section.	8	
Total Points		100	

CAAHEP Competencies Achieved

V. P. V (5)   Execute data management using electronic healthcare records such as the EMR

ABHES Competencies Achieved

7. b. (2) Apply computer application skills using a variety of different electronic programs including both practice management software and EMR software

8. (ll) Apply electronic technology

Patient Billing and Collections

Name_____ Class_____ Date_____

R E V I E W

Vocabulary Review

Matching

Match the key terms in the right column with the definitions in the left column by placing the letter of each correct answer in the space provided.

_____ 1. Another name for a patient bill

_____ 2. Patient account that receives periodic charges

_____ 3. Document that tracks accounts by the date of last payment

_____ 4. Patient billing where accounts are split in groups with staggered statement mailing dates

_____ 5. Money owed to other businesses by the practice

_____ 6. Document signed by the patient and practice when a payment agreement is met, consisting of four or more payments.

_____ 7. Company that tracks individuals' credit histories

_____ 8. Legal proceeding involving a group of individuals who were all wronged in the same way by a specific company

_____ 9. Account where services to be performed are written out and the document is signed by the person performing the service and the person receiving the services

_____ 10. Document revealing any service charge or interest payments to be charged when payments are to be spread out over a specific time frame; also known as TLS

_____ 11. Account consisting of only one charge or one date of service

_____ 12. Money or funds that are owed to the practice for services provided

_____ 13. Person who is responsible for a patient's debt

_____ 14. The balance resulting from an overpayment on a patient's account

_____ 15. Allowing a patient to pay for services at a time other than the time of service

a. accounts payable (A/P)
b. accounts receivable (A/R)
c. age analysis
d. class action lawsuit
e. credit
f. credit balance
g. single-entry account
h. statement
i. written-contract account
j. credit bureau
k. cycle billing
l. disclosure statement
m. guarantor
n. open-book account
o. Truth in Lending statement

Content Review

Multiple Choice

In the space provided, write the letter of the choice that best completes each statement or answers each question.

_____ 1. A superbill
   a. Includes the charges for services rendered on that day
   b. Is given to the doctor after he sees the patient
   c. Is inappropriate if the patient has insurance
   d. Is mailed to the patient when the account is 30 days past due
   e. Is always completed electronically

_____ 2. A practice may buy accounts receivable insurance to protect the practice from
   a. Welfare patients   d. Malpractice
   b. Employee theft   e. All of the above
   c. Lost income because of nonpayment

_____ 3. The Fair Debt Collection Practices Act of 1977
   a. Allows you to call patients at any time to get payment
   b. Permits you to threaten to turn the account over to collections
   c. Permits you to harass the patient daily for payment
   d. Governs the methods that can be used to collect unpaid debts
   e. Permits you to call a patient at work

_____ 4. Free treatment for hardship cases should be
   a. Up to the receptionist to allow
   b. Expected by all patients in all cases
   c. At the doctor's discretion
   d. Never permitted
   e. Based on the patient's financial statement

_____ 5. Acceptable form(s) of payment in many medical practices include
   a. Insurance   d. Credit card
   b. Debit card   e. All of the above
   c. Check

_____ 6. A hardship case is defined as a person who is
   a. Poor   d. Elderly
   b. Underinsured   e. a, b, and c
   c. Uninsured

_____ 7. The purpose of an age analysis is to
   a. Determine which accounts to turn over to collections
   b. Determine how much money is owed to the practice and how long it has been outstanding
   c. Classify and review past-due accounts
   d. All of the above
   e. a and b only

_____ 8. Most practices begin the collection process with
   a. Telephone calls, home visits, or letters
   b. Telephone calls, letters, or statements
   c. Credit checks, letters, or statements
   d. Credit checks or collection agencies
   e. Contracts or age analyses

_____ 9. The patient's first bill or "statement" occurs
    a. At the time of service with receipt of the superbill
    b. 7 days after service
    c. 14 days after service
    d. 30 days after service
    e. At the discretion of the practice

_____ 10. When sending a statement for the care of a minor, the statement should be addressed to
    a. The patient
    b. The patient only if he or she is not emancipated
    c. Either parent
    d. The guarantor
    e. Any of the above

Sentence Completion

In the space provided, write the word or phrase that best completes each sentence.

11. The Truth in Lending Act covers bilateral credit agreements that involve more than _____ payments.

12. A _____ provides information about the creditworthiness of a person seeking credit.

13. The _____ prevents creditors from calling the patient before 8 a.m. or after 9 p.m. to request payment.

14. When a physician treats other doctors for free, it is referred to as extending a _____.

15. If the physician and patient enter into a unilateral agreement about the patient's outstanding bill, the _____ currently owed will be billed to the patient monthly.

16. Age analysis is the process of _____ and _____ a past-due account by _____ from the _____ date of billing.

17. According to the AMA, it is appropriate to assess _____ or late charges on past-due accounts if the patient is notified _____.

18. Collection agencies typically keep _____ of collected funds as payment for their services.

19. The _____ states that if a patient is extended credit for any reason, any other patient in a similar circumstance must also be offered a similar credit arrangement.

20. A patient who moves before paying his debt and leaves no forwarding address or contact information is known as a _____.

11. _____
12. _____
13. _____
14. _____
15. _____
16. _____
_____
_____
_____
_____
17. _____
_____
18. _____
19. _____
20. _____

Short Answer

Write the answer to each question on the lines provided.

21. Describe what cycle billing means and give an example.

_____

_____

_____

22. Explain the "assumption" that should be made when a divorced parent brings a child in for treatment (if legal documentation of payment arrangements has not been provided to the office).

_____

_____

_____

23. In an open-book account, does the time limit for collection begin when the account is initiated? Why or why not?

_____

_____

_____

24. What "tone" should be used when making initial phone calls about a patient's overdue account? Why?

_____

_____

_____

25. Why is it important that collection proceedings not be threatened unless the proceedings will take place on the date given to the patient?

_____

_____

_____

A P P L I C A T I O N   WORK // DOC

Follow the directions for each application

1. Writing a Collection Letter

Using the guidelines described within the chapter, write a "payment is due" collection letter to Sharon Milford, who owes BWW Medical Associates $125, which is now over-due by 60 days. BWW Medical Associates letterhead is provided for your final document.

2. Making a Collection Phone Call

With a partner, role-play a scenario in which you, as the medical assistant, make an initial request for payment over the phone to a patient who is late in making a payment for her bill (balance is $225.00). Your partner should act as the patient, offering information or explanations as she chooses, and you must respond appropriately. Change places and let your partner act as the medical assistant and you act as the patient.

3. Accounts Receivable Age Analysis

Using the Accounts Receivable—Age Analysis Worksheet provided, enter the following patients' account information in the table. At the end of the entries, complete the total age analysis amounts for the practice.

a. Mary Simmons charged services on August 12 and has a balance of $300 with the entire amount over 120 days. She has been sent three notices by the office and was just sent a certified letter requesting payment on her account. She has made no payments to the account.

b. Frank Brown has a balance of $140, which was charged on September 30. He made a payment on October 5; $40 is 60 days past due and the remainder 90 days past due. An initial notice was sent to him requesting a payment on this account.

c. Harvey Jenson has a balance of $600 for services charged on November 8. He made four payments on the account, the last of which was received on November 30. He has not been sent a notice of payment due.

d. Theodore Thomas has a balance of $720 charged on September 18. He made a payment on October 15. His insurance company, Blue Cross Blue Shield, has been billed for the charges.

e. Adam Cooper has a balance of $1400 charged on June 1. He has made no payment on this account and has no insurance. This account was turned over to a collections agency on December 15.

f. Sally Carson has a balance of $75 charged on November 1. She has made no payment to the account, and a Medicare claim was filed.

Accounts Receivable–Age Analysis   Date:

Patient	Balance	Date of Charges	Most Recent Payment	30 days	60 days	90 days	120 days	Remarks
TOTAL								

Source: From Helen Houser and Terri Wyman, ADMINISTRATIVE MEDICAL ASSISTING: A WORKFORCE READINESS APPROACH, 1/e. © 2012 McGraw Hill Companies, Inc. Reprinted with permission.

C A S E   S T U D I E S

Write your response to each case study on the lines provided.

Case 1

A patient comes to you to pay for his office visit. He hands you the check and says he is in a hurry and cannot wait for a receipt. He leaves, and you notice he has not signed the check. What do you do?

_____

_____

_____

Case 2

Brenda is a new biller for the medical clinic where you are employed as the medical assistant. There are several patient accounts with large unpaid balances, and payments have not been made for weeks or, in some cases, several months. The physician has asked you to assist Brenda in contacting these patients about their delinquent accounts to try to collect some or all the money owed on these accounts. Brenda asks you to observe her first call to a patient who owes $250 on a bill that is over 3 months old. She threatens the patient that, if some payment is not made by the end of the week, the account will be turned over to a collection agency. She also tells the patient that the physician may not be able to treat her again until this bill is settled. You know that this is an inappropriate way to talk to a patient about this type of issue. You know that you should talk with Brenda about this approach to collecting bills.

1. What did Brenda say that was inappropriate as a method to collect the debt?

_____

_____

_____

2. What should you tell Brenda about the way she handled this call?

_____

_____

_____

Case 3

Maria Torres has come to the office today complaining of chest pain. After seeing the physician, you need to complete the superbill. Using the blank superbill provided for BWW Medical Associates, and following Procedure 20-1, complete the superbill using the following information.

Patient: Maria Torres   MRN: 001-564-879   DOB: 6/4/xx
Insurance: Aetna   Subscriber: Patient   Group: 56123

Procedures: 99213 - $82.00, 93000 - $45.00, 36415 - $15.00
Diagnoses: Chest wall pain, Anxiety syndrome
Payment Made: $25.00 copayment
Physician: Elizabeth Williams, MD   Return Appt: PRN

PROCEDURE 20-1 Using the Superbill as Bill/Receipt [WORK // DOC]

Goal
To complete a superbill accurately for use as the patient first bill or receipt.

OSHA Guidelines
This procedure does not involve exposure to blood, body fluids, or tissue.

Materials
Superbill, patient ledger card, patient information sheet, fee schedule, and a pen.

Method

Step Number	Procedure	Points Possible	Points Earned
1.	From the patient ledger card and information sheet, fill in the patient data, such as name, sex, date of birth, and insurance information.*	9	
2.	Fill in the date of service. If there are multiple practice locations, circle the location where the service is taking place.	9	
3.	Attach the superbill to the patient's medical record, and give both to the physician.	9	
4.	At the end of the visit, accept the completed superbill from the patient. Make sure the doctor has indicated the procedures performed and an appropriate diagnosis for each.*	9	
5.	If the physician has not already recorded the charges, refer to the fee schedule for marked procedures. Then fill in the charges next to those procedures.	9	
6.	In the appropriate blanks, list the total charges for the visit and the previous balance (if any).*	9	
7.	Calculate the subtotal.	9	
8.	Fill in the amount and type of payment (cash, check, money order, debit or credit card) made by the patient during this visit.	9	
9.	Calculate and enter the new balance.	10	
10.	If not already on file, have the patient sign the authorization-and-release section of the superbill.	9	
11.	Keep a copy of the superbill for the practice records. Give the original to the patient along with one copy to file with the insurer.	9	
Total Points		100	

CAAHEP Competencies Achieved
VI. P (2b) Perform billing procedures

ABHES Competencies Achieved
8. (i) Perform billing and collection procedures

8. (k) Perform accounts receivable procedures

PROCEDURE 20-2 Preparing an Age Analysis   【WORK // DOC】

Goal
To create and examine an age analysis of practice accounts.

OSHA Guidelines
This procedure does not involve exposure to blood, body fluids, or tissue.

Materials
Computer, patient accounts, ledger cards (if a manual system is used), accounts receivable age analysis form or template (Figure 20-5), policy and procedure manual, and a pen.

Method

Step Number	Procedure	Points Possible	Points Earned
1.	Using the reporting section of your billing computer program, create an age analysis report for patients and insurance companies. This also can be done manually by pulling patient ledger cards and noting balances due and dates of last payments. Use Figure 20-5 as a guide to create a spreadsheet for your findings.	10	
2.	Review the accounting report—highlight each account for proposed actions according to your office policy.*	10	
3.	Mark the accounts that are under 31 days as "No action to be taken at this time."	10	
4.	Bills that are unpaid at more than 31 days should be marked as "Contact or follow up with insurance company."	10	
5.	Accounts that are 31–60 days old should be marked according to your office policy. An initial phone call may be made inquiring as to payment arrangements.	10	
6.	Accounts that are 61–90 days old should be marked according to your office policy. Make notations such as "Account Past Due." A follow-up phone call and/or more insistent statement message letter for payment may be in order.	10	
7.	Accounts that are 91–120 days old should be marked according to your office policy. A last phone call to attempt discussing the account and a more insistent collection statement/letter should be sent.	10	
8.	For accounts older than 120 days, make sure you review previous collection attempts. At this point, after discussion with the physician, produce a letter stating that the account will be turned over to the collection agency on a specific date listed in the letter. This letter should be mailed by certified, return receipt mail.	10	
9.	Record all actions that have been taken beside each account.*	10	
10.	Finally, write follow-up letters to patients and document any agreements you and the patient have discussed via telephone. Be sure to keep a copy of any correspondence mailed to the patient in the financial record.*	10	
Total Points		100	

CAAHEP Competencies Achieved
VI. P (2)   Perform accounts receivable procedures

ABHES Competencies Achieved
8. (k) Perform accounts receivable procedures

PROCEDURE 20-3 Referring an Account to Collection Agency and Posting the Payment from the Agency

Goal
To follow the correct procedure in turning an account over to a collection agency and posting the payment from them when received.

OSHA Guidelines
This procedure does not involve exposure to blood, body fluids, or tissue.

Materials
Computer, patient accounts, ledger cards (if a manual system is used), patient's financial record containing demographic information, collection agency's phone number, pen.

Method

Step Number	Procedure	Points Possible	Points Earned
1.	Make sure all attempts made to collect the debt per office policy have been documented, including the return receipt from the letter sent to the patient stating the account would be turned over to the collection agency by a specific date (today).	11	
2.	Verify that the following information is in the patient's financial file to be turned over to the collection agency:* • Last known phone number and address for the patient • Employer (if any) name and phone number • Name of spouse, if applicable • Total amount of debt, with last payment amount and date • If there has been no payment, the last date a service was provided • Description of office actions to collect debt • Any patient response to those actions	13	
3.	Place a call to the agency, identifying yourself and the office, explaining you are calling to turn accounts over to them.	11	
4.	For each account to be turned over, supply the information listed in step 2.*	13	
5.	When a payment arrives from the agency, each account will be identified with the total amount of the debt collected. The agency will also deduct their fee from this amount.	13	
6.	When posting the payment, post the actual amount of the payment sent to the office from the collection agency to the patient's account, not the full amount of the payment made by the patient.*	13	
7.	Make an adjustment (write off) on the patient's account in the amount kept by the agency as their fee.	13	
8.	Subtract both the payment and the adjustment from the patient's balance. If the payment is noted by the agency as being the full payment on the account, the payment and adjustment should result in a zero balance on the patient's account.*	13	
Total Points		100	

CAAHEP Competencies Achieved

VI. P (2c)   Perform collection procedure

VI. P (2h)   Post collection agency payments

ABHES Competencies Achieved

8. (i) Perform billing and collection procedures

8. (k) Perform accounts receivable procedures

8. (m) Post collection agency payments

PROCEDURE 20-4 Completing a Truth in Lending Statement (Agreement)

Goal
To create an accurate and complete Truth in Lending Statement.

OSHA Guidelines
This procedure does not involve exposure to blood, body fluids, or tissue.

Materials
Computer, paper, patient financial record, the name of the procedure or service to be financed, total cost of procedure or service to be financed, amount of down payment, number of payments, amount of each payment, date of month for each payment, pen.

Method

Step Number	Procedure	Points Possible	Points Earned
1.	Create a document (or use a template) similar to that of Figure 20-7 to use as the Truth in Lending Statement.	16	
2	Make sure the following information is included: • Patient name and address • Price for service or procedure • Amount of down payment received • Unpaid balance • Amount financed • Finance charge (if applicable) • Finance charge as a percentage rate (if applicable) • Total amount to be financed • Number of payments and the amount of each • Date payments are due, including final payment date*	20	
3.	Once the template is completed, fill in the information for the patient's agreement. Make calculations carefully and check your work.	16	
4.	After going over the statement with the patient, have the patient sign and date the agreement.*	16	
5.	Give a copy of the signed agreement to the patient and keep a copy in the patient's financial record for future reference.*	16	
6.	If desired, a master document, such as that found in Figure 20-8, may be created outlining the agreement and listing the actual date and payment amount for each month of the agreement.	16	
Total Points		100	

CAAHEP Competencies Achieved

VI. P (2c)   Perform collection procedure

ABHES Competencies Achieved

8. (i) Perform billing and collection procedures

Financial Management

Name_____ Class_____ Date_____

Vocabulary Review

Matching

Match the key terms in the right column with the definitions in the left column by placing the letter of each correct answer in the space provided.

_____ 1. A financial instrument of guaranteed payment, which may be purchased from a bank, a post office, or some convenience stores

_____ 2. A person who receives a check in payment

_____ 3. The term for the legal right to act as the attorney or agent of another person, including handling that person's financial matters

_____ 4. The process of logging charges and receipts in a chronological list in the daily log

_____ 5. A monthly comparison of the office's financial records with bank records to ensure that they are consistent and accurate

_____ 6. A payer's check written and signed by the payer, and stamped by the bank, indicating the bank has already withdrawn money from the payer's account to guarantee that the check will be paid

_____ 7. Document or instrument that is legally transferable from one person to another.

_____ 8. A check made out to one recipient and given in payment to another, for instance, an insurance check made out to a patient which is then signed over to the medical practice

_____ 9. The systematic recording of business transactions

_____ 10. A person who pays a bill or writes a check

._____ 11. A business check with an attached stub, which is kept as a receipt

_____ 12. A special bank check that allows a depositor to draw funds from his own account, as when he has forgotten his checkbook

_____ 13. The signing or stamping of the back of a check with the proper identification of the person or organization to whom the check is written, to prevent the check from being cashed if it is stolen or lost

_____ 14. A check of preprinted denominations, purchased and signed at a bank and later signed over to a payee

_____ 15. A check purchased in a bank and signed by a bank representative, usually purchased for large purchases requiring guaranteed payment or by those without personal checking accounts

a. bookkeeping
b. cash flow statement
c. cashier's check
d. certified check
e. counter check
f. endorsement
g. journalizing
h. limited check
i. money order
j. negotiable
k. third-party check
l. tracking
m. traveler's check
n. voucher check
o. payee
p. payer
q. power of attorney
r. reconciliation
s. write-it-once (pegboard) system

_____ 16. The bookkeeping system that uses a lightweight board with pegs on which forms can be stacked, allowing each transaction to be entered and recorded on four bookkeeping forms simultaneously

_____ 17. A check that is valid to a maximum amount or is void after a certain amount of time

_____ 18. A periodic document that shows the cash on hand at the beginning of a period, the income and disbursements made during the period, and the new amount of cash on hand at the end of the period

_____ 19. Watching for changes in expenses or disbursement patterns

True or False

Decide whether each statement is true or false. In the space at the left, write T *for true or* F *for false. On the lines provided, rewrite the false statements to make them true.*

_____ 20. Medical assistants should obtain information for the daily log from word of mouth from patients.

_____

_____ 21. Reconciliation means to compare the records of the medical practice with the records of the patient.

_____

_____ 22. To help with the practice's bookkeeping and banking, you need to understand basic accounting systems and have certain financial management skills.

_____

_____ 23. After accepting a check, you should set it carefully aside for the endorsement process, which should be done in a batch with other checks.

_____

_____ 24. All bookkeeping systems include records of income, charges (money owed to the practice), and disbursements (money paid out by the practice).

_____

_____ 25. A check will be nonnegotiable if it is signed.

_____

_____ 26. Information on a patient ledger card includes the patient's name, address, phone number(s), and the name of the guarantor (if different from the patient).

_____

_____ 27. Patient accounting methods within a medical practice may be computerized or manual, with the manual method being the most commonly used type of system.

_____

_____ 28. The face, or front, of every check contains two important items: the ABA number and the endorsement area.

_____

_____ 29. Electronic banking can improve productivity, cash flow, and accuracy.

_____

_____ 30. The statement of income and expense, also known as a *cash flow statement,* highlights the practice's profitability.

_____

Content Review

Multiple Choice

In the space provided, write the letter of the choice that best completes each statement or answers each question.

_____ 1. An example of an accounts payable item is
   a. The monthly lease due on the office space
   b. The outstanding balance on a patient's ledger card
   c. The employees' biweekly salary
   d. The insurance premium for professional liability
   e. a, c, and d

_____ 2. If a patient's check does not clear due to nonsufficient funds (NSF), the practice should
   a. Not allow the patient to be seen by the physician
   b. Abandon the patient by not providing future care
   c. Adjust the account accordingly, adding the amount back to the account
   d. Send a collections letter to the patient
   e. Write off the amount of the check

_____ 3. When a check for payment from a patient is received some time after the patient's visit, the medical assistant should
   a. Hold it until the end of the week and do a batch entry of all checks received that week
   b. Deposit it in the bank and wait for it to clear, then post it to the patient's ledger card
   c. Place it with all the other checks received that day and post them the following day after the checks have been deposited
   d. Staple the envelope to the check and hold it until the end of the week
   e. Record it on the patient's ledger card and day sheet on the day received

_____ 4. The ABA number on a check appears
   a. As a fraction in the top-right side of the check
   b. Next to the routing number on the bottom of the check
   c. Below the signature line on the front of the check
   d. On the back of the check above the endorsement line
   e. Adjacent to the account number on the check

_____ 5. A third-party check
   a. Should never be accepted under any circumstances
   b. Is always written to the practice
   c. May be accepted if it is from the patient's health insurance company
   d. May be accepted as payment in full on the patient's account
   e. Should be deposited and credited to the patient's account when it clears the bank

_____ 6. Medical practices prefer electronic banking because
   a. It improves productivity
   b. Cash flow is usually increased
   c. There is improved accuracy in banking records
   d. Answers a and c only
   e. a, b, and c

_____ 7. What is the reconciled ending balance for a checking account with a balance of $1,800.00 on the month-end statement from the bank, with $3,200.00 deposited during that month, which is not yet showing, and $600.00 in outstanding checks that have not yet posted to the account?
    a. $4,400.00
    b. $2,600.00
    c. $2,000.00
    d. $1,800.00
    e. $1,200.00

_____ 8. A patient's beginning account balance is $30.00. The charge for medical services today is $40.00. A payment is made on the account today in the amount of $50.00. What is the current balance due on this account?
    a. $0.00
    b. $10.00
    c. $20.00
    d. $30.00
    e. $40.00

_____ 9. When an insurance company makes a payment to a medical practice for services rendered to a patient and the patient also makes a payment on the account, causing it to exceed the allowed charges, it is called
    a. Account imbalance
    b. Excessive billing
    c. Payment reconciliation
    d. Overpayment
    e. Incorrect billing

_____ 10. Sequentially, the first step in reconciling a bank account is to
    a. Check the closing balance on the previous bank statement against the opening statement balance on the new bank statement
    b. Place all the redeemed checks in numerical order
    c. Ensure that all deposits have posted
    d. Place a check mark on all checks if they are listed on the bank statement
    e. Subtract any service charges from the ending balance on the bank statement

_____ 11. A best practice for depositing checks is to
    a. Send all checks collected in one envelope through the mail to the bank
    b. Collect all checks for a 1-week period of time and deposit them all at one time
    c. Deposit checks on a daily basis in person at the bank
    d. Endorse all the checks at the end of the week and make a single deposit
    e. Mail the checks individually to the bank so if lost, only one check is missing

_____ 12. Which of the following features is not available with all medical office electronic banking software programs?
    a. Record deposits
    b. Manage payroll
    c. Pay bills
    d. Display a checkbook
    e. Balance a checkbook

_____ 13. A patient's ledger card would *not* include the
  a. Patient's insurance policy number
  b. Physician's DEA number
  c. Physician's practice name and address
  d. Patient's full name
  e. Patient's work phone number

_____ 14. Which of the following conditions should be met in order for a check to be negotiable?
  a. The check must be written and signed by the payer
  b. The check must be payable to the payee
  c. The check must include the amount of money to be paid
  d. The check must have the name of the bank on the check
  e. All of the above

_____ 15. Which formula would be used to balance a day sheet or a patient's ledger?
  a. Previous balance + Today's charges − (Payments − Adjustments) = Current balance
  b. Current balance + Today's charges + (Payments − Adjustments) = Previous balance
  c. Previous balance − Today's charges + (Payments − Adjustments) = Current balance
  d. Current balance − Today's charges + (Payments − Adjustments) = Current balance
  e. Previous balance − Today's charges   (Payments − Adjustments) = Current balance

_____ 16. The purpose of the daily log is to
  a. Provide a list of all disbursements made
  b. List appointments
  c. Reconcile all finances
  d. Provide a record of each patient seen
  e. None of the above

_____ 17. In which of the following denominations are travelers' checks printed?
  a. $5, $10, $20, $50, $100
  b. $5, $10, $20, $50
  c. $5, $10, $20, $50, $100, $500
  d. $10, $20, $50, $100
  e. $10, $20, $50, $100, $500

_____ 18. If you make an error when writing a check, you should
  a. Use correction fluid to cover up the error and insert the correction
  b. Tear up the check and throw it away
  c. Write VOID in ink across the front of the check and file it in numerical order with the returned checks
  d. Scratch out the error and fill in the correction above it
  e. Any of the above

_____ 19. Which of the following checks could be used by the physician if she forgot her checkbook and wished to make a withdrawal from her account?
  a. Counter check
  b. Voucher check
  c. Limited check
  d. Cashier's check
  e. Travelers' check

_____ **20.** Which item of a check identifies the bank from which the check originated?

    a. The ABA number

    b. The payer

    c. The MICR number

    d. All of the above

    e. a and c only

Sentence Completion

In the space provided, write the word or phrase that best completes each sentence.

21. An accounts payable record shows the amounts the practice owes to _____.

22. _____ shows how much cash is available to cover expenses, invest, or take as profits.

23. Whereas assets are goods or properties that are part of the worth of a practice, liabilities are amounts owed by the practice on a(n) _____.

24. A person who receives a check is known as a _____.

25. In the daily log you enter the name of each patient seen that day. Across from the name, you record the _____ provided, the fee _____, and the _____ received.

26. To prevent theft of checks, always put the checkbook in a _____ place when it is not in use and file deposit receipts promptly. If they are lost, you have no _____ of the deposit.

27. Every day, you must update the accounts receivable record, which shows the total _____ to the practice.

28. A check that is _____ is legally transferable from one person to another.

29. A physician is likely to have three different types of checking accounts: a(n) _____ account, a(n) _____ account for office expenses, and a(n) _____ earning account.

30. The _____ endorsement is the safest type of endorsement to use because it will allow the check to be deposited only in a specified account.

21. _____

22. _____

23. _____

24. _____

25. _____

_____

_____

26. _____

_____

27. _____

28. _____

29. _____

_____

_____

30. _____

Short Answer

Write the answer to each question on the lines provided

31. Describe the importance of accuracy in bookkeeping and banking.

_____

_____

_____

32. List the three main types or groups of accounts payable and give one example of an accounts payable item for each group.

_____

_____

_____

33. Why is it advantageous to make frequent bank deposits?

_____

_____

_____

34. Explain why it is important to reconcile the monthly bank statement with your checkbook balance.

_____

_____

_____

35. What is the purpose of a deposit slip?

_____

_____

_____

A P P L I C A T I O N   WORK // DOC

Follow the directions for each application.

1. Create Ledger Cards and Post Payments on a Daysheet

   a. Create a ledger card for each of the following patients:

Name	Address	Phone	Wk Phone	SSN	Employer	Insurance	Policy #	Guarantor
Caryn Cooper	12 Smythe Ave Carver, YZ 54321	555-234-9012	555-789-6321	111223333	Comcast	Aetna	456321	Self
Jorge Cruz	102 Main Trail Port Snead, YZ 12345	555-432-9857	555-321-6547	222445555	Cruz Imports	BCBS	B332546	Self
Yolanda Yaz	21A Clough Street Port Snead, YZ 12345	555 432-6541	None	123543212	Retired	Medicare	123543212A	Self
Terry Ward	2 Old Main Road Carver, YZ 54321	555-234-3578	None	234565891	Student	Travelers	4567892	Dad Gerald
Dale Johnson	15 Vermont Road Port Snead, YZ 12345	555-432-8958	5558958951	231456897	State of YZ	HNE	879564	Self

b. Post charges, payments, and adjustments on the ledger cards and on the daysheet provided, using the information given below. You may use today's date.

- Caryn Cooper: No previous balance. Today's Services: 99202 & 81000. Total Charge $85.00. Copayment of $15.00 received.
- Jorge Cruz: Previous balance $128. Today's Service 99214. Total Charge $100.00. Payment $100.
- Yolanda Yaz: Previous balance 72.16. Today's Service 99213 & 85025. Total Charge $90.00. No payment today.
- Terry Ward: No previous balance. Today's Services 99243. Total Charge $145.00. Payment of $50.00 today.
- Dale Johnson: Previous balance 85.14. Today's Services 99212, 93000. Total Charge $95.00. Copayment of $25.00 received.
- Jorge Cruz: Insurance check arrives in the mail for $80.00. Insurance adjustment required of $22.50.
- Caryn Cooper: Notice received from bank that check received last week for $20.00 is returned for NSF. Office charge for NSF checks is $15.00.

BWW

BWW Medical Associates, PC
305 Main Street, Port Snead YZ 12345-9876
Tel: 555-654-3210, Fax: 555-987-6543
Web: BWWAssociates.com

Paul F. Buckwalter, MD
Alexis N. Whalen, MD
Elizabeth H. Williams, MD

Date: Today

Patient	Services	Chg	Paymt	Adj	Cur. Bal	Prev. Bal
Totals						

c. Balance the daysheet using formula given in the textbook.

2. Creating a Record of Office Disbursements

a. Using the form provided, complete a monthly Record of Office Disbursements using the following transactions for the month of July 20xx. Ensure that the entries are in order of occurrence and start with Check #106.

- 7/01 – Payment to La Jolla Property Management for rent, $1700.00.
- 7/01 – Payment to Anderson Janitorial for monthly office cleaning, $850.00.

- 7/01 – Payment to Office Depot for fax machine paper, $37.89.
- 7/01 – Payment to Pacific Telephone for monthly telephone services, $384.57.
- 7/01 – Payment to Pacific Gas Company for monthly gas and electric, $683.84.
- 7/01 – Cash for stamps at the post office, $32.00.
- 7/02 – Payment to Uni Lab for blood work, $55.00.
- 7/02 – Payment to Harris Medical Supply for general medical supplies, $75.00.
- 7/05 – Payment to Medi Quik X-Ray, $32.50.
- 7/06 – Payment to Staples Office Supply for general office supplies, $68.24.
- 7/12 – Payment to City Laundry (uniforms and towels), $125.00.
- 7/15 – Payment to Toni Guzzi (payroll), $176.08.
- 7/15 – Payment to Terri Smart (payroll), $289.84.
- 7/15 – Payment to Janet Garcia (payroll), $125.00.
- 7/15 – Payment to James Smith (payroll), $278.76.
- 7/17 – Payment to Toni Guzzi (reimbursement for travel expenses), $12.50.
- 7/20 – Stamps at post office from petty cash, $64.00.
- 7/23 – Payment to Medi Quik X-Ray, $35.87.
- 7/25 – Payment to World Wide Insurance, $189.00
- 7/30 – Payment to IRS, $537.00.

Record of Office Disbursements
_____ 20____

TYPES OF EXPENSES

DATE	PAYEE	CK. NO.	TOTAL AMOUNT	RENT	UTILITIES	POSTAGE	LAB./ X-RAY	MEDICAL SUPPLIES	OFFICE SUPPLIES	WAGES	INSURANCE	TAXES	TRAVEL	MISC.

Total

Source: From Helen Houser and Terri Wyman, ADMINISTRATIVE MEDICAL ASSISTING: A WORKFORCE READINESS APPROACH, 1/e. © 2012 McGraw Hill Companies, Inc. Reprinted with permission.

3. Reconciling Bank Statement

Use the bank reconciliation form provided.

The balance of the bank statement is $1326.00. The balance that is showing on your transaction journal is $1807.00.

Outstanding Deposits: 7/27/xx – $ 57.00; 7/28/xx – 163.00; 7/29/xx – 786.00

Checks outstanding: #98 – $115.00; #101 – 78.00; #103 – 18.00; #105 – 236.00

Auto deposit from BCBS: $103.00

Bank Fees: $25.00

BANK RECONCILIATION

CLIENT NAME: _____ MONTH OF: _____

BANK: _____ ACCOUNT NO. : _____

GENERAL LEDGER	BALANCE PER BANK STATEMENT
ACCOUNT BALANCE............................	AS OF:
ADD DEBITS:	ADD DEPOSITS IN TRANSIT:
TOTAL DR..............	
TOTAL...........................	TOTAL IN TRANSIT
	TOTAL................
LESS CREDITS:	
Checks	
Auto Withdrawals	
Bank Fees	
	LESS CHECKS OUTSTANDING:
	(SEE LIST BELOW)
TOTAL CR..............	TOTAL................
BANK BAL PER GENERAL LEDGER..	BANK BALANCE PER REC.................

CHECKS:

NUMBER	AMOUNT	NUMBER	NUMBER	NUMBER	AMOUNT
					TOTAL
TOTAL		TOTAL		GRAND TOTAL	

Source: From Helen Houser and Terri Wyman, ADMINISTRATIVE MEDICAL ASSISTING: A WORKFORCE READINESS APPROACH, 1/e. © 2012 McGraw Hill Companies, Inc. Reprinted with permission.

4. Making a Bank Deposit

The patients for today, July 22, 20xx, have all been seen and payments have been posted. It is now time to prepare the daily deposit slip. Complete the deposit slip blank provided using the following scenario:

Cash: 125.84

Checks:	25.00	653.99	145.75
	45.00	25.00	357.21
	18.72	58.10	15.00

DEPOSIT TICKET

BWW Medical Associates, PC

305 Main St.
Port Snead, YZ 12345-9876

DATE _____ **20**____
DEPOSITS MAY NOT BE AVAILABLE FOR IMMEDIATE WITHDRAWAL

_____

CASH	CURRENCY		
	COIN		
LIST CHECKS SINGLY			
TOTAL			
LESS CASH RECEIVED			
NET DEPOSIT			

89-852
———
622

BE SURE EACH ITEM IS
PROPERLY ENDORSED

FIRST NATIONAL BANK

CLINTON BRANCH

⑆062208525⑆ 526 6612 1⑈ 0789

CHECKS AND OTHER ITEMS ARE RECEIVED FOR DEPOSIT SUBJECT TO THE PROVISIONS OF THE UNIFORM COMMERCIAL CODE OR ANY APPLICABLE COLLECTION AGREEMENT

CHECKS LIST SINGLY	DOLLARS	CENTS
1		
2		
3		
4		
5		
6		
7		
8		
9		
10		
11		
12		
13		
14		
15		
TOTAL		

ENTER TOTAL ON THE FRONT SIDE OF THIS TICKET

C A S E   S T U D I E S

Write your response to each case study on the lines provided.

Case 1

You are assigned the task of completing the office monthly disbursement journal, and this is the first time you have been asked to do this. As you enter the numerous monthly expenditures on the log sheet, you realize there are some items that are ordered frequently and in greater quantity than expected. These expenses include office and administrative supplies such as printed letterhead, business envelopes, copy and fax paper, pens, notebooks, and file folders. It was not apparent until now that the office consumed so many administrative supplies each month.

a. Why is it important to be concerned about the expenditures for the practice?

_____

_____

_____

b. What are some recommendations you might make to the practice manager to better control the use of administrative supplies?

_____

_____

_____

Case 2

Your bank statement has arrived in the mail and the balance from the bank does not agree with the balance in your check register. Outline the steps you will take to reconcile this bank statement.

_____

_____

_____

Case 3

You are a senior medical assistant in a physician's office in charge of all the bookkeeping and banking tasks. You decided to take a couple of days off and handed your duties off to a less experienced medical assistant. All she needed to do was make the Friday deposit at the bank, and you were supposed to call her on Friday to be sure it was done. You wake up in the middle of the night and are startled to remember that you forgot to call and help her through the process. What methods would you use to determine if the deposit had been made correctly?

_____

_____

_____

PROCEDURE 21-1 Posting Charges, Payments, and Adjustments

WORK // DOC

Goal
To post charges, payments, and adjustments to the patient account.

OSHA Guidelines
This procedure does not involve exposure to blood, body fluids, or tissue.

Materials
Daily log sheets, patient ledger cards, and check register or computerized bookkeeping system; summaries of charges, receipts, and disbursements.

Method

Step Number	Procedure	Points Possible	Points Earned
1.	Create a ledger card (patient account) for each new patient, and maintain a ledger card for each existing patient. Include the following information on each ledger:*	12	
	a. Patient name **b.** Patient address **c.** Patient home and work phone numbers **d.** Insurance carrier with policy number and guarantor information	12	
2.	Update the ledger card every time the patient incurs a charge or makes a payment. Be sure to adjust the account balance after every transaction. In a computerized system, a patient record contains the same information as a ledger card. This record also must be maintained and updated.	12	
3.	Use a new log (day) sheet each day. For each patient seen that day:	4	
	a. Record the following: patient name, the relevant charges, and any payments received **b.** Calculate any necessary adjustments and new balances. **c.** When using a computerized system, enter the patient's name or account number, the relevant charges, along with any payments received and adjustments made in the appropriate areas. The computer program will calculate the new balances.*	12	
4.	Record all deposits accurately in the check register	12	
5.	File the deposit receipt—with a detailed listing of checks, cash, and money orders deposited—for later use in reconciling the bank statement.	12	
6.	The deposit amount should match the amount of money collected by the practice for that day.*	12	
7.	Prepare, or if using a computerized program, print a summary of charges, receipts, and disbursements every month, quarter, or year, as directed. Double-check all entries and calculations from the monthly summary before posting them to the quarterly summary. Also, double-check the entries and calculations from the quarterly summary before posting them to the yearly summary..	12	
Total Points		100	

CAAHEP Competencies Achieved

VI. P (2)   Perform accounts receivable procedures, including

a. Post entries on a day sheet

d. Post adjustments

VI. P (3)   Utilize computerized office billing systems

ABHES Competencies Achieved

8. (h) Post entries on a day sheet

8. (m) Post adjustments

Name_____   Date_____

Evaluated by_____   Score_____

PROCEDURE 21-2 Posting a Nonsufficient Funds (NSF) Check

`WORK // DOC`

Goal
To post a nonsufficient funds (NSF) check amount and any applicable fees to the patient account.

OSHA Guidelines
This procedure does not involve exposure to blood, body fluids, or tissue.

Materials
Computer, returned check, patient ledger, calculator (optional), daily log sheet.

Method

Step Number	Procedure	Points Possible	Points Earned
1.	Locate the patient's account on the computer or pull the patient's ledger card for manual processes.	25	
2.	Use your medical facility code for NSF check (if used) and, using today's date, create a new charge log for the patient. Use the code and the description *Check returned by bank* in the description column.	25	
3.	In the payment/adjustment column, place the amount of the check in parentheses to indicate that the amount is debited as an *adjustment*. Add the amount of the returned check to the old balance and enter it in the *current balance* column.*	25	
4.	On the next line, also using today's date, enter the medical facility's code for the NSF charge allowed by the office. Enter the charge amount in the *charge column* and add this amount to the patient's current balance.*	25	
Total Points		100	

CAAHEP Competencies Achieved

VI. P (2)   Perform accounts receivable procedures, including

   a. Post entries on a day sheet

   g. Post nonsufficient fund (NSF) checks

ABHES Competencies Achieved

8. (h) Post entries on a day sheet

8. (p) Post nonsufficient funds (NSF)

8. (w) Use manual or computerized bookkeeping systems

PROCEDURE 21-3 Processing a Payment Resulting in a Credit Balance

[WORK//DOC]

Goal
To process a payment that results in a credit balance on the patient account.

OSHA Guidelines
This procedure does not involve exposure to blood, body fluids, or tissue.

Materials
Daily log or day sheet, patient ledger card, computer, calculator, patient explanation of benefits (EOB) or remittance advice (RA) if applicable, and patient or insurance payment.

Method

Step Number	Procedure	Points Possible	Points Earned
1.	Locate the patient's account in the computer or pull the patient's ledger card for paper-based systems.	20	
2.	Post the total amount of the payment received to the patient's account by writing (or keying) the remittance amount in the paid column.*	20	
3.	Subtract the payment amount from the previous balance and insert the new balance in the balance column. If the balance created is a credit balance, insert the figure in the current balance column within parentheses.*	20	
4.	Review the account thoroughly, checking to see if any more receipts are expected on the patient's account.	20	
5.	If a credit balance is verified, adjust the credit balance off the patient's account by issuing a refund (see Procedure 21-4).	20	
Total Points		100	

CAAHEP Competencies Achieved

VI. P (2)   Perform accounts receivable procedures, including

       a. Post entries on a day sheet

       e. Process a credit balance

ABHES Competencies Achieved

   8. (h) Post entries on a day sheet

   8. (n) Process credit balances

PROCEDURE 21-4 Processing Refunds to Patients `WORK // DOC`

Goal
To process a patient refund due to a credit balance.

OSHA Guidelines
This procedure does not involve exposure to blood, body fluids, or tissue.

Materials
Payment (check), ledger card, computer, calculator, Remittance Advice (RA) or Explanation of Benefits (EOB), if applicable.

Method

Step Number	Procedure	Points Possible	Points Earned
1.	Calculate and determine the amount to be refunded (from Procedure 21-3). If the amount to be refunded is determined by the EOB or RA, verify the amount listed.	20	
2.	Record the check number and amount in the disbursements journal or checkbook and write a check to the patient for the amount to be refunded.*	20	
3.	Ask the physician or business manager to sign the check so that it can be given or mailed to the patient.	20	
4.	Post the refund as a negative payment (credit) to the patient's ledger card or to the patient's account if a computerized system is being used. Using parentheses around the figure is a common way to record the credit.*	20	
5.	Make a copy of the check, retaining a copy in the patient's financial record. Give or mail the check to the patient. If the check is being mailed, be sure to verify the patient's address prior to mailing and utilize certified return receipt mail to be sure the patient receives the check.	20	
Total Points		100	

CAAHEP Competencies Achieved

VI. P (2)   Perform accounts receivable procedures, including

a. Post entries on a day sheet

f. Process refunds

ABHES Competencies Achieved

8. (h) Post entries on a day sheet

8. (o) Process refunds

8. (w) Use manual or computerized bookkeeping systems

PROCEDURE 21-5 Making a Bank Deposit

WORK // DOC

Goal
To prepare cash and checks for deposit and to deposit them properly into a bank account.

OSHA Guidelines
This procedure does not involve exposure to blood, body fluids, or tissue.

Materials
Bank deposit slip and items to be deposited, such as checks, cash, and money orders.

Method

Step Number	Procedure	Points Possible	Points Earned
1.	Divide the bills, coins, checks, and money orders into separate piles.	10	
2.	Sort the bills by denomination, from largest to smallest. Then, stack them—portrait side up—in the same direction. Total the amount of the bills, and write this amount on the deposit slip on the line marked "currency" or cash.*	10	
3.	If you have enough coins to fill coin wrappers, put them in wrappers of the proper denomination. If not, count the coins, and put them in the deposit bag. Total the amount of coins, and write this amount on the deposit slip on the line marked "Coin."*	10	
4.	Review all checks and money orders to be sure they are properly endorsed with a restrictive endorsement. List each check on the deposit slip, including the check number and amount.*	10	
5.	List each money order on the deposit slip. Include the notation "money order" or "MO" and the name of the writer.	10	
6.	Calculate the total deposit (total of amounts or currency, coin, checks, and money orders). Write this amount on the deposit slip on the line marked "Total." If you do not use deposit slips that record a copy for the office, photocopy the deposit slip for your office records.	10	
7.	Record the total amount of the deposit in the office checkbook register.*	10	
8.	If you plan to make the deposit in person, place the currency, coins, checks, and money orders in a deposit bag. If you cannot make the deposit in person, put the checks and money orders in a special bank-by-mail envelope, or put all deposit items in an envelope and send it via registered mail.	10	
9.	Make the deposit in person or by mail.	10	
10.	Obtain a deposit receipt from the bank. File it with the copy of the deposit slip in the office for later use when reconciling the bank statement.	10	
Total Points		100	

CAAHEP Competencies Achieved

VI. P (1)   Prepare bank deposits

ABHES Competencies Achieved

8. (g) Prepare and reconcile a bank statement and deposit record

PROCEDURE 21-6 Reconciling the Bank Statement WORK//DOC

Goal
To ensure that the bank record of deposits, payments, and withdrawals agrees with the practice record of deposits, payments, and withdrawals.

OSHA Guidelines
This procedure does not involve exposure to blood, body fluids, or tissue.

Materials
Previous month's bank statement, current month's bank statement, reconciliation worksheet (if not part of current bank statement), deposit receipts, red pencil, check stubs or checkbook register, returned checks or listing of checks returned.

Method

Step Number	Procedure	Points Possible	Points Earned
1.	Check the closing balance on the previous month's statement against the opening balance on the current month's statement. The balances should match. If they do not, call the bank.*	9	
2.	Record the closing balance from the current statement on the reconciliation worksheet (Figure 21–9). This worksheet usually appears on the back of the bank statement.	9	
3.	Check each deposit receipt against the bank statement	3	
	a. Place a red check mark in the upper right corner of each receipt recorded on the statement.	6	
	b. Also place a check mark next to each deposit recorded in the checkbook to be sure none was skipped in this record.		
4.	Total the amount of deposits that do *not* appear on the statement. Add this amount to the closing balance from the bank on the reconciliation worksheet.	9	
5.	Compare each redeemed check with the bank statement, making sure that the amount on the check agrees with the amount on the statement.	3	
	a. Place a red check mark in the upper-right corner of each redeemed check recorded on the statement	6	
	b. Also, place a check mark on the check stub or check register entry.		
	c. Any checks that were written but that do not appear on the statement and were not returned as redeemed are considered "outstanding" checks. You can find these easily on the check stubs or checkbook register because they have no red check mark next to them.		
6.	List each outstanding check separately on the worksheet, including its check number and amount. Total the outstanding checks and subtract this total from the bank statement balance.	9	
7.	Record the ending balance found in the office checkbook in the appropriate area of the reconciliation worksheet˟	9	
8.	If the statement shows that the checking account earned interest, add this amount to the checkbook balance.	9	
9.	If the statement lists such items as service charge, check printing charge, or automatic payment, subtract them from the checkbook balance and add these charges to the checkbook register itself.	9	

(continued)

Step Number	Procedure	Points Possible	Points Earned
10.	Compare the new checkbook balance with the new bank statement balance. They should match. If they do not, repeat the process, rechecking all calculations. Double-check the addition and subtraction in the checkbook register. Review the checkbook register to make sure you did not omit any items. Ensure that you carried the correct balance forward from one register page to the next. Double-check that you made the correct additions or subtractions for all interest earned and charges incurred.*	10	
11.	If you have double-checked your work, and the balances still do not agree, ask a coworker to check your figures. If the coworker also finds no error or omission, call the bank to determine if a bank error has been made. Contact the bank promptly because the bank may have a time limit for corrections and may otherwise consider the bank statement correct if you do not point out an error within a specified time. Check with your individual bank for their policy.	9	
Total Points		100	

CAAHEP Competencies Achieved

VI. P (1)　　Prepare bank deposits

ABHES Competencies Achieved

8. (g) Prepare and reconcile a bank statement and deposit record

Name_____ Date_____

Evaluated by_____ Score_____

PROCEDURE 21-7 Setting Up the Disbursements Journal

`WORK // DOC`

Goal
To set up the office disbursements journal.

OSHA Guidelines
This procedure does not involve exposure to blood, body fluids, or tissue.

Materials
Disbursements journal (either paper or electronic), pen (if journal is in a paper format), listing of the headings required for the disbursements journal.

Method

Step Number	Procedure	Points Possible	Points Earned
1.	Write in or key column headings for the basic information required for each check: date, payee's name, check number, and check amount.	20	
2.	Enter column headings for each type of business expense, such as utilities, payroll, and taxes.*	20	
3.	Write in column headings (if space is available) for deposits and the account balance.	20	
4.	Record the data from completed checks under the appropriate column headings.*	20	
5.	Be sure to subtract payments from the balance and add deposits to it.*	20	
Total Points		100	

CAAHEP Competencies Achieved

VI. C (6)   Differentiate between accounts payable and accounts receivable

ABHES Competencies Achieved

8. (j) Perform accounts payable procedures

Organization of the Body

Name_____ Class_____ Date_____

REVIEW

Vocabulary Review

Matching

Match the key terms in the right column with the definitions in the left column by placing the letter of each correct answer in the space provided.

_____ 1. Matter that generally contains carbon and hydrogen

_____ 2. Combination of two or more atoms from different elements

_____ 3. Chemical combination of two or more atoms

_____ 4. Segment of DNA that determines a bodily trait

_____ 5. Anything that takes up space and has weight

_____ 6. Positively and negatively charged particles

_____ 7. Simplest unit of all matter

_____ 8. Results when errors occur during DNA duplication

_____ 9. Substance that releases ions in water

_____ 10. Matter that does not contain carbon and hydrogen

_____ 11. Contains base meaning of a medical term

_____ 12. Comes at beginning of a term; alters the meaning

_____ 13. Eases pronunciation of a term; does not change the meaning

_____ 14. Comes at the end of a term; alters the meaning

_____ 15. Smallest living unit

a. gene
b. combining vowel
c. mutations
d. organic
e. inorganic
f. cell
g. ions
h. suffix
i. compound
j. matter
k. word root
l. molecule
m. atoms
n. electrolytes
o. prefix

True or False

Decide whether each statement is true or false. In the space at the left, write T for true or F for false. On the lines provided, rewrite the false statements to make them true.

_____ 16. Diffusion is an active mechanism.

_____

_____ 17. PCR is the technique used to make multiple copies of even a fragment of DNA.

_____

_____ 18. Connective tissue covers the body and lines body cavities.

_____

_____ **19.** The ventral body cavity contains the brain and spinal cord.

_____ **20.** In anatomical position, the body is erect, with the head, feet, and palms all facing anteriorly.

_____ **21.** The shoulder is distal to the elbow.

_____ **22.** The abdominal and pelvic cavities are separated by the diaphragm.

_____ **23.** Organs are created by the combination of two or more tissue types.

_____ **24.** The iliac region is also known as the inguinal region.

_____ **25.** The appendix is found in the RUQ.

_____ **26.** Household detergents have a pH that is acidic.

_____ **27.** Oxygen is the most abundant inorganic compound in the body.

_____ **28.** The cell membrane contains three layers of phospholipid.

_____ **29.** A cell's energy comes from the nucleus.

_____ **30.** A sagittal plane divides the body into right and left portions.

Content Review

Multiple Choice
In the space provided, write the letter of the choice that best completes each statement or answers each question.

_____ **1.** The cavity that contains the heart, lungs, aorta, esophagus, and trachea
   a. Dorsal   **d.** Pelvic
   b. Abdominal   **e.** Ventral
   c. Thoracic

_____ **2.** If a characteristic is carried on the female chromosome, the disease produced is known as a(n) _____ disease.
   a. Recessive   **d.** Y-linked
   b. X-linked   **e.** Mutated
   c. Dominant

_____ 3. The plane that divides the body into inferior and superior portions
- **a.** Transverse
- **b.** Frontal
- **c.** Sagittal
- **d.** Midsagittal
- **e.** Coronal

_____ 4. Different forms of genes are called
- **a.** Traits
- **b.** Ribosomes
- **c.** Chromosomes
- **d.** DNA
- **e.** Alleles

_____ 5. Which organelles perform the digestive function of the cell?
- **a.** Ribosomes
- **b.** Golgi apparatus
- **c.** Lysosomes
- **d.** Centrioles
- **e.** Mitochondria

_____ 6. Which type of gland secretes its product directly into the bloodstream?
- **a.** Endocrine
- **b.** Exocrine
- **c.** Ductal
- **d.** Sweat
- **e.** Sebaceous

_____ 7. Which one of the following terms describes organs working together?
- **a.** Organelles
- **b.** Tissues
- **c.** Organisms
- **d.** Systems
- **e.** Cells

_____ 8. The ankle is _____ to the foot.
- **a.** Distal
- **b.** Inferior
- **c.** Proximal
- **d.** Lateral
- **e.** Superficial

_____ 9. Which directional term is used to describe front to back?
- **a.** Mediolateral
- **b.** Anteroposterior
- **c.** Posteroanterior
- **d.** Anterolateral
- **e.** Anteroinferior

_____ 10. A cell carrying out its everyday function is said to be in which of the following phases?
- **a.** Interphase
- **b.** Mitosis
- **c.** Meiosis
- **d.** Cytokinesis
- **e.** Prophase

Sentence Completion

In the space provided, write the word or phrase that best completes each sentence.

11. _____ is defined as the relative consistency of the body's internal environment.

12. _____ is the process that uses pressure to separate substances in a solution.

13. The diffusion of water across a semipermeable membrane is called _____.

14. _____ is the movement of a substance to an area of low concentration from an area of higher concentration.

15. The study of matter and chemical reactions in the body is known as _____.

16. The most abundant tissue in the body is _____ tissue.

17. During mitosis the splitting of cytoplasm is called _____.

18. _____ describes the overall chemical functioning of the body.

19. _____ is the study of matter composition and how it changes.

20. _____ describes the study of the body structures.

21. The study of each structure's function describes _____.

11. _____

12. _____

13. _____

14. _____

15. _____

16. _____

17. _____

18. _____

19. _____

20. _____

21. _____

Short Answer

Write the answer to each question on the lines provided.

22. Using the figure provided, label the cell organelles appropriately and also give the main function of each organelle.

Organelle	Organelle's Function
a. _____	_____
b. _____	_____
c. _____	_____
d. _____	_____
e. _____	_____
f. _____	_____
g. _____	_____
h. _____	_____
i. _____	_____
j. _____	_____
k. _____	_____

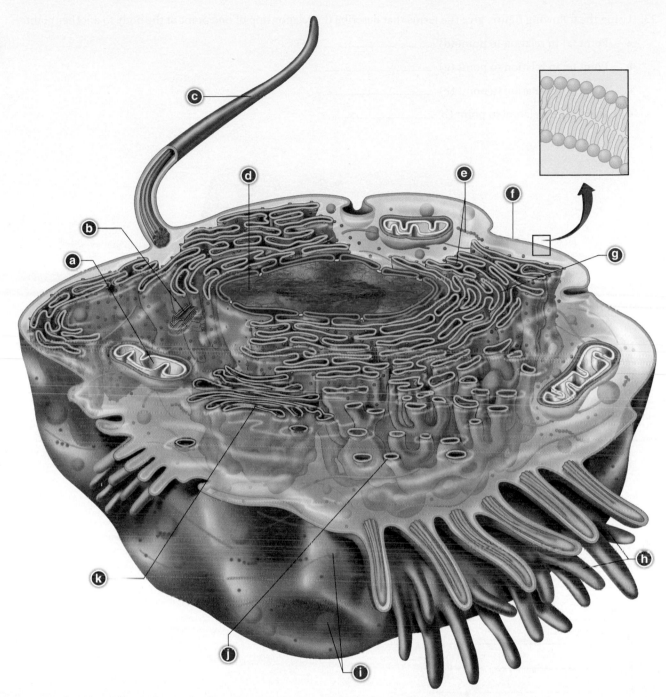

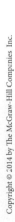
Source: From David Shier et al., HOLE'S HUMAN ANATOMY & PHYSIOLOGY, 12/e. © 2010 McGraw Hill Companies, Inc. Reprinted with permission.

23. Using the following figure, give the terms that describe the relationship of one point of the body to another point.

    a.   Point (a) in relation to point (d) _____

    b.   Point (e) in relation to point (g) _____

    c.   Point (e) in relation to point (b) _____

    d.   Point (d) in relation to point (b) _____

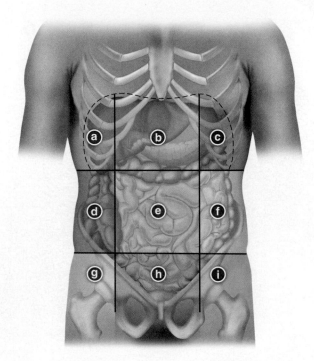

24. Using the previous figure, label each of the abdominal regions.

    a. _____

    b. _____

    c. _____

    d. _____

    e. _____

    f. _____

    g. _____

    h. _____

    i. _____

25. What are the four most common elements in the human body?

_____

_____

26. The following illustration shows the planes into which the body can be divided. Write the correct spatial terms on the blank lines in the illustration.

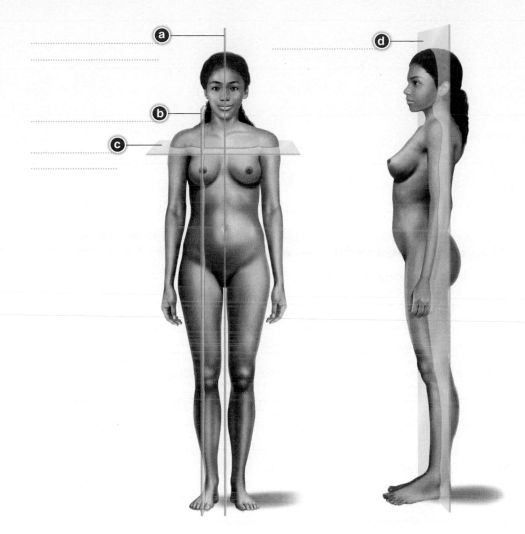

27. For each body cavity below, give its major divisions.

a. Dorsal cavity

_____

_____

_____

b. Ventral cavity

_____

_____

_____

c. Abdominopelvic cavity

_____

_____

_____

28. Give the locations of the following types of connective tissues.

a. Osseous tissue

_____

b. Blood

_____

c. Cartilage

_____

d. Dense connective tissue

_____

e. Adipose tissue

_____

Critical Thinking

Write the answer to each question on the lines provided.

1. Why are anatomy and physiology commonly studied together?

_____

_____

_____

2. As a medical assistant, why is it important for you to have a basic understanding of chemistry?

_____

_____

_____

3. How is mitosis different from meiosis? What is the importance of each?

_____

_____

_____

4. What are the clinical uses of PCR?

_____

_____

_____

5. If both parents have blonde hair, why can their children have brown, red, or very dark hair?

_____

_____

_____

A P P L I C A T I O N

Follow the directions for each application.

Major Tissue Types

The four major tissue types in the body are epithelial, connective, muscle, and nervous. They are the components used to make organs. For each organ listed, give the probable role of each tissue type.

a. Stomach _____

b. Heart _____

c. Urinary bladder _____

d. Biceps brachii (the muscle on the anterior surface of your arm) _____

C A S E   S T U D I E S

Write your response to each case study on the lines provided.

Case 1

Sickle-cell anemia is a disease that occurs when a person inherits two recessive alleles for this disease. If a man and a woman who both have the sickle-cell trait conceive a child, what is the chance that the child will have the disease?

_____

_____

_____

Case 2

What are some of the signs and symptoms of Down syndrome?

_____

_____

_____

Case 3

A baby has been diagnosed with PKU. What is this disorder and how must this baby's diet be modified?

_____

_____

_____

Case 4

You have been told that your child may have thalassemia. What tests may be used to test for this disorder?

_____

_____

_____

The Integumentary System

Name_____ Class_____ Date_____

REVIEW

Vocabulary Review

Matching

Match the key terms in the right column with the definitions in the left column by placing the letter of each correct answer in the space provided.

_____ 1. Also known as the subcutaneous layer

_____ 2. Epidermal cells that produce pigment

_____ 3. The term for hair loss (baldness)

_____ 4. The muscle that allows hair to stand erect

_____ 5. Cells that produce and accumulate protein in the epidermis

_____ 6. Sudoriferous glands that produce a watery type of sweat

_____ 7. A wart

_____ 8. The skin area innervated by a nerve

_____ 9. Sweat glands commonly activated by stress or nerves

_____ 10. A fungal infection

a. alopecia
b. apocrine
c. eccrine
d. keratinocyte
e. melanocyte
f. dermatome
g. arrector pili
h. hypodermis
i. tinea
j. verruca

True or False

Decide whether each statement is true or false. In the space at the left, write T for true or F for false. On the lines provided, rewrite the false statements to make them true.

_____ 11. The integumentary system is composed of skin, hair, and nails.

_____

_____ 12. The body needs vitamin A for calcium absorption.

_____

_____ 13. The stratum germinativum is also known as *stratum basale*.

_____

_____ 14. The stratum corneum is the epidermal layer that contains melanin.

_____

_____ 15. The subcutaneous layer is largely made of adipose tissue.

_____

_____ **16.** All people have about the same number of melanocytes regardless of their skin color.

_____

_____ **17.** Skin rashes that cause itching are known as purpura.

_____

_____ **18.** According to the rule of nines, one entire arm equals 18% of the body surface area.

_____

_____ **19.** A partial-thickness (second-degree) burn involves the epidermis and dermis.

_____

_____ **20.** A macule is any variation in the skin's surface or appearance.

_____

Content Review

Multiple Choice

In the space provided, write the letter of the choice that best completes each statement or answers each question.

_____ **1.** Which of the following is *not* a function of skin?

   a. Vitamin C production   **d.** Sensation

   b. Body temperature regulation   **e.** Melanin production

   c. Protection

_____ **2.** Which of the following is a pigment that traps UV radiation?

   a. Hemoglobin   **d.** Carotene

   b. Keratin   **e.** Melanoma

   c. Melanin

_____ **3.** A(n) _____ is a loss of the epidermis.

   a. Ulcer   **d.** Wheal

   b. Excoriation   **e.** Cicatrix

   c. Fissure

_____ **4.** Which of the following makes the skin waterproof?

   a. Melanin   **d.** Cyanosis

   b. Hemoglobin   **e.** Collagen

   c. Keratin

_____ **5.** Which of the following terms means blister?

   a. Pustule   **d.** Vesicle

   b. Papule   **e.** Ecchymosis

   c. Wheal

_____ **6.** Which of the following is a chronic skin disorder that is thought to be connected to an underlying inflammatory condition?

   a. Eczema   **d.** Folliculitis

   b. Psoriasis   **e.** Purpura

   c. Impetigo

_____ **7.** In addition to chickenpox, the varicella virus also causes

   a. Herpes simplex   **d.** Herpes zoster

   b. Dermatitis   **e.** Eczema

   c. Rosacea

_____ 8. Which inflammatory skin disorder is caused by excess sebum production?

    a. Rosacea   **d.** Herpes simplex

    b. Folliculitis   **e.** Psoriasis

    c. Acne vulgaris

_____ 9. The medical term for ringworm is

    a. Pediculosis   **d.** Verrucae

    b. Tinea   **e.** Keloid

    c. Herpes

_____ 10. An inflamed area includes all of the following characteristics except

    a. Redness   **d.** Scar formation

    b. Swelling   **e.** Warmth

    c. Pain

Sentence Completion

In the space provided, write the word or phrase that best completes each sentence.

11. The _____ layer is the support layer for the skin and is composed largely of adipose tissue.

12. Within the epidermis is the protein _____, which gives this layer of skin its protective properties.

13. The _____ glands are most concentrated in the axillary and groin areas of the body.

14. The topmost layer of the epidermis is the _____.

15. The _____ is the layer of "living" skin and is composed of all major tissue types.

16. The _____ is made up of the stratum corneum and the stratum germinativum.

17. The _____ glands are a type of sweat gland that responds to heat.

18. _____ refers to the bluish tint that skin gets from cold and the illnesses that result in decreased oxygen in the tissues.

19. The _____ is the layer of the epidermis that produces new skin cells.

20. A _____ is the skin area along a central nerve pathway.

21. The half-moon-shaped area at the base of the nail is called the _____.

22. _____ gives skin and hair their coloring.

23. The hair _____ contains the blood vessel that nourishes the hair.

24. _____ glands secrete sebum or oil for the hair and skin.

25. The sweat or _____ glands are part of the body's cooling system.

11. _____

12. _____

13. _____

14. _____

15. _____

16. _____

17. _____

18. _____

19. _____

20. _____

21. _____

22. _____

23. _____

24. _____

25. _____

Short Answer

Write the answer to each question on the lines provided.

26. The following figure shows structures and the layers of the skin. Label the figure using the following terms: hair shaft, hair follicle, arrector pili muscle, sebaceous gland, blood vessels, dermis, epidermis, hypodermis, sweat gland pore, stratum corneum, capillary, stratum germinativum, dermal papilla, basement membrane, touch receptor, sweat gland, sweat gland duct, nerve fiber, adipose tissue.

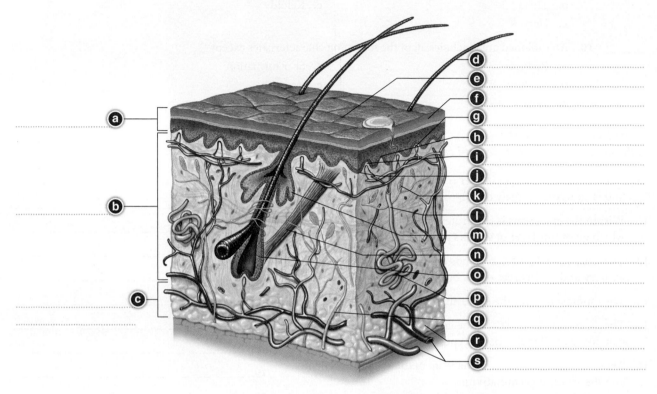

Source: From David Shier et al., HOLE'S HUMAN ANATOMY & PHYSIOLOGY, 12/e. © 2010 McGraw Hill Companies, Inc. Reprinted with permission.

27. Describe the following stages of melanoma.

   a. Stage 0 _____

   b. Stage I _____

   c. Stage II _____

   d. Stage III _____

   e. Stage IV _____

28. Briefly describe the following skin disorders.

   a. Fissure _____

   b. Eczema _____

   c. Herpes simplex _____

   d. Wheal _____

   e. Impetigo _____

   f. Psoriasis _____

    g. Rosacea _____

    h. Scabies _____

    i. Verrucae _____

    j. Nodule _____

29. Fill in the meanings for the American Cancer Society's Cancer Warning Signs using the acronym CAUTION:

    C _____

    A _____

    U _____

    T _____

    I _____

    O _____

    N _____

Critical Thinking

Write the answer to each question on the lines provided.

1. Describe how the skin regulates body temperature.

_____

_____

_____

2. Describe the structure of the stratum corneum. How is this structure important for the function of the epidermis?

_____

_____

_____

3. Why is skin cancer more common in people with lighter skin tones?

_____

_____

_____

4. What conditions are likely to result in a person with underactive sebaceous glands?

_____

_____

_____

5. How does washing your face and hair help to prevent acne?

_____

_____

_____

A P P L I C A T I O N

Follow the directions for each application.

1. **Skin Cancer**

   Describe the appearances and treatments of the following types of skin cancer. Also name the cells that are cancerous in each type.

   a. Basal cell carcinoma

   _____

   b. Squamous cell carcinoma

   _____

   c. Melanoma

   _____

2. **Inflammation of Skin**

   When skin is injured, it becomes inflamed. Describe what produces each of the following signs of inflammation.

   a. Redness

   _____

   b. Swelling

   _____

   c. Pain

   _____

C A S E   S T U D I E S

Write your response to each case study on the lines provided.

Case 1

A 35-year-old female recently had her family physician look at her moles during a routine yearly exam. The doctor asks you to explain to the patient the ABCDE rule to determine if a mole is suspected of being cancerous. How would you explain this rule?

_____

_____

_____

Case 2

Two boys are hospitalized for burns. The first boy has third-degree burns on his right hand and arm. The second boy has third-degree burns on his lower face. Why are the injuries of the second boy more life-threatening?

_____

_____

_____

Case 3
A 60-year-old diabetic woman comes to the office with a deepening sore on her left heel. It started as a blister from new shoes but is not healing. Why might this be of concern?

_____

_____

_____

Case 4
A 24-year-old woman comes to the office with a scrape over her left knee. She is concerned that the wound may cause a scar. What information can you give her about preventing the scar formation of a lasting scar?

_____

_____

_____

The Skeletal System

Name_____ Class_____ Date_____

REVIEW

Vocabulary Review

Matching
Match the key terms in the right column with the definitions in the left column by placing the letter of each correct answer in the space provided.

_____ 1. Attaches the finger to the hand

_____ 2. Bones of the extremities are included in this skeletal type

_____ 3. The opening for the spinal cord and brain attachment

_____ 4. Bone depression that allows for bones to join, as with the elbow

_____ 5. The baby's "soft spot"

_____ 6. The division of the skeleton including the cranium, vertebrae, and rib cage

_____ 7. The term used to describe the finger joints

_____ 8. Nonmoveable joints, such as those within the skull

_____ 9. Large bony projection, such as at the proximal end of the femur

_____ 10. Attaches the tongue to the pharynx

_____ 11. Ridge-like bony projection

_____ 12. Cartilaginous tip of the sternum

_____ 13. The location of red bone marrow

_____ 14. A rounded bone process often found near a joint

_____ 15. A large rounded process at the end of a long bone

a. appendicular
b. axial
c. fontanel
d. foramen magnum
e. suture
f. MCP joints
g. PIP/DIP
h. hyoid
i. cancellous bone
j. xiphoid process
k. condyle
l. fossa
m. trochanter
n. head
o. crest

True or False
Decide whether each statement is true or false. In the space at the left, write T for true or F for false. On the lines provided, rewrite the false statements to make them true.

_____ 16. The femur is an example of a long bone.

_____

_____ 17. An expanded end of a long bone is called a diaphysis.

_____

_____ 18. The periosteum is a membrane that lines the medullary cavity.

_____

_____ 19. The osteon is also known as the Haversian system.

_____ 20. Yellow bone marrow produces new blood cells.

_____ 21. The mastoid process is located on each temporal bone.

_____ 22. Ear ossicles are the smallest bones of the body.

_____ 23. The scapulae form the collarbone.

_____ 24. The first cervical vertebra is called the axis.

_____ 25. The thoracic segment of the spine includes seven vertebrae.

_____ 26. The ilium is one of the hip bones.

_____ 27. The humerus is the lower arm bone on the thumb (lateral) side of the arm.

_____ 28. Once growth stops, osteoclasts and osteoblasts cease their functioning.

_____ 29. Weight-bearing exercises are essential for bone health.

_____ 30. A synovial joint is the most moveable of the joints.

Content Review

Multiple Choice

In the space provided, write the letter of the choice that best completes each statement or answers each question.

_____ 1. Which of the following is an example of short bones?
- **a.** Carpal bones
- **b.** Humerus
- **c.** Ribs
- **d.** Sternum
- **e.** Tibia

_____ 2. The growth plate is also known as the
- **a.** Articular cartilage
- **b.** Diaphysis
- **c.** Epiphyseal plate
- **d.** Lamella
- **e.** Lacunae

_____ 3. The term for a hole or opening in a bone for blood vessels and nerves is the
- **a.** Fossa
- **b.** Head
- **c.** Suture
- **d.** Process
- **e.** Foramen

_____ 4. The cartilage that attaches the ribs to the sternum is called the
   a. Articular cartilage
   b. Intervertebral disk
   c. Epiphyseal plate
   d. Costal cartilage
   e. Meniscal cartilage

_____ 5. Which of the following bones is located at the base of the skull?
   a. Occipital bone
   b. Parietal bone
   c. Frontal bone
   d. Temporal bone
   e. Ethmoid bones

_____ 6. Which of the following bones creates the roof of the mouth?
   a. Maxilla
   b. Vomer
   c. Palatine
   d. Sphenoid
   e. Mandible

_____ 7. The rib cage is composed of
   a. 24 ribs and the scapula
   b. 12 ribs and the clavicle
   c. 12 pairs of ribs and the scapula
   d. 12 pairs of ribs and the sternum
   e. 12 ribs and the sternum

_____ 8. The membrane around the shaft of a long bone is the
   a. Endosteum
   b. Periosteum
   c. Paraosteum
   d. Osteocyte
   e. Medullary cavity

_____ 9. Which bone is the largest of the tarsal bones?
   a. Malleolus
   b. Femur
   c. Acetabulum
   d. Calcaneus
   e. Metatarsals

_____ 10. The coxal bones are more commonly known as the
   a. Sternal bones
   b. Hip bones
   c. Hand bones
   d. Wrist bones
   e. Shoulder bones

Sentence Completion

In the space provided, write the word or phrase that best completes each sentence.

11. _____ are immature bone cells that create new bone.

12. _____ are cells that digest old bone in preparation for new bone growth.

13. The process of bone hardening is called _____.

14. _____ is the process of blood formation.

15. The fibrous bands that attach bone to bone are _____.

16. The _____ is commonly known as the shaft of a long bone.

17. The rounded end of the long bone is called the _____.

18. Spongy or _____ bone is where red bone marrow is located.

19. Yellow bone marrow is located in the _____.

20. The _____ is the tough fibrous membrane that covers the shaft of the long bone.

11. _____

12. _____

13. _____

14. _____

15. _____

16. _____

17. _____

18. _____

19. _____

20. _____

Short Answer

Write the answer to each question on the lines provided.

21. The following figure shows the structure of a long bone. Label the figure using the following terms: diaphysis, articular cartilage, spongy bone, compact bone, medullary cavity, yellow marrow, periosteum, epiphyseal disks, proximal epiphysis, distal epiphysis, space occupied by red marrow.

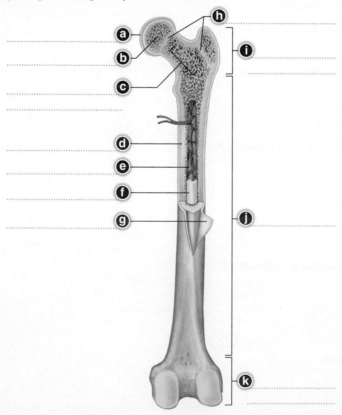

Source: From David Shier et al., HOLE'S HUMAN ANATOMY & PHYSIOLOGY, 12/e. © 2010 McGraw Hill Companies, Inc. Reprinted with permission.

22. Label the bones of the skeleton shown as follows appropriately.

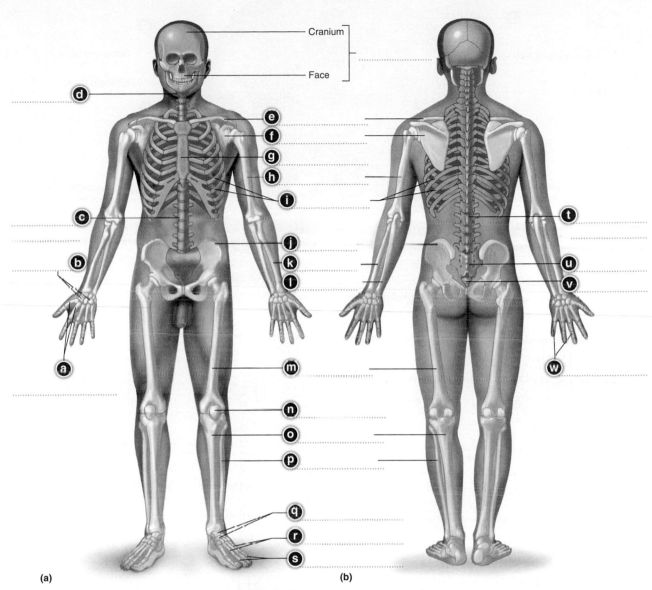

Cranium

Face

(a)

(b)

Source: From David Shier et al., HOLE'S HUMAN ANATOMY & PHYSIOLOGY, 12/e. © 2010 McGraw Hill Companies, Inc. Reprinted with permission.

23. Label the bones of the skull appropriately.

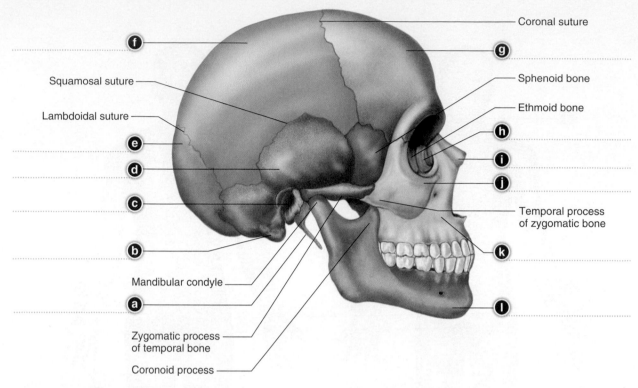

Coronal suture

Squamosal suture

Lambdoidal suture

Sphenoid bone

Ethmoid bone

Temporal process
of zygomatic bone

Mandibular condyle

Zygomatic process
of temporal bone

Coronoid process

24. Label the bones of the arm appropriately.

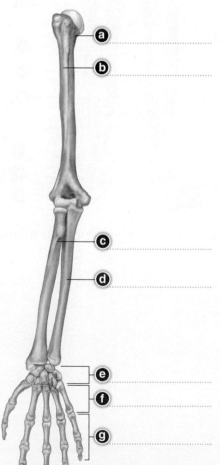

25. Describe the following disorders.

a. Osteoporosis

_____

_____

_____

b. Osteosarcoma

_____

_____

_____

c. Osteogenesis imperfecta

_____

_____

_____

Critical Thinking

Write the answer to each question on the lines provided.

1. What are the roles of osteoblasts and osteoclasts throughout life?

_____

_____

_____

2. Some sunlight exposure is necessary for bone growth and maintenance. What vitamin synthesis is aided by sunlight, and why is it important in bone health?

_____

_____

_____

3. Explain the importance of the pectoral and pelvic girdles. What bones are included in each?

_____

_____

_____

4. Describe the three common vertebral deformities and give at least one causative factor for each.

_____

_____

_____

5. Explain the difference between compact bone and cancellous (spongy) bone.

_____

_____

_____

A P P L I C A T I O N

Follow the directions for the application.

Inflammatory Diseases of Bones and Joints

Inflammation is an "enemy" of bones and joints. Explain how inflammation affects bones and joints in the following inflammatory diseases.

a. Bursitis_____

b. Osteoarthritis_____

c. Rheumatoid arthritis _____

d. Gouty arthritis _____

C A S E   S T U D I E S

Write your response to each case study on the lines provided.

Case 1

A 25-year-old woman is concerned that she may have osteoporosis because her mother has the disorder. Is the 25-year-old likely to have osteoporosis? What would you tell her about preventing the disease?

_____

_____

_____

Case 2

A young woman is pregnant and neglects to make sure that her diet has sufficient amounts of calcium. How is her diet likely to affect her bones and the bones of her fetus?

_____

_____

_____

Case 3

A 60-year-old man has just been diagnosed with gouty arthritis. What can you tell him about his condition and preventive measures he can take to prevent attacks?

_____

_____

_____

Case 4

Your 3-year-old has osteogenesis imperfecta type I. She is very prone to fractures and you are taking a trip to the shore for a week this summer. What special precautions might you need to take while vacationing? Why might it be a good idea to take a copy of your child's medical record with you?

_____

_____

_____

25

The Muscular System

Name_____ Class_____ Date_____

REVIEW

Vocabulary Review

Matching

Match the key terms in the right column with the definitions in the left column by placing the letter of each correct answer in the space provided.

_____ **1.** Helper muscle in skeletal muscle movement

_____ **2.** A structure that covers and separates skeletal muscles

_____ **3.** A condition produced by buildup of lactic acid in muscle

_____ **4.** A structure that connects groups of cardiac muscle

_____ **5.** Tough connective tissue that attaches muscle to bone

_____ **6.** A thin covering that surrounds the entire muscle

_____ **7.** The cell membrane of myocytes

_____ **8.** The muscle primarily responsible for skeletal muscle movement

_____ **9.** An energy-producing process for muscles that requires oxygen

_____ **10.** A muscle that works in opposition to a prime mover

a. tendon
b. prime mover
c. synergist
d. antagonist
e. fascia
f. aerobic respiration
g. muscle fatigue
h. epimysium
i. intercalated disc
j. sarcolemma

True or False

Decide whether each statement is true or false. In the space at the left, write T for true or F for false. On the lines provided, rewrite the false statements to make them true.

_____ **11.** When muscles contract, heat is released.

_____

_____ **12.** Striated muscle is found in the wall of blood vessels.

_____

_____ **13.** Muscle cells are the same things as muscle fibers.

_____

_____ **14.** The muscle in the iris of the eye is a voluntary muscle.

_____

_____ **15.** Groups of skeletal muscle are connected to each other through intercalated discs.

_____

_____ **16.** Muscle fatigue usually develops from an accumulation of hydrochloric acid.

_____

_____ 17. Epimysium surrounds an entire muscle.

_____ 18. Straightening a body part is called flexion.

_____ 19. Moving a body part anteriorly is called retraction.

_____ 20. The orbicularis oculi muscle puckers the lips.

_____ 21. The deltoid muscle acts to adduct the arm at the shoulder.

_____ 22. The biceps brachii muscle extends the arm at the elbow.

_____ 23. The external oblique muscle compresses the abdominal wall and flexes the vertebral column.

_____ 24. The contraction of the diaphragm causes inspiration.

_____ 25. The gastrocnemius acts in dorsiflexion of the foot.

_____ 26. Myasthenia gravis is one of the few muscular diseases in which rest temporarily alleviates or minimizes many of its symptoms.

_____ 27. An agonist works with a prime mover.

_____ 28. Rotation describes the movement of a body part in a circular motion.

_____ 29. Sprains involve joints, tendons, and ligaments; strains involve injuries to muscles.

_____ 30. Skeletal muscle is described as being both striated and involuntary.

Content Review

Multiple Choice
In the space provided, write the letter of the choice that best completes each statement or answers each question.

_____ 1. Which of the following is not a function of muscle?
   a. Production of body movement
   b. Stabilization of joints
   c. Control of body openings
   d. All of the above are functions of muscle
   e. None of the above are functions of muscle

_____ 2. Which of the following is true about visceral muscle?

      a. It is voluntary

      b. It is striated

      c. It is slow to contract and relax

      d. It is attached to bones

      e. It is connected by intercalated discs

_____ 3. Which of the following is a connective tissue that divides a muscle into fascicles?

      a. Fascia

      b. Epimysium

      c. Endomysium

      d. Perimysium

      e. Aponeurosis

_____ 4. Which disease is commonly called *lockjaw*?

      a. Botulism

      b. Tetanus

      c. Trichinosis

      d. Encephalitis

      e. Torticollis

_____ 5. Which disease can be caused by dented cans and undercooked or raw fish or pork?

      a. Botulism

      b. Tetanus

      c. Trichinosis

      d. Encephalitis

      e. Myasthenia gravis

_____ 6. Which of the following is the action of pointing the toes up?

      a. Inversion

      b. Eversion

      c. Plantar flexion

      d. Protraction

      e. Dorsiflexion

_____ 7. Which of the following is the action of moving a body part posteriorly?

      a. Elevation

      b. Retraction

      c. Protraction

      d. Depression

      e. Rotation

_____ 8. Which muscle closes the jaw?

      a. Platysma   **d.** Orbicularis oris

      b. Masseter   **e.** Mandible

      c. Sternocleidomastoid

_____ 9. Which of the following structures connect cardiac muscle fibers to each other?

      a. Tendons   **d.** Intercalated discs

      b. Ligaments   **e.** Perimysium

      c. Intracalated discs

_____ **10.** Which of the following terms is another name for *myocyte?*
   a. Muscle fiber
   b. Sarcolemma
   c. Sarcoplasm
   d. Myofibril
   e. Striation

_____ **11.** Peristalsis describes the contraction of which of the following muscle types?
   a. Skeletal
   b. Visceral (smooth)
   c. Multiunit (smooth)
   d. Cardiac
   e. Sphincter

_____ **12.** Which of the following terms refers to the loss of a muscle's ability to contract?
   a. Oxygen debt
   b. Lactic acid production
   c. Muscle fatigue
   d. Aerobic respiration
   e. Anaerobic respiration

Sentence Completion
In the space provided, write the word or phrase that best completes each sentence.

13. _____ is the pinkish pigment of muscle that stores oxygen.

14. The attachment of muscle to the more moveable bone is known as _____ .

15. The neurotransmitter _____ causes a skeletal muscle response.

16. The rhythmic movement of visceral muscle is called _____.

17. The attachment of a muscle to the least moveable bone is called the _____.

18. _____ is the enzyme responsible for skeletal muscle relaxation.

19. A ring of muscle known as a _____ is responsible for opening and closing body cavities and openings.

20. The _____ describes the aerobic process of creating ATP for muscle energy.

21. The byproduct of pyruvic acid conversion is _____, which occurs when muscle is low on oxygen.

22. _____ occurs during muscle fatigue, when oxygen supplies in muscles are low.

13. _____

14. _____

15. _____

16. _____

17. _____

18. _____

19. _____

20. _____

21. _____

22. _____

Short Answer

Write the answer to each question on the lines provided.

23. The following figure shows the muscular system. Write the names of the following muscles on the correct lines in the figure: biceps brachii, deltoid, external oblique, gastrocnemius, gluteus maximus, gluteus medius, hamstring group, latissimus dorsi, pectoralis major, quadriceps group, rectus abdominis, rectus femoris, sternocleidomastoid, trapezius, triceps brachii.

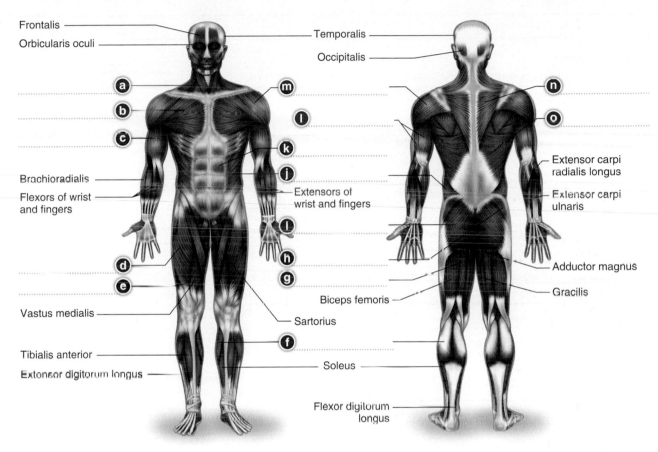

Frontalis
Orbicularis oculi
Temporalis
Occipitalis
Brachioradialis
Flexors of wrist and fingers
Extensors of wrist and fingers
Extensor carpi radialis longus
Extensor carpi ulnaris
Adductor magnus
Gracilis
Vastus medialis
Biceps femoris
Sartorius
Tibialis anterior
Extensor digitorum longus
Soleus
Flexor digitorum longus

Source: From David Shier et al., HOLE'S HUMAN ANATOMY & PHYSIOLOGY, 12/e. © 2010 McGraw Hill Companies, Inc. Reprinted with permission.

24. Briefly describe the following disorders:

a. Botulism

_____

_____

_____

b. Fibromyalgia

_____

_____

_____

c. Muscular dystrophy

_____

_____

_____

d. Myasthenia gravis

_____

_____

_____

e. Tendonitis

_____

_____

_____

f. Trichinosis

_____

_____

_____

g. Strains

_____

_____

_____

h. Sprains

_____

_____

_____

Critical Thinking

Write the answer to each question on the lines provided.

1. Norepinephrine works with the sympathetic nervous system. How does its presence in the bloodstream affect cardiac function?

_____

_____

_____

2. When a person is exercising, his breathing rate increases to ensure the adequate delivery of oxygen to skeletal muscle tissues. Why does the breathing rate stay increased for a period of time even after a person stops exercising?

_____

_____

_____

3. When a muscle is overworked, it often becomes sore. Why does massaging a muscle help reduce muscle soreness?

_____

_____

_____

4. In cooler weather, mothers often tell children to put on a sweater or "get up and move around" to warm up. Why do they think movement will warm up their children?

_____

_____

_____

5. Why do cardiac muscles have intercalated discs?

_____

_____

_____

_____

A P P L I C A T I O N

Follow the directions for each application.

Skeletal Muscle Actions
For each of the following actions, list the prime mover, at least one synergist, and the antagonist.

a. Bending the leg at the knee _____

b. Raising the arm laterally at the shoulder _____

c. Bending the hand at the wrist _____

C A S E   S T U D I E S

Write your response to each case study on the lines provided.

Case 1
Recently a patient at your office was diagnosed with botulism. He states that he enjoys sushi at the new restaurant in town. How might this information possibly affect his diagnosis and treatment?

_____

_____

_____

Case 2
A friend calls and tells you that she thinks she has a muscle strain. You tell her that immediate RICE treatment is recommended. What does this mean?

_____

_____

_____

Case 3

A young woman arrives in the office with an increasing lateral turning of her head and neck that seems to be worsening since a motor vehicle accident in which she was rear ended. What is her likely diagnosis and what treatment(s) should be tried?

_____

_____

_____

Case 4

A young man is hospitalized for seizures after running his first marathon. Tests reveal he has myoglobin in his blood and urine. Why does he have myoglobin in his blood and urine? How is this harmful to his kidneys?

_____

_____

_____

26

The Cardiovascular System

Name_____ Class_____ Date_____

R E V I E W

Vocabulary Review

Matching
Match the key terms in the right column with the definitions in the left column by placing the letter of each correct answer in the space provided.

_____ **1.** Part of the cardiac conduction system located just above the ventricles, between the atria

_____ **2.** A membrane that covers the heart and the large blood vessels attached to it

_____ **3.** The route blood takes from the heart to the lungs and back again

_____ **4.** Part of the cardiac conduction system that splits into right and left branches

_____ **5.** Thickest layer of the heart wall

_____ **6.** Measures blood pressure in the aorta and carotid arteries

_____ **7.** Structures that anchor the tricuspid valve to papillary muscles

_____ **8.** Part of the cardiac conduction system located in the lateral walls of the ventricles

_____ **9.** Pressure in the arteries when the ventricles relax

_____ **10.** The route blood takes from the heart to the body cells and back to the heart

_____ **11.** The innermost layer of the heart wall

_____ **12.** The smallest type of blood vessel

_____ **13.** The widening of blood vessel walls

_____ **14.** Part of the cardiac conduction system that generates the electrical impulse that initiates a heartbeat

_____ **15.** Another name for the visceral pericardium

_____ **16.** The blood vessel that empties blood from the cardiac veins into the right atrium

_____ **17.** Pressure in the arteries when the ventricles contract

_____ **18.** The total amount of blood pumped out of the heart in 1 minute

_____ **19.** The tightening of blood vessel walls

_____ **20.** The collection of veins that carries blood to the liver

a. myocardium
b. diastolic pressure
c. atrioventricular node
d. capillary
e. vasodilation
f. chordae tendineae
g. endocardium
h. hepatic portal system
i. pulmonary circulation
j. coronary sinus
k. sinoatrial node
l. baroreceptor
m. Purkinje fibers
n. systemic circulation
o. cardiac output
p. epicardium
q. systolic pressure
r. pericardium
s. vasoconstriction
t. bundle of His

True or False

Decide whether each statement is true or false. In the space at the left, write T for true or F for false. On the lines provided, rewrite the false statements to make them true.

_____ **21.** A membrane called the endocardium covers the heart.

_____

_____ **22.** The myocardium is the inner layer of the heart wall.

_____

_____ **23.** The upper chambers of the heart are the ventricles.

_____

_____ **24.** The bicuspid valve is located between the right atrium and right ventricle.

_____

_____ **25.** Lubb is the first heart sound and occurs when the tricuspid and bicuspid valves snap shut.

_____

_____ **26.** The AV node is the pacemaker of the heart.

_____

_____ **27.** Venules are branches of veins.

_____

_____ **28.** Diastolic pressure is higher than systolic pressure.

_____

_____ **29.** Arteries carry blood away from the heart.

_____

_____ **30.** The phrenic artery carries blood to the intestines.

_____

_____ **31.** The radial artery carries blood to the forearm.

_____

_____ **32.** The azygous vein carries blood from the head and neck.

_____

_____ **33.** The bundle of His is also known as the AV node.

_____

_____ **34.** Myocardial infarction can be caused by a cerebral artery blockage.

_____

_____ **35.** Capillaries are known as exchange vessels.

_____

_____ **36.** Vasodilation increases blood pressure.

_____

_____ **37.** The hepatic portal system carries blood to the kidneys.

_____

_____ **38.** Angina can be caused by blockage of one or more coronary of the arteries.

_____

_____ **39.** Inflammation of the muscular layer of the heart is called endocarditis.

_____

_____ **40.** Substances move through capillary walls through diffusion, filtration, and osmosis.

_____

Content Review

Multiple Choice

In the space provided, write the letter of the choice that best completes each statement or answers each question.

_____ **1.** In an ECG, what does the QRS complex represent?
   a. Origination of the electrical impulse
   b. Atrial depolarization
   c. Ventricular depolarization
   d. Atrial repolarization
   e. Ventricular repolarization

_____ **2.** Which of the following is the wall between the upper and lower chambers of the heart?
   a. Interventricular septum
   b. Intraventricular septum
   c. Interatrial septum
   d. Intra-atrial septum
   e. Atrioventricular septum

_____ **3.** Which of the following is the heart's natural pacemaker?
   a. AV septum   **d.** SA node
   b. AV node   **e.** SV septum
   c. SV node

_____ **4.** Which of the following conditions involves hardening of the fatty plaque within arteries?
   a. Atherosclerosis   **d.** Otosclerosis
   b. Multiple sclerosis   **e.** Phlebosclerosis
   c. Arthrosclerosis

_____ **5.** Which of the following best describes a heart murmur?
   a. Titanic contraction   **d.** Normal cardiac blood flow
   b. Electrical impulse   **e.** Abnormal heart rate
   c. Abnormal heart sound

_____ **6.** In which order do electrical impulses flow through the cardiac conduction system?
   a. SA node, AV node, Purkinje fibers, bundle of His
   b. SA node, AV node, bundle of His, Purkinje fibers
   c. Purkinje fibers, AV node, SA node, bundle of His
   d. AV node, Purkinje fibers, bundle of His, SA node
   e. Bundle of His, Purkinje fibers, SA node, AV node

_____ **7.** From which vein, other than the venae cavae, does blood flow into the right atrium?
   a. Jugular vein   **d.** Femoral vein
   b. Subclavian vein   **e.** Coronary sinus
   c. Axillary vein

_____ 8. Which area of the body receives oxygen and nutrients through the lingual artery?
    a. Maxillary artery   d. Ophthalmic artery
    b. Lingual artery   e. Facial artery
    c. Popliteal artery

_____ 9. Which of the following veins carries oxygen-rich blood?
    a. Ulnar veins   d. Hepatic portal veins
    b. Radial veins   e. Saphenous veins
    c. Pulmonary veins

_____ 10. Which of the following terms refers to a ballooned, weakened area on an arterial wall?
    a. Aneurysm   d. Murmur
    b. Hemorrhoid   e. Stenosis
    c. Arrhythmia

Sentence Completion

In the space provided, write the word or phrase that best completes each sentence.

11. The path of blood from the heart through the lungs and back to the heart is _____ circulation.

12. An abnormal heart sound caused by faulty valve closure is a(n) _____.

13. The path of blood from the heart through the body cells and back to the heart is _____ circulation.

14. The space between the parietal pericardium and the visceral pericardium is known as the pericardial _____.

15. The walled membrane that separates the atria of the heart is the _____.

16. The valve between the right atrium and right ventricle is the _____ valve, or right AV valve.

17. Physicians use a test called a(n) _____ to determine whether the cardiac conduction system is working properly.

18. The strongest blood vessels are the _____.

19. The presence of _____ in the veins prevents blood from flowing backward.

20. The amount of blood that flows into a capillary is controlled by openings known as _____.

11. _____

12. _____

13. _____

14. _____

15. _____

16. _____

17. _____

18. _____

19. _____

20. _____

Short Answer

Write the answer to each question on the lines provided.

21. The following illustration shows the structure of the heart wall. Label the figure using the following terms: epicardium, myocardium, endocardium, fibrous pericardium, parietal pericardium, pericardial cavity, coronary blood vessel.

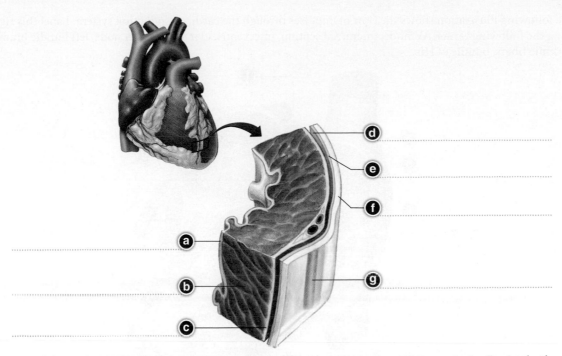

Source: From David Shier et al., HOLE'S HUMAN ANATOMY & PHYSIOLOGY, 12/e. © 2010 McGraw Hill Companies, Inc. Reprinted with permission.

22. The following illustration shows a sectional view of the heart. Label this figure using the following terms: right ventricle, left ventricle, right atrium, left atrium, superior vena cava, inferior vena cava, aorta, tricuspid valve, bicuspid valve, pulmonary semilunar valve, aortic semilunar valve, left pulmonary veins, right pulmonary veins, left pulmonary artery, right pulmonary artery, chordae tendineae, papillary muscles, interventricular septum, pulmonary trunk, opening of coronary sinus.

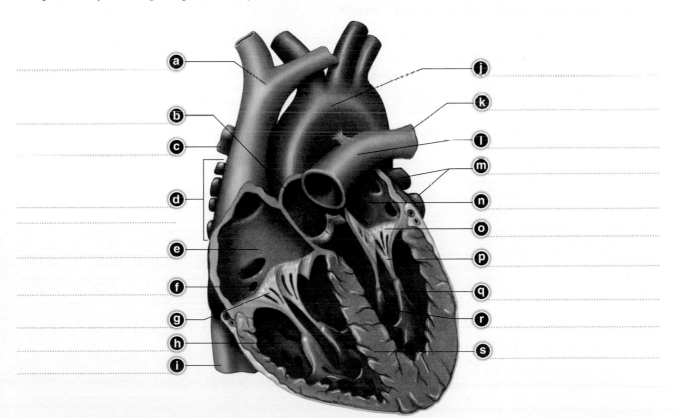

Source: From David Shier et al., HOLE'S HUMAN ANATOMY & PHYSIOLOGY, 12/e. © 2010 McGraw Hill Companies, Inc. Reprinted with permission.

23. The following illustration shows the flow of impulses through the cardiac conduction system. Label this figure using the following terms: AV node, interatrial septum, interventricular septum, SA node, left bundle branch, Purkinje fibers, bundle of His.

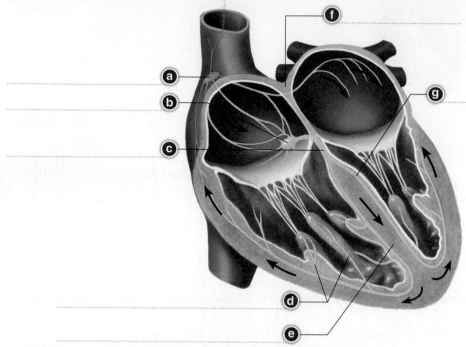

Source: From David Shier et al., HOLE'S HUMAN ANATOMY & PHYSIOLOGY, 12/e. © 2010 McGraw Hill Companies, Inc. Reprinted with permission.

24. Answer the following questions about chest pain.

  a. What are four common cardiac causes of chest pain?

  _____

  _____

  _____

  _____

  b. What are eight common noncardiac causes of chest pain?

  _____

  _____

  _____

  _____

  _____

  _____

  _____

  _____

  c. What tests are used to determine the cause of chest pain?

  _____

  _____

  _____

d. What causes angina?

_____

_____

_____

Critical Thinking

Write the answer to each question on the lines provided.

1. The left ventricular wall is more muscular than the right ventricular wall. Why do you think this is necessary?

_____

_____

_____

2. Why is it important for tricuspid and bicuspid valves to close completely when the ventricles contract?

_____

_____

_____

3. Patients with angina pectoris are given sublingual nitroglycerin. Why is this medication helpful to them?

_____

_____

_____

A P P L I C A T I O N

Follow the directions for each application.

1. Systemic Circulation

Using the correct anatomical terms for the blood vessels, trace the blood's journey as it leaves the heart to bring oxygen to the body cells and then back to the heart again. (Hint: Start with the largest artery.)

_____

_____

_____

2. Interpreting Blood Pressure

Your patient's BP is 126/82. What does each of these numbers represent within the cardiac cycle?

_____

_____

_____

3. Layers of the Heart

List each of the three layers of the heart wall and describe the function of each.

_____

_____

_____

_____

_____

4. Cardiac Diseases and Disorders

Briefly describe each of the following cardiac diseases or disorders, including treatment options.

a. Aneurysm

_____

_____

_____

b. Pericarditis

_____

_____

_____

c. Congestive heart failure

_____

_____

_____

d. Thrombophlebitis

_____

_____

_____

C A S E   S T U D I E S

Write your response to each case study on the lines provided.

Case 1

The left side of the heart in a 79-year-old patient is failing. How will this patient's lungs be affected if the condition is not treated?

_____

_____

_____

Case 2

A 28-year-old man thinks he is having a heart attack. He has just eaten a spicy Italian meal, and his chest pains seem to get worse when he bends forward or lies down. What would you tell him?

_____

_____

_____

Case 3

Your 80-year-old patient states she can "see and feel" her heartbeat in her upper abdomen. The physician has ordered an abdominal ultrasound. What is the diagnosis? What should her treatment be?

_____

_____

_____

The Blood

Name_____ Class_____ Date_____

R E V I E W

Vocabulary Review

Matching

Match the key terms in the right column with the definitions in the left column by placing the letter of each correct answer in the space provided.

_____	**1.** Control bleeding	**a.** agglutination
_____	**2.** Cells releasing heparin and histamines	**b.** agranulocyte
_____	**3.** Stimulates bone marrow to produce RBCs	**c.** basophil
_____	**4.** WBC	**d.** coagulation
_____	**5.** RBC	**e.** embolus
_____	**6.** Cells assisting in blood clotting	**f.** eosinophil
_____	**7.** Plasma with cells and clotting factor removed	**g.** erythrocyte
_____	**8.** Measures percentage of RBCs in blood	**h.** erythropoietin
_____	**9.** Clumping of cells	**i.** fibrinogen
_____	**10.** Blood proteins	**j.** globulins
_____	**11.** Blood clot "on the move"	**k.** granulocyte
_____	**12.** Fights viruses and parasitic infections	**l.** hematocrit
_____	**13.** WBC with no cytoplasmic granules	**m.** hemostasis
_____	**14.** WBCs of the immune system	**n.** leukocyte
_____	**15.** Neutrophils, eosinophils, and basophils	**o.** lymphocyte
_____	**16.** The other term for platelets	**p.** monocyte
_____	**17.** A blood clot	**q.** neutrophil
_____	**18.** Destroys bacteria, viruses, and toxins in the blood	**r.** platelets
_____	**19.** Plasma substance important in blood clotting	**s.** serum
_____	**20.** Process of blood clotting	**t.** thrombocytes
_____	**21.** Phagocytes destroying bacteria, viruses, and toxins	**u.** thrombus

True or False

Decide whether each statement is true or false. In the space at the left, write T for true or F for false. On the lines provided, rewrite the false statements to make them true.

_____ **22.** When agglutination occurs, there is a match between blood types and Rh factor.

_____

_____ **23.** Platelets are fragments of cells that keep blood from clotting.

_____

_____ **24.** A monocyte is an example of an agranulocyte.

_____

_____ **25.** A white blood cell count above normal is termed leukocytosis.

_____

_____ **26.** The gases dissolved in plasma include oxygen, carbon dioxide, and nitrogen.

_____

_____ **27.** If an embolus blocks a cerebral artery, the result may be a myocardial infarction.

_____

_____ **28.** Blood type O (negative) is the universal donor.

_____

_____ **29.** Erythoblastosis fetalis could develop if an Rh positive woman and Rh negative man produce a child.

_____

_____ **30.** One cause of anemia is the production of too few WBCs in the blood.

_____

_____ **31.** Leukemia is a cancer of too many RBCs in the blood.

_____

_____ **32.** Hemolytic anemias result from RBC destruction.

_____

_____ **33.** Plasma is the blood fluid after all clotting factor has been removed.

_____

_____ **34.** Diapedesis is the squeezing of a cell through the blood vessel wall.

_____

_____ **35.** A normal RBC count is between 5000–10,000 cells per mm of blood.

_____

Content Review

Multiple Choice

In the space provided, write the letter of the choice that best completes each statement or answers each question.

_____ **1.** The control of bleeding is called
   a. Homeostasis
   b. Hemostasis
   c. Agglutination
   d. Vasospasm
   e. Deoxygenation

_____ 2. Which antigen(s) is present on red blood cells of type A blood?
   a. Antigen A   **d.** Antigen A and antigen B
   b. Antigen B   **e.** Neither antigen A nor antigen B
   c. Antigen O

_____ 3. Which antibody is found in the plasma of someone with blood type AB?
   a. Antigen A and antigen B
   b. No antigens
   c. Antibody A and antibody B
   d. No antibodies
   e. Both antigens and antibodies

_____ 4. Which vitamin is given to treat pernicious anemia?
   a. Iron   **d.** Vitamin D
   b. Vitamin B_6 **e.** Folate
   c. Vitamin B_{12}

_____ 5. Which of the following terms describes cell clumping?
   a. Coagulation   **d.** Cluster emboli
   b. Erythropoiesis   **e.** Agglutination
   c. Thrombosis

_____ 6. Which of the following terms refers to hemoglobin when it carries carbon dioxide?
   a. Oxyhemoglobin
   b. Deoxyhemoglobin
   c. Anemia
   d. Carboxyhemoglobin
   e. Erythrocytosis

_____ 7. Which cells are described as being biconcave?
   a. Platelets   **d.** RBCs
   b. WBCs   **e.** Antigens and antibodies
   c. Thrombocytes

_____ 8. Erythropoietin is created in which organ?
   a. Bone marrow   **d.** Liver
   b. Stomach   **e.** Kidneys
   c. Pancreas

_____ 9. In addition to iron, what compounds are necessary for the creation of RBCs?
   a. Vitamin B_{12} **d.** a and c
   b. Vitamin C   **e.** All of the above
   c. Vitamin B_9

_____ 10. When bilirubin builds up in the blood, the condition of _____ develops.
   a. Anemia   **d.** Jaundice
   b. Icterus   **e.** b or d
   c. Hepatitis

Sentence Completion

In the space provided, write the word or phrase that best completes each sentence.

11. The largest percentage of blood volume, approximately 55%, is _____.

12. The greatest number of WBCs, the phagocytes, are known as _____.

13. _____ is a WBC count that is above normal.

14. A WBC count that is below normal is called _____.

15. A diagnosis of _____ would be given if a patient's hemoglobin level or RBC level is abnormally low.

16. _____ is characterized by *sickle-shaped* RBCs.

17. Patients of Mediterranean descent are more likely to develop this type of anemia, _____.

18. The blood neoplasm resulting in an elevated WBC level is _____.

19. The Rh antigen is named after the _____.

20. If a patient with B+ blood is accidentally given an A+ donation, _____ will result.

21. _____ is the medical term for control of bleeding.

22. The squeezing of a blood cell through a vessel wall is called _____.

23. A _____ lists the percentages of the different types of leukocytes in a sample of blood.

24. As RBCs age, _____ in the liver and spleen destroy them.

25. When whole blood is spun in a centrifuge, the WBCs and platelets form a layer known as the _____.

11. _____

12. _____

13. _____

14. _____

15. _____

16. _____

17. _____

18. _____

19. _____

20. _____

21. _____

22. _____

23. _____

24. _____

25. _____

Short Answer

Write the answer to each question on the lines provided.

26. Explain how the kidneys have an important role in the body's ability to create adequate red blood cells.

_____

_____

_____

27. Describe the functions of each of the following proteins found in blood plasma.

   a. Albumins

_____

_____

_____

b. Globulins

_____

_____

_____

c. Fibrinogens

_____

_____

_____

In the space given, label each figure with the correct WBC type.

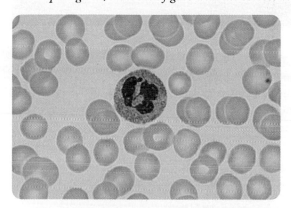

28. _____

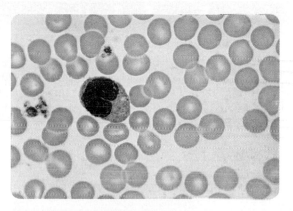

31. _____

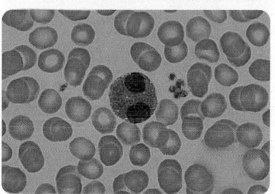

29. _____

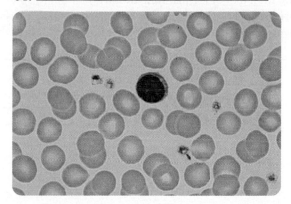

32. _____

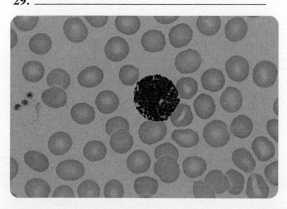

30. _____

Source for all art on page: © Ed Reschke.

33. Complete the following table so that each row contains the blood type and its appropriate antigens and antibodies as well as the blood type the patient can receive.

Blood Type	Antigen Present	Antibody Present	Blood Type That Can be Received
A			A and O
	B	A	
AB		None	
	None		O only

C A S E   S T U D I E S

Write your response to each case study on the lines provided.

Case 1
A patient is being prepped for surgery, but the surgeon notices that the patient has a platelet count of 90,000 platelets per mL of blood. Is this normal? Why might the surgeon want to postpone the surgery?

_____

_____

_____

Case 2
Mr. and Mrs. Ramey are planning to start their family soon. Mrs. Ramey has made an appointment to discuss her concerns regarding her planned pregnancy because her blood type is O– and her husband's is B+. Why is Mrs. Ramey concerned about the differences in their blood types, and what can be done to alleviate some of her fears?

_____

_____

_____

Case 3
Irene Stork has just been diagnosed with polycythemia vera. What can you tell her about this condition and the treatment that may be undertaken to help her with this condition?

_____

_____

_____

The Lymphatic and Immune Systems

Name_____ Class_____ Date_____

REVIEW

Vocabulary Review

Matching
Match the key terms in the right column with the definitions in the left column by placing the letter of each correct answer in the space provided.

_____ 1. Located in the LUQ; filters blood to remove old and diseased RBCs

_____ 2. Found in the mediastinum; stimulates lymphocyte production

_____ 3. Areas that house macrophages and lymphocytes

_____ 4. A disease-causing substance

_____ 5. The other name for tissue fluid

_____ 6. Foreign substances in the body

_____ 7. Small foreign substances that join with proteins to trigger an immune response

_____ 8. Produced by the body in response to an antigen

_____ 9. The other term for body fluids

_____ 10. Cells that primarily target cancer cells

_____ 11. IgA, IgD, IgE, IgG, IgM

_____ 12. Occurs with the first exposure to an antigen

_____ 13. Responsible for the secondary immune response

_____ 14. A type of disease in which the body attacks itself

_____ 15. The other term for *cancerous*

a. interstitial fluid
b. humors
c. haptens
d. immunoglobulins
e. thymus
f. antibodies
g. NK cells
h. pathogen
i. primary immune response
j. autoimmune
k. spleen
l. memory cells
m. malignant
n. antigens
o. lymph nodes

True or False
Decide whether each statement is true or false. In the space at the left, write T for true or F for false. On the lines provided, rewrite the false statements to make them true.

_____ 16. An infection is the presence of an allergen in or on the body.

_____

_____ 17. Salt in sweat is an example of a mechanical barrier that the body uses for protection.

_____

_____ 18. Fever causes the liver and spleen to take iron out of the bloodstream.

_____

_____ **19.** Lymphocytes are phagocytes.

_____ **20.** Nonspecific defenses are called immunities.

_____ **21.** Antibodies are defined as foreign substances in the body.

_____ **22.** T cells respond to antigens by secreting complements.

_____ **23.** T cells respond to antigens by becoming plasma cells.

_____ **24.** Helper B cells make antibodies.

_____ **25.** Memory cells trigger relatively slow primary immune responses.

_____ **26.** IgD triggers allergic reactions.

_____ **27.** Antibodies are also called immunoglobulins.

_____ **28.** The spleen decreases in size as a person ages.

_____ **29.** A person who receives an immunization develops an artificially acquired active immunity.

_____ **30.** Epinephrine causes vasodilation to increase blood pressure (BP).

Content Review

Multiple Choice

In the space provided, write the letter of the choice that best completes each statement or answers each question.

_____ **1.** Which of the following is a nonspecific mechanism used to protect the body against pathogens?

   a. Antibodies   **d.** Haptens

   b. Antigens   **e.** Phagocytosis

   c. Cytokines

_____ **2.** Which of the following does *not* occur during inflammation?

   a. Blood vessels dilate

   b. More blood enters the area that is inflamed

   c. Blood vessels become leaky

   d. Fewer proteins are delivered to the areas that are inflamed

   e. The skin over the inflamed area becomes warm

_____ 3. Which of the following cells are involved in specific defenses?
   a. Monocytes   d. Neutrophils
   b. T cells   e. Erythrocytes
   c. Lysozymes

_____ 4. Which of the following is *not* needed to activate a T cell?
   a. An eosinophil   d. Macrophages
   b. An antigen   e. An allergen
   c. MHC proteins

_____ 5. Which type of cell targets primarily cancer cells but also protects the body against other types of pathogens?
   a. A helper T cell   d. A plasma cell
   b. A memory cell   e. A cytotoxic T cell
   c. A natural killer cell

_____ 6. Which of the following antibodies is found in breast milk, sweat, tears, saliva, and mucus?
   a. IgA   d. IgD
   b. IgG   e. IgE
   c. IgM

_____ 7. Exposure to a viral illness causes the formation of a(n)
   a. Naturally acquired active immunity
   b. Naturally acquired passive immunity
   c. Artificially acquired active immunity
   d. Artificially acquired passive immunity
   e. Artificially acquired local immunity

_____ 8. Which of the following terms is used to describe an illness that occurs when the body attacks its own antigens?
   a. Immune disease   d. Allergies
   b. Malignancy   e. Autoimmune disorders
   c. Benign growth

_____ 9. The stage of cancer in which the malignancy has spread but is still within the primary site is
   a. Stage 0   d. Stage III
   b. Stage I   e. Stage IV
   c. Stage II

_____ 10. Which of the following organs takes over many functions of the spleen after a splenectomy has been performed?
   a. Thymus   d. Gallbladder
   b. Pancreas   e. Appendix
   c. Liver

Sentence Completion

In the space provided, write the word or phrase that best completes each sentence.

11. When interstitial fluid enters lymphatic capillaries, it becomes _____.

12. Two major types of _____ are B cells and T cells.

13. Once activated, _____ divide to make plasma cells and memory cells.

14. _____ are chemicals secreted by T cells in response to antigens.

15. Some activated T cells form _____ cells to help protect the body from cancers and some viral infections.

16. A(n) _____ reaction is an immune response to a substance, such as pollen, that is not normally harmful to the body.

17. _____ is a life-threatening condition in which severe allergic reactions result from a usually harmless antigen.

18. _____ are cells that recognize, engulf, and destroy invading pathogens.

19. The uncontrolled growth of abnormal cells characterizes the disease _____.

20. _____, caused by the cytomegalovirus, is a highly contagious viral illness that is spread by saliva.

21. _____ is the blockage of lymphatic vessels, which causes tissue swelling.

22. _____ is a multisystem autoimmune disorder that may affect the integumentary, renal, and nervous systems.

11. _____

12. _____

13. _____

14. _____

15. _____

16. _____

17. _____

18. _____

19. _____

20. _____

21. _____

22. _____

Short Answer

Write the answer to each question on the lines provided.

23. Explain the differences among the following types of immunity:

   a. Naturally acquired active immunity _____

   _____

   b. Artificially acquired active immunity _____

   _____

   c. Naturally acquired passive immunity _____

   _____

   d. Artificially acquired passive immunity _____

   _____

24. What are three treatments used by persons with allergies?

   _____

   _____

   _____

Critical Thinking

Write the answer to each question on the lines provided.

1. Why is mononucleosis nicknamed "the kissing disease"?

_____

_____

_____

2. Penicillin is an example of a hapten. How does penicillin trigger an immune response in some people?

_____

_____

_____

3. Why do some allergens produce runny noses while others produce diarrhea?

_____

_____

_____

4. What is the difference between a cancer cell and a normal cell?

_____

_____

_____

A P P L I C A T I O N

Follow the directions for each application.

1. Nonspecific Defenses

Explain how the following nonspecific defenses help protect the body from pathogens.

a. Mechanical barriers _____

b. Chemical barriers _____

c. Fever _____

d. Inflammation _____

2. Immune Disorders

Immune disorders develop for various reasons. Give the causes of the following conditions.

a. Chronic fatigue syndrome _____

b. Systemic lupus erythematosus _____

c. Lymphedema _____

d. Mononucleosis _____

3. Lymphatic Pathway

Complete the chart of the lymphatic pathway by inserting the following labels in the proper order:

Collecting duct

Lymphatic vessel

Lymphatic vessel

Lymph node

Lymphatic trunk

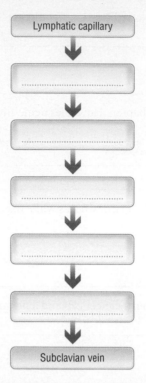

Lymphatic capillary

⬇

....

⬇

....

⬇

....

⬇

....

⬇

....

⬇

Subclavian vein

C A S E   S T U D I E S

Write your response to each case study on the lines provided.

Case 1

A patient with cuts and scrapes is treated with antibiotic creams. Why is this treatment important?

_____

_____

_____

Case 2

A 15-month-old child received his MMR (mumps, measles, rubella) immunization yesterday. Today, his mother calls, stating he is fussy and has a runny nose and a slight temperature. Is it likely the child's symptoms are related to yesterday's immunization? Why or why not?

_____

_____

_____

Case 3

A woman has a "butterfly" rash on her face, joint pain, fatigue, and headaches. What autoimmune disease should she be tested for?

_____

_____

_____

The Respiratory System

Name_____ Class_____ Date_____

R E V I E W

Vocabulary Review

Matching

Match the key terms in the right column with the definitions in the left column by placing the letter of each correct answer in the space provided.

_____ 1. Commonly referred to as the vocal cords, it is actually the space between them

_____ 2. A structure that consists of three lobes

_____ 3. The main branch from the trachea

_____ 4. Cartilaginous covering for the vocal cords

_____ 5. The voice box

_____ 6. Pulmonary parenchyma

_____ 7. A structure that consists of two lobes

_____ 8. A structure that contains the esophagus, the windpipe, and the voice box

_____ 9. The protective membrane (sac) around the lungs

_____ 10. The windpipe

a. alveoli
b. pharynx
c. larynx
d. trachea
e. bronchus
f. pleura
g. right lung
h. left lung
i. epiglottis
j. glottis

True or False

Decide whether each statement is true or false. In the space at the left, write T for true or F for false. On the lines provided, rewrite the false statements to make them true.

_____ 11. The exchange of oxygen and carbon dioxide at the cellular level is known as external respiration.

_____

_____ 12. The trachea splits into two main tubes known as bronchi.

_____

_____ 13. The medical term for the nostrils is nares.

_____

_____ 14. The internal membrane of the pleura is the parietal pleura.

_____

_____ 15. The diaphragm relaxes during inspiration.

_____

_____ **16.** The respiratory center is a group of neurons in the thalamus.

_____ **17.** Expiratory reserve volume is the amount of air that moves in or out of the lungs during a normal breath.

_____ **18.** Carboxyhemoglobin is hemoglobin-carrying oxygen.

_____ **19.** Bronchitis is a chronic condition that damages the alveoli of the lungs.

_____ **20.** The most common malignant neoplasm in the United States is lung cancer.

_____ **21.** A pulmonary embolism is a blocked artery in the heart.

_____ **22.** The pharynx plays a dual role in the digestive and respiratory systems.

_____ **23.** Grade III snoring is heard outside of the bedroom with the door open.

_____ **24.** The tidal volume is the volume of air that remains in the lungs at all times.

_____ **25.** Pneumonia is the inflammation of the lung(s).

Content Review

Multiple Choice

In the space provided, write the letter of the choice that best completes each statement or answers each question.

_____ **1.** Structures that extend from the lateral walls of the nasal cavity are called nasal
    a. Conchae   **d.** Microvilli
    b. Septa   **e.** Trachea
    c. Sinuses

_____ **2.** Lungs are divided into sections called
    a. Septa   **d.** Lobules
    b. Segments   **e.** Bronchioles
    c. Lobes

_____ **3.** Which of the following is *not* a type of pneumoconiosis?
    a. Silicosis   **d.** Halitosis
    b. Asbestosis   **e.** Kyphosis
    c. Anthracosis

_____ **4.** Which of the following is the volume of air moved in and out of the lungs during a respiratory cycle?
    a. Tidal volume   **d.** Expiratory reserve volume
    b. Residual volume   **e.** Forced expiratory volume
    c. Vital capacity

_____ 5. Once oxygen gets into the bloodstream, most of it
   a. Stays dissolved in plasma
   b. Reacts with water to form bicarbonate ions
   c. Binds to hemoglobin
   d. Binds to platelets
   e. Binds to leukocytes

_____ 6. Which of the following is a condition in which the membranes covering the lungs become inflamed?
   a. Bronchitis
   b. Pericarditis
   c. Pleuritis
   d. Pneumonitis
   e. Tracheobronchitis

_____ 7. The structures at the ends of the bronchioles in the lungs are
   a. Alveoli
   b. Bronchioles
   c. Bronchi
   d. Tracheoles
   e. Pleura

_____ 8. The respiratory disease that causes abnormal dilation of the alveolar spaces is
   a. RDS
   b. Pneumoconiosis
   c. SARS
   d. Empyema
   e. Emphysema

_____ 9. Many respiratory conditions are linked to which of the following?
   a. Exposure to cigarette smoke
   b. Family history
   c. Obesity
   d. Alcohol abuse
   e. Pollution and other environmental factors

_____ 10. In which of the following conditions does fluid fill spaces within the lungs?
   a. Pleural effusion
   b. Pulmonary edema
   c. Pulmonary embolism
   d. Hydrothorax
   e. Pleurisy

Sentence Completion

In the space provided, write the word or phrase that best completes each sentence.

11. A treatment for pneumothorax, hemothorax, or hydrothorax, a(n) _____ removes air, blood, or fluid from the chest cavity.

12. The pulmonary parenchyma are more commonly known as the _____.

13. _____ is the medical term for a collapsed lung.

14. Common in many cardiac and respiratory illnesses, _____ is excessive sweating due to illness.

15. Insertion of a chest tube or _____ is done to provide continuous drainage.

16. The inflammation of the pleura is known as _____.

17. _____ describes the inflammation of the spaces within the cranium.

18. Formerly known as hyaline membrane disease, _____ mostly affects premature infants.

19. A symptom of TB and some respiratory neoplasms, _____ is the expectoration of blood.

20. The condition in which the bronchial tree becomes obstructed as a result of inflammation is _____.

11. _____

12. _____

13. _____

14. _____

15. _____

16. _____

17. _____

18. _____

19. _____

20. _____

Short Answer
Write the answer to each question on the lines provided.

21. The following figure shows the structures of the respiratory system. Label each structure using the following terms: nasal cavity, nostril, pharynx, larynx, trachea, bronchus, lung, epiglottis, glottis, alveolar sac, diaphragm.

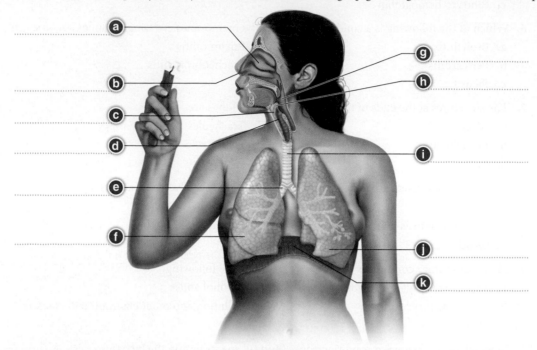

22. The following figures show anterior and posterior views of the larynx. Label the figures using the following terms: hyoid bone, epiglottic cartilage, thyroid cartilage, cricoid cartilage, trachea. (Hint: Each term is used twice.)

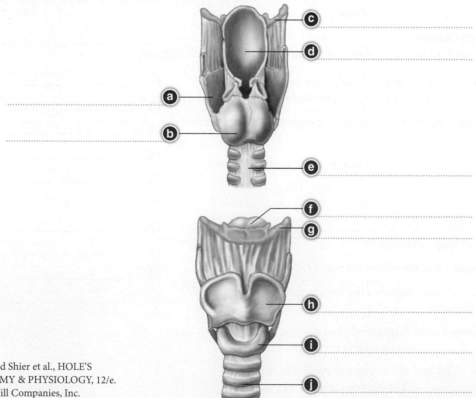

Source: From David Shier et al., HOLE'S
HUMAN ANATOMY & PHYSIOLOGY, 12/e.
© 2010 McGraw Hill Companies, Inc.
Reprinted with permission.

23. Answer the following questions about snoring.

a. What are common causes of snoring? _____

_____

b. What is grade 4 snoring? _____

_____

c. What are the treatments of snoring? _____

_____

24. Briefly describe the following disorders, including typical signs and symptoms:

a. Asthma _____

_____

b. Laryngitis _____

_____

c. SARS _____

_____

d. COPD _____

_____

e. TB _____

_____

f. RDS _____

Critical Thinking

Write the answer to each question on the lines provided.

1. What causes the formation of the Adam's apple in a male? What causes the deepening of the male voice?

_____

_____

_____

2. Explain the function of the diaphragm and the intercostal muscles in the respiratory process.

_____

_____

_____

3. How do carbon dioxide levels in blood affect breathing?

_____

_____

_____

4. Why is carbon monoxide poisonous whereas carbon dioxide is not?

_____

_____

_____

5. Give an overview of the four different classifications of lung cancer.

_____

_____

_____

6. Explain the meaning of the five stages of cancer.

_____

_____

_____

A P P L I C A T I O N

Follow the directions for the application.

1. **Respiratory Diseases**

   Many respiratory diseases produce similar symptoms. Give the meanings for each of the following:

   a. Dyspnea _____   **d.** Diaphoresis _____

   b. Orthopnea _____   **e.** Hemoptysis _____

   c. Dysphonia _____

2. **Disorders of the Respiratory System**

   Explain why the following symptoms are produced.

   a. Difficulty breathing in asthma _____

   b. Pale skin in pulmonary edema _____

   c. Fever in bronchitis or pneumonia _____

   d. Fatigue in emphysema _____

   e. Grunting in RDS _____

   f. Barrel chest in emphysema _____

C A S E   S T U D I E S

Write your response to each case study on the lines provided.

Case 1

A mother brought her 5-year-old son to the doctor's office because he had had a runny nose for the past month. After several tests, it was determined that the boy had enlarged adenoids. How does this condition produce a runny nose? Recall that the adenoids (pharyngeal tonsils) sit at the back of the nasal cavity where it opens into the oral cavity.

_____

_____

_____

Case 2

A 36-year-old smoker constantly sees her doctor for the treatment of bronchitis. What other respiratory diseases is she at high risk for because she smokes?

_____

_____

_____

30

The Nervous System

Name_____ Class_____ Date_____

R E V I E W

Vocabulary Review

Matching

Match the key terms in the right column with the definitions in the left column by placing the letter of each correct answer in the space provided.

_____ 1. Governs organs such as the heart, stomach, and intestines

_____ 2. Prepares the body for resting and digesting food

_____ 3. Insulates axons and allows them to send impulses quickly

_____ 4. The control center for the neuron

_____ 5. The brain and spinal cord

_____ 6. Brings impulses to the cell body

_____ 7. Releases neurotransmitters to provide transmission between neurons

_____ 8. Produces the "fight-or-flight" response

_____ 9. Consists of the nerves outside of the brain and spinal cord

_____ 10. Carries impulses away from the cell body

a. central nervous system (CNS)
b. peripheral nervous system
c. autonomic nervous system
d. sympathetic division
e. parasympathetic division
f. axon
g. dendrite
h. cell body
i. synaptic bulb
j. myelin sheath

True or False

Decide whether each statement is true or false. In the space at the left, write T for true or F for false. On the lines provided, rewrite the false statements to make them true.

_____ 11. The decision-making function of the nervous system takes place in the CNS.

_____

_____ 12. The autonomic nervous system is part of the CNS.

_____

_____ 13. Motor neurons carry information from the periphery to the CNS.

_____

_____ 14. Another term for sensory neurons is afferent nerves.

_____

_____ 15. An unmyelinated axon does not conduct a nerve impulse as quickly as a myelinated axon.

_____

_____ 16. Pia mater is the area in the meninges that contains cerebrospinal fluid (CSF).

_____

_____ 17. The cervical enlargement of the spinal cord contains motor neurons that control muscles of the legs.

_____

_____ 18. The cerebrum is the largest part of the brain.

_____

_____ 19. The midbrain includes the thalamus and hypothalamus.

_____

_____ 20. Oculomotor nerves carry visual information to the brain for interpretation.

_____

_____ 21. The trigeminal nerves innervate muscles of facial expression.

_____

_____ 22. The somatic nervous system consists of nerves that connect the CNS to the skin and skeletal muscle.

_____

_____ 23. Ganglia are collections of neuron cell bodies in the CNS.

_____

_____ 24. The efferent nerves transmit impulses from the CNS to the peripheral nervous system.

_____

_____ 25. The trochlear nerves are tested by asking a patient to smell various substances.

_____

Content Review

Multiple Choice

In the space provided, write the letter of the choice that best completes each statement or answers each question.

_____ 1. Which of the following neuroglial cells is a phagocyte?

    a. Oligodendrocyte   **d.** Neurocyte

    b. Microglia   **e.** Macroglia

    c. Astrocyte

_____ 2. Which lobe of the cerebrum contains the primary visual areas that interpret what a person sees?

    a. Temporal   **d.** Parietal

    b. Occipital   **e.** Brainstem

    c. Frontal

_____ 3. Which of the following areas of the brain contains CSF?

    a. Gyri   **d.** Medulla oblongata

    b. Sulci   **e.** Ventricles

    c. Blood-brain barrier

_____ 4. Which of the following is a function of the cerebellum?

    a. The interpretation of hearing

    b. The regulation of breathing

    c. The coordination of fine movements such as writing

    d. The secretion of hormones

    e. The regulation of blood pressure

_____ 5. Which of the following acts as an "interpreter" for afferent and efferent neurons?

    a. Interneurons   d. Myelin

    b. Microglia   e. Oligodendrocytes

    c. Neurotransmitters

_____ 6. Which procedure involves the use of a needle to remove CSF from the subarachnoid space?

    a. Cerebral angiography   d. CT scan

    b. X-ray   e. Lumbar puncture

    c. MRI

_____ 7. Which cranial nerve does *not* control the eyes or visual functioning?

    a. II   d. V

    b. III   e. VI

    c. IV

Sentence Completion

In the space provided, write the word or phrase that best completes each sentence.

8. _____ are the neuroglial cells that anchor blood vessels to nerves.

9. The _____ is formed by a tight network of capillaries that protect the delicate tissues of the CNS.

10. The myelin sheath is created by the _____.

11. _____ wrap themselves around some axons, forming what is known as white matter.

12. Neuron cell membranes are polarized; the term for this is _____.

13. Chemicals called _____ are released from the synaptic knob.

14. Unmyelinated axons of the CNS are referred to as _____.

15. The _____ tracts of the spinal cord carry sensory information to the brain.

16. A predictable, automatic response to a stimulus is called a(n) _____.

17. The cerebrum is split into four sections called _____.

18. The _____ consists of the midbrain, the pons, and the medulla oblongata.

19. The area of skin innervated by a single spinal or cranial nerve is called a(n) _____.

20. The _____ is the outermost layer of the cerebrum.

21. _____ refers to the loss of feeling in the extremities associated with neurological disorders.

22. A(n) _____ is an x-ray of the blood vessels of the brain after an infusion of contrast media.

8. _____

9. _____

10. _____

11. _____

12. _____

13. _____

14. _____

15. _____

16. _____

17. _____

18. _____

19. _____

20. _____

21. _____

22. _____

Short Answer
Write the answer to each question on the lines provided.

23. Use the following terms to label the following illustration of a synapse: synaptic vesicle, neurotransmitter, axon membrane, synaptic knob, vesicle releasing neurotransmitter, cell body or dendrite of postsynaptic structure, polarized membrane, depolarized membrane, synaptic cleft.

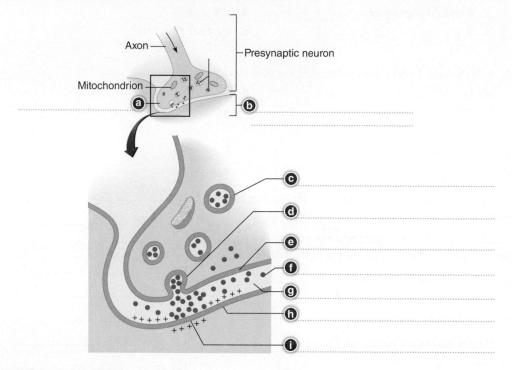

24. Use the following terms to label the following illustration of a reflex arc: flexor contracts, motor neurons, interneuron, extensor contracts, sensory neuron, motor neurons, extensor relaxes, flexor relaxes.

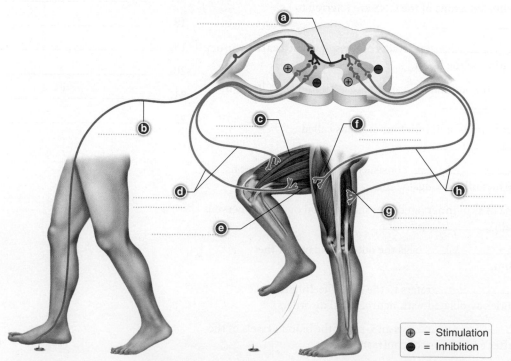

⊕ = Stimulation
● = Inhibition

Source for all art on page: From David Shier et al., HOLE'S HUMAN ANATOMY & PHYSIOLOGY, 12/e. © 2010 McGraw Hill Companies, Inc. Reprinted with permission.

25. Use the following terms to label the following illustration of the spinal nerves and plexuses: lumbar nerves, thoracic nerves, coccygeal plexus, brachial plexus, cervical nerves, lumbosacral plexus, sacral nerves, sacral plexus, coccygeal nerves, cervical plexus, lumbar plexus.

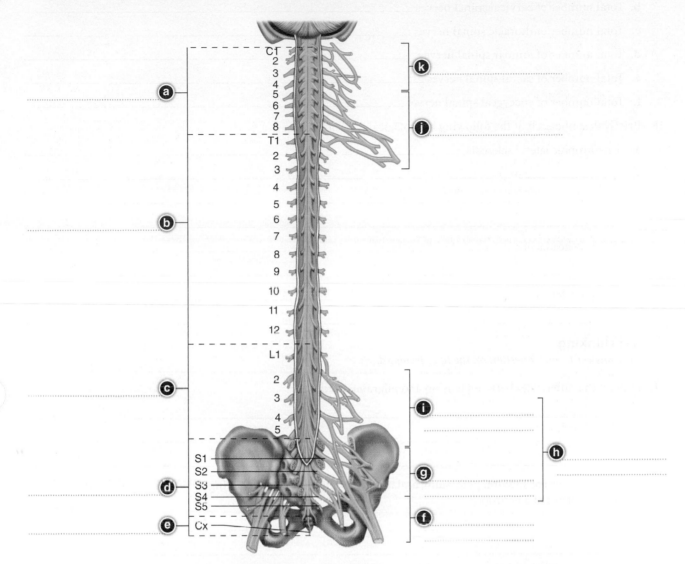

26. Fill in the following table with information about the cranial nerves.

Cranial Nerve Number	Name of Cranial Nerve	Function of Cranial Nerve
II		
V		
VI		
X		
XII		

27. Give the correct number for each of the following.

    a. Total number of spinal nerves _____

    b. Total number of cervical spinal nerves _____

    c. Total number of thoracic spinal nerves _____

    d. Total number of lumbar spinal nerves _____

    e. Total number of sacral spinal nerves _____

    f. Total number of coccygeal spinal nerves _____

28. Briefly describe each of the following neurological disorders.

    a. Amyotrophic lateral sclerosis _____

    _____

    b. Bell's palsy _____

    _____

    c. Migraine headaches _____

    _____

    d. Multiple sclerosis _____

    _____

Critical Thinking

Write the answer to each question on the lines provided.

1. Explain the differences between tension and migraine headaches.

    _____

    _____

    _____

2. Describe the roles of sodium, potassium, and negatively charged ions in creating polarized, depolarized, and repolarized states of a neuron.

    _____

    _____

    _____

3. Explain why diseases that destroy the myelin sheath cause muscle weakness and paralysis.

    _____

    _____

    _____

4. Explain the major differences between the somatic nervous system and autonomic nervous system.

    _____

    _____

    _____

A P P L I C A T I O N

Follow the directions for each application.

1. Nerve Plexuses
Describe the nerves branching off each of the following plexuses.

a. Cervical _____

b. Brachial _____

c. Lumbosacral _____

d. Coccygeal _____

2. Evaluation of Cranial Nerves
Disorders of cranial nerves can be determined by using various tests. Name what tests might be used to evaluate the following nerves.

a. Oculomotor, trochlear, and abducens nerves _____

b. Trigeminal nerves _____

c. Hypoglossal nerves _____

3. Reflex Testing
Name the nerves that may be damaged if the following reflexes are abnormal.

a. Biceps reflex _____

b. Knee reflex _____

c. Abdominal reflexes _____

C A S E   S T U D I E S

Write your response to each case study on the lines provided.

Case 1
A patient has a bacterial infection in the brain. Why will this patient need a higher concentration of antibiotics than a patient with the same bacterial infection in the lungs?

_____

_____

_____

Case 2
An EEG on your patient shows spikes of electrical activity in the brain. What condition may cause this finding?

_____

_____

_____

Case 3

A mother is concerned that her 12-month-old baby has not started walking yet. The pediatrician explains that the baby's peripheral nerves are probably not yet fully myelinated. How does this explain why the baby cannot walk?

_____

_____

_____

Case 4

Your patient's wife calls very concerned that her husband may have had a stroke during the night. His face looks lopsided and he is drooling. Strangely, he has no other symptoms. Is it likely that the patient had a stroke? If not, what disease or disorder might he be experiencing?

_____

_____

_____

31

The Urinary System

Name_____ Class_____ Date_____

REVIEW

Vocabulary Review

Matching
Match the key terms in the right column with the definitions in the left column by placing the letter of each correct answer in the space provided.

_____ 1. The working tissue of kidney that filters the blood

_____ 2. The structure that consists of the proximal convoluted tubule, the loop of Henle, and the distal convoluted tubule

_____ 3. The triangle formed by the three openings in the bladder

_____ 4. Small arteries that bring blood to the glomerulus

_____ 5. The tubes that bring urine to the bladder

_____ 6. Tightly coiled capillaries of the nephron that begin the filtration process

_____ 7. The position of the kidneys

_____ 8. Smooth muscle of the bladder wall

_____ 9. The hormone that assists with blood pressure regulation

_____ 10. Vessels that carry blood to the peritubular capillaries

_____ 11. Muscular contractions that move urine through the ureters

_____ 12. The tube leading from the bladder to the outside of the body

_____ 13. Composed of the glomerulus and the Bowman's capsule

_____ 14. The hormone that helps the body retain fluid

_____ 15. An alternate term for urination

a. afferent arteriole
b. antidiuretic hormone
c. detrusor muscle
d. efferent arteriole
e. glomerulus
f. micturition
g. nephron
h. peristalsis
i. renal corpuscle
j. renal tubule
k. renin
l. retroperitoneal
m. trigone
n. urethra
o. ureter

True or False
Decide whether each statement is true or false. In the space at the left, write T for true or F for false. On the lines provided, rewrite the false statements to make them true.

_____ 16. The kidneys lie outside the peritoneal cavity.

_____

_____ 17. Inside a kidney, the ureter expands as a renal pyramid.

_____

_____ 18. The outer portion of the kidney is called the renal medulla.

_____

_____ **19.** Erythropoietin stimulates the kidney to produce red blood cells.

_____ **20.** The loop of Henle is between a distal convoluted tubule and a collecting duct.

_____ **21.** The ureter enters the kidney at the hilum.

_____ **22.** Glomerular filtration takes place in the renal corpuscles of nephrons.

_____ **23.** In tubular secretion, substances move out of the peritubular capillaries and into the renal tubules.

_____ **24.** Urine is composed mostly of urea.

_____ **25.** The ureter empties the bladder to the outside.

_____ **26.** The external urethral sphincter is under voluntary control.

_____ **27.** Renal calculi are stones in the bladder.

_____ **28.** Retention is a condition in which a person cannot control urination.

_____ **29.** Pyelonephritis is considered a hereditary condition.

_____ **30.** Diuretics help the body retain fluid.

Content Review

Multiple Choice

In the space provided, write the letter of the choice that best completes each statement or answers each question.

_____ **1.** Which of the following are the tubes inside the kidney?
   a. Pelvis   **d.** Ureters
   b. Calyces   **e.** Hilum
   c. Column

_____ **2.** The triangular-shaped areas of the renal medulla are the
   a. Renal pelvis   **d.** Trigones
   b. Calices   **e.** Renal pyramids
   c. Renal columns

_____ **3.** Which of the following is part of a renal corpuscle?
   a. The glomerular capsule   **d.** The proximal convoluted tubule
   b. The distal convoluted tubule   **e.** The renal cortex
   c. The loop of Henle

_____ 4. Which of the following delivers blood to the glomerulus?
  a. The afferent arterioles
  b. The efferent arterioles
  c. The glomerulus
  d. The interlobular arteries
  e. The renal vein

_____ 5. Which of the following is responsible for tubular reabsorption?
  a. The glomerulus
  b. The ureters
  c. The collecting tubules
  d. The Bowman's capsule
  e. The proximal convoluted tubules

_____ 6. The three openings of the floor of the bladder are
  a. One opening for the ureter and two for each urethra
  b. One opening for the urethra and two for the ureters
  c. One opening for the urethra and two for the urinary arteries
  d. One opening for the ureter and two for the urinary arteries
  e. One opening for the urinary arteries and two for each ureter

_____ 7. The trigone refers to
  a. The proximal convoluted tubule, the loop of Henle, and the distal convoluted tubule
  b. The afferent arterioles, glomerulus, and efferent arterioles
  c. The "jobs" of the kidney, which are filtration, reabsorption, and secretion
  d. The area of the bladder that encompasses the ureteral and urethral openings
  e. The shape of the renal pyramids

_____ 8. Secretion refers to
  a. The formation and release of erythropoietin
  b. The formation of filtrate
  c. The removal of urine from the bladder
  d. A substance that forms urine
  e. A substance moving out of the peritubular capillaries and into the renal tubules

_____ 9. The inability of kidneys to create urine is called
  a. Renal failure
  b. Incontinence
  c. Retention
  d. Renal calculi
  e. Glomerulonephritis

_____ 10. The detrusor muscle is responsible for
  a. Moving urine from the ureters to the bladder
  b. Retaining urine in the bladder
  c. Expelling urine from the bladder
  d. Controlling the filtration rate
  e. Sensing that the bladder is full

Sentence Completion

In the space provided, write the word or phrase that best completes each sentence.

11. The innermost layer of the kidney is called the renal _____.

12. A nephron consists of a renal corpuscle and a _____.

13. When more glomerular filtrate is formed, _____ urine is ultimately formed.

14. Erythropoietin causes the formation of _____.

15. _____ is a condition in which the kidneys slowly lose their ability to function.

16. _____ is an inflammation of the glomeruli.

17. _____ is a disorder in which the kidneys enlarge because of the presence of many cysts within them.

18. _____ is a complicated urinary tract infection.

19. _____ is commonly known as a bladder infection.

20. _____ describes the condition in which "stones" are found within the kidney.

11. _____

12. _____

13. _____

14. _____

15. _____

16. _____

17. _____

18. _____

19. _____

20. _____

Short Answer

Write the answer to each question on the lines provided.

21. The following figure illustrates the organs of the urinary system. Label the illustration using the following terms: kidney, bladder, ureter, aorta, inferior vena cava, hilum of kidney, renal artery, renal vein, urethra.

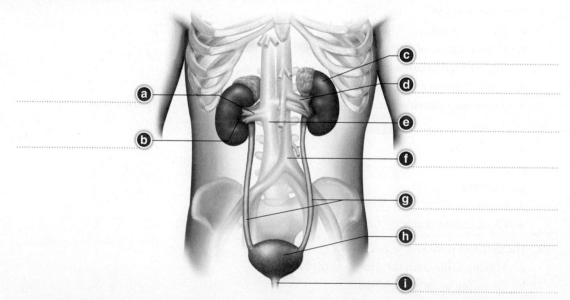

Source: From David Shier et al., HOLE'S HUMAN ANATOMY & PHYSIOLOGY, 12/e. © 2010 McGraw Hill Companies, Inc. Reprinted with permission.

22. The following figure illustrates a section of a kidney. Label the illustration using the following terms: renal corpuscle, renal pelvis, calyx (major), calyx (minor), renal cortex, renal medulla, renal pyramid, renal papilla, ureter, renal column.

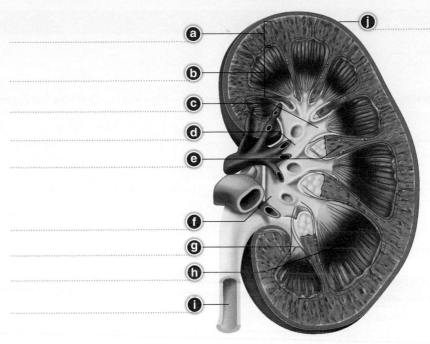

....

....

....

....

....

....

....

....

Source: From David Shier et al., HOLE'S HUMAN ANATOMY & PHYSIOLOGY, 12/e. © 2010 McGraw Hill Companies, Inc. Reprinted with permission.

Critical Thinking

Write the answer to each question on the lines provided.

1. How does blood pressure affect glomerular filtration?

   _____

   _____

   _____

2. How do the hormones ADH and aldosterone decrease urine production?

   _____

   _____

   _____

3. Explain the difference between acute and chronic renal failure.

   _____

   _____

   _____

4. What is the difference between glomerulonephritis and pyelonephritis?

   _____

   _____

   _____

5. What is the relationship between chronic renal failure and anemia?

   _____

   _____

   _____

A P P L I C A T I O N

Follow the directions for each application.

1. **Kidney Hormones**

   Besides filtering blood and forming urine, the kidneys also release important hormones. Describe the functions of the following kidney hormones.

   a. Renn _____

   _____

   b. Erythropoietin _____

   _____

2. **Nephrons**

   Nephrons are the functional units of the kidneys. Describe the functions of the following parts of a nephron.

   a. Glomerulus _____

   _____

   b. Bowman's capsule _____

   _____

   c. Renal tubule _____

   _____

C A S E   S T U D I E S

Write your response to each case study on the lines provided.

Case 1

A young female patient complains that she has had three urinary tract infections in the last 5 years, but her brothers haven't had any. How would you explain to her why females are more likely to develop urinary tract infections than males?

_____

_____

_____

Case 2

A young female patient has frequent urinary tract infections. What would you tell her to do to help prevent these frequent infections?

_____

_____

_____

Case 3

How would you explain to a pregnant patient why she may develop incontinence?

_____

_____

_____

32

The Reproductive Systems

Name_____ Class_____ Date_____

REVIEW

Vocabulary Review

Matching

Match the key terms in the right column with the definitions in the left column by placing the letter of each correct answer in the space provided.

_____ 1. The area within the testes responsible for sperm production

_____ 2. Tissue responsible for male hormone production

_____ 3. The process that reduces the number of chromosomes in a cell from 46 to 23

_____ 4. A male fluid that alkalinizes the female vagina

_____ 5. The process of ovum formation

_____ 6. The monthly release of a mature ovum from an ovary

_____ 7. The neck of the uterus

_____ 8. The innermost layer of the uterus

_____ 9. The muscular layer of the uterus

_____ 10. The outermost layer of the uterus

_____ 11. The oviducts

_____ 12. The area between the vagina and the anus

_____ 13. The milk glands of the female breast

_____ 14. A cell formed by a fertilized ovum

_____ 15. The rapid mitosis of a zygote

_____ 16. The hormone released that confirms pregnancy

_____ 17. The communication organ between a pregnant woman and the developing embryo or fetus

_____ 18. The product of conception, weeks 2–8

_____ 19. Week 9 through the delivery of the neonate

_____ 20. The act of giving birth

a. prostate fluid
b. endometrium
c. embryo
d. interstitial cells
e. parturition
f. placenta
g. perimetrium
h. cleavage
i. fetus
j. seminiferous tubules
k. meiosis
l. perineum
m. fallopian tubes
n. ovulation
o. myometrium
p. HCG
q. mammary glands
r. cervix
s. zygote
t. oogenesis

True or False

Decide whether each statement is true or false. In the space at the left, write T for true or F for false. On the lines provided, rewrite the false statements to make them true.

_____ **21.** The other name for the bulbourethral glands is the Bartholin's glands.

_____

_____ **22.** The epididymis is a tube in which sperm cells mature.

_____

_____ **23.** A zygote contains 46 chromosomes.

_____

_____ **24.** In a transurethral resection of the prostate (TURP), the vas deferens are cut and tied.

_____

_____ **25.** Cryptorchidism is the term for undescended testicles.

_____

_____ **26.** FSH and LH are released by the hypothalamus.

_____

_____ **27.** The prepuce is the glans penis.

_____

_____ **28.** The fringed part of a fallopian tube is the fimbriae.

_____

_____ **29.** The cleavage is the female erectile tissue.

_____

_____ **30.** Menarche refers to the end of the menstrual period for women.

_____

_____ **31.** All fetal organs are formed by the primary germ layers.

_____

_____ **32.** The yolk sac makes new blood cells for the fetus.

_____

_____ **33.** The ovaries or testes are formed in the abdominopelvic cavity of a developing fetus.

_____

_____ **34.** The foramen ovale is a connection between the pulmonary trunk and the aorta.

_____

_____ **35.** The prenatal period is the 6-week time frame after birth.

_____

Content Review

Multiple Choice

In the space provided, write the letter of the choice that best completes each statement or answers each question.

_____ 1. The portion of a sperm cell that contains the genetic information from the biological father is the

     a. Head   **d.** Acrosome

     b. Tail   **e.** Flagellum

     c. Midpiece

_____ 2. Which of the following is the muscular gland at the base of the male urethra?

     a. Seminal vesicle   **d.** Bulbourethral gland

     b. Epididymis   **e.** Prostate

     c. Seminiferous tubules

_____ 3. The domed portion of the uterus is called the

     a. Body   **d.** Myometrium

     b. Fundus   **e.** Cervix

     c. Peristalsis

_____ 4. To which of the following organs does the term effacement apply?

     a. Uterus   **d.** Cervix

     b. Ovary   **e.** Fallopian tube

     c. Vagina

_____ 5. Which of the following structures releases progesterone to increase the vascularity of the uterine lining?

     a. Follicle   **d.** Anterior pituitary

     b. Oocyte   **e.** Corpus luteum

     c. Ovary

_____ 6. Which of the following organ systems are the last to develop in a fetus?

     a. Reproductive and urinary   **d.** Integumentary and muscular

     b. Respiratory and digestive   **e.** Cardiovascular and respiratory

     c. Nervous and endocrine

_____ 7. Which of the following connects the pulmonary trunk and the aorta in the developing fetus?

     a. Hepatic portal vein   **d.** Ductusvenosus

     b. Foramen ovale   **e.** Umbilical arteries

     c. Ductusarteriosus

_____ 8. Which hormone stimulates uterine contractions for the birth process?

     a. PTH   **d.** Relaxin

     b. Progesterone   **e.** Aldosterone

     c. Oxytocin

_____ 9. Which stage is known as afterbirth?

     a. Postnatal   **d.** Postpartum

     b. Placental   **e.** Delivery

     c. Expulsion

_____ 10. The term breech refers to

     a. A fetus who is in the head-down position

     b. A pregnancy of twins

     c. A cesarean delivery

     d. A fetus in the buttocks or feet-first position

     e. A premature delivery

_____ 11. Which of the following forms of contraception requires surgery?
     a. Tubal ligation
     b. Insertable contraceptives
     c. Implantable contraceptives
     d. Intrauterine devices
     e. Ingestible contraceptives

_____ 12. The inability to conceive after trying for 12 consecutive months is termed
     a. Impotence   **d.** Infection
     b. Conception   **e.** Infertility
     c. Contraception

_____ 13. Which of the following STIs has been implicated in cervical cancer?
     a. Gonorrhea
     b. Herpes simplex virus
     c. Human immunodeficiency virus (HIV)
     d. Human papilloma virus (HPV)
     e. Chlamydia

_____ 14. Which of the following STIs is caused by a parasite?
     a. Gonorrhea   **d.** Genital warts
     b. Trichomoniasis   **e.** Syphilis
     c. Pediculosis pubis

_____ 15. Gonorrhea and chlamydia can cause infertility due to which of the following diseases?
     a. HIV   **d.** Syphilis
     b. PID   **e.** HSV
     c. HPV

Sentence Completion

In the space provided, write the word or phrase that best completes each sentence.

16. The _____ gland provides mucus for lubrication for the penis.

17. The process of _____ occurs when semen is forced out of the male urethra.

18. When in a nonerect state, the penis is said to be _____.

19. _____ is the malignant neoplasm (cancer) of the male sex organs.

20. The _____ are the lubricating glands of the vagina.

21. A(n) _____ is the surgical procedure done to remove the uterus.

22. The protective sac around the developing embryo or fetus is the _____.

23. The _____ carries oxygenated blood to the developing fetus.

24. _____ barrier forms of birth control include the diaphragm, condoms, and the cervical cap.

25. _____ is defined as the inability to conceive a child after 12 months of trying.

16. _____

17. _____

18. _____

19. _____

20. _____

21. _____

22. _____

23. _____

24. _____

25. _____

Short Answer
Write the answer to each question on the lines provided.

26. The following figure illustrates the male reproductive system with some structures unlabeled. Label the rest of the illustration using the following terms: scrotum, testis, penis, prostate gland, seminal vesicle, vas deferens, urethra, bulbourethral gland, epididymis.

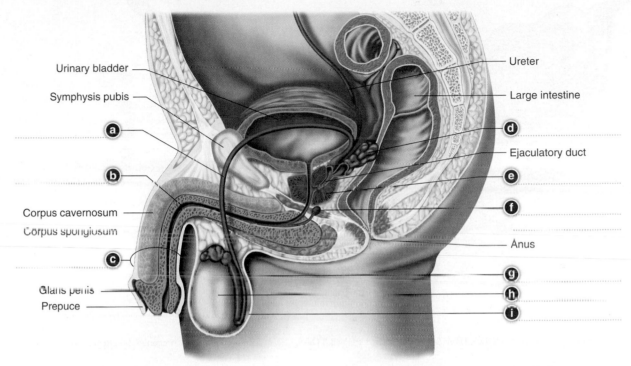

Urinary bladder
Symphysis pubis
a
b
Corpus cavernosum
Corpus spongiosum
c
Glans penis
Prepuce

Ureter
Large intestine
d
Ejaculatory duct
e
f
Anus
g
h
i

27. The following figure illustrates the female reproductive system with some structures unlabeled. Label the rest of the figure using the following terms: ovary, uterus, fallopian tube, clitoris, vagina, cervix.

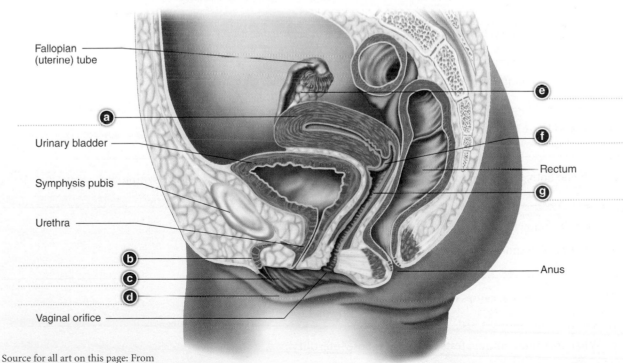

Fallopian (uterine) tube
a
Urinary bladder
Symphysis pubis
Urethra
b
c
d
Vaginal orifice

e
f
Rectum
g
Anus

Source for all art on this page: From David Shier et al., HOLE'S HUMAN ANATOMY & PHYSIOLOGY, 12/e. © 2010 McGraw Hill Companies, Inc. Reprinted with permission.

28. The following figure illustrates the internal female reproductive organs and ovulation. Label the figure using the following terms: cervical orifice, fimbriae, body of uterus, uterine tube, cervix, endometrium, infundibulum, perimetrium, vagina, oocyte, ovary, myometrium, follicle.

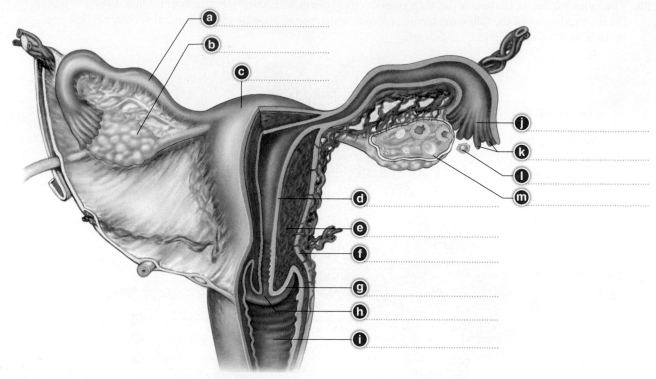

a _____

b _____

c

j _____

k _____

l _____

m _____

d _____

e _____

f _____

g _____

h _____

i _____

Source: From David Shier et al., HOLE'S HUMAN ANATOMY & PHYSIOLOGY, 12/e. © 2010 McGraw Hill Companies, Inc. Reprinted with permission.

29. Answer the following questions about STIs.

a. Which STI has three distinct stages?

_____

b. Which viral STI has been found to increase the risk of cervical cancer?

_____

c. What three common signs or symptoms are found in a woman with an STI?

_____

d. What STIs are known to cause pelvic inflammatory disease?

_____

e. Why do both partners need to be treated for any STI, even if only one partner has symptoms?

_____

30. Answer the following questions about infertility.

a. What are common causes of infertility due to male factors?

_____

b. What are common causes of infertility due to female factors?

_____

c. What are some common tests used to diagnose infertility?

_____

Critical Thinking

Write the answer to each question on the lines provided.

1. Why must sperm cells and oocytes have only 23 chromosomes instead of 46 like most body cells?

_____

_____

_____

2. Explain the differences between fetal circulation and normal circulation.

_____

_____

_____

3. Why is it possible for an egg to be fertilized in the pelvic cavity of a female instead of her reproductive tract?

_____

_____

_____

4. Explain why STIs are more readily passed from a male to a female than from a female to a male.

_____

_____

_____

5. Why can a woman not feel her fetus move before the fifth month of pregnancy?

_____

_____

_____

A P P L I C A T I O N

Follow the directions for the application.

1. Male Reproductive Organs

Describe the functions of the following male reproductive organs.

a. Penis _____

b. Scrotum _____

c. Epididymis _____

d. Prostate gland _____

e. Vas deferens _____

2. **Female Reproductive Organs**

   Describe the functions of the following female reproductive organs.

   a. Uterus _____

   b. Vagina _____

   c. Fallopian tubes _____

   d. Bartholin's glands _____

   e. Ovaries _____

C A S E   S T U D I E S

Write your response to each case study on the lines provided.

Case 1

A 20-year-old man is reluctant to perform testicular self-exams. What can you tell him to persuade him about the importance of this exam?

_____

_____

_____

Case 2

Why is ovarian cancer harder to detect in its early stages than other types of reproductive cancers?

_____

_____

_____

Case 3

A 6-month-old baby is diagnosed with having a hole in his heart. The doctor explains that this hole is normal during fetal development but should close after the birth of the baby. How would you explain to the mother the function of this hole during fetal development?

_____

_____

_____

33

The Digestive System

Name_____ Class_____ Date_____

R E V I E W

Vocabulary Review

Matching

Match the key terms in the right column with the definitions in the left column by placing the letter of each correct answer in the space provided.

_____	**1.** A necessary food substance	**a.** bile
_____	**2.** The term for food mixed with saliva and mucus	**b.** chyme
_____	**3.** The hole in the diaphragm through which the esophagus extends	**c.** esophageal hiatus
_____	**4.** The duct that delivers bile to the duodenum	**d.** chemical digestion
_____	**5.** A substance created in the liver that is used in the digestion of fats	**e.** feces
_____	**6.** The roof of the mouth	**f.** glycogen
_____	**7.** Abnormal dilations in the intestinal wall	**g.** lipid
_____	**8.** Breakdown of food by chemicals such as enzymes	**h.** mechanical digestion
_____	**9.** The structure that anchors the tongue to the floor of the mouth	**i.** nutrient
_____	**10.** Sugar stored in the liver and skeletal muscle cells	**j.** sphincters
_____	**11.** A structure that covers the opening of the larynx to prevent food from entering	**k.** triglycerides
		l. palate
_____	**12.** Projections that increase the surface area of the small intestine	**m.** salivary glands
_____	**13.** A mixture of food and gastric juices	**n.** alimentary canal
_____	**14.** The part of the soft palate that hangs down into the throat	**o.** lingual frenulum
_____	**15.** Circular bands of muscle located at the openings of many tubes in the body	**p.** uvula
		q. intrinsic factor
_____	**16.** A substance from parietal cells that is needed for B_{12} absorption	**r.** cholesterol
_____	**17.** Fats that are used by the body to make energy when glucose levels are low	**s.** epiglottis
_____	**18.** The folds of the stomach lining	**t.** bolus
_____	**19.** Leftover chyme after water and electrolytes are reabsorbed into the body	**u.** hepatic portal vein
_____	**20.** Breakdown of food by chewing	**v.** diverticula
_____	**21.** The most abundant dietary lipids	**w.** rugae
_____	**22.** The parotid, submandibular, and sublingual glands	**x.** microvilli
_____	**23.** The structure that carries blood from the digestive organs to the liver	**y.** common bile duct
_____	**24.** The tube or pathway that extends from the mouth to the anus	
_____	**25.** A dietary lipid that is essential to cell growth and function	

True or False

Decide whether each statement is true or false. In the space at the left, write T for true or F for false. On the lines provided, rewrite the false statements to make them true.

_____ **26.** The visceral peritoneum is the lining of the abdominal cavity.

_____

_____ **27.** The serosa is the innermost layer of the alimentary canal and is responsible for absorbing nutrients.

_____

_____ **28.** The serosa is also known as the visceral peritoneum.

_____

_____ **29.** Amylase begins the digestion of fats.

_____

_____ **30.** The pharynx extends from the back of the nasal cavity to the esophagus.

_____

_____ **31.** The palatine tonsils are known as the adenoids.

_____

_____ **32.** The epiglottis covers the opening of the trachea.

_____

_____ **33.** The main part of the stomach is called the cardiac region.

_____

_____ **34.** The first portion of the small intestine is the duodenum.

_____

_____ **35.** If a patient's stomach has been removed, a G tube may be placed for feeding him.

_____

_____ **36.** The cardiac sphincter keeps food boluses from reentering the esophagus once they are inside the stomach.

_____

_____ **37.** The liver is located in the lower left quadrant of the abdomen.

_____

_____ **38.** The ascending colon becomes the sigmoid colon.

_____

_____ **39.** The gallbladder makes bile, which is then stored in the liver.

_____

_____ **40.** The fat-soluble vitamins are vitamins A, D, E, and K.

_____

Content Review

Multiple Choice

In the space provided, write the letter of the choice that best completes each statement or answers each question.

_____ 1. Which of the following is *not* an organ of the alimentary canal?
   a. The mouth
   b. The stomach
   c. The liver
   d. The anal canal
   e. The small intestine

_____ 2. Which layer of the alimentary canal contracts in order to move materials through the canal?
   a. The mucosa
   b. The serosa
   c. The muscular layer
   d. The submucosa
   e. The mesentery

_____ 3. Which of the following is a component of saliva?
   a. Glucose
   b. Amylase
   c. Pepsin
   d. Gastrin
   e. Sucrase

_____ 4. Which sphincter separates the stomach from the small intestine?
   a. Cardiac sphincter
   b. Esophageal sphincter
   c. Ileocecal sphincter
   d. Pyloric sphincter
   e. Anal sphincter

_____ 5. Which of the following lists the large intestine segments in order from the small intestine to the rectum?
   a. Descending colon, transverse colon, ascending colon, sigmoid colon, cecum
   b. Cecum, ascending colon, descending colon, transverse colon, sigmoid colon
   c. Cecum, descending colon, transverse colon, ascending colon, sigmoid colon
   d. Sigmoid colon, ascending colon, transverse colon, descending colon, cecum
   e. Cecum, ascending colon, transverse colon, descending colon, sigmoid colon

_____ 6. Which of the following is part of the small intestine?
   a. The jejunum
   b. The cecum
   c. The cardiac region
   d. The fundus
   e. The pylorus

_____ 7. Which disease occurs when normal liver tissue is replaced by scar tissue?
   a. Hepatitis
   b. Colitis
   c. Cirrhosis
   d. Jaundice
   e. Crohn's disease

_____ 8. Which of the following is a screening test used to determine the presence of colon polyps and colon cancer?

     a. Colectomy

     b. Colonoscopy

     c. Endoscopy

     d. Colostomy

     e. Enterectomy

_____ 9. What common gastrointestinal disorder is also known as *GERD*?

     a. Constipation

     b. Hemorrhoids

     c. Diarrhea

     d. Hernia

     e. Heartburn

_____ 10. Which of the following foods is not a good source of protein?

     a. Eggs

     b. Cheese

     c. Fish

     d. Carrots

     e. Beans

Sentence Completion

In the space provided, write the word or phrase that best completes each sentence.

11. The _____ glands are the largest of the salivary glands.

12. If chyme moves too quickly through the small intestine, nutrients are not absorbed and _____ results.

13. The _____ is the area where the esophagus goes through the diaphragm.

14. _____ are defined as necessary food substances.

15. _____ from the parietal cells of the stomach is necessary for vitamin B_{12} absorption.

16. Vitamin _____ is needed for blood clotting.

17. Pancreatic _____ produce pancreatic juices for digestion.

18. _____ is the condition of difficult defecation.

19. Acidic chyme is neutralized in the duodenum by _____ from the pancreas.

20. The _____ is primarily responsible for most of the nutrient absorption.

11. _____

12. _____

13. _____

14. _____

15. _____

16. _____

17. _____

18. _____

19. _____

20. _____

Short Answer

Write the answer to each question on the lines provided.

21. The following illustration shows the organs of the digestive system. Label the figure using the following terms: stomach, mouth, large intestine, esophagus, small intestine, pharynx, salivary glands, liver, gallbladder, pancreas, rectum, anus.

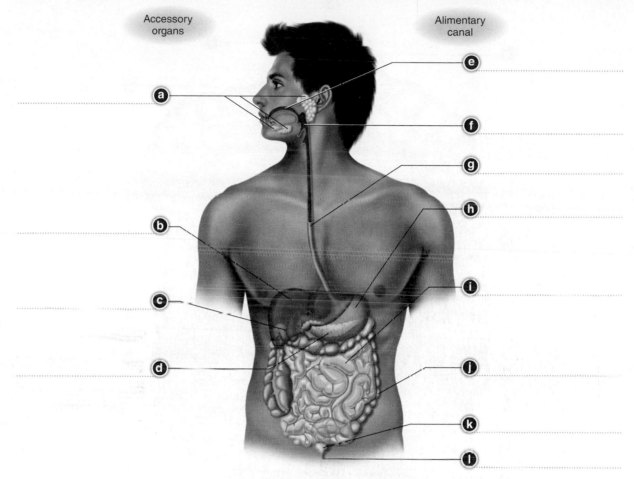

22. The following illustration shows the different regions of the stomach. Label the figure using the following terms: fundus, cardiac region, body, pylorus, pyloric canal, duodenum, pyloric sphincter, esophagus, rugae.

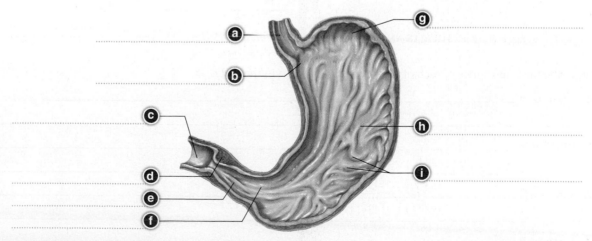

Source for all art on this page: From David Shier et al., HOLE'S HUMAN ANATOMY & PHYSIOLOGY, 12/e. © 2010 McGraw Hill Companies, Inc. Reprinted with permission.

23. The following illustration shows the various parts of the large intestine and the layers in the wall of the alimentary canal. Label the figure using the following terms: mucus membrane, serous layer, muscular layer, vermiform appendix, cecum, ascending colon, descending colon, transverse colon, sigmoid colon, rectum, anal canal, orifice of appendix, ileocecal sphincter.

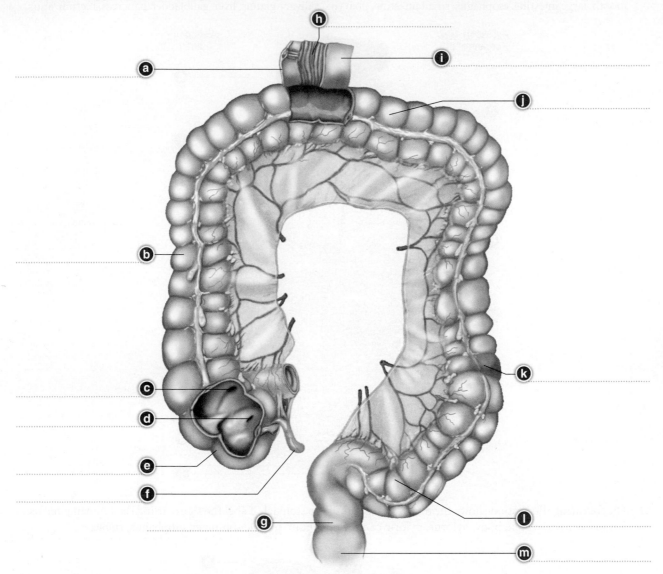

Source: From David Shier et al., HOLE'S HUMAN ANATOMY & PHYSIOLOGY, 12/e. © 2010 McGraw Hill Companies, Inc. Reprinted with permission.

24. Describe the importance of each of the following vitamins in the body.

a. Vitamin A _____

_____

b. Riboflavin _____

_____

c. VitaminC_____

_____

d. Vitamin B$_{12}$ _____

_____

e. Folic acid _____

_____

f. Vitamin E _____

_____

Critical Thinking
Write the answer to each question on the lines provided.

1. Why is it impossible to breathe and swallow at the same time?

_____

_____

_____

2. Why are oral and dental health important in good nutrition?

_____

_____

_____

3. What sphincter must open to permit vomiting?

_____

_____

_____

4. Why would a lack of fiber (roughage) in the diet be implicated in colon diseases, including colon cancer?

_____

_____

_____

5. What is the difference between a hiatal hernia and an inguinal hernia?

_____

_____

_____

A P P L I C A T I O N

Follow the directions for each application.

1. Pharynx

The pharynx has three divisions. Describe the location and functions of each of these divisions.

a. Nasopharynx _____

_____

b. Oropharynx _____

_____

c. Laryngopharynx _____

_____

2. **Nutrients**

Nutrients are necessary food substances. Tell how the body uses each of the following types of nutrient.

a. Carbohydrates_____

_____

b. Proteins_____

_____

c. Lipids_____

_____

d. Vitamins_____

_____

e. Minerals_____

_____

CASE STUDIES

Write your response to each case study on the lines provided.

Case 1

A patient with cancer is having surgery to remove a portion of his small intestine. What digestive complications is this patient likely to have?

_____

_____

_____

Case 2

A young man has been diagnosed with hepatitis. When he is advised that he should stop alcohol consumption, he objects. What reasons can you give him for stopping the use of alcohol?

_____

_____

_____

Case 3

A young girl has a diet that lacks dairy products. What nutrients are missing from her diet, and what conditions might result?

_____

_____

_____

Case 4

The physician has informed a patient that she has polyps in her colon. He explains that although they are not cancerous, they should be removed. Why should they be removed if they are not cancerous?

_____

_____

_____

34

The Endocrine System

Name_____ Class_____ Date_____

Vocabulary Review

Matching
Match the key terms in the right column with the definitions in the left column by placing the letter of each correct answer in the space provided.

_____ 1. Any stimulus that produces stress

_____ 2. A chemical secreted by a cell that affects the functions of other cells

_____ 3. A substance that is activated by a hormone-receptor complex and causes enzymes inside a cell to be turned on

_____ 4 The gland that produces calcitonin

_____ 5. A hormone made of amino acids or proteins

_____ 6. A mechanism that controls hormone levels

_____ 7. A gland that lies between the lungs and secretes thymosin.

_____ 8. The ovaries and testes

_____ 9. A hormone derived from steroids

_____ 10. Local hormones that typically do not travel in the bloodstream

_____ 11. Small glands embedded in the posterior surface of the thyroid gland

_____ 12. A small gland located between the cerebral hemispheres that secretes melatonin

_____ 13. A type of ductless gland that secretes substances directly into the bloodstream or target tissue

_____ 14. Structures in the pancreas that secrete hormones into the bloodstream

_____ 15. A type of gland that secretes substances through a duct

a. thyroid gland
b. islets of Langerhans
c. gonads
d. hormone
e. nonsteroidal hormone
f. parathyroid glands
g. endocrine gland
h. thymus gland
i. pineal body
j. G-protein
k. prostaglandins
l. steroidal hormone
m. feedback loop
n. exocrine gland
o. stressor

True or False
Decide whether each statement is true or false. In the space at the left, write T for true or F for false. On the lines provided, rewrite the false statements to make them true.

_____ 16. A hormone must target cells that have a receptor for it.

_____

_____ 17. Steroid hormones use G-proteins to activate enzymes within a cell.

_____

_____ 18. Labor and delivery are examples of a negative feedback loop.

_____

_____ **19.** The hypothalamus produces oxytocin and ADH.

_____ **20.** TSH stimulates the testes to release their hormones.

_____ **21.** Osteoclasts build up bone by removing calcium from the blood.

_____ **22.** The adrenal cortex secretes cortisol.

_____ **23.** Insulin promotes the uptake of glucose by cells.

_____ **24.** Epinephrine and norepinephrine decrease the heart rate.

_____ **25.** Too much thyroid hormone produces cretinism in children.

_____ **26.** Diabetes mellitus is the chronic condition of elevated blood glucose levels.

_____ **27.** Diabetes insipidus is caused by hypersecretion of ADH.

_____ **28.** Exophthalmos is a symptom of hypothyroidism.

_____ **29.** Addison's disease is a condition caused by the adrenal medulla.

_____ **30.** Somatotropin deficiency causes acromegaly.

_____ **31.** A goiter is caused by a dietary iodine deficiency.

_____ **32.** The thymus is considered both an endocrine gland and an exocrine gland.

_____ **33.** Luteinizing hormone stimulates the testes to produce testosterone.

_____ **34.** Follicle-stimulating hormone has no function in males.

_____ **35.** The anterior lobe of the pituitary gland is also known as the neurohypophysis.

_____ **36.** The body's physiologic response to stress is primarily caused by the release of hormones.

Content Review

Multiple Choice

In the space provided, write the letter of the choice that best completes each statement or answers each question.

_____ 1. Which of the following is the bony structure that protects the pituitary gland?

a. Optic chiasm

b. Sella turcica

c. Paranasal sinus

d. Larynx

e. Hypophysis

_____ 2. The alpha cells in the pancreas secrete

a. Pancreatic acid

b. Lipase

c. Insulin

d. Glycogen

e. Glucagon

_____ 3. Which of the following are small glands that are embedded within another gland?

a. Adrenal glands

b. Ovaries

c. Parathyroid glands

d. Pituitary glands

e. Testes

_____ 4. Which of the following hormones is *not* produced by a digestive organ?

a. Gastrin

b. Secretin

c. Cortisol

d. Insulin

e. Cholecystokinin

_____ 5. Which of the following is also known as hypercortisolism?

a. Cushing's syndrome

b. Graves' disease

c. Acromegaly

d. Dwarfism

e. Addison's disease

_____ 6. Which hormones are also known as tissue hormones?

a. Steroidal hormones

b. Nonsteroidal hormones

c. Lipid hormones

d. Prostaglandins

e. Amino acid hormones

_____ 7. Hormones from which of the following glands are responsible for T lymphocyte production?

a. Thymus

b. Thyroid

c. Pancreas

d. Parathyroid

e. Hypothalamus

_____ 8. Which of the following diseases may be congenital in nature?

a. Myxedema

b. Graves' disease

c. Cretinism

d. Addison's disease

e. Acromegaly

_____ 9. Which of the following symptoms is *not* associated with general stress syndrome?

a. Increased blood pressure

b. Increased blood glucose

c. Increased breathing rate

d. Increased heart rate

e. Weight gain

_____ 10. Parathyroid hormone is an agonist to which of the following hormones?

a. Calcitonin

b. Oxytocin

c. Thymosin

d. Cortisol

e. Prolactin

Sentence Completion

In the space provided, write the word or phrase that best completes each sentence.

11. The target cells of a hormone are the cells that contain the _____ for the hormone.

12. A stimulus that produces a physiological change in the body is a(n) _____.

13. Glucagon is produced by the _____ cells of the pancreas.

14. Stimulating milk production in females, _____ enhances the actions of LH in males.

15. Hormone levels are controlled by _____.

16. Cretinism is caused by a _____ deficiency.

17. A "moon face" and "buffalo hump" are symptoms of _____.

18. _____ occurs when blood sugar levels rise during a woman's pregnancy.

19. _____ is an extreme form of hypothyroidism in adults.

20. The _____ gland is located between the lungs.

11. _____

12. _____

13. _____

14. _____

15. _____

16. _____

17. _____

18. _____

19. _____

20. _____

Short Answer

Write the answer to each question on the lines provided.

21. Describe the following disorders and the signs and symptoms of each.

    a. Acromegaly _____

    _____

    b. Cushing's syndrome _____

    _____

    c. Graves' disease _____

    _____

    d. Myxedema _____

    _____

    e. Diabetes mellitus _____

    _____

22. Answer the following questions about diabetes mellitus.

    a. What is the difference between type 1 and type 2 diabetes? _____

    _____

    b. What is gestational diabetes? _____

    _____

c. What are the causes of diabetes? _____

_____

d. What are some treatments for diabetes? _____

_____

23. The following illustration shows the endocrine glands and organs that produce hormones throughout the body. Label the figure using the following terms: pineal gland, testes, parathyroid glands, heart, gastrointestinal tract, ovaries, thymus, adrenal glands, thyroid gland, hypothalamus, pancreatic islets, pituitary gland, kidney.

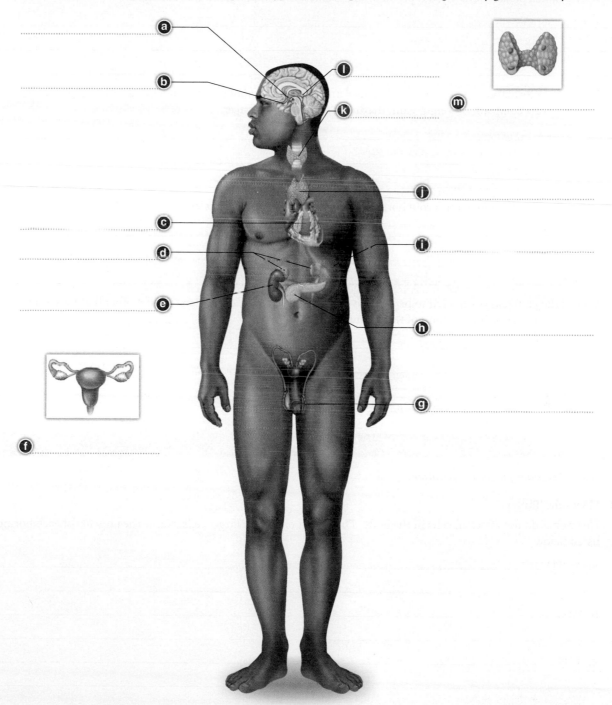

Source: From Michael McKinley and Valerie O'Loughlin, HUMAN ANATOMY, 1/e. © 2006 McGraw Hill Companies, Inc. Reprinted with permission.

Critical Thinking

Write the answer to each question on the lines provided.

1. Why must the receptors for nonsteroidal hormones be located on cell surfaces rather than inside the cells?

_____

_____

_____

2. Why would a person have thyroid problems if his anterior pituitary gland was damaged?

_____

_____

_____

3. Given the information you know about cortisol and steroidal hormones, explain why patients taking steroids such as prednisone complain of weight gain, tiredness, and extreme hunger.

_____

_____

_____

4. How do calcitonin and parathyroid hormones work together to control calcium levels in the blood?

_____

_____

_____

5. Why is the pancreas considered to be both an endocrine and an exocrine gland? What other body system is affected by the exocrine function of this gland?

_____

_____

_____

A P P L I C A T I O N

Follow the directions for each application.

1. **Hormone Targets**

   Hormones do not affect all cells in the body. They affect only their target cells. Name the target(s) of each hormone listed below.

   a. ACTH _____

   _____

   b. Insulin _____

   _____

   c. TSH _____

   _____

   d. Calcitonin _____

   _____

      e. FSH and LH _____

_____

      f. MSH _____

_____

2. Endocrine Disorders

Endocrine disorders can produce too many or too few hormones. Name the disorders that may result from the following conditions.

      a. Hypersecretion of GH in adults _____

_____

      b. Hyposecretion of GH in children _____

_____

      c. Hypersecretion of thyroid hormone in adults _____

_____

      d. Hyposecretion of thyroid hormone in adults _____

_____

      e. Hyposecretion of thyroid hormone in children _____

_____

      f. Hyposecretion of ACTH in adults or children _____

_____

CASE STUDIES

Write your response to each case study on the lines provided.

Case 1

A female patient has a diet that is totally lacking in lipids. How does her diet affect hormone production in her body?

_____

_____

_____

Case 2

A male patient wants you to explain to him how the use of steroid hormones can adversely affect his body. What would you tell him?

_____

_____

_____

Case 3

A 35-year-old woman is pregnant with her first child. Her glucose tolerance test (GTT) is elevated and she has been put on a diabetic diet. She is relieved that her diabetes is gestational and that she will return to normal blood sugar levels after her pregnancy. What information might you share with her?

_____

_____

_____

35

Special Senses

Name_____ Class_____ Date_____

REVIEW

Vocabulary Review

Matching
Match the key terms in the right column with the definitions in the left column by placing the letter of each correct answer in the space provided.

_____ 1. Receptors such as those found in the nose and on the tongue

_____ 2. "Bumps" on the tongue that contain taste buds

_____ 3. Fluids of the labyrinth

_____ 4. The part of the external ear also known as the pinna

_____ 5. A benign tumor of the cranial nerve

_____ 6. Function to detect the body's balance

_____ 7. Visual receptors responsible for night vision

_____ 8. Visual receptors responsible for color vision

_____ 9. The watery fluid of the anterior chamber of the eye

_____ 10. The jelly-like fluid of the posterior chamber of the eye

_____ 11. A waxlike substance commonly called earwax

_____ 12. The snail-shaped structure in the ear that contains hearing receptors

_____ 13. Mucous membrane that lines the inner surface of the eyelids

_____ 14. An inner ear infection

_____ 15. A condition commonly known as swimmer's ear

_____ 16. An enzyme in tears that can destroy bacteria and viruses

_____ 17. The middle layer of the eye

_____ 18. Malleus, incus, and stapes

_____ 19. Helps maintain equal pressure on both sides of the eardrum

_____ 20. The system of communicating chambers and tubes of the inner ear

a. auricle
b. cerumen
c. chemoreceptors
d. choroid
e. conjunctiva
f. lysozyme
g. eustachian tube
h. perilymph/endolymph
i. papillae
j. cochlea
k. aqueous humor
l. acoustic neuroma
m. otitis externa
n. rods
o. ossicles
p. otitis interna
q. cones
r. labyrinth
s. semicircular canals
t. vitreous humor

True or False
Decide whether each statement is true or false. In the space at the left, write T *for true or* F *for false. On the lines provided, rewrite the false statements to make them true.*

_____ 21. Smell receptors are located in the olfactory organ, which is in the lower part of the nasal cavity.

_____

_____ **22.** Taste cells that respond to sweet chemicals are concentrated at the back of the tongue.

_____

_____ **23.** The external ear is composed of the auricle and the external auditory canal.

_____

_____ **24.** The cornea is part of the middle layer of the eye.

_____

_____ **25.** The middle ear is connected to the pharynx by the eustachian tube.

_____

_____ **26.** The tiny bones of each eye are called ossicles.

_____

_____ **27.** The semicircular canals contain hearing receptors.

_____

_____ **28.** In the process of seeing, the image is projected onto the retina upside down.

_____

_____ **29.** The pupil is the colored part of the eye.

_____

_____ **30.** The clear covering over the iris and pupil is the sclera.

_____

Content Review

Multiple Choice

In the space provided, write the letter of the choice that best completes each statement or answers each question.

_____ **1.** Which of the following is *not* a special sense?
  a. Smell
  b. Taste
  c. Hearing
  d. Vision
  e. Touch

_____ **2.** Taste cells that respond to sour chemicals are concentrated on what part of the tongue?
  a. The tip
  b. The back
  c. The sides
  d. The bottom
  e. The entire tongue

_____ **3.** Where is the organ of Corti located?
  a. The cochlea
  b. The vestibule
  c. The tympanic membrane
  d. The semicircular canals
  e. The auditory meatus

_____ 4. The optic nerves cross at the optic
    a. Angle
    b. Chiasm
    c. Canal
    d. Lobe
    e. Chamber

_____ 5. The taste sensation often described as meaty or brothy is
    a. Sweet
    b. Salty
    c. Bitter
    d. Sour
    e. Umami

_____ 6. The auricle begins the hearing process by collecting sound waves and channeling them to
    a. The labyrinth
    b. The tympanic membrane
    c. The cochlea
    d. The pinna
    e. The auditory nerve

_____ 7. The area in the brain responsible for interpreting taste is known as the
    a. Brocca's area
    b. Gustatory cortex
    c. Temporal cortex
    d. Occipital area
    e. Olfactory bulbs

_____ 8. The shape of the eye's lens is controlled by muscles in the
    a. Cornea
    b. Optic nerve
    c. Ciliary body
    d. Pupil
    e. Iris

_____ 9. The area where the optic nerve enters the retina is known as the
    a. Optic disc
    b. Limbus
    c. Optic chiasma
    d. Choroid
    e. Scleral junction

_____ 10. The process of bending or focusing light is known as
    a. Constriction
    b. Tracking
    c. Inversion
    d. Refraction
    e. Accommodation

Sentence Completion

In the space provided, write the word or phrase that best completes each sentence.

11. When you eat spicy foods, you are activating _____ receptors on the tongue.

12. The fifth acknowledged taste sensation is _____.

13. The _____ controls the amount of light entering the eye.

14. _____ is a loss of hearing due to aging.

15. The _____ carries odor impulses to the cerebrum for interpretation.

16. _____ is an eversion of the lower eyelid.

17. The muscles of the _____ control the shape of the lens.

18. The corneal-scleral junction is also called the _____.

19. Tears are produced by the _____.

20. The job of the _____ is to equalize pressure within the ears.

11. _____

12. _____

13. _____

14. _____

15. _____

16. _____

17. _____

18. _____

19. _____

20. _____

Short Answer

Write the answer to each question on the lines provided.

21. Identify the taste associated with the darkened area on each of the following illustrations of the tongue.

(a) .... (b) .... (c) .... (d) ....

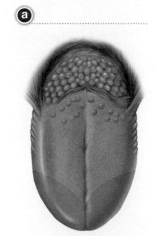 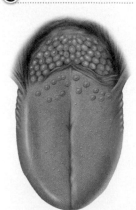 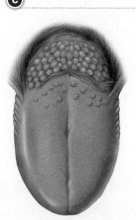 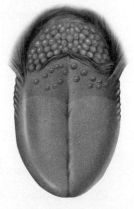

22. The following illustration shows a horizontal section of the eye. On the lines provided, label each structure.

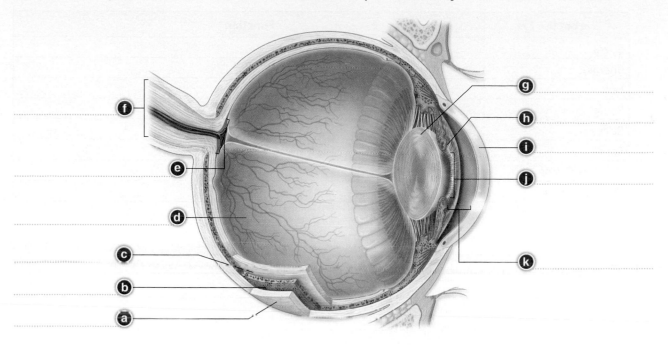

23. The following figure illustrates the outer, middle, and inner ear. On the lines provided, label each structure.

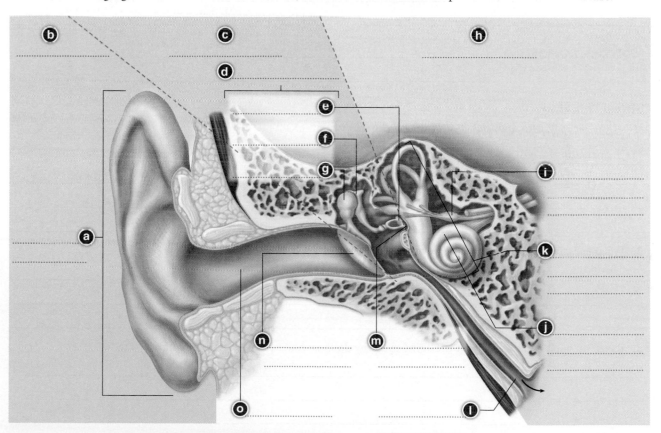

Source for all art on page: From Michael McKinley and Valerie O'Loughlin, HUMAN ANATOMY, 1/e. © 2006 McGraw Hill Companies, Inc. Reprinted with permission.

24. Fill in the following table, identifying the functions of the parts of the eye.

Part of the Eye	Function
Sclera	
Choroid	
Lens	
Retina	
Rods	
Cones	
Aqueous humor	
Vitreous humor	

25. Briefly describe the following disorders.

a. Nystagmus _____

_____

b. Entropion _____

_____

c. Dry eye syndrome _____

_____

d. Retinal detachment _____

_____

Critical Thinking

Write the answer to each question on the lines provided.

1. If a person is on a drug that causes his nasal membranes to become dry, why might he have trouble smelling?

_____

_____

_____

2. What ear care instructions would you give a person with repeated cerumen impactions?

_____

_____

_____

3. Based on what you know about the aging eye, why do most older people need more light to read?

_____

_____

_____

4. Why do people who work in a perfume factory no longer smell the perfume after a certain amount of time?

_____

_____

_____

A P P L I C A T I O N

Follow the directions for each application.

1. Hearing Problems in Babies

Hearing problems in babies are not easy to recognize. For each age group listed below, give some general guidelines parents can use to identify hearing problems.

a. In babies up to 4 months of age

_____

_____

_____

b. In babies 4 to 8 months of age

_____

_____

_____

c. In babies 8 to 12 months of age

_____

_____

_____

_____

2. Eye Safety

The overwhelming majority of eye injuries can be avoided by using eye safety practices. Name some eye safety practices for each situation.

a. At home _____

_____

b. While playing sports _____

_____

c. In the workplace _____

_____

C A S E   S T U D I E S

Write your response to each case study on the lines provided.

Case 1

A 52-year-old woman has a sudden onset of the following symptoms: light flashes, wavy vision, a sudden loss of vision (particularly of peripheral vision), and a larger amount of floaters. She asked if she should be seen or if she can wait until she returns from her vacation. What should you tell her?

_____

_____

_____

Case 2

A 79-year-old man recently suffered a stroke in his left primary visual area. Why did he lose some vision in both eyes?

_____

_____

_____

Case 3

Your friend Angela, a 46-year-old, tells you she has just been diagnosed with an acoustic neuroma and she is worried that she has brain cancer. What can you tell her about acoustic neuromas?

_____

_____

_____

Case 4

Mrs. Westerholm, an 89-year-old, has just moved in with her daughter. Her daughter tells you she is afraid that her mother will fall in her house. What actions can the daughter take to help keep her mother safe from falls?

_____

_____

_____

Patient Interview and History

Name_____ Class_____ Date_____

REVIEW

Vocabulary Review

Matching

Match the key terms in the right column with the definitions in the left column by placing the letter of each correct answer in the space provided.

_____ 1. Stating what you think has been suggested

_____ 2. Formed as a result of deeper thought

_____ 3. Restating what is said in your own words

_____ 4. Term that describes the patient's most significant symptoms

_____ 5. Using agents in a way that is not medically approved

_____ 6. A physical or psychological dependence

_____ 7. Asking questions that provide an increase in understanding of a problem

_____ 8. Thoughts, feelings, and perceptions

_____ 9. Apparent and measurable

_____ 10. A way of organizing information so that the most recent information is featured on top

_____ 11. Repeating something back to a patient in your own words

a. addiction
b. chief complaint
c. substance abuse
d. reverse chronological
e. subjective
f. objective
g. mirroring
h. verbalizing
i. restatement
j. reflection
k. clarification

True or False

Decide whether each statement is true or false. In the space at the left, write T for true or F for false. On the lines provided, rewrite the false statements to make them true.

_____ 12. The chief complaint is the physician's diagnosis of a patient's problem.

_____

_____ 13. The Health Insurance Portability and Accountability Act (HIPAA) is part of the patient's responsibilities when receiving health care.

_____

_____ 14. Sitting back and just hearing the patient is part of active listening.

_____

_____ 15. The patient's tone of voice, facial expression, and body language are signs of nonverbal communication.

_____

_____ 16. The statement "I think you probably just have the flu" is an example of making a diagnosis and should be said by the medical assistant.

_____ 17. A patient who has white-coat syndrome is anxious about visiting the physician.

_____ 18. If a patient is using the drug Ecstasy, you may notice an increase in her heart rate and blood pressure.

Content Review

Multiple Choice

In the space provided, write the letter of the choice that best completes each statement or answers each question.

_____ 1. During a patient interview, repeating in your own words what the patient has said is an important part of
   a. Effective questioning
   b. Being aware of nonverbal clues
   c. Using a broad knowledge base
   d. Summarizing to form a general picture
   e. Effective listening

_____ 2. "Have you had this pain long?" is an example of a(n)
   a. Hypothetical question
   b. Open-ended question
   c. Encouragement for the patient to take the lead
   d. Closed-ended question
   e. Focus on the patient

_____ 3. "This pain seems to be causing you more problems than it did last week" is an example of which of the following interviewing skills?
   a. Verbalizing the implied
   b. Asking a hypothetical question
   c. Challenging the patient
   d. Asking a closed-ended question
   e. Being aware of nonverbal clues

_____ 4. "What activities seem to make the pain worse?" is an example of which of the following interviewing skills?
   a. Asking a hypothetical question
   b. Encouraging the patient to provide more information
   c. Mirroring the patient's responses
   d. Asking a leading question
   e. Challenging the patient

_____ 5. Where would you look on the patient's chart for information about a previous hospitalization?
   a. Laboratory report
   b. Discharge summary
   c. Patient medical history form
   d. Consent form
   e. Physician's treatment plan

_____ 6. Which of the following is an example of *subjective* data?

      a. Pain in the right arm

      b. A blood pressure reading of 138/88

      c. A height measurement of 5'6" and a weight measure of 138 lbs.

      d. A reddened rash on the left arm

      e. Elevated blood glucose

_____ 7. Which of the following is an example of *objective* data?

      a. Dizziness

      b. Pain

      c. Swollen feet

      d. Weakness

      e. Tiredness

Sentence Completion

In the space provided, write the word or phrase that best completes each sentence.

8. An elderly patient who seems to be senile may actually be _____.

9. Abuse can be physical, _____, or both.

10. _____ combine SOMR and POMR and are easily accessible to healthcare workers.

11. _____ are used more extensively in large medical offices than any other type of medical record.

12. The _____ is the reason the patient came to the healthcare facility.

13. The _____ includes information about the level of stress, exposure to hazardous substances, and heavy lifting.

14. The _____ includes information about allergies.

15. A medical assistant should obtain information about the parents, siblings, and grandparents to complete the _____.

8. _____

9. _____

10. _____

11. _____

12. _____

13. _____

14. _____

15. _____

Short Answer

Write the answer to each question on the lines provided.

16. What are the six Cs of charting?

_____

_____

_____

17. Name seven kinds of standard information that should appear in a patient's chart.

_____

_____

_____

_____

18. To what does the acronym SOAP refer? What does each letter represent?

_____

_____

_____

19. Why might depression be called a hidden illness?

_____

_____

_____

20. What are six signs of possible physical or psychological abuse?

_____

_____

_____

_____

Critical Thinking

Write the answer to each question on the lines provided.

1. What are important guidelines to consider when using progress notes?

_____

_____

_____

2. Why is it important to consider a patient's polypharmacy when obtaining a chief complaint or medical history?

_____

_____

_____

3. Name two general kinds of errors in taking a patient's history that could affect a physician's ability to care for the patient.

_____

_____

_____

4. Which of the following is a definite sign of depression in an adolescent patient: problems in sleeping, problems in eating, sudden mood changes, or illogical thought patterns?

_____

_____

_____

5. Name two abbreviations that have been banned by the JCAHO. Why are these abbreviations banned from patient charting?

_____

_____

_____

6. Analyze each of the following and decide whether it is objective (O) or subjective (S) data. In the space provided, mark an "O" for objective or an "S" for subjective data.

_____ **a.** Stiff neck in the morning

_____ **b.** Ankle pain

_____ **c.** Rash on right forearm

_____ **d.** Nausea

_____ **e.** Lesion on lower lip

_____ **f.** Total cholesterol of 190 mg/dL

_____ **g.** Lethargy

_____ **h.** Oral temperature of 99.6°F

_____ **i.** Irregular pulse

_____ **j.** Anxiety

APPLICATION   WORK // DOC

Follow the directions for each application.

1. Conducting a Patient Interview

a. In groups of three or four, discuss and record on index cards appropriate open-ended questions for the following chief complaints:

  1. Low back pain

  2. Diabetes follow-up

  3. Insomnia

b. As a class, discuss the questions each group prepared. Formulate a list of interview questions for each of the patient complaints.

c. In pairs or groups of three, role-play each scenario, interviewing and documenting the chief complaint on the progress note provided in the documentation section in the back of the workbook.

2. Charting Patient Data

a. You have collected the following information during a client interview. Use a progress note example in the documentation section in the back of the workbook.

A 14-year-old girl comes to the client because she has had a sore throat and fever for the past 2 days. Her vital signs are TPR 99.8-88-24, BP 110/70. She describes the pain as burning and says she has just not felt like eating lately.

b. You have collected the following information during a client interview. Use a progress note example in the documentation section in the back of the workbook.

Robert Greenwood, a 70-year-old male, arrives at the client for a blood pressure checkup. He denies pain. His vital signs are TPR 97.4-66-20, BP 158/90, O_2 Sat 96%. He is 69¾ inches tall and 165 lbs. His previous records indicate that he is allergic to "sulfa drugs." He states that he is currently taking Lipitor, 20 mg, one every day; Atenolol, 50 milligrams, one every day; and 81 mg of aspirin daily. He denies using alcohol, tobacco, and recreational drugs and does not know when he had his last tetanus shot.

c. You have collected the following information during a client interview. Use a progress note example in the documentation section in the back of the workbook.

Peter Todman, a 28-year-old male, is returning to the office today for a post-op visit after his appendectomy 1 week ago. He says he "feels pretty good except for the soreness on the right side of his abdomen." His vital signs are TPR 99.2°F, tympanic-78-19. BP 118/74. He states he is currently taking two 325-mg acetaminophen twice a day for the pain because the hydrocodone made him too sleepy.

C A S E   S T U D I E S

Write your response to each case study on the lines provided.

Case 1

As you interview a patient before he sees the physician, he points out a mysterious rash that developed during the night. He asks what you think it is. You explain that he needs to talk to the doctor about it. The patient insists that you know him because you were assisting the physician during his last visit. He is sure you can tell him what caused his rash. You know this patient has many allergies and probably touched something that caused his rash. What should you tell the patient?

_____

_____

_____

Case 2

A 17-year-old girl arrives alone for an appointment with the doctor. She seems tense and stiff; she avoids looking at you. When you ask why she has come to the doctor's office today, she whispers that she will tell the doctor. What should you do?

_____

_____

_____

Case 3

You are interviewing a 25-year-old woman who is being seen for a general physical exam. Her husband insists that he come in to the room with the patient. You notice several bruises on the patient's arm in various stages of healing. When you inquire about the bruises, the patient gives you a vague answer and the husband says she is just accident prone. What should you do?

_____

_____

_____

Case 4

While reviewing Mr. Ortega's health history form, you notice that he did not fill out the Social and Occupational History part of the form. Why might Mr. Ortega not have filled out this part of the form? What should you do?

_____

_____

_____

PROCEDURE 36-1 Using Critical Thinking Skills During an Interview

WORK // DOC

Goal

To be able to use verbal and nonverbal clues and critical thinking skills to optimize the process of obtaining data for the patient's chart.

OSHA Guidelines

This procedure does not involve exposure to blood, body fluids, or tissues.

Materials

Patient chart or electronic health record, pen (if using a paper record).

Method

Step Number	Procedure*	Points Possible	Points Earned
Getting at an Underlying Meaning			
1.	Use open-ended questions, allowing the patient to explain the situation in her own words.	25	
2.	Encourage the patient to verbalize her concerns more clearly by mirroring her response or restating her comments in your own words.	25	
3.	Verbalize the implied.	25	
4.	After determining the specific problem, address it in the interview or note it in the patient's chart for the doctor's attention.	25	
Total Points		100	
Dealing with a Potentially Violent Patient			
1.	Pay attention to body language clues that the patient may be angry.	25	
2.	Explain to the patient that you need to ask him some questions so that the doctor can provide proper medical care.	25	
3.	Recognize signs that the patient may become violent, such as the patient raising his voice in anger.	25	
4.	Do not try to handle the patient alone; leave the room and ask for assistance.	25	
Total Points		100	
Gathering Symptom Information About a Child			
1.	Ask the child various questions so that he feels his view of the problem is important.	25	
2.	Confirm the child's answers with the parent or guardian using open-ended questions.	25	
3.	Ask the child to confirm the parent's answers, allowing them to provide additional information if possible.	25	
4.	Document the information in the patient's chart.	25	
Total Points		100	

*Note: Each section may be treated as a separate procedure depending on the patient scenario.

Name_____ Date_____

Evaluated by_____ Score_____

CAAHEP Competencies Achieved

I. A (1)   Apply critical thinking skills in performing patient assessment and care

IV. C (4)   Identify techniques for overcoming communication barriers

ABHES Competencies Achieved

5. (b) Identify and respond appropriately when working/caring for patients with special needs

5. (e) Advocate on behalf of family/patients, having ability to deal and communicate with family

Copyright © 2014 by The McGraw-Hill Companies, Inc.

PROCEDURE 36-2 Using a Progress Note

WORK // DOC

Goal
To accurately record a chief complaint on a progress note.

OSHA Guidelines
This procedure does not involve exposure to blood, body fluids, or tissues.

Materials
Progress note, patient chart or electronic health record, pen (if using a paper record).

Method

Step Number	Procedure	Points Possible	Points Earned
1.	Wash your hands.	10	
2.	Review the patient's chart notes from the patient's previous office visit. Verify that all results for any previously ordered laboratory work or diagnostics are in the chart.	10	
3.	Greet the patient and escort her to a private exam room.	10	
4.	Introduce yourself and identify the patient.	10	
5.	Use open-ended questions to find out why the patient is seeking medical care today.	15	
6.	Accurately document the chief complaint on the progress note. Document vital signs. Initial or sign the chart entry according to office policy.	15	
7.	File the progress note in chronological order within the patient's chart if the record is a paper record.	10	
8.	Thank the patient and offer to answer any questions she may have. Explain that the physician will come in soon to examine her.	10	
9.	Wash your hands.	10	
Total Points		100	

CAAHEP Competencies Achieved

IX. P (7)   Document accurately in the patient record

ABHES Competencies Achieved

4. (a) Document accurately

8. (jj) Perform fundamental writing skills, including correct grammar, spelling, and formatting techniques when writing prescriptions, documenting medical records, etc.

PROCEDURE 36-3 Obtaining a Medical History   WORK // DOC

Goal
To obtain a complete medical history with accuracy and professionalism.

OSHA Guidelines
This procedure does not involve exposure to blood, body fluids, or tissues.

Materials
Medical history form, patient chart, pen or electronic medical record.

Method

Step Number	Procedure	Points Possible	Points Earned
1.	Wash your hands.	10	
2.	Assemble the necessary materials. Review the medical history form and plan your interview.	10	
3.	Invite the patient to a private exam room and correctly identify the patient by introducing yourself and asking his or her name and date of birth.	10	
4.	Explain the medical history form while maintaining eye contact. Make the patient feel at ease.	10	
5.	Using language that the patient can understand, ask appropriate, open-ended questions related to the medical history form. Listen actively to the patient's response.	10	
6.	Accurately document the patient's responses.	10	
7.	Thank the patient for his or her participation in the interview. Offer to answer any questions.	10	
8.	Sign or initial the medical history form and file it in the patient's chart.	10	
9.	Inform the physician that you are finished with the medical history according to the physician's office policy.	10	
10.	Wash your hands.	10	
Total Points		100	

CAAHEP Competencies Achieved

I. P (6)	Perform patient screening using established protocols
I. A (1)	Apply critical thinking skills in performing patient assessment and care
I. A (2)	Use language/verbal skills that enable patients' understanding
IV. C (4)	Identify techniques for overcoming communication barriers
IV. C (6)	Differentiate between subjective and objective information
IV. C (7)	Identify resources and adaptations that are required based on individual needs, i.e., culture and environment, developmental life stage, language, and physical threats to communication
IV. P (3)	Use medical terminology, pronouncing medical terms correctly, to communicate information, patient history, data, and observations
IV. A (2)	Apply active listening skills
IV. A (3)	Use appropriate body language and other nonverbal skills in communicating with patients, family, and staff

ABHES Competencies Achieved

    4. (a) Document accurately

    8. (ff) Interview effectively

    9. (a) Obtain chief complaint, recording patient history

Vital Signs and Measurements

Name_____ Class_____ Date_____

REVIEW

Vocabulary Review

Matching

Match the key terms in the right column with the definitions in the left column by placing the letter of each correct answer in the space provided.

_____ **1.** Difficult or painful breathing

_____ **2.** An exceptionally high fever

_____ **3.** A slow heart rate of fewer than 60 beats per minute

_____ **4.** A fast heart rate of more than 100 beats per minute

_____ **5.** Having a body temperature within the normal range

_____ **6.** Crackling sounds indicating fluid in the lung

_____ **7.** Instrument that amplifies body sounds

_____ **8.** A measure of blood pressure taken when the heart relaxes

_____ **9.** A measure of blood pressure taken when the left ventricle contracts

_____ **10.** Deep, rapid breathing

_____ **11.** Pulse at the lower left corner of the heart

_____ **12.** Temperature scale on which a healthy adult's temperature would be 98.6°

_____ **13.** High blood pressure

_____ **14.** Low blood pressure

_____ **15.** To make sure an instrument is measuring correctly

_____ **16.** The bend of the elbow

_____ **17.** The lower left corner of the heart, where the strongest heart sounds can be heard

_____ **18.** Having a body temperature above the normal range

_____ **19.** A breathing pattern that includes shallow and deep breaths and apnea

_____ **20.** A device used to measure the temperature on the forehead

a. Fahrenheit
b. hypotension
c. rales
d. diastolic pressure
e. febrile
f. systolic pressure
g. stethoscope
h. dyspnea
i. hypertension
j. apical
k. hyperpnea
l. calibrate
m. antecubital space
n. apex
o. afebrile
p. hyperpyrexia
q. Cheyne-Stokes respirations
r. temporal scanner
s. bradycardia
t. tachycardia

True or False

Decide whether each statement is true or false. In the space at the left, write T for true or F for false. On the lines provided, rewrite the false statements to make them true.

_____ **21.** An adult will have his weight, head circumference, and height measured once a year.

_____

_____ **22.** A patient is febrile if her body temperature is above normal.

_____

_____ **23.** On a Fahrenheit scale, the normal oral temperature in a healthy adult is about 98.6°.

_____

_____ **24.** A patient with tachypnea breathes slowly.

_____

_____ **25.** A tympanic temperature is taken in the ear canal.

_____

_____ **26.** A tympanic thermometer measures the temperature of a patient's inner ear.

_____

_____ **27.** You should measure an adult's pulse at the radial artery.

_____

_____ **28.** The temporal artery is located at the side of the neck.

_____

_____ **29.** A sphygmomanometer is used to measure blood pressure.

_____

_____ **30.** Using the palpatory method, a medical assistant can take an estimate of a patient's systolic blood pressure before measuring it exactly.

_____

_____ **31.** The axilla is the armpit.

_____

_____ **32.** Auscultated blood pressure is determined by palpation.

_____

_____ **33.** Hypertension is also known as low blood pressure.

_____

_____ **34.** Body temperature is affected by numerous factors including the patient's weight.

_____

Content Review

Multiple Choice

In the space provided, write the letter of the choice that best completes each statement or answers each question.

_____ **1.** BMI calculations are based on
   a. pulse and respirations.
   b. height and weight.
   c. weight and abdominal girth.
   d. blood pressure and pulse.
   e. average blood pressure over last three visits.

2. An adult patient has started taking a medication for hypertension since his last visit. Which of the following would you most likely expect at this visit?

   a. A blood pressure within the normal range

   b. A blood pressure result higher than normal

   c. A blood pressure result lower than normal

   d. A blood pressure result lower than the results from the previous visit

   e. A blood pressure result unchanged from the previous visit

3. Review the following vital sign results for an adult patient older than age 65 and determine which set is considered out of the normal range.

   a. BP 118/78, T 98.6°F, P 98, R 14

   b. BP 116/68, T 98.6°F, P 98, R 17

   c. BP 108/78, T 37°C, P 88, R 18

   d. BP 116/74, T 98.2°F, P 106, R 20

   e. BP 114/76, T 97.8°F, P 98, R 20

4. A patient enters the facility with open lesions on his arms and hands. What *special* OSHA precautions should you take while measuring his vital signs?

   a. Wear a mask and gown

   b. Wear gloves and wash your hands

   c. Clean the exam area before the patient arrives

   d. Take a rectal temperature to ensure accurate results

   e. Isolate the patient from other patients

5. Which of the following would most likely cause rales?

   a. Congestive heart failure   d. Brain tumor

   b. Head injury   e. Influenza

   c. Asthma

6. Blood pressure and pulse are taken in different positions to assess for

   a. Obesity

   b. Heart disease

   c. Hypertension

   d. Orthostatic hypotension

   e. Lymphedema

7. Which of the following is generally *not* a health problem?

   a. Apnea   d. Hyperpnea

   b. Hypertension   e. Hypotension

   c. Dyspnea

8. Which of the following is the best way to weigh a toddler?

   a. Ask the toddler to stand very still on the scale

   b. Weigh the parent and the toddler together, and then subtract the weight of the parent from the result

   c. Lay the toddler on the infant scale

   d. Have the toddler hold the height bar during the weighing process to encourage him to stand still

   e. Ask the parent what the child's last weight was

9. Which of the following is an internal factor that affects the blood pressure?

   a. Papilledema   d. Hyperpyrexia

   b. Blood viscosity   c. Renal failure

   c. Malignant hypertension

Sentence Completion

In the space provided, write the word or phrase that best completes each sentence.

10. On the top moveable bar of the height scale, the numbers _____ as you go down the bar.

11. To ensure the proper size cuff when taking the blood pressure, the bladder inside the cuff should encircle _____ to _____ of the distance around the arm or leg being used.

12. Deep and rapid respirations associated with hysteria or excitement are called _____.

13. Severe _____ is usually associated with shock.

14. A person's axillary temperature is usually about 1° lower than her _____ temperature.

15. The eardrum was selected as a location to measure body temperature because it has the same blood supply as the _____.

16. If a patient's pulse rate is high, his _____ rate is also likely to be high.

17. Electronic sphygmomanometers are _____ likely to provide more accurate readings than other types of sphygmomanometers.

10. _____

11. _____

12. _____

13. _____

14. _____

15. _____

16. _____

17. _____

Short Answer

Write the answer to each question on the lines provided.

18. Name the five vital signs.

_____

_____

_____

19. Name and describe the parts of a stethoscope.

_____

_____

_____

20. Explain why pulse and respirations should be taken together.

_____

_____

_____

21. Name five methods for taking temperature, and discuss the circumstances under which each method might be used.

_____

_____

_____

22. How can you ensure that a tympanic temperature is accurate?

_____

_____

_____

23. Why is it necessary to hold the thermometer in place when taking a rectal temperature?

_____

_____

_____

24. When you are taking a blood pressure measurement, how do you determine how high to inflate the cuff to determine the patient's systolic reading?

_____

_____

_____

25. Identify the blood pressure values on the illustration of aneroid gauges below. Write your answers on the lines in the figure.

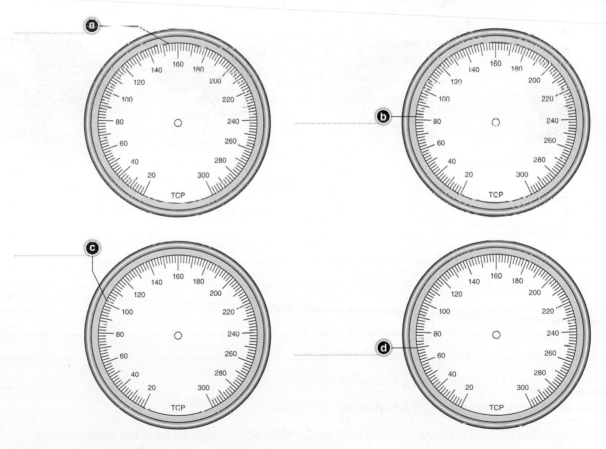

Using the illustrations above, write the patient's blood pressure reading if the systolic pressure is represented by the reading in (a) and the diastolic reading is represented in (b). _____

26. Explain why it is important for a physician to keep a record of how much a patient weighs.

_____

_____

_____

27. The following illustrations show sites for taking a patient's pulse rate. Identify and label the artery used for each measurement.

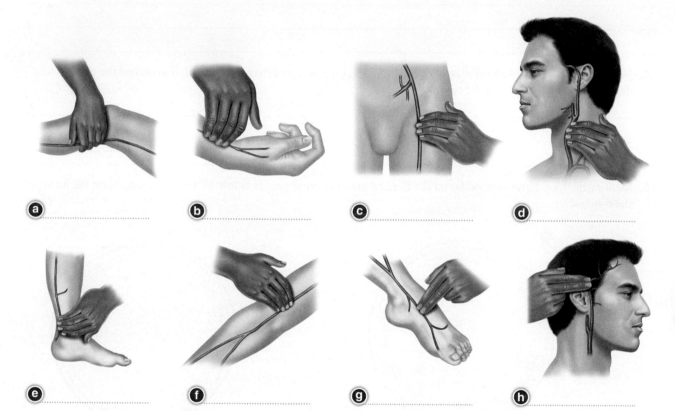

a ....
b ....
c ....
d ....

e ....
f ....
g ....
h ....

28. Name and describe the five phases of Korotkoff sounds.

_____

_____

_____

_____

_____

Critical Thinking

Write the answer to each question on the lines provided.

1. Discuss at least three ways that you can ensure accuracy when performing vital signs and measurements.

_____

_____

_____

2. What should you do if you suspect an incorrect digital blood pressure reading?

_____

_____

3. Explain why you should not take a blood pressure in a patient who has lessened circulation in his or her arm.

_____

_____

4. What will you do if a patient has just had a cup of coffee and you need to take his temperature?

_____

_____

5. How long should you measure a patient's pulse if it is irregular?

_____

_____

_____

A P P L I C A T I O N `WORK // DOC`

Follow the directions for each application.

1. Using Procedure Checklist 37-1, Measuring and Recording Temperature

Review and practice taking temperatures. Use the following circumstances during your practice:

a. Taking turns as the patient, role-play the sequence of taking a temperature. Be certain to use proper communication with the patient and document your results.

b. Obtain various types of thermometers—electronic, tympanic, temporal, and disposable—and compare the results of the temperatures among them, and then document your results.

2. Using Procedure Checklist 37-2, Measuring and Recording Pulse and Respirations

Review and practice taking pulse and respirations. Use the following circumstances during your practice:

a. On yourself, find and count at least 4 of the pulse sites found in Figure 37-7 in the text. Determine if the results are the same.

b. Find and count each of the same pulse sites on a partner. Compare your results.

c. Count a classmate's respirations while she is not aware that you are doing so. Then count the respirations when she is aware. Is there a difference?

d. Obtain and record the radial pulse on five different classmates. Keep your results confidential. Once completed, compare your results with other classmates. If the difference in one person's rate is greater than 5 beats per minute, recheck the pulse of that classmate at the same time that the classmate himself does to ensure an accurate measurement.

3. Using Procedure Checklist 37-3, Taking the Blood Pressure of Adults and Older Children

Review and practice taking blood pressure. Use the following circumstances during your practice:

a. In groups of three, practice taking blood pressure readings. With one student as the patient, the other two students should take the blood pressure and record the results without telling them to the other students. Each student should have her blood pressure taken by the other two team members. Once all the blood pressure readings have been taken, compare your results. Repeat the blood pressure readings until all the results on one student are within 10 mm Hg for the systolic measure and 4 mm Hg for the diastolic measure.

4. Using Procedure Checklist 37-4, Measuring Adults and Children

Review and practice measuring adults and children. Use the following circumstances during your practice:

a. Obtain the height and weight of at least three other students. Do not disclose your results while measuring. Compare your results with other classmates who have measured the same students. If the results are different, retake the measurements until they are the same.

b. Using the Body Mass Index chart in the textbook, calculate the BMI of each student.

5. Take at Least One Complete Set of Vital Signs

Record vital signs correctly on the medical record example found at the end of the workbook.

6. Measure the Forearm Circumference of at Least Three Students

You should take the measurement of the forearm at the area just below the elbow. Compare the measurement of each student's right arm with that of the left. Which is bigger? If the student is left handed, does that make a difference?

7. Use the Formulas Provided in the Textbook

Convert each of the following measurements. Write your answers in the space provided. Convert

a. 25 kg to lb _____

b. 57 kg to lb _____

c. 124 lb to kg _____

d. 188 lb to kg _____

e. 124 cm to in _____

f. 54 cm to in _____

g. 64 in to cm _____

h. 50 in to cm _____

C A S E   S T U D I E S

Write your response to each case study on the lines provided.

Case 1

A female patient arrives at the clinic and you must take her blood pressure. During the patient interview, you discover that she has had a double mastectomy. What should you do when taking her blood pressure?

_____

_____

_____

Case 2
The physician has asked you to get a pulse oximetry reading on a 35 year-old male patient with suspected pneumonia. The patient was recently injured in an accident and has broken his fingers on both hands. What should you do?

_____

_____

_____

Case 3
An adult patient who uses a wheelchair comes in for his annual checkup. How would you weigh him? How would you check his height?

_____

_____

_____

Case 4
An overweight 13-year-old girl comes in for an annual checkup. Her mother waits for her in the reception area. The patient seems nervous, and she refuses to get on the scales when it is time to weigh her. She says she does not want anyone to know how much she weighs, not even you. You and the patient both know that another girl from her school was in the office last week, and you are sure the other patient weighed much more than this patient does. The patient asks you how much the other girl weighed. Maybe telling the patient would make her feel better, and she would let you weigh her. What should you do?

_____

_____

_____

PROCEDURE 37-1   Measuring and Recording Temperature

WORK // DOC

Goal

To accurately measure the temperature of patients while preventing the spread of infection.

OSHA Guidelines

Materials

Thermometer, probe cover if required by thermometer, lubricant for rectal temperature, gloves, trash receptacle, patient's chart, a black pen if recording in a paper record.

Method

Step Number	Procedure	Points Possible	Points Earned
1.	Gather the equipment and make sure the thermometer is in working order.	5	
2.	Identify the patient and introduce yourself.	5	
3.	Wash your hands and explain the procedure to the patient.	10	
4.	Prepare the patient for the temperature.* **a.** Oral—If the patient has had anything to eat or drink, or has been smoking, wait at least 15 minutes before measuring the temperature orally. **b.** Rectal—Have the patient remove the appropriate clothing; assist as needed. Have the patient lie on his or her left side and drape for comfort. **c.** Axillary—Assist the patient to expose the axilla. Provide for privacy and comfort. Pat dry the axilla. **d.** Temporal or Tympanic—Remove the patient's hat if necessary.	15	
5.	Prepare the equipment.* **a.** Prepare an electronic thermometer by inserting the probe into the probe cover if necessary. **b.** Prepare the disposable thermometer by removing the wrapper to expose the handle end. Avoid touching the part of the thermometer that goes in the mouth or on the skin. **c.** Prepare the temporal scanner by removing the protective cap and making sure the lens is clean.	15	
6.	Measure the temperature.* **a.** Oral—Place the thermometer under the tongue in the back of the mouth on one side. Have the patient hold it in place with his or her lips and tongue. Wait for the electronic thermometer to beep or indicate completion. For a disposable thermometer, wait the required time, usually 60 seconds.	15	

(continued)

Step Number	Procedure	Points Possible	Points Earned
	b. Rectal—Put on gloves. Lubricate the thermometer tip. Raise the buttock to expose the anus with one hand and insert the thermometer into the anal canal, 1½ inches for adults and ½ to 1 inch for infants and children. Hold the thermometer securely in place until the indicator beeps or blinks. **c.** Axillary—Place the thermometer into the axilla, making sure the tip is in direct contact with the top of the axilla and is touching skin on all sides. Hold the arm firmly against the body until the indicator light blinks or beeps or the proper amount of time has passed. **d.** Tympanic—Hold the outer edge of the ear (pinna) with your free hand. Gently pull the pinna up for adults and down for children. Insert the probe into the ear canal directed to the eardrum and sealing the ear canal. Press the scan button. **e.** Temporal—Position the probe flat on the center of the exposed forehead. Press and hold the SCAN button and then slide the thermometer straight across the forehead until it beeps and the red light blinks.		
7.	Remove and read the measurement in the display or on the thermometer. Discard the disposable thermometer. Eject and discard the probe cover for an electronic thermometer. Replace the cap and/or place the thermometer into the charging base.*	15	
8.	Record the results.	5	
9.	Help the patient to replace clothing as necessary. Clear the area and provide for safety and comfort for the patient.	5	
10.	Wash your hands.	10	
Total Points		100	

CAAHEP Competencies Achieved

    I. P (1)   Obtain vital signs

    IV. P (2)   Report relevant information to others succinctly and accurately

ABHES Competencies Achieved

    9. (c) Take vital signs

    9. (i) Use Standard Precautions

PROCEDURE 37-2 Measuring and Recording Pulse and Respirations

WORK // DOC

Goal
To accurately measure the pulse and respirations of a patient while keeping the patient unaware the respirations are being counted.

OSHA Guidelines

Materials
Watch with a second hand, patient's chart, black pen if recording in a paper chart.

Method

Step Number	Procedure	Points Possible	Points Earned
1.	Gather the equipment and wash your hands.	5	
2.	Introduce yourself and identify the patient.	5	
3.	Explain that you will be taking the patient's vital signs. Do not tell them you are counting the respirations.*	15	
4.	Ask the patient to sit or lie in a comfortable position. Have the patient rest the arm on a table, palm facing downward.	5	
5.	Position yourself so you can observe and/or feel the chest wall movements.	5	
6.	Place two to three fingers on the radial pulse site.*	15	
7.	Count the pulse for 15 to 30 seconds if regular. Note the rhythm and volume. If irregular, count for a full minute.*	15	
8.	Without letting go of the wrist, observe and feel the respirations, counting for one full minute. Observe for rhythm, volume, and effort.*	15	
9.	Once you are certain of both numbers, release the wrist and record them. If the pulse was taken for less than one minute, obtain the number of beats per minute. Multiply the number of beats counted in 30 seconds by 2 or the number of beats counted in 15 seconds by 4.	10	
10.	Document results with the date and time.	5	
11.	Report any findings that are a significant change from a previous result or outside the normal values.	5	
Total Points		100	

CAAHEP Competencies Achieved

I. P (1)   Obtain vital signs

IV. P (2)   Report relevant information to others succinctly and accurately

ABHES Competencies Achieved

9. (c) Take vital signs

PROCEDURE 37-3 Taking the Blood Pressure of Adults and Older Children

Goal
To accurately measure blood pressure in adults and older children.

OSHA Guidelines

Materials
Aneroid or mercury sphygmomanometer, stethoscope, alcohol gauze squares, patient's chart, black pen if recording in a paper chart.

Method

Step Number	Procedure	Points Possible	Points Earned
1.	Gather the equipment and make sure the sphygmomanometer is in working order and is correctly calibrated.	2	
2.	Identify the patient and introduce yourself.	2	
3.	Wash your hands and explain the procedure to the patient.	2	
4.	Have the patient sit in a quiet area. If she is wearing long-sleeved clothing, have her loosely roll up one sleeve. If she cannot, have her change into a gown.	2	
5.	Have the patient rest her bared arm on a flat surface so that the midpoint of the upper arm is at the same level as the heart.	2	
6.	Select a cuff that is the appropriate size for the patient.*	10	
7.	Locate the brachial artery in the antecubital space.		
8.	Position the cuff so that the midline of the bladder is above the arterial pulsation. Wrap and secure the cuff snugly around the patient's bare upper arm, 1 inch above the antecubital.*	10	
9.	Place the manometer so that the center of the aneroid dial is at eye level and easily visible and so that the tubing from the cuff is unobstructed.	2	
10.	Close the valve of the pressure bulb until it is finger-tight.	2	
11.	Inflate the cuff rapidly to 70 mm Hg with one hand, and increase this pressure by 10 mm Hg increments while palpating the radial pulse with your other hand. Note the level of pressure at which the pulse disappears and subsequently reappears during deflation.*	10	
12.	Open the valve to release the pressure, deflate the cuff completely, and wait 30 seconds or remove and replace the cuff.	2	
13.	Properly place the earpieces of the stethoscope in your ear canals, and adjust them to fit snugly and comfortably. Confirm that the stethoscope setting is correct by listening as you tap the stethoscope head gently.	3	
14.	Place the head of the stethoscope over the brachial artery pulsation; hold the stethoscope firmly in place between the index and middle fingers, making sure the head is in contact with the skin around its entire circumference.	3	

(continued)

Step Number	Procedure	Points Possible	Points Earned
15.	Inflate the bladder rapidly and steadily to a pressure 20 to 30 mm Hg above the level previously determined by palpation. Partially open the valve and deflate the bladder at approximately 2 mm per second while you listen for the appearance of the Korotkoff sounds.*	10	
16.	As the pressure in the bladder falls, note the level of pressure on the manometer at the first appearance of repetitive sounds. This reading is the systolic pressure.*	10	
17.	Continue to deflate the cuff gradually, noting the point at which the sound changes from strong to muffled.	2	
18.	Continue to deflate the cuff, and note when the sound disappears. This reading is the diastolic pressure.*	10	
19.	Continue to listen for an additional 10 mm Hg, listening carefully for a return of the repetitive sounds.	3	
20.	Deflate the cuff completely, and remove it from the patient's arm.	2	
21.	Record the numbers, separated by slashes, in the patient's chart. Chart the date and time of the measurement, the arm on which the measurement was made, the subject's position, and the cuff size when a nonstandard size is used.	3	
22.	Fold the cuff and replace it in the holder.	2	
23.	Inform the patient that you have completed the procedure.	2	
24.	Disinfect the earpieces and diaphragm of the stethoscope with gauze squares moistened with alcohol.	2	
25.	Properly dispose of the used gauze squares and wash your hands.	2	
Total Points		100	

CAAHEP Competencies Achieved

I. P (1)   Obtain vital signs

IV. P (2)   Report relevant information to others succinctly and accurately

ABHES Competencies Achieved

9. (c) Take vital signs

Name_____ Date_____

Evaluated by_____ Score_____

PROCEDURE 37-4 Measuring Adults and Children

Goal
To accurately measure weight and height of adults and children.

OSHA Guidelines

Materials
For an adult or older child, adult scale with height bar, disposable towel; for toddler, adult scale with height bar or height chart, disposable towel.

Method

Step Number	Procedure	Points Possible	Points Earned
Adult or Older Child: Weight			
1.	Identify the patient and introduce yourself.	4	
2.	Wash your hands and explain the procedure to the patient.	4	
3.	Check to see whether the scale is in balance.*	8	
4.	Place a disposable towel on the scale or have the patient leave her socks on.	5	
5.	Ask the patient to remove her shoes, if that is the standard office policy.	4	
6.	Ask the patient to step on the center of the scale, facing forward. Assist as necessary.	3	
7.	Place the lower weight at the highest number that does not cause the balance indicator to drop to the bottom.*	8	
8.	Move the upper weight slowly to the right until the balance bar is centered at the middle mark, adjusting as necessary.*	8	
9.	Add the two weights together to get the patient's weight.*	8	
10.	Record the patient's weight in the chart to the nearest quarter of a pound or tenth of a kilogram.	4	
11.	Return the weights to their starting positions on the left side.	3	
Adult or Older Child: Height			
12.	With the patient off the scale, raise the height bar well above the patient's head and swing out the extension.	4	
13.	Ask the patient to step on the center of the scale and to stand up straight and look forward.	3	
14.	Gently lower the height bar until the extension rests on the patient's head.*	8	
15.	Have the patient step off the scale while you hold the height bar before reading the measurement.	5	
16.	Read the height in the right direction.*	8	
17.	Record the patient's height.	5	

(continued)

Step Number	Procedure	Points Possible	Points Earned
18.	Have the patient put her shoes back on, if necessary.	4	
19.	Properly dispose of the used towel and wash your hands.	4	
Total Points		100	
Toddler: Weight			
1.	Identify the patient and obtain permission from the parent to weigh the toddler.	5	
2.	Wash your hands and explain the procedure to the parent.	5	
3.	Check to see whether the scale is in balance, and place a disposable towel on the scale or have the patient wear shoes or socks, depending upon the facility's policy.*	15	
4.	Ask the parent to hold the patient and to step on the scale. Follow the procedure for obtaining the weight of an adult. *	15	
5.	Have the parent put the child down or hand the child to another staff member.	3	
6.	Obtain the parent's weight.*	15	
7.	Subtract the parent's weight from the combined weight to determine the child's weight.*	15	
8.	Record the patient's weight in the chart to the nearest quarter of a pound or tenth of a kilogram.	5	
Toddler: Height			
9.	Measure the child's height in the same manner as you measure adult height, or have the child stand with his back against the height chart. Measure height at the crown of the head.*	15	
10.	Record the height in the patient's chart.	5	
11.	Properly dispose of the towel (if used) and wash your hands.	2	
Total Points		100	

CAAHEP Competencies Achieved

II. C (7)   Analyze charts, graphs, and/or tables in the interpretation of health-care results

II. P (3)   Maintain growth charts

IV. P (2)   Report relevant information to others succinctly and accurately

ABHES Competencies Achieved

2. (c) Assist the physician with the regimen of diagnostic and treatment modalities as they relate to each body system

Assisting with a General Physical Examination

Name_____ Class_____ Date_____

REVIEW

Vocabulary Review

Matching

Match the key terms in the right column with the definitions in the left column by placing the letter of each correct answer in the space provided.

_____ 1. Objective information about a disorder that can be detected by a person other than the affected person

_____ 2. The systematic moving of a patient's body parts

_____ 3. A patient covering that has a special opening that provides access to the area to be examined

_____ 4. An exam in which the physician uses an index finger to palpate the rectum for lesions or irregularities

_____ 5. Touching to assess characteristics such as texture, temperature, and shape

_____ 6. The process of measuring

_____ 7. Determining the correct diagnosis when two or more diagnoses are possible

_____ 8. The process of listening to body sounds

_____ 9. A pattern of assumptions, beliefs, and practices that shape the way people think and act

_____ 10. Visual exam of the patient's entire body and overall appearance

_____ 11. Forecast of the probable course and outcome of a disorder and prospects of recovery

_____ 12. The degree to which one side is the same as the other

_____ 13. An initial diagnosis based on the patient's signs and symptoms

_____ 14. The four equal sections of the abdominal region

_____ 15. Subjective information about a disorder supplied by the patient

_____ 16. Tapping or striking the body to hear sounds or feel vibrations

a. mensuration
b. clinical diagnosis
c. sign
d. culture
e. differential diagnosis
f. auscultation
g. inspection
h. manipulation
i. symmetry
j. palpation
k. digital exam
l. percussion
m. prognosis
n. quadrants
o. fenestrated drape
p. symptom

True or False

Decide whether each statement is true or false. In the space at the left, write T for true or F for false. On the lines provided, rewrite the false statements to make them true.

_____ **17.** A clinical diagnosis is based on the signs and symptoms of a disease.

_____

_____ **18.** Culture is based on a person's race.

_____

_____ **19.** Nasal mucosa is the lining of the nose.

_____

_____ **20.** Hyperventilation is shallow breathing that leads to a loss of carbon dioxide in the blood.

_____

_____ **21.** An example of a digital exam is palpating for breast lumps.

_____

_____ **22.** A lateral curvature of the spine is referred to as kyphosis.

_____

_____ **23.** The proper medical term for earwax is cerumen.

_____

_____ **24.** Mensuration is the probable course or outcome of a disease.

_____

_____ **25.** Patients should be instructed on proper respiratory hygiene and cough etiquette.

_____

Content Review

Multiple Choice

In the space provided, write the letter of the choice that best completes each statement or answers each question.

_____ **1.** Which of the following is *not* an example of a safety measure you would take while assisting a physician with a patient's general physical exam?

    a. Performing a thorough hand washing before and after each procedure

    b. Cleaning and disinfecting the exam room after the exam

    c. Consulting the list of OSHA safety rules

    d. Wearing gloves whenever there is a possibility of contact with blood or body fluids

    e. Instructing symptomatic patients to maintain respiratory hygiene/cough etiquette

_____ **2.** When you prepare a patient for a physical exam, you will

    a. Explain to the patient what will occur during the exam

    b. Request that the patient pay his copayment before the exam

    c. Ask the patient to wash his hands thoroughly

    d. Auscultate the patient's breath sounds

    e. Schedule the patient for future visits at the office

_____ **3.** One of the six methods for examining a patient during a general physical exam is

    a. Supination   **d.** Pronation

    b. Positioning   **e.** Palpation

    c. Draping

_____ 4. Most physicians perform the general physical exam in the same order, starting with an exam of the patient's
   a. Chest and lungs
   b. Head
   c. Overall appearance and skin condition
   d. Abdomen
   e. Musculoskeletal system

_____ 5. At the physician's request, you have positioned a male patient in a sitting position. The drape should be placed
   a. Across the patient's chest and lap
   b. Across the patient's lap
   c. From the patient's neck to his hips
   d. From the patient's neck to his feet
   e. From the patient's knees to his feet

_____ 6. Which of the following is *not* included in the role of the medical assistant during a general physical exam?
   a. Ensuring that the patient is comfortable during the exam
   b. Ensuring that all instruments and supplies are readily available
   c. Helping the patient into the required exam positions
   d. Suturing a wound after the licensed practitioner cleans it
   e. Observing the patient for signs of distress

_____ 7. In which of the following positions does the patient lie flat on her back during a procedure?
   a. Prone
   b. Sims'
   c. Fowler's
   d. Dorsal recumbent
   e. Supine

_____ 8. Which of the following positions is most commonly used for gynecological exam procedures?
   a. Knee-chest
   b. Sims'
   c. Proctologic
   d. Lithotomy
   e. Fowler's

_____ 9. In which exam method does the physician assess characteristics such as texture, temperature, shape, and the presence of vibrations or movements by touching the skin surface and pressing against underlying tissues?
   a. Inspection
   b. Manipulation
   c. Palpation
   d. Auscultation
   e. Percussion

_____ 10. Which exam method allows the physician to determine the location, size, and density of organs?
   a. Percussion
   b. Inspection
   c. Mensuration
   d. Auscultation
   e. Manipulation

Sentence Completion

In the space provided, write the word or phrase that best completes each sentence.

11. One of the best positions for examining patients who are experiencing shortness of breath, the _____ position has the patient on his back with his head elevated.

12. When checking a patient's general appearance, a physician looks at the patient's skin, hair, and _____.

13. By using a(n) _____, the physician can view a patient's retinas and other internal structures of the eyes.

14. To auscultate the heart sounds, a physician uses an instrument known as a(n) _____.

15. You should pay special attention to educating patients about _____ for diseases such as breast cancer.

11. _____

12. _____

13. _____

14. _____

15. _____

Short Answer

Write the answer to each question on the lines provided.

16. What are the two reasons why physicians perform general physical exams?

_____

_____

_____

17. Why do physicians use six different exam methods during a general physical exam?

_____

_____

_____

18. Write the name of the exam position on the line below each illustration.

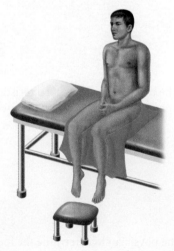

a. _____

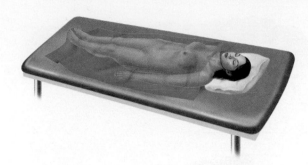

b. _____

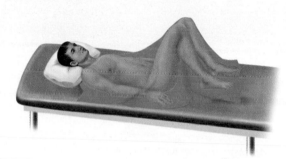

c. _____

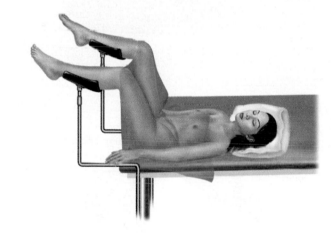

d. _____

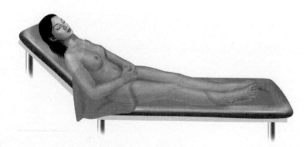

e. _____

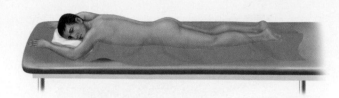

f. _____

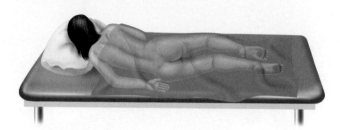

g. _____

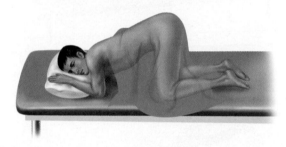

h. _____

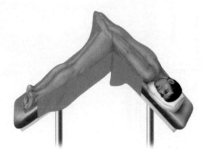

i. _____

19. Label the instruments and supplies used for a physical exam and identify what component of the exam each is used for.

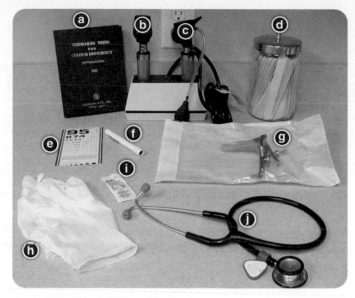

Source: © Total Care Programming Inc.

a. _____

b. _____

c. _____

d. _____

e. _____

f. _____

g. _____

h. _____

i. _____

j. _____

20. What are the six methods of examining a patient during a general physical exam?

_____

_____

_____

_____

_____

_____

21. During an exam of the lungs, what does the stethoscope allow the physician to do?

_____

_____

_____

22. For each of the following types of infection, indicate the appropriate PPE to wear.

    a. Gastroenteritis_____

    b. Hepatitis A_____

    c. Chickenpox_____

    d. AIDS_____

    e. Meningitis_____

    f. Mumps_____

    g. Streptococcal infection_____

    h. Influenza_____

23. List at least four examples of tests and procedures the doctor might order following a general physical exam.

_____

_____

_____

_____

24. What can you do to ensure that patients understand the instructions you give them?

_____

_____

_____

25. List three examples of patient follow-up that might be done after a physical exam.

_____

_____

_____

26. List two behaviors that a medical assistant should observe for when screening for visual acuity.

_____

_____

_____

Critical Thinking

Write the answer to each question on the lines provided.

  1. Why is it particularly important to prepare children emotionally for a physical exam?

_____

_____

_____

  2. Why is it important to avoid making any assumptions about patients from other cultures?

_____

_____

_____

3. Why is it necessary to assist patients into a variety of positions during a physical exam?

_____

_____

_____

4. Why is it important to help patients with disabilities during a physical exam, and what are some of the ways this can be accomplished?

_____

_____

_____

5. How would you prepare a patient for a diabetes follow-up? What testing may be ordered?

_____

_____

_____

A P P L I C A T I O N

Follow the directions for each application.

1. **Assisting During a Physical Exam**

    Working with two partners, role-play the procedures for assisting with the eyes, ears, nose and sinuses, and mouth and throat portions of a general physical exam. One partner should take the role of the medical assistant, one that of the patient, and the third should act as observer and evaluator. Your instructor can play the role of the physician.

    a. The medical assistant should first prepare the instruments for the exam: penlight, ophthalmoscope, vision charts, color charts, otoscope, audiometer, nasal speculum, and tongue depressor. The instruments should be organized in the order of the exam: eyes, ears, nose and sinuses, mouth and throat.

    b. The assistant should wash her hands thoroughly and observe appropriate safety precautions throughout.

    c. The assistant should prepare the patient emotionally and physically by explaining the procedure, what the patient will feel, and so on. She should then direct the patient to take the appropriate sitting position on the examining table.

    d. The assistant should put on gloves, protective clothing, and a face mask.

    e. While the physician conducts the exam, the assistant should hand the doctor the instruments as needed as well as provide assistance to the patient.

    f. After the exam, the observer should critique the medical assistant's role in the exam. Comments should concern the emotional and physical preparation given the patient, the observance of all safety precautions, aid given to the physician, and assistance given to the patient during the exam. All three students should discuss the procedure and the observer's comments.

    g. Exchange roles and have the new medical assistant assist with another portion of the exam, assembling equipment and supplies, preparing and positioning the patient, and assisting the physician. Critique and discuss the exam at its conclusion.

    h. Exchange roles one more time so that each partner has the opportunity to play each role during one portion of the exam.

2. Educating the Patient

Work with a partner. One partner should take the role of a medical assistant, the other the role of a patient who is at risk for breast cancer.

a. The medical assistant should review the information on the patient's chart. This patient is 42 years old. Both a sister and her mother have had breast cancer. The patient began menstruating at age 12 and has never had children. The medical assistant knows that breast cancer is the most commonly cancer diagnosed in women. With early detection, however, breast cancer can be successfully managed. Regular, routine screening, which includes a clinical breast exam and a mammogram, is essential for early detection and prompt treatment.

b. The medical assistant should use the foregoing information to educate the patient about breast cancer. The medical assistant should explain to the patient that she is at risk for breast cancer and why and should explain the need for regular screening. The assistant should periodically assess the patient's understanding of what is being discussed by questioning her and should then clarify misunderstandings.

c. The medical assistant should carefully explain the mammography procedure. The patient should ask questions. The medical assistant should answer all questions as fully as possible. If the assistant does not know the answer, she should tell the patient she will check with the physician and provide the information later.

d. Following the educational discussion, assess the interview with your partner. Was all pertinent information covered? Was the mammography procedure accurately and completely explained? Check the textbook for details.

3. Patients with Special Needs

Two clinical situations that require special considerations when conducting physical examinations are described as follows. In the space provided, complete each sentence.

A young female Middle Eastern patient is here for a complete physical exam.

a. Ensure cooperation by _____.

b. If necessary, use a _____.

c. If the patient understands some English you can _____.

d. Techniques you can use when dealing with patients from other cultures include _____.

The husband of a 73-year-old woman with Alzheimer's disease has brought his wife to the office for a general physical exam.

e. Before the test, make the patient feel more comfortable by _____.

f. When explaining procedures to the patient, _____.

g. During the exam, help the patient by _____.

h. If the patient's memory and language skills are impaired, _____.

i. If the patient seems to have trouble with one part of the exam, _____.

C A S E   S T U D I E S

Write your response to each case study on the lines provided.

Case 1

You normally place patients in the prone position to allow the physician to examine the back, feet, and musculoskeletal system. The patient being examined is extremely obese and has had some respiratory difficulties. Would you place him in this position? If not, what position(s) would you recommend?

_____

_____

_____

Case 2

A patient presents with symptoms of low back pain. What questions should you ask about the symptoms when obtaining the chief complaint? What supplies will be needed by the physician? When asking the patient to disrobe, what do you tell the patient to remove? Per the style of the practice, what testing can you perform before the physician's examination of the patient?

_____

_____

_____

Name_____ Date_____

Evaluated by_____ Score_____

PROCEDURE 38-1 Positioning a Patient for an Exam

Goal
To effectively assist a patient in assuming the various positions used in a general physical exam.

OSHA Guidelines

Materials
Adjustable examining table or gynecologic table, stepstool, exam gown, drape.

Method

Step Number	Procedure	Points Possible	Points Earned
1.	Identify the patient and introduce yourself.	5	
2.	Wash your hands.	10	
3.	Explain the procedure to the patient.	10	
4.	Provide a gown or drape if the physician has requested one, and instruct the patient in the proper way to wear it after disrobing. Allow the patient privacy while disrobing, and assist only if the patient requests help.*	15	
5.	Explain to the patient the necessary exam and the position required.	10	
6.	Ask the patient to step on the stool or the pullout step of the examining table. If necessary, assist the patient onto the examining table.	5	
7.	Assist the patient into the required position: **a.** Sitting **b.** Supine (recumbent) **c.** Dorsal recumbent **d.** Lithotomy **e.** Fowler's **f.** Prone **g.** Sims' **h.** Knee-chest **i.** Proctologic	10	
8.	Drape the client to prevent exposure and avoid embarrassment. Place pillows for comfort as needed.*	15	
9.	Adjust the drapes during the exam.	10	
10.	On completion of the exam, assist the patient out of the position as necessary and provide privacy as the patient dresses.	10	
Total Points		100	

CAAHEP Competencies Achieved

    I. P (10)   Assist physician with patient care

    IV. P (6)   Prepare a patient for procedures and/or treatments

ABHES Competencies Achieved

    9. (l) Prepare patient for examinations and treatments

    9. (m) Assist physician with routine and specialty examinations and treatments

PROCEDURE 38-2 Communicating Effectively with Patients from Other Cultures and Meeting Their Needs for Privacy

Goal
To ensure effective communication with patients from other cultures while meeting their needs for privacy.

OSHA Guidelines
This procedure does not involve exposure to blood, body fluids, or tissue.

Materials
Exam gown, drapes.

Method

Step Number	Procedure	Points Possible	Points Earned
Effective Communication			
1.	When it is necessary to use a translator, direct conversation or instruction to the translator.*	10	
2.	Direct conversation and demonstrations of what to do, such as putting on an exam gown, to the patient.*	10	
3.	Confirm with the translator that the patient has understood the instruction or demonstration.*	10	
4.	Allow the translator to be present during the exam if that is the patient's preference.	5	
5.	If the patient understands some English, speak slowly, use simple language, and demonstrate instructions whenever possible.	10	
Meeting the Need for Privacy			
6.	Before the procedure, thoroughly explain to the patient or translator the reason for disrobing. Indicate that you will allow the patient privacy and ample time to undress.	10	
7.	If the patient is reluctant, reassure him that the physician respects the need for privacy and will look at only what is necessary for the exam.*	10	
8.	Provide extra drapes if you think doing so will make the patient feel more comfortable.	10	
9.	If the patient is still reluctant, discuss the problem with the physician; the physician may be able to negotiate a compromise with the patient.	5	
10.	During the procedure, ensure that the patient is undraped only as much as necessary.	10	
11.	Whenever possible, minimize the amount of time the patient remains undraped.	10	
Total Points		100	

CAAHEP Competencies Achieved

I. P (10)   Assist physician with patient care

I. A (2)   Use language/verbal skills that enable patients' understanding

IV. P (6)   Prepare a patient for procedures and/or treatments

ABHES Competencies Achieved

5. (b) Identify and respond appropriately when working/caring for patients with special needs

5. (e) Advocate on behalf of family/patients, having ability to deal and communicate with family

8. (cc) Communicate on the recipient's level of comprehension

9. (l) Prepare patient for examinations and treatments

PROCEDURE 38-3 Transferring a Patient in a Wheelchair for an Exam

Goal
To assist a patient in transferring from a wheelchair to the examining table safely and efficiently.

OSHA Guidelines

Materials
Adjustable examining table or gynecologic table, stepstool (optional), exam gown, drape.

Method
Caution: Never risk injuring yourself; call for assistance when in doubt. As a rule, you should not attempt to lift more than 35% of your body weight.

Step Number	Procedure	Points Possible	Points Earned
Preparation for Transfer			
1.	Identify the patient and introduce yourself.	4	
2.	Wash your hands.	4	
3.	Explain the procedure in detail.	4	
4.	Position the wheelchair at a right angle to the end of the examining table.	4	
5.	Lock the wheels of the wheelchair.*	5	
6.	Lift the patient's feet and fold back the foot and leg supports of the wheelchair.	4	
7.	Place the patient's feet on the floor. The patient should have shoes or slippers with nonskid soles. Place your feet in front of the patient's feet.*	5	
8.	If needed, place a stepstool in front of the table, and place the patient's feet flat on the stool.	4	
Transferring the Patient by Yourself			
9.	Face the patient, spread your feet apart, align your knees with the patient's knees, and bend your knees slightly.*	5	
10.	Have the patient hold onto your shoulders.	3	
11.	Place your arms around the patient, under the patient's arms.	3	
12.	Tell the patient that you will lift on the count of 3, and ask the patient to support as much of her own weight as possible (if she is able).	4	
13.	At the count of 3, lift the patient.	4	
14.	Pivot the patient to bring the back of the patient's knees against the table.	4	
15.	Gently lower the patient into a sitting position on the table. If the patient cannot sit unassisted, help her move into a supine position.	4	
16.	Move the wheelchair out of the way.	3	
17.	Assist the patient with disrobing as necessary, providing a gown and drape.	3	

(continued)

Copyright © 2014 by The McGraw-Hill Companies, Inc.

Step Number	Procedure	Points Possible	Points Earned
Transferring the Patient with Assistance			
18.	Working with your partner, both of you face the patient, spread your feet apart, position yourselves so that one of each of your knees is aligned with the patient's knees, and bend your knees slightly.*	5	
19.	Have the patient place one hand on each of your shoulders and hold on.	4	
20.	Each of you places your outermost arm around the patient, one under each of the patient's arms. Then interlock your wrists.	4	
21.	Tell the patient that you will lift on the count of 3, and ask the patient to support as much of her own weight as possible (if she is able).	4	
22.	At the count of 3, you should lift the patient together.	4	
23.	The stronger of the two of you should pivot the patient to bring the back of the patient's knees against the table.	3	
24.	Working together, gently lower the patient into a sitting position on the table. If the patient cannot sit unassisted, help her move into a supine position.	3	
25.	Move the wheelchair out of the way.	3	
26.	Assist the patient with disrobing as necessary, providing a gown and drape.	3	
Total Points		100	

CAAHEP Competencies Achieved

IV. P (6)   Prepare a patient for procedures and/or treatments

ABHES Competencies Achieved

9. (l) Prepare patient for examinations and treatments

PROCEDURE 38-4 Assisting with a General Physical Exam

WORK // DOC

Goal
To effectively assist the physician with a general physical exam.

OSHA Guidelines

Materials
Supplies and equipment will vary depending on the type and purpose of the exam and the physician's practice preferences. Supplies may include the following: gown, drape, adjustable examining table, gloves, laryngeal mirror, lubricant, nasal speculum, otoscope and ophthalmoscope, pillow, reflex hammer, tuning fork, sphygmomanometer, stethoscope, tape measure, tongue depressors, penlight.

Method

Step Number	Procedure	Points Possible	Points Earned
1.	Wash your hands and adhere to Standard Precautions throughout the procedure.*	6	
2.	Gather and assemble the equipment and supplies.	3	
3.	Arrange the instruments and equipment in a logical sequence for the physician's use.	3	
4.	Greet and properly identify the patient, using at least two patient identifiers.*	6	
5.	Review the patient's medical history with the patient if office policy requires it.	3	
6.	Obtain vital statistics per the physician's preference.	3	
7.	Obtain the patient's weight and height (with shoes removed).	3	
8.	Obtain a urine specimen before the patient undresses for the exam.	3	
9.	Explain the procedure and exam to the patient.*	6	
10.	Obtain blood specimens or other laboratory tests per the chart or verbal order.	3	
11.	Provide the patient with an appropriate gown and drape, and explain where the opening for the gown is placed.	3	
12.	Obtain the ECG if ordered by the physician.	3	
13.	Assist patient to a sitting position at the end of the table with the drape placed across her legs.	3	
14.	Inform the physician that the patient is ready, and remain in the room to assist the physician.	3	
15.	You may be asked to shut off the light in the exam room to allow the patient's pupils to dilate sufficiently for a retinal exam.	2	
16.	Hand the instruments to the physician as requested.	3	
17.	Assist the patient to a supine position and drape her for an exam of the front of the body.	3	
18.	If a gynecological exam is needed, assist and drape the patient in the lithotomy position.	3	

(continued)

Step Number	Procedure	Points Possible	Points Earned
19.	If a rectal exam is needed, assist and drape the patient in the Sims' position.	3	
20.	Assist the patient to a prone position for a posterior body exam.	3	
21.	When the exam is complete, assist the patient to a sitting position and ask the patient to sit for a brief period of time.*	6	
22.	Ask the patient if he or she needs assistance in dressing.	3	
23.	After the patient has left, dispose of contaminated materials in an appropriate container.	3	
24.	Remove the table paper and pillow covering, and dispose of them in the proper container.	4	
25.	Disinfect and clean counters and the examining table with a disinfectant.	4	
26.	Sanitize and sterilize the instruments, if needed.	4	
27.	Prepare the room for the next patient by replacing the table paper, pillowcase, equipment, and supplies.	2	
28.	Document the procedure.*	6	
Total Points		100	

CAAHEP Competencies Achieved

I. P (10)   Assist physician with patient care

IV. P (6)   Prepare a patient for procedures and/or treatments

IX. P (7)   Document accurately in the patient record

ABHES Competencies Achieved

2. (c) Assist the physician with the regimen of diagnostic and treatment modalities as they relate to each body system

9. (l) Prepare patient for examinations and treatments

9. (m) Assist physician with routine and specialty examinations and treatments

Name_____ Class_____ Date_____

R E V I E W

Vocabulary Review

Matching
Match the key terms in the right column with the definitions in the left column by placing the letter of each correct answer in the space provided.

_____ 1. An instrument that permits the viewing of the vagina and cervix by expanding the vagina

_____ 2. Absence of menstruation

_____ 3. Bleeding between menstrual periods

_____ 4. The natural cessation of the menstrual cycle between ages 45 and 55

_____ 5. The first day of a patient's last menstrual period

_____ 6. "Morning after" or after sexual intercourse

_____ 7. Prolonged menstrual period or excessive menstrual flow

_____ 8. Painful menstruation

_____ 9. A woman's normal cycle of preparation for conception

_____ 10. A procedure in which a doctor removes a section of each tube that carries sperm from the testicles to the penis

_____ 11. The beginning of menstruation between ages 10 and 15

a. metrorrhagia
b. LMP
c. menarche
d. amenorrhea
e. menorrhagia
f. menstruation
g. menopause
h. speculum
i. vasectomy
j. dysmenorrhea
k. postcoital

True or False
Decide whether each statement is true or false. In the space at the left, write T for true or F for false. On the lines provided, rewrite the false statements to make them true.

_____ 12. As an optional cancer screening tool, women can perform a CBE monthly, just after their menstrual period ends.

_____

_____ 13. The prone and lithotomy exam positions are not recommended for pregnant patients.

_____

_____ 14. Abruptio placenta is a painless, bright red vaginal bleeding during the prenatal period.

_____

_____ 15. Gestational diabetes is indicated by a decrease in blood or urine glucose levels.

_____

_____ **16.** Nägele's rule is used to estimate the delivery date for a pregnant woman.

_____

_____ **17.** Human chorionic gonadotropin is the first milk the mother produces after delivery.

_____

_____ **18.** Ultrasonography is avoided while a woman is pregnant due to the dangers of radiation to the fetus.

_____

_____ **19.** Hysterosalpingography is an X-ray exam of the fallopian or uterine tubes and the uterus that uses a contrast medium, such as dye or air.

_____

_____ **20.** Alpha fetoprotein is a protein that is produced by an unborn child and passes into the mother's blood.

_____

_____ **21.** Colposcopy consists of dilating the cervix and scraping the uterine lining.

_____

_____ **22.** Cystometry is used to measure urinary bladder capacity and pressure.

_____

_____ **23.** Testicular biopsy is an invasive procedure.

_____

_____ **24.** The absence of menstruation is known as menorrhagia.

_____

_____ **25.** Reduction of labor is the process of giving medication to start uterine contractions for childbirth.

_____

Content Review

Multiple Choice

In the space provided, write the letter of the choice that best completes each statement or answers each question.

_____ **1.** Which of the following would *not* be included in your teaching to patients who have STIs?
  a. Importance of completing the course of therapy
  b. Avoiding sexual contact while the infection is active
  c. Dietary restrictions until the infection subsides
  d. Treating all sexual partners concurrently
  e. Methods of preventing STIs

_____ **2.** Which of the following licensed practitioners treats disorders of the male reproductive system?
  a. Gerontologist   **d.** Oncologist
  b. Urologist   **e.** Obstetrician
  c. Gynecologist

_____ **3.** A Pap smear is used to determine
  a. Pregnancy
  b. Menopause
  c. The presence of abnormal or precancerous cells
  d. The presence of an embolism
  e. Menarche

_____ 4. A digital exam is done during the gynecological exam to
   a. Check the position of the internal organs
   b. Test for cancer of the cervix
   c. Obtain a smear for cytologic exam
   d. Check for abnormalities in the cervix
   e. Check the rectum for polyps

_____ 5. During her pelvic exam, you notice that Sonya seems nervous and uncomfortable. To help her relax, you suggest that she
   a. Move closer to the end of the table
   b. Pull her knees together
   c. Hold her breath
   d. Take her feet out of the stirrups
   e. Take several deep breaths

_____ 6. The American Cancer Society recommends that men perform a testicular self-exam every
   a. Day
   b. Week
   c. Month
   d. Year
   e. Decade

_____ 7. The type of diabetes that is usually diagnosed between the 24th and 28th weeks of pregnancy is known as _____ diabetes.
   a. Gestational
   b. Postpartum
   c. Type I
   d. Type II
   e. Temporary

_____ 8. The most common test ordered in a urology practice is a(n)
   a. Cystogram
   b. Semen analysis
   c. Urinalysis
   d. Cystometry
   e. Pyelogram

_____ 9. Which diagnostic test involves using a needle to vacuum a sample of tissue from a cyst or tumor in the breast?
   a. Laparoscopy
   b. Cystometry
   c. Cystoscopy
   d. Fine-needle aspiration
   e. Chorionic villus sampling

_____ 10. Which diagnostic test involves using a needle guided by ultrasonography to remove a sample of the fluid that surrounds the fetus in the uterus?
   a. Cystometry
   b. Amniocentesis
   c. Chorionic villus sampling
   d. Stereotactic core biopsy
   e. Colposcopy

Sentence Completion

In the space provided, write the word or phrase that best completes each sentence.

11. A physician may order an AFP test to rule out _____ defects.

12. During _____, a woman may experience irregular periods, hot flashes, and vaginal dryness.

13. The image, or _____, produced by an ultrasound can help identify cysts and tumors in the abdominal cavity.

14. A special type of X-ray of the breast, called a(n) _____, detects cancer and other breast abnormalities.

15. If a woman cannot deliver a baby vaginally, the physician may perform a(n) _____ section.

16. FAS is a condition caused by consuming _____ during pregnancy.

17. A KOH test is often used to determine the presence of _____ in the vagina or cervix.

18. Surgical removal of the uterus and ovaries can cause women to experience _____ at any age.

19. Commonly called trich, _____ is a vaginal infection that is caused by a microscopic organism and is transferred during sexual intercourse.

20. Menstrual cycles are regulated by the hormones estrogen and _____.

11. _____

12. _____

13. _____

14. _____

15. _____

16. _____

17. _____

18. _____

19. _____

20. _____

Short Answer

Write the answer to each question on the lines provided.

21. The figure below illustrates a woman and fetus just before delivery. Label the rest of the illustration using the following terms: placenta, urethra, mucus plug, vagina, umbilical cord, urinary bladder, rectum, symphysis pubis.

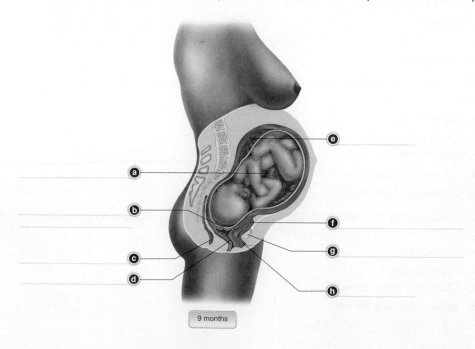

9 months

22. What are the three general guidelines to offer victims of domestic violence?

_____

_____

_____

23. Describe the guidelines for breast cancer screening.

_____

_____

_____

24. Describe the basic procedure for testicular self-exam.

_____

_____

_____

Critical Thinking

Write the answer to each question on the lines provided.

1. Two days after a cervical biopsy, a patient calls to tell you that she is experiencing some bleeding and does not know what she should do. What would you tell her?

_____

_____

_____

2. Using Nägele's rule, estimate the delivery date of a pregnant woman whose last menstrual period was July 16, 2013.

_____

_____

_____

3. Write three questions you might ask when taking a patient's history for a urologist.

_____

_____

_____

_____

A P P L I C A T I O N   WORK // DOC

Follow the directions for the application.

1. Preparing for a Gynecological Exam

Describe how you would prepare the patient for and assist with an annual gynecological exam with follow-up. Use Procedure Competency Sheet 39-1 to practice the procedure.

_____

_____

2. Reproductive and Urologic Diseases and Disorders

Briefly describe each of the following disorders.

a. Ectopic pregnancy _____

_____

b. Endometriosis_____

_____

c. Pelvic inflammatory disease _____

_____

d. Hydrocele _____

_____

e. Prostatic hypertrophy_____

_____

C A S E   S T U D I E S

Write your response to each case study on the lines provided.

Case 1

Megan Thomas's annual Pap smear reveals high-grade changes in the cervix. How might the physician decide to proceed?

_____

_____

_____

Case 2

You have just given Mr. Arturas instructions for performing a testicular self-exam. He questions you about having to do this monthly, stating that he doesn't think it is necessary to do it that often. What will you say to Mr. Arturas?

_____

_____

_____

Case 3

Jeanette Carson, a long-time patient at the OB/GYN practice where you work, is just past her eighth month of pregnancy. During her regular prenatal visit, Jeanette asks about classes she can take on breast-feeding. She then tells you that her sister lost her 4-month-old son to SIDS. Jeanette wants to know what she can do to avoid having the same thing happen to her baby. She wonders whether genetic factors play a role in SIDS cases. What can you tell Jeanette?

_____

_____

_____

PROCEDURE 39-1 Assisting with a Gynecological Exam

WORK // DOC

Goal
To assist the licensed practitioner and maintain the client's comfort and privacy during a gynecological exam.

OSHA Guidelines

Materials
Gown and drape; vaginal speculum; specimen collection equipment, including cervical brush, cervical broom, and/or scraper; cotton-tipped applicator; potassium hydroxide solution (KOH); exam gloves; tissues; laboratory requisition; water-soluble lubricant; examining table with stirrups; exam light; microscopic slide(s); thin layer collection vial (or slides if used); tissues; spray fixative; pen; and pencil.

Method

Step Number	Procedure	Points Possible	Points Earned
1.	Gather equipment and make sure all items are in working order. Correctly label the slide and/or the collection vials.*	8	
2.	Identify the patient and explain the procedure. The patient should remove all clothing, including underwear, and put the gown on with the opening in the front.	5	
3.	Ask the patient to sit on the edge of the examining table with the drape until the licensed practitioner arrives.	4	
4.	Place patient in lithotomy position when the licensed practitioner is ready.	7	
5.	Provide the licensed practitioner with gloves and an exam lamp as she examines the genitalia by inspection and palpation. Put on gloves per standard precautions guidelines.	8	
6.	Pass the speculum to the licensed practitioner. To increase patient comfort, you may place it in warm water before handing it to the licensed practitioner. Lubricant is not typically recommended prior to the Pap smear because it may interfere with the test results. A light speculum may be used.*	8	
7.	For the Pap (Papanicolaou) smear, be prepared to pass a cotton-tipped applicator and cervical brush, broom, or scraper for the collection of the specimens. Have the labeled slide or vial available for the licensed practitioner to place the specimen on the slide. Label containers or slides correctly depending upon procedure type.*	7	
8.	Once the specimen is on the slide, a cytology fixative must be applied immediately. A spray fixative is common, and it should be held 6 inches from the slide and sprayed lightly with a back and forth motion. Allow the slide to dry completely.*	8	
9.	After the licensed practitioner removes the speculum, a digital exam is performed to check the position of the internal organs. Provide the licensed practitioner with additional lubricant as needed.	5	
10.	Upon completion of the exam, help the patient switch from the lithotomy position to a supine or sitting position.	7	

(continued)

Step Number	Procedure	Points Possible	Points Earned
11.	Provide tissues or moist wipes for the patient to remove the lubricant, and ask the patient to get dressed. Assist as necessary or provide for privacy. Explain the procedure for communicating the laboratory results.	5	
12.	After the patient has left, don gloves and clean the exam room and equipment. Dispose of the disposable speculum, specimen collection devices, and other contaminated waste in a biohazardous waste container.	5	
13.	Store the supplies, straighten the room, and discard the used exam paper on the table.	4	
14.	Prepare the requisition slip and place the specimen and requisition slip in the proper place for transport to an outside laboratory.	7	
15.	Remove your gloves and wash your hands.	5	
16.	Document the specimen and complete the laboratory log if needed.*	7	
Total Points		100	

CAAHEP Competencies Achieved

I. P (10)   Assist physician with patient care

IV. P (6)   Prepare a patient for procedures and/or treatments

IV. P (8)   Document patient care

IX. P (7)   Document accurately in the patient record

ABHES Competencies Achieved

4. (a) Document accurately

9. (l) Prepare patient for examinations and treatments

9. (m) Assist physician with routine and specialty examinations and treatments

Name_____ Date_____

Evaluated by_____ Score_____

PROCEDURE 39-2 Assisting During the Exam
of a Pregnant Patient

Goal
To assist the licensed practitioner and meet the special needs of the pregnant woman during the general physical exam.

OSHA Guidelines

Materials
Patient education materials, examining table, exam gown, drape.

Method

Step Number	Procedure	Points Possible	Points Earned
Providing Patient Information			
1.	Identify the patient and introduce yourself.	6	
2.	Assess the patient's need for education by asking appropriate questions and having the patient describe what she already knows about the information you are providing.	7	
3.	Provide any appropriate instructions or materials.	6	
4.	Ask the patient whether she has any special concerns or questions about her pregnancy that she might want to discuss with the licensed practitioner.	7	
5.	Communicate the patient's concerns or questions to the licensed practitioner; include all pertinent background information on the patient.	7	
Ensuring Comfort during the Exam			
6.	Identify the patient and introduce yourself.	6	
7.	Wash your hands.	6	
8.	Explain the procedure to the patient.	6	
9.	Provide a gown or drape, and instruct the patient in the proper way to wear it after disrobing. (Allow the patient privacy while disrobing, and assist only if she requests help.)	6	
10.	Assist the patient onto the examining table. Ask the patient to step on either the stool or the pullout step of the examining table.	6	
11.	Help the patient into the position requested by the licensed practitioner, observing the patient for any difficulties she may have in achieving the requested position.	8	
12.	Provide and adjust additional drapes as needed.	6	
13.	Minimize the time the patient must spend in uncomfortable positions by making sure that the licensed practitioner has all supplies and equipment for the exam before it begins.	7	

(continued)

Name_____ Date_____

Evaluated by_____ Score_____

Step Number	Procedure	Points Possible	Points Earned
14.	If the patient appears to be uncomfortable during the procedure, ask whether she would like to reposition herself or take a break; assist as necessary.	8	
15.	To prevent pelvic pooling of blood and subsequent dizziness or hyperventilation, allow the patient time to adjust to sitting before standing after she has been lying on the examining table. Assist the patient off the exam table if needed.	8	
Total Points		100	

CAAHEP Competencies Achieved

I. P (10)   Assist physician with patient care

IV. P (6)   Prepare a patient for procedures and/or treatments

ABHES Competencies Achieved

5. (b) Identify and respond appropriately when working/caring for patients with special needs

9. (l) Prepare patient for examinations and treatments

9. (m) Assist physician with routine and specialty examinations and treatments

PROCEDURE 39-3 Assisting with a Cervical Biopsy [WORK // DOC]

Goal
To assist the physician in obtaining a sample of cervical tissue for analysis.

OSHA Guidelines

Materials
Gown and drape, tray or Mayo stand, disposable cervical biopsy kit (disposable forceps, curette, and spatula in a sterile pack), transfer forceps, vaginal speculum, biopsy specimen container, clean basin, sterile cotton balls, sterile gauze squares, sanitary napkin.

Method

Step Number	Procedure	Points Possible	Points Earned
1.	Identify the patient and introduce yourself.	5	
2.	Look at the patient's chart, and ask the patient to confirm information or explain any changes. Specific patient information you need to ask about and note in the chart includes the following: • Date of birth and Social Security number (verify that you have the correct chart for the correct patient) • Date of last menstrual period • Method of contraception, if any • Previous gynecologic surgery • Use of hormone replacement therapy or other steroids	5	
3.	If within your scope of practice, describe the biopsy procedure to the patient, noting that a piece of tissue will be removed to diagnose the cause of her problem. Explain that it may be painful but only for the brief moment during which tissue is taken.	5	
4.	Give the patient a gown, if needed, and a drape. Direct her to undress from the waist down and to wrap the drape around herself. Tell her to sit at the end of the examining table.	5	
5.	Wash your hands and put on exam gloves.	5	
6.	Using sterile method, open the sterile pack to create a sterile field on the tray or Mayo stand, and arrange the instruments with transfer forceps. Add the vaginal speculum and sterile supplies to the sterile field.*	8	
7.	When the physician arrives in the exam room, ask the patient to lie back, place her heels in the stirrups of the table, and move her buttocks to the edge of the table.	5	
8.	Assist the physician by arranging the drape so that only the genitalia are exposed, and place the light so that the genitalia are illuminated.	5	

(continued)

Step Number	Procedure	Points Possible	Points Earned
9.	Use transfer forceps to hand instruments and supplies to the physician as he requests them. You may don sterile gloves and hand the physician supplies and instruments directly.	5	
10.	When the licensed practitioner is ready to obtain the biopsy, tell the patient that it may hurt. If she seems particularly fearful, instruct her to take a deep breath and let it out slowly.	6	
11.	When the physician hands you the instrument with the tissue specimen, place the specimen in the specimen container and discard the instrument in the appropriate container.	7	
12.	Label the specimen container with the patient's name, the date and time, cervical or endocervical (as indicated by the physician), the physician's name, and your initials.	7	
13.	Place the container and the cytology laboratory requisition form in the envelope or bag provided by the laboratory.	6	
14.	When the physician has completed the procedure and removed the speculum, properly clean instruments as needed and dispose of used supplies and disposable instruments.	6	
15.	Remove the gloves and wash your hands.	6	
16.	Tell the patient that she may get dressed. Inform her that she may have some vaginal bleeding for a couple of days, and provide her with a sanitary napkin. Instruct her not to take tub baths or have intercourse and not to use tampons for 2 days. Encourage her to call the office if she experiences problems or has questions.	7	
17.	Document the procedure as appropriate.	7	
Total Points		100	

CAAHEP Competencies Achieved

    I. P (10)   Assist physician with patient care

    IV. P (6)   Prepare a patient for procedures and/or treatments

ABHES Competencies Achieved

    2. (c) Assist the physician with the regimen of diagnostic and treatment modalities as they relate to each body system

    9. (l) Prepare patient for examinations and treatments

    9. (m) Assist physician with routine and specialty examinations and treatments

40

Assisting in Pediatrics

Name_____ Class_____ Date_____

R E V I E W

Vocabulary Review

Matching
Match the key terms in the right column with the definitions in the left column by placing the letter of each correct answer in the space provided.

_____ 1. The onset of menstruation

_____ 2. A yellowish color of the skin caused by an accumulation of bilirubin

_____ 3. A vaccine or toxoid administered to protect people from infectious diseases

_____ 4. Soft spots on an infant's skull made of tough cartilage

_____ 5. A physical or psychological dependence on a substance

_____ 6. Nocturnal bed-wetting

_____ 7. Use of a substance in a way that is not medically approved

_____ 8. A known risk or reason not to give an immunization or medication

_____ 9. Physiological changes that make a person capable of sexual reproduction

_____ 10. A waste product from the normal breakdown of red blood cells

a. fontanels
b. menarche
c. puberty
d. substance abuse
e. bilirubin
f. enuresis
g. addiction
h. contraindication
i. jaundice
j. immunization

True or False
Decide whether each statement is true or false. In the space at the left, write T for true or F for false. On the lines provided, rewrite the false statements to make them true.

_____ 11. Psychiatry is a specialty area of medicine that involves the care of children up to the age of 18, or in some cases 21.

_____

_____ 12. Intellectual-cognitive development refers to the way a person relates to other people.

_____

_____ 13. An infant is called a toddler from birth to 1 month of age.

_____

_____ 14. One treatment for jaundice in an infant is to place the infant under infrared light.

_____

_____ 15. Infants develop in a cephalocaudal fashion, from the head and upper extremities down to the feet.

_____

Name_____ Class_____ Date_____

_____ **16.** Pediatricians examine the interior of a child's eyes with an instrument called a stethoscope.
_____

_____ **17.** Aspirin use in children has been associated with Reye syndrome.
_____

_____ **18.** Impetigo is a parasitic infestation caused by swallowing worm eggs or putting infested sand or dirt into the mouth.
_____

_____ **19.** Cerebral palsy is the most frequent crippling disease in children.
_____

_____ **20.** Congenital heart disease is a genetic disorder resulting from one extra chromosome in each of the millions of cells formed during development of the fetus.
_____

Content Review

Multiple Choice

In the space provided, write the letter of the choice that best completes each statement or answers each question.

_____ **1.** Infants typically triple their birth weight by the age of
    a. 1 month   **d.** 3 years
    b. 3 months   **e.** 5 years
    c. 1 year

_____ **2.** Girls usually reach half their adult height between the ages of
    a. 1½ to 2 years   **d.** 6 to 8 years
    b. 2 to 3 years   **e.** 10 to 12 years
    c. 3 to 5 years

_____ **3.** To help keep toddlers safe, parents should set the temperature of the household hot water tank at
    a. 80°F   **d.** 120°F
    b. 90°F   **e.** 145°F
    c. 100°F

_____ **4.** In the United States, females experience puberty at about _____ years of age.
    a. 6 to 8   **d.** 15 to 16
    b. 8 to 9   **e.** 16 to 18
    c. 12 to 13

_____ **5.** Children should have a well-child exam annually starting at age
    a. 6 months   **d.** 3 years
    b. 1 year   **e.** 5 years
    c. 2 years

_____ **6.** Keeping careful immunization records and ensuring proper vaccine storage and handling are generally the responsibility of the
    a. Receptionist
    b. Medical assistant
    c. Patient
    d. County courthouse
    e. Physician

_____ 7. The DTP vaccine immunizes children against
   a. Diphtheria, tetanus, and pneumonia
   b. Diarrhea, typhoid, and poliomyelitis
   c. Down syndrome, tuberculosis, and pertussis
   d. Diarrhea, tuberculosis, and pneumonia
   e. Diphtheria, tetanus, and pertussis

_____ 8. When taking vital signs on a child, which should you measure last?
   a. Temperature   d. Respirations
   b. Blood pressure   e. Oxygen
   c. Pulse

_____ 9. A major cause of lower respiratory disease in children is
   a. Respiratory syncytial virus   d. Herpes simplex virus
   b. Hepatitis B   e. Impetigo
   c. Viral gastroenteritis

_____ 10. Which of the following guidelines may help reduce the risk of sudden infant death syndrome?
   a. Place the baby on her stomach to sleep
   b. Avoid breast-feeding the baby
   c. Allow the baby to sleep in the parents' bed
   d. Place bumper pads around the sides of the crib
   e. Avoid exposing the baby to smoke

Sentence Completion

In the space provided, write the word or phrase that best completes each sentence.

11. Single parenthood and financial problems are among the risk factors for _____.

12. Pressure from media and peers may lead teens to develop abnormal eating behaviors such as _____ or bulimia nervosa.

13. A defect of spinal development called _____ results when tissues fail to close properly around the spinal cord during fetal development.

14. Cardiovascular malformation in the fetus before birth leads to _____ heart disease.

15. The risk of _____ syndrome increases as maternal age increases.

16. A contagious fungal disease called _____ may cause bald patches if the scalp is infected.

17. One reason children have frequent ear infections is that the _____ in children are more horizontal than they are in adults, allowing fluid to collect more easily.

18. The _____ of a child's head is measured to evaluate for diseases such as hydrocephalus.

19. Before administering an immunization to a child, you must obtain _____ from the parent or guardian.

20. Males experience _____ at about age 14, which is generally a few years later than females.

11. _____

12. _____

13. _____

14. _____

15. _____

16. _____

17. _____

18. _____

19. _____

20. _____

Short Answer
Write the answer to each question on the lines provided.

21. Describe the symptoms of viral gastroenteritis.

_____

_____

_____

22. What signs in a child might prompt you to alert the physician to possible child abuse?

_____

_____

_____

23. Why is viral gastroenteritis of concern in young children?

_____

_____

_____

24. What test might a doctor order to confirm a negative rapid strep test?

_____

_____

_____

25. Compare the aspects of care for preadolescents and adolescents.

_____

_____

_____

_____

Critical Thinking
Write the answer to each question on the lines provided.

1. In what ways would you handle readying a child for a general physical exam differently than readying an adult for this exam?

_____

_____

_____

2. Why is it important to obtain the parent's informed consent before administering an immunization to a child?

_____

_____

_____

A P P L I C A T I O N

Follow the directions for each application.

1. Describe how you would prepare the patient for and assist with each of these exams and procedures.

   a. A physical exam for a toddler

   _____

   _____

   b. A physical exam for an adolescent

   _____

   _____

2. Briefly describe each of the following childhood diseases.

   a. Cerebral palsy

   _____

   b. Impetigo

   _____

   c. Juvenile rheumatoid arthritis

   _____

   d. ADHD

   _____

3. Using Procedure Checklist 40-1 Measuring Infants, practice measuring the weight, length and head circumference of infants and children. You could visit a daycare center or bring infants and children to class to measure. Practice on at least one child, one toddler, and one infant. Check your results with another student.

4. Using the Procedure Checklist 40-2 Maintaining Growth Charts, and the measurements obtained in #3 above, complete the appropriate growth chart(s).

5. On his first visit to your clinic, an 18-month-old male infant was 33 inches in length and weighed 33 pounds. His head circumference was 19 inches. Using Procedure Checklist 40-2 and the correct growth chart, plot these examples and note the percentiles for the following:

   a. Length for age _____

   b. Weight for age _____

   c. Head circumference for age _____

   d. Weight for length _____

CASE STUDIES

Write your response to each case study on the lines provided.

Case 1

Austin, a 6-year-old male, is seen at the pediatrician's office today. He complains of a severe sore throat. His throat is red, and he has a fever of 102.8°F. The doctor orders a rapid strep test, which is negative. Why might the doctor order a throat culture for Austin?

_____

_____

_____

Case 2

An 18-year-old female patient has just been diagnosed with an STI. What general information should you ensure that the patient knows before she leaves the clinic? How would you go about telling her?

_____

_____

_____

Case 3

A 2-month-old infant arrives at the clinic for a well-child visit. During the exam by the physician, the infant is crying and agitated. What should you do?

_____

_____

_____

Case 4

A patient calls because he has found a small tick behind his son's ear. What would you advise him to do?

_____

_____

_____

Case 5

A mother calls your office and tells you her son is scheduled to come in for routine immunizations but he has a mild cold. What should you tell the patient?

_____

_____

_____

PROCEDURE 40-1 Measuring Infants

Goal
To accurately measure weight and length of infants and infant head circumference.

OSHA Guidelines

Materials
Pediatric examining table or infant scale, cardboard, pencil, yardstick, tape measure, disposable towel, growth chart or progress note of patient chart.

Method

Step Number	Procedure	Points Possible	Points Earned
Weight			
1.	Identify the patient and obtain permission from the parent to weigh the infant.	4	
2.	Wash your hands and explain the procedure to the parent.	4	
3.	Ask the parent to undress the infant.	3	
4.	Check to see whether the infant scale is in balance, and place a disposable towel on it.	4	
5.	Have the parent place the child face-up on the scale (or on the examining table if the scale is built into it). Keep one hand over the infant at all times, and hold a diaper over a male patient's penis to catch any urine the infant might void.	4	
6.	Place the lower weight at the highest number that does not cause the balance indicator to drop to the bottom.	5	
7.	Move the upper weight slowly to the right until the balance bar is centered at the middle mark, adjusting as necessary.	5	
8.	Add the two weights together to get the infant's weight.	5	
9.	Record the infant's weight in the chart or on the growth chart in pounds and ounces or to the nearest tenth of a kilogram.	4	
10.	Return the weights to their starting positions on the left side.	3	
Length: Scale with Length (Height) Bar			
11.	If the scale has a height bar, move the infant toward the head of the scale or examining table until her head touches the bar.	4	
12.	Have the parent hold the infant by the shoulders in this position.	3	
13.	Holding the infant's ankles, gently extend the legs, and slide the bottom bar to touch the soles of the feet.	4	
14.	Note the length and release the infant's ankles.	4	
15.	Record the length in the patient's chart or on the growth chart.	4	

(continued)

Step Number	Procedure	Points Possible	Points Earned
Length: Scale or Examining Table without Length (Height) Bar			
16.	If neither the scale nor the examining table has a height bar, have the parent position the infant close to the head of the examining table and hold the infant by the shoulders in this position.	4	
17.	Place a stiff piece of cardboard against the crown of the infant's head, and mark a line on the paper.	4	
18.	Hold the infant's ankles and gently extend the legs and draw a line on the paper to mark the heel, or note the measure on the yardstick.	4	
19.	Release the infant's ankles and measure the distance between the two markings on the towel or paper using the yardstick or a tape measure.	4	
20.	Record the length in the patient's chart or on the growth chart.	4	
Head Circumference			
21.	With the infant in a sitting or the supine position, place the tape measure around the infant's head at the forehead.	4	
22.	Adjust the tape so that it surrounds the infant's head at its largest circumference.	4	
23.	Overlap the ends of the tape, and read the measure at the point of overlap.	5	
24.	Remove the tape, and record the circumference in the patient's chart or on the growth chart.	4	
25.	Properly dispose of the used towel and wash your hands.	3	
Total Points		100	

CAAHEP Competencies Achieved

I. P (6)   Perform patient screening using established protocols

ABHES Competencies Achieved

2. (c) Assist the physician with the regimen of diagnostic and treatment modalities as they relate to each body system

Name_____ Date_____

Evaluated by_____ Score_____

PROCEDURE 40-2 Maintaining Growth Charts [WORK//DOC]

Goal
To accurately document the height, weight, and head circumference of a pediatric patient on a growth chart.

OSHA Guidelines
This procedures does not require exposure to blood or body fluids.

Materials
Appropriate growth chart, calculator or BMI calculator, pencil and pen.

Method

Step Number	Procedure	Points Possible	Points Earned
1.	Obtain accurate measurements.	10	
2.	Select the growth chart to use based on the age and gender of the child being weighed and measured.	10	
3.	Record the patient's name and record number at the top of the form	10	
4.	Record the mother's and father's stature (height) and the gestational age (pregnancy week) that the infant was born.	10	
5.	Record the date of birth, birth weight, length, and head circumference, and add notable comments, for example, breastfeeding. Note: This data is not included for growth charts for children aged 2 to 20 years.	10	
6.	Determine the age based upon the date of birth.* Round to the nearest month or the nearest ¼ of year based upon age.	13	
7.	Record the date, age, weight, height (stature), and head circumference. Add comments as appropriate such as "patient uncooperative."	10	
8.	Use a BMI calculator or a regular calculator and the formulas below to calculate the BMI. • BMI = Weight (kg) ÷ Stature (cm) ÷ Stature (cm) × 10,000 Or • BMI = Weight (lb) ÷ Stature (in) ÷ Stature (in) × 703	12	
9.	Accurately plot the measurement on the graph using the data you entered on the chart from the current visit.	15	
Total Points		100	

CAAHEP Competencies Achieved

II. P (3)   Maintain growth charts

IX. P (7)   Document accurately in the patient record.

ABHES Competencies Achieved

4. (a) Document accurately

PROCEDURE 40-3 Collecting a Urine Specimen from a Pediatric Patient

WORK // DOC

Goal
To collect a urine specimen from an infant or a child who is not toilet-trained.

OSHA Guidelines

Materials
Urine specimen bottle or container, label, sterile cotton balls, soapy water, sterile water, plastic disposable urine collection bag, laboratory requisition form.

Method

Step Number	Procedure	Points Possible	Points Earned
1.	Confirm the patient's identity, and be sure all forms are correctly completed.	5	
2.	Explain the procedure to the child (if age-appropriate) and to the parents or guardians.	5	
3.	Wash your hands, and put on exam gloves.	5	
4.	Have the parent(s) pull the child's pants down and take off the diaper.	5	
5.	Position the child with the genitalia exposed.	5	
6.	Clean the genitalia. For a male patient, wipe the tip of the penis with a soapy cotton ball, and then rinse it with a cotton ball saturated with sterile water. Allow to air-dry. For a female patient, use soapy cotton balls to clean the labia majora from front to back, using one cotton ball for each wipe. Again, use cotton balls saturated in sterile water to rinse the area, and allow it to air dry.	7	
7.	Remove the paper backing from the plastic urine collection bag, and apply the sticky, adhesive surface over the penis and scrotum (in a male patient) or vulva (in a female patient). Seal tightly to avoid leaks. Do not include the child's rectum within the collection bag or cover it with the adhesive surface.	7	
8.	Diaper the child.	5	
9.	Remove the gloves and wash your hands.	5	
10.	Check the collection bag every half-hour for urine. You must open the diaper to check; do not just feel the diaper.	7	
11.	If the child has voided, wash your hands and put on exam gloves.	5	
12.	Remove the diaper, take off the urine collection bag very carefully so that you do not irritate the child's skin, wash off the adhesive residue, rinse, and pat dry.	7	
13.	Diaper the child.	5	
14.	Place the specimen in the specimen container and cover it.	5	
15.	Label the urine specimen container with the patient's name, ID number, and date of birth; the physician's name, the date and time of collection; and your initials.	7	

(continued)

Step Number	Procedure	Points Possible	Points Earned
16.	Remove the gloves and wash your hands.	5	
17.	Complete the laboratory request form.	5	
18.	Record the collection in the patient's chart.	5	
Total Points		100	

CAAHEP Competencies Achieved

I. P (6)   Perform patient screening using established protocols

ABHES Competencies Achieved

2. (c) Assist the physician with the regimen of diagnostic and treatment modalities as they relate to each body system

41

Assisting in Geriatrics

Name_____ Class_____ Date_____

R E V I E W

Vocabulary Review

Matching
Match the key terms in the right column with the definitions in the left column by placing the letter of each correct answer in the space provided.

_____ 1. Measures taken to prevent illness

_____ 2. Brown spots caused by melanocytes gathering together

_____ 3. Curvature of the spine

_____ 4. Taking several medications concurrently

_____ 5. Involuntary leakage of urine

_____ 6. Decreased bone density

_____ 7. Specialist who cares for patients over age 65

_____ 8. Movement of the uterus down the vaginal canal

_____ 9. Obedience in following the physician's orders

_____ 10. Excessive nighttime urination

_____ 11. Degenerative joint disease

a. kyphosis
b. prolapse
c. osteoarthritis
d. osteoporosis
e. geriatrician
f. preventive medicine
g. polypharmacy
h. lentigos
i. nocturia
j. incontinence
k. patient compliance

True or False
Decide whether each statement is true or false. In the space at the left, write T for true or F for false. On the lines provided, rewrite the false statements to make them true.

_____ 12. Elderly patients are patients over 65 years of age.

_____

_____ 13. Thinning and wrinkling of the skin as a person ages are due to decreased amounts of estrogen and progesterone.

_____

_____ 14. Decreased blood flow to the brain in older people is often due to a thickening of the artery walls, called osteoporosis.

_____

_____ 15. A sign of aging in the cardiovascular system is increased cardiac output, especially during exercise.

_____

_____ 16. Alzheimer's disease is characterized by an abnormal growth of cells that are able to invade other tissues.

_____

_____ 17. Hypertension is a condition in which lipid (fat) levels are above normal.

_____ 18. Therapeutic touch is based on an ancient therapy called the laying on of hands.

_____ 19. Nocturia is a condition that can interfere with collecting a 24-hour urine specimen.

_____ 20. Elderly patients are usually less sensitive than younger patients to cold and heat.

Content Review

Multiple Choice
In the space provided, write the letter of the choice that best completes each statement or answers each question.

_____ 1. Which of the following is a risk factor for elder abuse?
   a. Isolation of the victim from family members and friends
   b. Presence of a child in the household
   c. History of divorce in the family
   d. History of heart disease in the family
   e. Presence of a pet in the household

_____ 2. Which of the following statements is true regarding the process of aging?
   a. Everyone experiences the same changes due to aging
   b. Aging rarely affects the integumentary system
   c. Aging makes people more prone to diseases and disorders
   d. The needs of geriatric patients are the same as those of other adult patients
   e. Elderly patients may take longer to process information

_____ 3. A common sign of aging in the endocrine system is
   a. Loss of voluntary control of urination
   b. Loss of estrogen production in postmenopausal women
   c. Susceptibility to autoimmune diseases
   d. Loss of elasticity in the lungs
   e. Slower reaction time and thought processing

_____ 4. Which of the following is *not* a sign of aging in the nervous system?
   a. Shrinkage of the temporal lobes
   b. Impaired vision and hearing
   c. Slower reaction times
   d. Shortened attention span
   e. Decreased inflammatory response

_____ 5. Which of the following is true regarding the cognitive-intellectual development of elderly patients?
   a. They can no longer learn
   b. Their wealth of experiences make them great teachers
   c. Their long-term memory becomes less acute
   d. Their short-term memory remains intact
   e. They process information quickly

_____ 6. Which of the following statements might you include in patient education for an 82-year-old female patient?
   a. It is no longer necessary to get regular exercise
   b. Volunteer work is generally a bad idea for elderly people
   c. It is not necessary to "exercise" your brain
   d. Continue to get regular health and dental care checkups
   e. You probably need only 2 or 3 hours of sleep each night

_____ 7. Weight-bearing and aerobic exercise benefits elderly people by
   a. Helping to prevent bone loss
   b. Preventing osteoarthritis
   c. Increasing their attention span
   d. Preventing atrophy of the subcutaneous layer of the skin
   e. Relieving congestive heart failure

_____ 8. The condition that causes cloudiness of the lens of the eye, decreasing vision, is
   a. Hypertension   d. Hyperlipidemia
   b. Myopia   e. Hyperopia
   c. Cataract

_____ 9. A patient complains of fatigue, hunger, increased thirst, and increased urination. You might suspect that this patient is suffering from
   a. Hyperlipidemia   d. Diabetes mellitus
   b. Cataracts   e. Cancer
   c. Congestive heart failure

_____ 10. Which of the following guidelines or techniques should you use when educating elderly patients?
   a. Understand that all elderly patients are frail and confused and treat them accordingly
   b. Do not provide written instructions because many elderly patients can no longer read them
   c. Adjust procedures as needed to accommodate any physical limitations the patient has
   d. Speak in high-pitched tones so elderly patients can hear you better
   e. Avoid embarrassing patients by asking them to perform a procedure you have just taught them

Sentence Completion

In the space provided, write the word or phrase that best completes each sentence.

11. When elderly patients see several different specialists for different health problems, one negative result can be drug-drug interactions caused by _____.

12. Treatment for _____ generally combines a course of medication with psychotherapy.

13. Changes in the semicircular canals in the inner ear can cause equilibrium or _____ problems, which may make an elderly person more prone to falling.

14. "Floaters" in the eyes are the result of the breakdown of the _____ in the eyes.

15. Some elderly people are concerned about the potential side effects of _____, or vaccination against diseases such as influenza.

11. _____

12. _____

13. _____

14. _____

15. _____

Short Answer

Write the answer to each question on the lines provided.

16. There are several signs of neglect of an elderly patient. Name four.

_____

_____

_____

17. Why are extra precautions needed when drawing blood from elderly patients?

_____

_____

_____

18. Why should sleep disturbances or excessive fatigue in an elderly patient be reported to the physician?

_____

_____

_____

19. What are the possible effects of retirement on a mature adult?

_____

_____

_____

20. Why is it important to stay with an elderly patient during the application of hot or cold therapy?

_____

_____

_____

Critical Thinking

Write the answer to each question on the lines provided.

1. Why is therapeutic touch sometimes an important part of caring for elderly patients?

_____

_____

_____

2. Why are elderly people more prone to falling than younger adults?

_____

_____

_____

A P P L I C A T I O N

Follow the directions for each application.

1. Atherosclerosis

The following figure illustrates a blood vessel affected by atherosclerosis. Label the illustration using the following terms: intima, lumen of vessel, fat, damaged area, media, smooth muscle cells, cholesterol crystals.

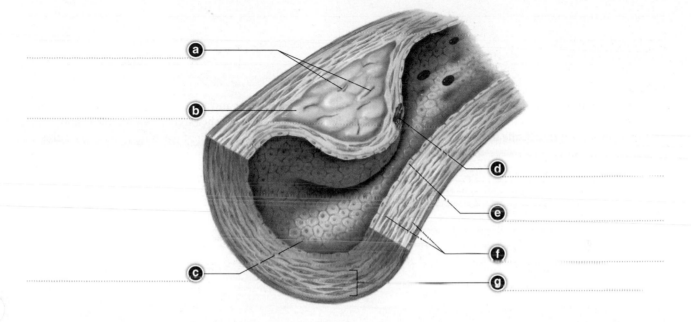

2. Malnutrition

List four types of factors that should be reported to the physician because they may interfere with an elderly person's ability to eat, causing the potential for malnutrition.

a. _____

b. _____

c. _____

d. _____

C A S E   S T U D I E S

Write your response to each case study on the lines provided.

Case 1

Mr. Felder is an 81-year-old patient who has several disorders that require medication. When you ask Mr. Felder about taking his medications, he tells you, "Yes, I take them, when I remember." What can you tell Mr. Felder to help increase his compliance with his medication schedule?

_____

_____

_____

Case 2

An elderly female patient arrives at your office for a check-up. She is underweight and appears to be dehydrated. When you ask about her food and fluid intake, she states that cooking is such a bother that she rarely eats a full meal, and since she doesn't eat much, she doesn't need to drink much to "wash it down." What patient teaching is needed for this patient?

_____

_____

_____

PROCEDURE 41-1 Educating Adult Patients about Daily Water Requirements

WORK // DOC

Goal
To teach patients how much water their bodies need to maintain health.

OSHA Guidelines
This procedure does not involve exposure to blood, body fluids, or tissues.

Materials
Patient education literature, patient's chart with Progress Note, and device to document education.

Method

Step Number	Procedure	Points Possible	Points Earned
1.	Explain the importance of water to the body. Point out the water content of the body and the many functions of water in the body, including maintaining the body's fluid balance, lubricating the body's moving parts, and transporting nutrients and secretions.*	15	
2.	Add any comments applicable to an individual patient's health status, such as issues related to medication use, physical activity, fluid limitation, or increased fluid needs.	15	
3.	Explain that people obtain water by drinking water and other fluids and by eating foods that contain water. On average, an adult should drink six to eight glasses of water a day to maintain a healthy water balance in which intake equals excretion. People's daily need for water varies with size and age, the temperatures to which they are exposed, the degree of physical exertion, and the water content of foods eaten. Make sure you reinforce the physician's or dietitian's recommendations for a particular patient's water needs.	10	
4.	Caution patients that soft drinks, coffee, and tea are not good substitutes for water and that it would be wise to filter out any harmful chemicals contained in the local tap water or to drink bottled water, if possible. A good rule of thumb is that for every soft drink, coffee, or tea, the patient should drink the same amount of water to ensure hydration.	10	
5.	Provide patients with tips about reminders to drink the requisite amount of water. Some patients may benefit from using a water bottle of a particular size, so they know they have to drink, say, three full bottles of water each day. Another helpful tip is to make a habit of drinking a glass of water at certain points in the daily routine, such as first thing in the morning and after lunch or right before bedtime.	10	
6.	Provide patients with printed materials documenting the amount of water to drink and methods to ensure that their fluid intake is adequate.	10	
7.	Remind patients that you and the physician are available to discuss any problems or questions.	10	
8.	Document any formal patient education sessions or significant exchanges with a patient in the patient's chart, noting whether the patient understood the information presented.*	20	
Total Points		100	

Name_____ Date_____

Evaluated by_____ Score_____

CAAHEP Competencies Achieved

IV. P (5)   Instruct patients according to their needs to promote health maintenance and disease prevention

ABHES Competencies Achieved

9. (r) Teach patients methods of health promotion and disease prevention

42

Assisting in Other Medical Specialties

Name_____ Class_____ Date_____

REVIEW

Vocabulary Review

Matching
Match the key terms in the right column with the definitions in the left column by placing the letter of each correct answer in the space provided.

_____ 1. Procedure in which reflected sound waves are used to test the structure and function of the heart

_____ 2. Procedure that enables an orthopedist to see inside a joint

_____ 3. Diagnostic exam in which the patient's skin is examined under ultraviolet light

_____ 4. Radiographic exam that produces a three-dimensional, cross-sectional view of the brain

_____ 5. X-ray examination of a blood vessel after injection of a contrast medium

_____ 6. Procedure that records the electrical activity of the brain

_____ 7. Surgical procedure in which a blood vessel from another area is used to bypass blocked coronary vessels

_____ 8. Gallbladder function test performed by X-ray with a contrast agent

_____ 9. X-ray visualization of the spinal cord after injection of a radioactive contrast medium or air into the spinal subarachnoid space

_____ 10. A metal mesh tube placed in an artery to keep it open

_____ 11. Viewing technique that uses a magnetic field to produce an image of internal body structures

_____ 12. Procedure that records nerve impulses and measures conduction time

_____ 13. Diagnostic test that allows physicians to study blood flow and metabolic activity in the brain

_____ 14. Procedure that provides direct visualization of the large intestine

_____ 15. Any procedure in which a scope is used to visually inspect a canal or cavity within the body

_____ 16. Procedure in which a catheter is inserted into the blood vessels of the heart

_____ 17. Procedure in which a balloon is inflated to compress arterial blockage

a. arthroscopy
b. echocardiography
c. cholecystography
d. colonoscopy
e. electroencephalography
f. balloon angioplasty
g. stent
h. positron emission tomography
i. angiography
j. magnetic resonance imaging
k. coronary artery bypass graft
l. Wood's light examination
m. electromyography
n. myelography
o. cardiac catheterization
p. computed tomography
q. endoscopy

True or False

Decide whether each statement is true or false. In the space at the left, write T for true or F for false. On the lines provided, rewrite the false statements to make them true.

_____ **18.** Another name for Holter monitoring is ambulatory cardiography.

_____

_____ **19.** An intradermal test is more sensitive than a scratch test.

_____

_____ **20.** A stress test is usually performed with the patient lying down.

_____

_____ **21.** Cardiac catheterization is a diagnostic method in which a catheter is inserted into a vein or an artery in the arm or leg and passed through the blood vessels into the lungs.

_____

_____ **22.** During a whole-body skin exam, a doctor examines the visible top layer of the entire surface of the skin.

_____

_____ **23.** Tumors are classified as benign or hostile.

_____

_____ **24.** Squamous cell carcinoma is the most dangerous type of skin cancer.

_____

_____ **25.** Sigmoidoscopy is an exam of the S-shaped segment of the large intestine.

_____

_____ **26.** Myelography is an X-ray visualization of the spinal cord after injection of a contrast medium or air into the spinal subarachnoid space.

_____

_____ **27.** Neuromuscular disorders or nerve damage can be detected through a lumbar puncture.

_____

_____ **28.** Gastroenterologists may use a Wood's light examination to visually inspect the esophagus, stomach, and duodenum.

_____

_____ **29.** A barium swallow is used to detect abnormalities in the large intestine.

_____

_____ **30.** Arthroscopy enables an orthopedist to see inside a muscle.

_____

Content Review

Multiple Choice

In the space provided, write the letter of the choice that best completes each statement or answers each question.

_____ **1.** A test using sound waves to examine the structure and function of the heart is known as a(n)

    a. Electrocardiogram   **d.** Angiogram

    b. Echocardiogram   **e.** Stress test

    c. Ultrasound

_____ **2.** A patient with a suspected hormonal imbalance is likely to be referred to a(n)

    a. Oncologist

    b. Gastroenterologist

    c. Cardiologist

    d. Endocrinologist

    e. Dermatologist

_____ **3.** An electroencephalogram can be used to detect

    a. Brain injuries   **d.** Neuromuscular disorders

    b. Bone injuries   **e.** Hormonal abnormalities

    c. Cardiac abnormalities

_____ **4.** A medical assistant in an oncologist's office might assist with a(n)

    a. Scratch test   **d.** Colonoscopy

    b. Electrocardiogram   **e.** Needle biopsy

    c. Ultrasound

_____ **5.** A type of diabetes that occurs in pregnant women is known as _____ diabetes.

    a. Type 1   **d.** Gestational

    b. Type 2   **e.** Temporal

    c. Postpartum

_____ **6.** Neuromuscular disorders or nerve damage can be detected through

    a. Lumbar puncture   **d.** Electromyography

    b. Cerebral angiography   **e.** Electrocardiography

    c. Electroencephalography

_____ **7.** A diagnostic procedure that uses strong magnets and radio waves to produce images of the heart is known as

    a. PET scanning   **d.** Balloon angioplasty

    b. Heart CT   **e.** Encephalography

    c. Heart MRI

_____ **8.** A diagnostic test in which a square of linen or paper is soaked with a suspected allergen and is applied to a patient's skin is a(n)

    a. Patch test   **d.** Intradermal test

    b. Paper test   **e.** Linen test

    c. Scratch test

_____ **9.** Two cardiology procedures often performed together are cardiac catheterization and

    a. Angiography   **d.** ECG

    b. Stress test   **e.** Angioplasty

    c. CABG

_____ **10.** Paralysis on one side of the body is known as

    a. Paraplegia   **d.** Quadriplegia

    b. Hemiplegia   **e.** Paraparesis

    c. Hemiparesis

_____ **11.** An instrument used to view inside a joint and guide surgical procedures is an

    a. Arthroscope   **d.** Arthrography

    b. Arthrogram   **e.** Arthrocentesis

    c. Arthroscopy

_____ 12. A procedure in which a scope is used to view a patient's lower rectum and anal canal is
   a. Arthroscopy
   b. Peroral endoscopy
   c. Proctoscopy
   d. Colonoscopy
   e. Sigmoidoscopy

_____ 13. Which of the following is *not* an indication of anaphylactic shock?
   a. Hives
   b. Difficulty breathing
   c. Convulsions
   d. Sharp increase in blood pressure
   e. Flushing

_____ 14. A medical assistant who is asked to assist with electroencephalography probably works for a(n)
   a. Gastroenterologist
   b. Cardiologist
   c. Oncologist
   d. Endocrinologist
   e. Neurologist

_____ 15. A disease of the brain that alters brain function or structure is known as
   a. Cardiomyopathy
   b. Encephalopathy
   c. Neuropathy
   d. Adenopathy
   e. Retinopathy

_____ 16. On which two body systems does an orthopedist concentrate?
   a. Skeletal and digestive systems
   b. Endocrine and reproductive systems
   c. Muscular and endocrine systems
   d. Skeletal and muscular systems
   e. Digestive and muscular systems

Sentence Completion
In the space provided, write the word or phrase that best completes each sentence.

17. Some gastrointestinal exams involve spraying the patients throat with a(n) _____ to inhibit the gag reflex.

18. During a needle biopsy, a surgeon removes _____ with a needle inserted through the skin and into a growth.

19. When a severe allergic reaction called _____ occurs, immediate medical intervention is needed to save the patient's life.

20. When cells become malignant, they are capable of _____, the transfer of abnormal cells to body sites other than the original tumor.

17. _____

18. _____

19. _____

20. _____

Short Answer
Write the answer to each question on the lines provided.

21. List four categories of chemotherapy drugs and describe their mechanism of action.

_____

_____

_____

_____

_____

_____

22. List three types of skin cancer, and identify the most dangerous type.

_____

_____

_____

23. Which medical specialties use imaging techniques such as X-ray, CT scan, and MRI as diagnostic tests?

_____

_____

_____

24. What are the five categories of neurological function evaluated in a complete neurological exam?

_____

_____

_____

25. List four procedures used to detect and diagnose cancer.

_____

_____

_____

26. When might joint replacement surgery be indicated?

_____

_____

_____

27. What is the purpose of myelography?

_____

_____

_____

28. When might a gastroenterologist perform an ultrasound on a patient?

_____

_____

_____

Critical Thinking

Write the answer to each question on the lines provided.

1. Why is the medical assistant's role in educating a cardiology patient about diet and exercise important?

_____

_____

_____

2. What advice might you give to a patient in her teens who has fair skin and hair and who is planning to work outdoors during the coming summer months?

_____

_____

_____

3. Compare and contrast an incisional biopsy and a needle biopsy.

_____

_____

_____

4. Write three questions you might ask when taking a patient's history for a gastroenterologist.

_____

_____

_____

_____

5. How might pretest instructions for a peroral endoscopy be different from those for a colonoscopy? Why might they be the same?

_____

_____

_____

_____

6. Why are diagnostic urine and blood tests essential in endocrine exams?

_____

_____

_____

A P P L I C A T I O N   WORK // DOC

Follow the directions for each application.

1. **Interviewing a Patient before a Specialized Exam**

    Work with two partners. While you assume the role of a medical assistant, have one partner play the role of a patient who is about to have a gastrointestinal exam performed by a gastroenterologist. Have the second partner act as an observer and evaluator.

    a. Using the Medical History Form and the Physical Examination Form take the patient's history, recording your questions and the patient's responses. On the basis of the responses, ask appropriate follow-up questions.

    b. Explain to the patient what the doctor is likely to do and why. Allow the patient to interrupt at any time with questions, which you should answer to the best of your ability. Record your statements, the patient's questions, and your responses.

    c. Have the observer present a critique of your patient interview. The critique should involve your approach and attitude as well as the appropriateness and accuracy of your questions and responses. The observer should also evaluate the order in which you took the history and its completeness.

d. You and your partners should then discuss the observer's critique, noting the strengths and weaknesses of your interview. Comments should include both positive feedback and suggestions for improvement.

e. Exchange roles and repeat the exercise with a patient who has an appointment for a general orthopedic, dermatology, or cardiology exam. The student playing the observer chooses the specialty exam for the patient.

f. Exchange roles again so that each group member has the opportunity to play the medical assistant, the patient, and the observer once.

g. Repeat this role-playing exercise with your partners, this time with a group member playing a patient who has an appointment for treatment of a specific disease or disorder. The disease or disorder may be chosen by the student who is playing the observer.

2. **Educating Patients**

Work with a partner to plan a health-awareness booth for a community health fair.

a. You and your partner choose one disease or disorder (such as heart disease, cancer, a thyroid gland dysfunction, or a common gastrointestinal disorder) about which to educate the public. Brainstorm to decide what information to provide in the booth. Ask yourselves these questions: What are some important issues associated with this disease or disorder? Can these issues be organized into general categories?

b. Decide whether you will use printed materials, an oral presentation, audiovisual materials, or a combination of these. Discuss with your partner interesting and appealing ways to present the information. What resources might be available in the community to increase awareness of the causes, diagnosis, treatment, and management of this disease or disorder?

c. Outline your plan for the booth. Gather information on resources available in your community about the disease or disorder. If your plan includes posters, brochures, or flyers, make a sketch of these to demonstrate the type of information that would appear on them. If your plan includes an oral presentation, write it on paper and record it. If your plan includes audiovisual material, make or procure a videotape that demonstrates how the information would be presented.

d. You and your partner prepare your booth.

e. Present your booth to the class. Have your classmates critique your presentation. The critique should focus on the appropriateness of the content as well as its accuracy and clarity. Comments should include both positive feedback and suggestions for improvement.

f. Continue until all pairs of students have had the opportunity to present their booths to the class.

CASE STUDIES

Write your response to each case study on the lines provided.

Case 1

You are assisting a cardiologist in administering a treadmill stress test to a patient when the physician is suddenly called out of the room. It becomes apparent that the physician will not return for several minutes. What should you do? Why?

_____

_____

_____

Case 2

Marge is a patient in your office who has recently been diagnosed with type 2 diabetes. She asks you why it is so important for her to monitor her blood sugar and diet so carefully if she is feeling fine. What can you tell her about the long-term complications of diabetes?

_____

_____

_____

Case 3

Jenna is a 17-year-old patient who is allergic to bee stings. She wants to go on a camping trip with her family in a wilderness area. What advice might you give Jenna? What might the physician prescribe?

_____

_____

_____

Case 4

David is a 42-year-old patient with a history of high blood pressure and high cholesterol. He is seeing the physician today because a friend told him he is at risk for a heart attack. You notice that he has gained 12 pounds since his last exam. What advice might you give David?

_____

_____

_____

PROCEDURE 42-1 Assisting with a Scratch Test Examination

WORK // DOC

Goal
To assist a licensed practitioner in determining substances to which a patient has an allergic reaction.

OSHA Guidelines

Materials
Disposable sterile needles or lancets, allergen extracts, control solution, cotton balls, alcohol, timer, adhesive tape, ruler, cold packs or ice bag.

Method

Step Number	Procedure	Points Possible	Points Earned
1.	Wash your hands and assemble the necessary materials.	5	
2.	Identify the patient and introduce yourself.	5	
3.	Show the patient into the treatment area. Explain the procedure and discuss any concerns. Confirm whether the patient followed pretesting procedures such as discontinuing medications.*	10	
4.	Assist the patient into a comfortable position and put on exam gloves.	5	
5.	Swab the test site, usually the upper arm or back, with an alcohol prep pad.	5	
6.	Identify the sites with tape labels.*	10	
7.	Apply small drops of the allergen extracts and control solution onto the test site at evenly spaced intervals, about 1½ to 2 inches apart.	5	
8.	Open the package containing the first needle or lancet, making sure you do not contaminate the instrument.	5	
9.	Assist the physician with the scratch procedure, or perform the procedure if it is within your scope of practice. Using a new sterile needle or lancet for each site, scratch the skin beneath each drop of allergen, no more than $1/_8$ inch deep.	5	
10.	Start the timer for the 20-minute reaction period.	5	
11.	After the reaction time has passed, cleanse each site with an alcohol prep pad. (Do not remove identifying labels until the physician has checked the patient.)	5	
12.	Assist the physician, or examine and measure the sites.	5	
13.	Apply cold packs or an ice bag to sites as needed to relieve itching.	5	
14.	Properly dispose of used materials and instruments.	5	
15.	Clean and disinfect the area according to OSHA guidelines.	5	
16.	Remove the gloves and wash your hands.	5	
17.	Document the test results in the patient's chart on a Progress Note, if required, and initial your entries.*	10	
Total Points		100	

CAAHEP Competencies Achieved

    I. P (10)   Assist physician with patient care

    IV. P (6)   Prepare a patient for procedures and/or treatments

    IX. P (7)   Document accurately in the patient record

ABHES Competencies Achieved

    4. (a) Document accurately

    9. (l) Prepare a patient for examinations and treatments

    9. (m) Assist physician with routine and specialty examinations and treatments

PROCEDURE 42-2 Assisting with a Sigmoidoscopy

Goal

To assist the physician during the examination of the rectum, anus, and sigmoid colon using a sigmoidoscope.

OSHA Guidelines

Materials

Sigmoidoscope, suction pump, lubricating jelly, drape, patient gown, tissues.

Method

Step Number	Procedure	Points Possible	Points Earned
1.	Wash your hands and assemble and position materials and equipment according to the physician's preference.	5	
2.	Test the suction pump.	5	
3.	Identify the patient and introduce yourself.	5	
4.	Show the patient into the treatment room. Explain the procedure and discuss any concerns the patient may have.*	10	
5.	Instruct the patient to empty the bladder, take off all clothing from the waist down, and put on the gown with the opening in the back.	5	
6.	Put on exam gloves and assist the patient into the knee-chest or Sims' position. Immediately cover the patient with a drape.*	5	
7.	Use warm water to bring the sigmoidoscope to slightly above body temperature; lubricate the tip.*	5	
8.	Assist as needed, including handing the doctor the necessary instruments and equipment.	5	
9.	Monitor the patient's reactions during the procedure, and relay any signs of pain to the doctor.	5	
10.	Clean the anal area with tissues after the exam.	5	
11.	Properly dispose of used materials and disposable instruments.	5	
12.	Remove the gloves and wash your hands.	5	
13.	Help the patient gradually assume a comfortable position.*	10	
14.	Instruct the patient to dress.	5	
15.	Put on clean gloves.	5	
16.	Sanitize reusable instruments and prepare them for disinfection and/or sterilization, as necessary.	5	
17.	Clean and disinfect the equipment and the room according to OSHA guidelines.	5	
18.	Remove the gloves and wash your hands.	5	
Total Points		100	

CAAHEP Competencies Achieved

I. P (10)   Assist physician with patient care

IV. P (6)   Prepare a patient for procedures and/or treatments

ABHES Competencies Achieved

9. (l) Prepare a patient for examinations and treatments

9. (m) Assist physician with routine and specialty examinations and treatments

PROCEDURE 42-3 Assisting with a Needle Biopsy

Goal
To assist the licensed practitioner to remove tissue from a patient's body so that it can be examined in a laboratory.

OSHA Guidelines

Materials
Sterile drapes, tray or Mayo stand, antiseptic solution, cotton balls, local anesthetic, disposable sterile biopsy needle or disposable sterile syringe and needle, sterile sponges, specimen bottle with fixative solution, laboratory packaging, sterile wound-dressing materials.

Method

Step Number	Procedure	Points Possible	Points Earned
1.	Identify the patient and introduce yourself.	5	
2.	Instruct the patient as needed, and discuss any concerns the patient may have.*	10	
3.	Wash your hands and assemble the necessary materials.	5	
4.	Prepare the sterile field and instruments.	5	
5.	Put on exam gloves.	5	
6.	Position and drape the patient.	5	
7.	Cleanse the biopsy site. Prepare the patient's skin.	10	
8.	Remove the gloves, wash your hands, and put on clean exam gloves.	5	
9.	Assist the doctor as needed when she injects anesthetic.	5	
10.	Perform a surgical scrub and put on sterile gloves if you will be handing the physician sterile instruments.	5	
11.	Place the sample in a properly labeled specimen bottle, complete the laboratory requisition form, and package the specimen for immediate transport to the laboratory.*	10	
12.	Apply a dressing to the patient's wound site.	5	
13.	Properly dispose of used supplies and instruments.	5	
14.	Clean and disinfect the room according to OSHA guidelines.	5	
15.	Remove the gloves and wash your hands.	5	
16.	Document as needed.*	10	
Total Points		100	

CAAHEP Competencies Achieved

I. P (10)   Assist physician with patient care

IV. P (6)   Prepare a patient for procedures and/or treatments

IX. P (7)   Document accurately in the patient record

ABHES Competencies Achieved

4. (a) Document accurately

9. (l) Prepare a patient for examinations and treatments

9. (m) Assist physician with routine and specialty examinations and treatments

Assisting with Eye and Ear Care

43

Name_____ Class_____ Date_____

R E V I E W

Vocabulary Review

Matching

Match the key terms in the right column with the definitions in the left column by placing the letter of each correct answer in the space provided.

_____ 1. An instrument used to measure intraocular pressure

_____ 2. Using a device with multiple lenses to verify the need for corrective lenses

_____ 3. The number of complete fluctuations of energy that pass a specific point in 1 second

_____ 4. The type of hearing loss that results when sound waves are blocked

_____ 5. The type of hearing loss that results when neural tissues are damaged

_____ 6. Ringing in the ears

_____ 7. A handheld instrument with a light used to view the inner eye structures

_____ 8. A specialist who focuses on evaluating and correcting hearing problems

_____ 9. An electronic device that stimulates the auditory nerve

_____ 10. A specialist who treats diseases and disorders of the ears

_____ 11. A condition produced by increased intraocular pressure

_____ 12. An inner ear disease that causes bouts of vertigo, nausea, and tinnitus

_____ 13. Clouding and hardening of the lens of the eye, which causes visual disturbance

_____ 14. A condition commonly referred to as nearsightedness

_____ 15. Hearing loss due to aging

_____ 16. A visual impairment in near vision

_____ 17. The bacterial form of this condition is known as pink eye

_____ 18. An electronic device that measures hearing acuity by producing sounds in specific frequencies and intensities

_____ 19. The process of the eye focusing on objects

_____ 20. A unit used to measure the relative intensity of sound

a. conductive
b. glaucoma
c. tonometer
d. conjunctivitis
e. cataract
f. hyperopia
g. accommodation
h. frequency
i. refraction exam
j. Meniere's disease
k. cochlear implant
l. sensorineural
m. presbycusis
n. ophthalmoscope
o. audiometer
p. myopia
q. audiologist
r. decibel
s. tinnitus
t. otologist

Copyright © 2014 by The McGraw-Hill Companies, Inc.

True or False

Decide whether each statement is true or false. In the space at the left, write T for true or F for false. On the lines provided, rewrite the false statements to make them true.

_____ **21.** A slit lamp is used to examine the eye's posterior structures.

_____

_____ **22.** Fluorescein dye is used to check for problems with the retina.

_____

_____ **23.** The most common chart used to test near vision is the Jaegar chart.

_____

_____ **24.** Applying pressure to the outer corner of the eye helps prevent systemic absorption of an eye medication.

_____

_____ **25.** The medical term for "swimmer's ear" is otitis externa.

_____

_____ **26.** Mastoiditis is an infection of the bone located just in front of the ear.

_____

_____ **27.** The innermost of the ossicles is the stapes.

_____

_____ **28.** A cerumen impaction can cause sensorineural hearing loss.

_____

_____ **29.** Ménière's disease is caused by increased fluid in the middle ear.

_____

_____ **30.** Drooping of the upper eyelid is known as ptosis.

_____

_____ **31.** A sty is usually caused by *Staphylococcus aureus*.

_____

_____ **32.** Color blindness occurs more often in males.

_____

_____ **33.** An M.D. who examines and treats eye diseases is the specialist called an optometrist.

_____

_____ **34.** In otosclerosis, the malleus becomes immobilized.

_____

_____ **35.** Ear irrigation is contraindicated in someone who has had a mastoidectomy.

_____

Content Review

Multiple Choice

In the space provided, write the letter of the choice that best completes each statement or answers each question.

_____ 1. Macular degeneration causes
   a. Loss of peripheral vision
   b. Conductive hearing loss
   c. Sensorineural hearing loss
   d. Loss of central vision
   e. Ringing in the ears

_____ 2. The term for the condition caused when the brain "ignores" a lazy eye is
   a. Strabismus
   b. Amblyopia
   c. Esotropia
   d. Retinopathy
   e. Hypermetropia

_____ 3. Presbycusis is
   a. Sudden hearing loss
   b. Loss of vision due to aging
   c. Loss of hearing due to aging
   d. Loss of peripheral vision
   e. Nearsightedness

_____ 4. What is the term for the physician who specializes in treating diseases and conditions of the eye?
   a. Optician
   b. Otologist
   c. Audiologist
   d. Optometrist
   e. Ophthalmologist

_____ 5. The medical term for nearsightedness is
   a. Myopia
   b. Hyperopia
   c. Hypermetropia
   d. Presbyopia
   e. Amblyopia

_____ 6. Eyeglasses with concave lenses are used to correct
   a. Presbyopia
   b. Amblyopia
   c. Myopia
   d. Hyperopia
   e. Strabismus

_____ 7. Physicians use tuning forks to
   a. Measure air pressure in the ear
   b. Treat hearing loss
   c. Determine the extent of hearing loss
   d. Determine if the patient has hearing loss
   e. Check for cerumen impaction

_____ 8. A myringotomy is a procedure done to treat
   a. Glaucoma
   b. Conjunctivitis
   c. Otitis media
   d. Tympanic membrane rupture
   e. Tinnitus

_____ 9. The most common cause for vision loss in the United States is
   a. Cataracts   d. Presbyopia
   b. Glaucoma   e. Macular degeneration
   c. Retinitis

_____ 10. An abnormally shaped cornea or lens causes the condition of
   a. Astigmatism   d. Entropion
   b. Amblyopia   e. Ectropion
   c. Strabismus

Sentence Completion

In the space provided, write the word or phrase that best completes each sentence.

11. During accommodation, the _____ muscles contract, changing the shape of the lens.

12. The area that is visible when the patient looks at an object straight ahead is the visual _____.

13. The way light from objects is focused through the eye to form an image on the retina is _____.

14. Aqueous humor diffuses into a vascular channel known as the _____ canal.

15. Loss of visual acuity due to aging is called _____.

16. A(n) _____ is used to measure hearing acuity.

17. The eye's _____ structures include the eyelids, iris, lens, and cornea.

18. _____ is an inflammation of the eyelid.

19. The test that is done to measure fluid pressure within the eye is _____.

20. A(n) _____ is used to visualize the internal structures of the eye.

11. _____

12. _____

13. _____

14. _____

15. _____

16. _____

17. _____

18. _____

19. _____

20. _____

Short Answer

Write the answer to each question on the lines provided.

21. What are some common causes of conjunctivitis?

_____

_____

_____

22. What is the medical term for a sty?

_____

_____

23. Name two common treatments for retinal detachment.

_____

_____

24. Describe the type of exam performed with a retinoscope.

_____

_____

25. Name the two most common tests used to evaluate color vision.

_____

_____

Critical Thinking
Write the answer to each question on the lines provided.

1. When instilling eye medications, how might you keep them from being absorbed systemically?

_____

_____

2. How might a sore throat produce otitis media?

_____

_____

3. Why is it important to face a person with a hearing impairment instead of speaking directly into his ear?

_____

_____

4. How might the speech development of an infant with chronic otitis media be affected?

_____

_____

A P P L I C A T I O N

Follow the directions for each application.

1. Working with the Hearing Impaired

List six things you can do to improve communication with a patient who has a hearing impairment.

_____   _____

_____   _____

_____   _____

2. Eye Care Tips

Create a patient education brochure outlining specific eye care tips.

C A S E   S T U D I E S

Write your response to each case study on the lines provided.

Case 1

A 2-year-old is undergoing a procedure to place tubes in his ears. The doctor explains that this procedure is necessary because the toddler's auditory tubes are not functioning properly. What problems occur if auditory tubes do not function well?

_____

_____

_____

Case 2

You have been instructed to perform ear irrigation on a patient. What questions should you ask before the irrigation? What instructions should you give the patient after the procedure?

_____

_____

_____

Case 3

A 65-year-old woman has been diagnosed with glaucoma. The doctor prescribes eye drops to treat the condition. However, the woman complains she does not like putting medicines in her eyes and that her eyes do not hurt. How would you convince her that she needs to use the eye drops?

_____

_____

_____

Case 4

A 52-year-old woman has noticed that when she looks at straight lines, they sometimes become wavy. She also has noticed that she cannot see details very well and that her central vision is becoming worse. What condition does she most likely have?

_____

_____

_____

PROCEDURE 43-1 Preparing the Ophthalmoscope for Use

Goal
To ensure that the ophthalmoscope is ready for use during an eye exam.

OSHA Guidelines
This procedure does not involve exposure to blood, body fluids, or tissues.

Materials
Ophthalmoscope, lens, spare bulb, spare battery.

Method

Step Number	Procedure	Points Possible	Points Earned
1.	Wash your hands.	20	
2.	Take the ophthalmoscope out of its battery charger. In a darkened room, turn on the ophthalmoscope light.	20	
3.	Shine the large beam of white light on the back of your hand to check that the instrument's tiny lightbulb is providing strong enough light.	20	
4.	Replace the bulb or battery if necessary. (The battery is located in the ophthalmoscope's handle.)	20	
5.	Make sure the instrument's lens is screwed into the handle. If it is not, attach the lens.	20	
Total Points		100	

CAAHEP Competencies Achieved

I. P (10)　　Assist physician with patient care

ABHES Competencies Achieved

None

PROCEDURE 43-2 Performing Vision Screening Tests [WORK // DOC]

Goal
To screen a patient's ability to see distant or close objects, to determine contrast sensitivity, or to detect color blindness.

OSHA Guidelines

Materials
Occluder or card; alcohol; gauze squares; appropriate vision charts to test for distance vision, near vision, and color blindness.

Method

Step Number	Procedure	Points Possible	Points Earned
Distance Vision			
1.	Wash your hands, clean the occluder with a gauze square dampened in alcohol, identify the patient, introduce yourself, and explain the procedure.	2	
2.	Mount one of the following eye charts at eye level: Snellen letter or similar chart (for patients who can read), Snellen E, Landolt C, pictorial, or similar chart (for patients who cannot read). If using the Snellen letter chart, verify that the patient knows the letters of the alphabet. With children or nonreading adults, use demonstration cards to verify that they can identify the pictures or direction of the letters.	2	
3.	Make a mark on the floor 20 feet away from the chart.	2	
4.	Have the patient stand with his or her heels at the 20-foot mark, or sit with the back of the chair at the mark.	2	
5.	Instruct the patient to keep both eyes open and not to squint or lean forward during the test.*	5	
6.	Test both eyes first, then the right eye, and then the left eye. (Different offices may test in a different order. Follow your office policy.)*	5	
7.	Have the patient read the lines on the chart (or identify the picture/direction), beginning with the 20-foot line. If the patient cannot read this line, begin with the smallest line the patient can read.*	5	
8.	Note the smallest line the patient can read or identify with no more than two errors.	2	
9.	Record the results as a fraction (for example, each eye 20/40 −1 if the patient misses one letter on a line or each eye 20/40 −2 if the patient misses two letters on a line).	2	
10.	Show the patient how to cover the left eye with the occluder or card. Again, instruct the patient to keep both eyes open and not to squint or lean forward during the test.*	5	
11.	Have the patient read the lines on the chart.*	5	
12.	Record the results of the right eye (for example, Right Eye 20/30).	2	
13.	Have the patient cover the right eye and read the lines on the chart.*	5	
14.	Record the results of the left eye (for example, Left Eye 20/20).	2	

(continued)

Step Number	Procedure	Points Possible	Points Earned
15.	If the patient wears corrective lenses, record the results using c̄c̄ (if your office uses this abbreviation for "with correction") in front of the abbreviation (for example, c̄c̄ both eyes 20/20).	2	
16.	Note and record any observations of squinting, head tilting, excessive blinking, or tearing.	2	
17.	Ask the patient to keep both eyes open and to identify the two colored bars, and record the results in the patient's chart.	2	
18.	Clean the occluder with a gauze square dampened with alcohol.	2	
19.	Properly dispose of the gauze square and wash your hands.	2	
Near Vision			
1.	Wash your hands, identify the patient, introduce yourself, and explain the procedure.	2	
2.	Have the patient hold one of the following at normal reading distance (approximately 14 to 16 inches): Jaeger, Richmond pocket, or similar chart or card.*	5	
3.	Ask the patient to keep both eyes open and to read or identify the letters, symbols, or paragraphs.*	5	
4.	Record the smallest line read without error.*	5	
5.	If the card is laminated, clean it with a gauze square dampened with alcohol.	2	
6.	Properly dispose of the gauze square and wash your hands.	2	
Color Vision			
1.	Wash your hands, identify the patient, introduce yourself, and explain the procedure.	2	
2.	Hold one of the following color charts or books at the patient's normal reading distance (approximately 14 to 16 inches): Ishihara, Richmond pseudoisochromatic, or similar color-testing system.*	5	
3.	Ask the patient to tell you the number or symbol within the colored dots on each chart or page.*	5	
4.	Proceed through all the charts or pages, usually totaling 24.	2	
5.	Record the number correctly identified and failed with a slash between them (for example, 23 passed/1 failed).*	5	
6.	If the charts are laminated, clean them with a gauze square dampened with alcohol.	2	
7.	Properly dispose of the gauze square and wash your hands. Document the results after you have completed the procedure.	2	
Total Points		100	

CAAHEP Competencies Achieved

IV. P (8)   Document patient care

IX. P (7)   Document accurately in the patient record

ABHES Competencies Achieved

2. (c) Assist the physician with the regimen of diagnostic and treatment modalities as they relate to each body system

4. (a) Document accurately

9. (m) Assist physician with routine and specialty examinations and treatments

PROCEDURE 43-3 Administering Eye Medications   WORK // DOC

Goal

To instill (introduce) medication into the eye for treatment of certain eye disorders.

OSHA Guidelines

Materials

Medication (drops, cream, or ointment), tissues, eye patch (if applicable).

Method

Step Number	Procedure	Points Possible	Points Earned
1.	Identify the patient, introduce yourself, and explain the procedure.	3	
2.	Review the doctor's medication order. This should include the patient's name, drug name, concentration, number of drops (if a liquid), into which eye(s) the medication is to be administered, and the frequency of administration.*	7	
3.	Compare the drug with the medication order three times, checking the rights of medication administration.	7	
4.	Ask whether the patient has any known allergies to substances contained in the medication.*		
5.	Wash your hands and put on gloves.	3	
6.	Assemble the supplies.	3	
7.	Ask the patient to lie down or to sit back in a chair with the head tilted back.	3	
8.	Give the patient a tissue to blot excess medication as needed.	3	
9.	Remove an eye patch, if present.	3	
10.	Instruct the patient to look at the ceiling, and to keep both eyes open during the procedure.	3	
11.	With a tissue, gently pull the lower eyelid down by pressing downward on the patient's cheekbone just below the eyelid with your nondominant hand. This pressure will open a pocket of space between the eyelid and the eye.*	7	
Eyedrops			
12.	Resting your dominant hand on the patient's forehead, hold the filled eyedropper or bottle approximately ½ inch from the conjunctiva.	3	
13.	Drop the prescribed number of drops into the pocket. If any drops land outside the eye, repeat instilling the drops that missed the eye.*	7	
Creams or Ointments			
12.	Rest your dominant hand on the patient's forehead, and hold the tube or applicator above the conjunctiva.	3	
13.	Without touching the eyelid or conjunctiva with the applicator, evenly apply a thin ribbon of cream or ointment along the inside edge of the lower eyelid on the conjunctiva, working from the medial (inner) to the lateral (outer) side.*	7	

(continued)

Step Number	Procedure	Points Possible	Points Earned
All Medications			
14.	Release the lower lid and instruct the patient to gently close the eyes.*	7	
15.	Repeat the procedure for the other eye as necessary.	3	
16.	Remove any excess medication by wiping each eyelid gently with a fresh tissue from the medial to the lateral side.	3	
17.	Apply a clean eye patch to cover the entire eye, if ordered.	3	
18.	Ask whether the patient felt any discomfort and observe for any adverse reactions. Notify the doctor as necessary.*	7	
19.	Instruct the patient on self-administration of medication and patch application, if ordered.*	7	
20.	Ask the patient to repeat the instructions.	3	
21.	Provide written instructions.	3	
22.	Properly dispose of used disposable materials.	2	
23.	Remove gloves and wash your hands.	3	
24.	Document administration in the patient's chart. Include the drug, concentration, the number of drops or amount, the time of administration, and the eye(s) that received the medication.*	7	
Total Points		100	

CAAHEP Competencies Achieved

I. P (10)   Assist with patient care

IV. P (8)   Document patient care

IX. P (7)   Document accurately in the patient record

ABHES Competencies Achieved

4. (a) Document accurately

9. (m) Assist physician with routine and specialty examinations and treatments

PROCEDURE 43-4 Performing Eye Irrigation [WORK // DOC]

Goal
To flush the eye to remove foreign particles or relieve eye irritation.

OSHA Guidelines

Materials
Sterile irrigating solution, sterile basin, sterile irrigating syringe and kidney-shaped basin, tissues.

Method

Step Number	Procedure	Points Possible	Points Earned
1.	Identify the patient, introduce yourself, and explain the procedure.	5	
2.	Review the physician's order. This should include the patient's name, the irrigating solution, the volume of solution, and for which eye(s) the irrigation is to be performed.*	8	
3.	Compare the solution with the instructions three times, checking the rights of medication administration.*	8	
4.	Wash your hands and put on gloves, a gown, and a face shield.	5	
5.	Assemble supplies.	5	
6.	Ask the patient to lie down or to sit with the head tilted back and to the side that is being irrigated. The solution should not spill over into the other eye.	5	
7.	Place a towel or a disposable waterproof underpad over the patient's shoulder. Have the patient hold the kidney-shaped basin at the side of the head next to the eye to be irrigated.*	8	
8.	Pour the solution into the sterile basin.	5	
9.	Fill the irrigating syringe with solution (approximately 50 mL).	5	
10.	Hold a tissue on the patient's cheekbone below the lower eyelid with your nondominant hand, and press downward to expose the eye socket.	5	
11.	Holding the tip of the syringe ½ inch away from the eye, direct the solution onto the lower conjunctiva from the inner to the outer aspect of the eye. (Avoid directing the solution against the cornea because it is sensitive; do not use excessive force.)*	8	
12.	Refill the syringe and continue irrigation until the prescribed volume of solution is used.	5	
13.	Dry the area around the eye with tissues or gauze squares.	5	
14.	Properly dispose of used disposable materials.	5	
15.	Remove your gloves, gown, and face shield, and wash your hands.	5	

(continued)

Step Number	Procedure	Points Possible	Points Earned
16.	Record the following in the patient's chart: procedure, type of solution, amount of solution used, time of administration, and eye(s) irrigated.*	8	
17.	Put on gloves and clean the equipment and room according to OSHA guidelines.	5	
Total Points		100	

CAAHEP Competencies Achieved

I. P (10) Assist physician with patent care

IV. P (6) Prepare patient for procedures and/or treatments

IV. P (8) Document patient care

IX. P (7) Document accurately in the patient record

ABHES Competencies Achieved

4. (a) Document accurately

9. (m) Assist physician with routine and specialty examinations and treatments

PROCEDURE 43-5 Measuring Auditory Acuity   (WORK // DOC)

Goal
To determine how well a patient hears.

OSHA Guidelines

Materials
Audiometer, headset, graph pad (if applicable), alcohol, gauze squares.

Method

Step Number	Procedure	Points Possible	Points Earned
Infants and Toddlers			
1.	Identify the patient and introduce yourself.	8	
2.	Wash your hands.	8	
3.	Pick a quiet location.*	12	
4.	The patient can be sitting, lying down, or held by the parent.	8	
5.	Instruct the parent to be silent during the procedure.*	12	
6.	Position yourself so your hands are behind the child's right ear and out of sight.ˣ	12	
7.	Clap your hands loudly. Observe the child's response. (Never clap directly in front of the ear because this can damage the eardrum. As an alternative to clapping, use special devices, like rattles or clickers (which may be available in the office) to generate sounds of varying loudness.*	12	
8.	Record the child's response as positive or negative for loud noise.	5	
9.	Position one hand behind the child's right ear, as before.	8	
10.	Snap your fingers. Observe the child's response.	5	
11.	Record the response as positive or negative for moderate noise.	5	
12.	Repeat steps 6 through 11 for the left ear. Document the patient's results after you have completed the procedure.	5	
Total Points		100	
Adults and Children			
1.	Wash your hands, identify the patient, introduce yourself, and explain the procedure.	4	
2.	Clean the earpieces of the headset with a sanitizing wipe according to manufacturer's instructions.*	6	
3.	Have the patient sit with his back to you.*	6	
4.	Assist the patient in putting on the headset, and adjust it until it is comfortable.*	6	
5.	Tell the patient he will hear tones in the right ear.*	6	

(continued)

Step Number	Procedure	Points Possible	Points Earned
6.	Tell the patient to raise his finger or press the indicator button when he hears a tone.	4	
7.	Set the audiometer for the right ear.*	6	
8.	Set the audiometer for the lowest range of frequencies and the first degree of loudness (usually 15 decibels). (When using automated audiometers, follow the instructions printed in the user's manual.)*	6	
9.	Press the tone button or switch and observe the patient.	4	
10.	If the patient does not hear the first degree of loudness, raise it two or three times to greater degrees, up to 50 or 60 decibels.*	6	
11.	If the patient indicates that he has heard the tone, record the setting on the graph.*	6	
12.	Change the setting to the next frequency. Repeat steps 9, 10, and 11.	4	
13.	Proceed to the midrange frequencies. Repeat steps 9, 10, and 11.	4	
14.	Proceed to the high-range frequencies. Repeat steps 9, 10, and 11.	4	
15.	Set the audiometer for the left ear.*	6	
16.	Tell the patient that he will hear tones in the left ear, and ask him to raise his finger or press the indicator button when he hears a tone.*	6	
17.	Repeat steps 8 through 14.	4	
18.	Have the patient remove the headset.	4	
19.	Clean the earpieces with a sanitizing wipe.	4	
20.	Properly dispose of the used sanitizing wipe and wash your hands.	4	
Total Points		100	

CAAHEP Competencies Achieved

I. P (10)   Assist physician with patient care

ABHES Competencies Achieved

2. (c) Assist the physician with the regimen of diagnostic and treatment modalities as they relate to each body system

PROCEDURE 43-6 Administering Eardrops   [WORK // DOC]

Goal
To instill medication into the ear to treat certain ear disorders.

OSHA Guidelines

Materials
Liquid medication, cotton balls.

Method

Step Number	Procedure	Points Possible	Points Earned
1.	Identify the patient, introduce yourself, and explain the procedure.	2	
2.	Check the physician's medication order. It should include the patient's name, drug name, concentration, the number of drops, into which ear(s) the medication is to be administered, and the frequency of administration.*	10	
3.	Compare the drug with the instructions three times, checking the rights of medication administration.*	10	
4.	Ask whether the patient has any allergies to ear medications.*	10	
5.	Wash your hands and put on gloves.	2	
6.	Assemble supplies.	2	
7.	Warm the medication with your hands or by placing the bottle in a pan of warm water.ˣ	10	
8.	Have the patient lie on his or her side with the ear to be treated facing up.	2	
9.	Straighten the ear canal by pulling the auricle upward and outward for adults, down and back for infants and children.*	10	
10.	Hold the dropper ½ inch above the ear canal.	2	
11.	Gently squeeze the bottle or dropper bulb to administer the correct number of drops.*	10	
12.	Have the patient remain in this position for 10 minutes.	2	
13.	If ordered, loosely place a small wad of cotton in the outermost part of the ear canal.	2	
14.	Note any adverse reaction, notifying the physician as necessary.	2	
15.	Repeat the procedure for the other ear, if ordered.	2	
16.	Instruct the patient on how to administer the drops at home.*	10	
17.	Ask the patient to repeat the instructions.	2	
18.	Provide written instructions.	2	
19.	Remove the cotton after 15 minutes.	2	
20.	Properly dispose of used disposable materials.	2	

(continued)

Step Number	Procedure	Points Possible	Points Earned
21.	Remove gloves and wash your hands.	2	
22.	Record in the patient's chart the medication, concentration, the number of drops, the time of administration, and which ear(s) received the medication.	2	
Total Points		100	

CAAHEP Competencies Achieved

I. P (10)   Assist with patient care

IV. P (8)   Document patient care

IX. P (7)   Document accurately in the patient record

ABHES Competencies Achieved

4. (a) Document accurately

9. (m) Assist physician with routine and specialty examinations and treatments

PROCEDURE 43-7 Performing Ear Irrigation   『WORK // DOC』

Goal
To wash out the ear canal to remove impacted cerumen, relieve inflammation, or remove a foreign body.

OSHA Guidelines

Materials
Fresh irrigating solution, clean basin, clean irrigating syringe, towel or absorbent pad, kidney-shaped basin, cotton balls.

Method

Step Number	Procedure	Points Possible	Points Earned
1.	Identify the patient, introduce yourself, and explain the procedure.	4	
2.	Check the doctor's order. It should include the patient's name, the irrigating solution, the volume of solution, and for which ear(s) the irrigation is to be performed. If the doctor has not specified the volume of solution, use the amount needed to remove the wax.*	8	
3.	Compare the solution with the instructions three times, checking the rights of medication administration.*	8	
4.	Wash your hands and put on gloves, a gown, and a face shield.	4	
5.	Look into the patient's ear to identify cerumen or a foreign body needing to be removed. You will know when you have completed the irrigation when the cerumen or foreign body is removed.	4	
6.	Assemble the supplies.	4	
7.	If the solution is cold, warm it to body temperature by placing the bottle in a pan of warm water.*	8	
8.	Have the patient sit or lie on his or her back with the ear to be treated facing you.	4	
9.	Place a towel or disposable waterproof underpad over the patient's shoulder (or under the head and over the shoulder if the patient is lying down), and have the patient hold the kidney-shaped basin under the ear.	4	
10.	Pour the solution into the other basin.	4	
11.	If necessary, gently clean the external ear with cotton moistened with the solution.	4	
12.	Fill the irrigating syringe with solution (approximately 50 mL).	4	
13.	Straighten the ear canal by pulling the auricle upward and outward for adults.	4	
14.	Holding the tip of the syringe ½ inch from the opening of the ear and tilted toward the top of the ear canal, slowly instill the solution into the ear. Allow the fluid to drain out during the process.*	8	

(continued)

Step Number	Procedure	Points Possible	Points Earned
15.	Refill the syringe and continue irrigation until the canal is cleaned or the solution is used up.	4	
16.	Dry the external ear with a cotton ball, and, if ordered, leave a clean cotton ball loosely in place for 5–10 minutes.	4	
17.	If the patient becomes dizzy or nauseated, allow him or her time to regain balance before standing up. Assist patient as needed.	4	
18.	Properly dispose of used disposable materials.	4	
19.	Remove your gloves, gown, and face shield, and wash your hands.	4	
20.	Record the following in the patient's chart: procedure and result, amount of solution used, time of administration, and ear(s) irrigated.	4	
21.	Put on gloves and clean the equipment and room according to OSHA guidelines.	4	
Total Points		100	

CAAHEP Competencies Achieved

I. P (10)   Assist physician with patent care

IV. P (6)   Prepare patient for procedures and/or treatments

IV. P (8)   Document patient care

IX. P (7)   Document accurately in the patient record

ABHES Competencies Achieved

4. (a) Document accurately

9. (m) Assist physician with routine and specialty examinations and treatments

44

Assisting with Minor Surgery

Name_____ Class_____ Date_____

R E V I E W

Vocabulary Review

Matching

Match the key terms in the right column with the definitions in the left column by placing the letter of each correct answer in the space provided.

_____ 1. Applied directly to the skin

_____ 2. Initial phase of wound healing

_____ 3. During surgery

_____ 4. The removal of dead tissue

_____ 5. The elimination of all microorganisms

_____ 6. A sterile cloth with cutout section in the center

_____ 7. Suture materials

_____ 8. A collection of pus that forms as a result of infection

_____ 9. The use of extreme cold to destroy unwanted tissue

_____ 10. To bring the edges of a wound together

_____ 11. Surgical stitches used to close a wound

_____ 12. A dilute solution of formaldehyde

_____ 13. The third stage of wound healing, when scar tissue forms

_____ 14. After surgery

_____ 15. The process of removing fluid or tissue cells by aspiration with a needle and syringe

_____ 16. A jagged, open wound in the skin that can extend down into the underlying tissue

a. abscess
b. approximate
c. cryosurgery
d. debridement
e. fenestrated drape
f. formalin
g. intraoperative
h. inflammatory phase
i. laceration
j. ligature
k. maturation phase
l. needle biopsy
m. postoperative
n. surgical asepsis
o. sutures
p. topical

True or False

Decide whether each statement is true or false. In the space at the left, write T for true or F for false. On the lines provided, rewrite the false statements to make them true.

_____ 17. Surgical asepsis reduces the number of microorganisms but does not necessarily eliminate them.

_____

_____ 18. Anesthesia is a loss of sensation.

_____

_____ **19.** A sterile scrub assistant assists during a procedure by handling sterile equipment.

_____ **20.** During the maturation phase, scar tissue forms at the wound site.

_____ **21.** A medical assistant may be responsible for closing a wound after a surgical procedure.

_____ **22.** During debridement, a doctor surgically removes healthy tissue from a wound.

_____ **23.** During the inflammatory phase of wound healing, bleeding is reduced by constriction of the blood vessels.

_____ **24.** During a surgical procedure, a sterile field is used as a work area.

_____ **25.** During the preoperative stage in a procedure, the surgical room is prepared for surgery.

_____ **26.** A doctor may use a needle biopsy to aspirate fluid or tissue cells for examination.

_____ **27.** A minor surgical procedure is usually performed without an anesthetic.

_____ **28.** Bleeding from a blood vessel can be stopped by the use of a hemostat.

Content Review

Multiple Choice

In the space provided, write the letter of the choice that best completes each statement or answers each question.

_____ **1.** One event that occurs during the inflammatory phase of wound healing is
  a. The formation of a scab
  b. The clotting of the blood
  c. The formation of scar tissue
  d. The formation of new tissue
  e. Clot retraction

_____ **2.** When a patient's skin is prepared for surgery, how far should the prepped area extend beyond the surgical field?
  a. 1 inch   **d.** 4 inches
  b. 2 inches   **e.** 5 inches
  c. 3 inches

_____ **3.** Lidocaine is the most commonly used
  a. Anesthetic   **d.** Dressing
  b. Antiseptic   **e.** Preservative
  c. Disinfectant

_____ 4. The procedure using extreme cold to destroy tissues is known as
   a. Electrocautery
   b. Laser surgery
   c. Cryosurgery
   d. Approximation
   e. Thermotherapy

_____ 5. A collection of pus that forms as a result of an infection is a(n)
   a. Ligature
   b. Incision
   c. Wound
   d. Debris
   e. Abscess

_____ 6. A surgical wound created when a doctor cuts into body tissue is a(n)
   a. Laceration
   b. Incision
   c. Puncture
   d. Irrigation
   e. Biopsy

_____ 7. A ligature is a(n)
   a. Jagged, open wound
   b. Deep layer of tissue
   c. Absorbable suture material
   d. Surgical stitch used to close a wound
   e. Type of biopsy

_____ 8. Using a probe or needle heated by electric current to destroy tissue is known as
   a. Electrocauterization
   b. Cryosurgery
   c. Anesthesia
   d. Approximation
   e. A needle biopsy

_____ 9. A dilute solution of formaldehyde used to prevent tissue changes is
   a. Normal saline
   b. Lidocaine
   c. Povidone iodine
   d. Formalin
   e. Glutaraldehyde

_____ 10. Using a needle and syringe to withdraw tissue or fluid for examination is known as a(n)
   a. Debridement
   b. Needle biopsy
   c. Puncture
   d. Biopsy specimen
   e. Incision

_____ 11. An instrument used to hold back the sides of an incision to provide greater access and a better view is a
   a. Probe
   b. Curette
   c. Hemostat
   d. Dilator
   e. Retractor

_____ 12. A 0.9% solution of sodium chloride is also known as
   a. Zephiran chloride
   b. Normal saline
   c. Chlorhexidine gluconate
   d. Formalin
   e. Lidocaine

_____ 13. A sterile solution sometimes injected along with an anesthetic to constrict blood vessels and reduce bleeding is known as
   a. Lidocaine
   b. Tetracaine
   c. Zephiran chloride
   d. Epinephrine
   e. Normal saline

_____ 14. Sterilization tape that is used to secure autoclave wrap is also used to
   a. Identify and date the contents
   b. Prove that the sterility of the items has taken place
   c. Indicate that the pack has been exposed to the autoclave process
   d. a and c only
   e. All of the above

_____ 15. The proof that an instrument pack has been sterilized is achieved by using a
   a. Chemical indicator strip placed under the instruments
   b. Chemical indicator strip placed in the center of the pack
   c. Chemical indicator tape around the outside of the pack
   d. Biological monitor placed next to a pack
   e. Biological monitor placed in the load with the packs

_____ 16. The critical step of the autoclave cycle when the microorganisms are destroyed is when
   a. The greatest temperature is reached
   b. The water is changed into pressurized steam
   c. Heat is transferred to the items in the chamber
   d. The steam saturates items in the chamber
   e. The instruments are drying

_____ 17. While using an autoclave, the medical assistant must monitor
   a. Temperature-pressure combinations
   b. Time-temperature combinations
   c. Pressure-time combinations
   d. All of the above
   e. None of the above

_____ 18. When storing items removed from an autoclave, the major factor contributing to the integrity of the sterility is
   a. Preventing dust accumulation
   b. Maintaining the temperature of the environment
   c. The state of dryness when the pack is stored
   d. The shelf-life expectancy
   e. Whether there is a sterilization indicator in the pack

Sentence Completion

In the space provided, write the word or phrase that best completes each sentence.

19. A small wound may be approximated by using a(n) _____ or sterile strip.

20. With certain electrocautery units, a(n) _____ plate or pad will be placed somewhere on the patient's body during the procedure.

21. If a patient is allergic to _____, Hibiclens should be used as a preoperative antiseptic to swab the skin.

22. During surgery, scissors and clamps should be held by the _____ when you pass them to a surgeon.

23. Typically, suture removal takes place _____ days after minor surgery.

19. _____

20. _____

21. _____

22. _____

23. _____

Short Answer

Write the answer to each question on the lines provided.

24. The following illustration shows a variety of cutting and dissecting instruments used to perform minor surgery. Write the names of the instruments on the lines provided. Then explain the instruments' use.

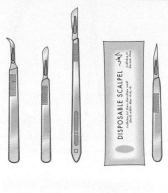

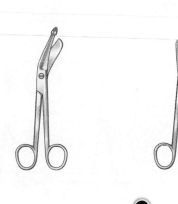

a ....

b ....

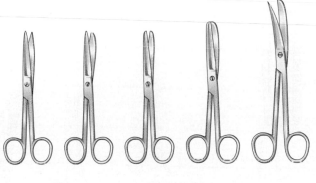

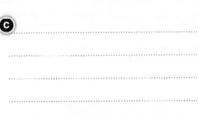

c ....
....
....
....
....

d ....
....

e ....
....

25. The following illustration shows a variety of grasping and clamping instruments used to perform minor surgery. Write the names of the instruments on the lines provided.

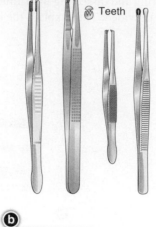
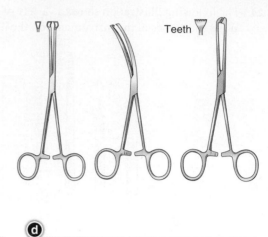

Teeth

Teeth

ⓐ ....

ⓑ ....

ⓒ ....

ⓓ ....

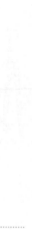
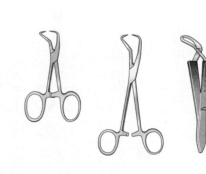

Serrated jaws

ⓔ ....

ⓕ ....

ⓖ ....

26. The following illustration shows a variety of retracting, dilating, and probing instruments used to perform minor surgery. Write the names of the instruments on the lines provided. Then explain the instruments' use.

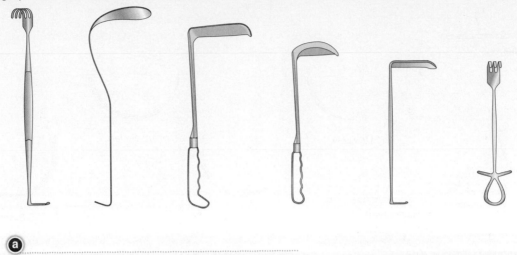

ⓐ ....

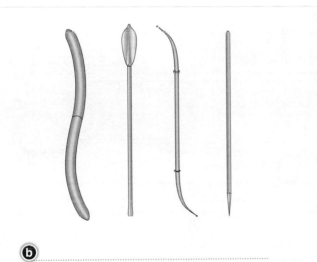

ⓑ ....

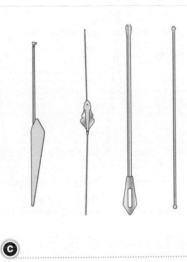

ⓒ ....

27. The following illustration shows a variety of instruments and materials used to suture. Write the names of the instruments on the lines provided. Then explain the instruments' use.

Needles

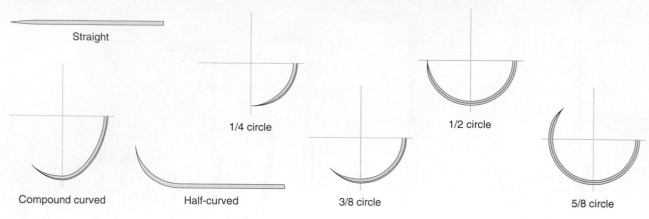

Straight

1/4 circle

1/2 circle

Compound curved

Half-curved

3/8 circle

5/8 circle

a ....

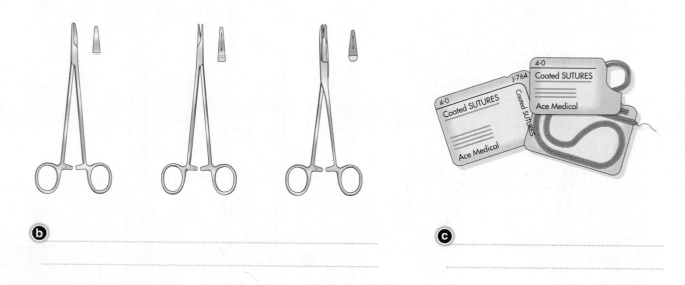

b ....
....
....

c ....
....
....

28. What are some potential side effects of local anesthetics?

_____

_____

_____

29. Instruments in a surgical tray should be arranged in the order in which they will be used. The following instruments are listed in random order. On the lines provided, rewrite the names of the instruments in the order the surgeon is *most likely* to use them.

Probes _____

Cutting instruments _____

Needle holders _____

Grasping instruments _____

Suture materials _____

Retractors _____

30. Why is epinephrine not used in areas such as the fingers, toes, or nose?

_____

_____

_____

31. Why is it important to place biopsy specimens in a formalin solution?

_____

_____

_____

32. Describe how a nonsurgical wound should be cleaned.

_____

_____

_____

Critical Thinking

Write the answer to each question on the lines provided.

1. While opening a sterile surgical instrument pack, you notice that the sterilization indicator has not been exposed. What should you do?

_____

_____

2. Following cryosurgery, a large, bloody, and painful blister often forms. Why is it important to avoid rupturing the blister?

_____

_____

3. Why is a sterile field considered contaminated if you turn your back to the field?

_____

_____

4. How does positioning the Mayo stand above waist height help prevent contamination?

_____

_____

_____

5. How can you avoid contaminating a sterile field when pouring liquids into a container on the field?

_____

_____

_____

6. How will you ease the fears of a patient who is about to have a minor surgical procedure?

_____

_____

_____

7. Describe how you should prepare the patient's skin before surgery.

_____

_____

_____

8. What should you do with a curette that a coworker says has "probably been sterilized"?

_____

_____

_____

9. Would you use transfer forceps during a procedure if you were wearing sterile gloves to handle instruments in a sterile field? Explain.

_____

_____

_____

A P P L I C A T I O N   WORK // DOC

Follow the directions for each application.

1. Interviewing Patients with Wounds

Work with two partners. One partner should assume the role of a patient with a wound. The second should play the role of a medical assistant, and the third should act as an observer and evaluator. Assume the wound is an infected laceration.

a. The medical assistant should take a history, noting his or her questions and the patient's responses. On the basis of the responses, the medical assistant should ask appropriate follow-up questions.

b. The medical assistant should explain to the patient what the doctor is likely to do and why, allowing the patient to interrupt with questions, which the assistant should answer to the best of his or her ability. Again, the medical assistant should note his or her statements, the patient's questions, and her responses.

c. Have the observer present a critique of what the medical assistant has done. The critique should involve the assistant's attitude, or approach, as well as the appropriateness and accuracy of his or her questions and responses.

d. The three of you should then discuss the observer's critique, noting the strengths and weaknesses of the interview.

e. Exchange roles and repeat with a patient who has an appointment for another minor surgical procedure. The new observer should choose the procedure.

f. Exchange roles one final time so that each member of the team gets to play medical assistant, patient, and observer once.

2. **Surgical Skin Preparation**

You must prepare a patient's skin prior to any surgical procedure. This reduces the number of microorganisms and the risk of infection. Working with two partners, practice preparing a patient's skin prior to surgery. One student should act as the patient, and one should observe and critique your performance.

a. Clean the area first with antiseptic soap and sterile water, using forceps and gauze sponges dipped in solution. Begin at the center of the site and work outward in a firm, circular motion. Discard the gauze sponge after each complete pass. Clean in concentric circles until you cover the full preparation area. Continue the process, repeating as necessary, for at least 2 minutes or the amount of time specified in the office's procedure manual. Cleaning takes more time if a wound is dirty or contains foreign materials. When procedures are performed on a hand or foot, clean the entire hand or foot.

b. Consider whether hair should be removed from the area and comment on the procedure used to remove the hair. *Do not remove the hair during this simulation.*

c. Apply antiseptic solution to the area. Swab an area 2 inches larger than the surgical field with the antiseptic solution in a circular outward motion, starting at the surgical site. For surgery on a hand or foot, swab the entire hand or foot. Allow the antiseptic to air-dry; do not pat it dry—that would remove some of the solution's antiseptic properties.

d. Cover the area with a sterile fenestrated drape, from front to back. Avoid reaching over the field. At this point, notify the physician that the patient is ready.

C A S E   S T U D I E S

Write your response to each case study on the lines provided.

Case 1

You are called away from the room while setting up a sterile surgical tray. What should you do?

_____

_____

_____

Case 2

A patient arrives at the office with a deep wound across the elbow. What type of suture should you make sure is at hand? Why?

_____

_____

_____

Case 3

You have just completed a surgical scrub and you are now donning sterile gloves. When lifting up the second glove, you think it touches the outer 1-inch margin of the sterile glove wrapper. What should you do?

_____

_____

_____

Case 4

Why is it important to use sterile solutions when irrigating a nonsurgical wound?

_____

_____

_____

Case 5

You are assisting the doctor during a minor surgical procedure. You are wearing sterile gloves and handling sterile items directly. The doctor knocks an instrument to the floor and needs a replacement. The instruments are in a supply cabinet next to you. What should you do?

_____

_____

_____

Name_____ Date_____

Evaluated by_____ Score_____

PROCEDURE 44-1 Creating a Sterile Field

Goal
To create a sterile field for a minor surgical procedure.

OSHA Guidelines
This procedure does not involve exposure to blood, body fluids, or tissues.

Materials
Tray or Mayo stand, sterile instrument pack, sterile transfer forceps, cleaning solution, sterile drape, and additional packaged sterile items as required.

Method

Step Number	Procedure	Points Possible	Points Earned
1.	Clean and disinfect the tray or Mayo stand.	5	
2.	Wash your hands and assemble the necessary materials.	5	
3.	Check the label on the instrument pack to make sure it is the correct pack for the procedure.*	10	
4.	Check the date and sterilization indicator on the instrument pack to make sure the pack is still sterile.*	15	
5.	Place the sterile pack on the tray or stand, and unfold the outermost fold away from yourself.	10	
6.	Unfold the sides of the pack outward, touching only the areas that will become the underside of the sterile field.	10	
7.	Open the final flap toward yourself, stepping back and away from the sterile field.	10	
8.	Place additional packaged sterile items on the sterile field.* • Ensure that you have the correct item or instrument and that the package is still sterile. • Stand away from the sterile field. • Grasp the package flaps and pull apart about halfway. • Bring the corners of the wrapping beneath the package, paying attention not to contaminate the inner package or item. • Hold the package over the sterile field with the opening down; with a quick movement, pull the flap completely open and snap the sterile item onto the field.	15	
9.	Place basins and bowls near the edge of the sterile field so you can pour liquids without reaching over the field.	10	
10.	Use sterile transfer forceps if necessary to add additional items to the sterile field.	5	
11.	If necessary, don sterile gloves after a sterile scrub to arrange items on the sterile field.	5	
Total Points		100	

CAAHEP Competencies Achieved

III. P (6)   Perform sterilization procedures

ABHES Competencies Achieved

9. (p) Perform sterilization techniques

PROCEDURE 44-2 Performing a Surgical Scrub

Goal
To remove dirt and microorganisms from under the fingernails and from the surface of the skin, hair follicles, and oil glands of the hands and forearms.

OSHA Guidelines
This procedure does not involve exposure to blood, body fluids, or tissues.

Materials
Dispenser with surgical soap, sterile surgical scrub brush or sponge, and sterile towels.

Method

Step Number	Procedure	Points Possible	Points Earned
1.	Remove all jewelry and roll up your sleeves to above the elbow.	5	
2.	Assemble the necessary materials.	5	
3.	Turn on the faucet using the foot or knee pedal.	5	
4.	Wet your hands from fingertips to elbows, keeping your hands higher than your elbows.*	15	
5.	Under running water, use a sterile brush to clean under your fingernails."	15	
6.	Apply surgical soap, and scrub your hands, fingers, areas between the fingers, wrists, and forearms with the scrub sponge, using a firm circular motion. Follow the manufacturer's recommendations to determine appropriate length of time (usually 2 to 6 minutes).*	15	
7.	Rinse from fingers to elbows, always keeping your hands higher than your elbows.*	15	
8.	Thoroughly dry your hands and forearms with sterile towels, working from the hands to the elbows.*	15	
9.	Turn off the faucet with the foot or knee pedal. Use a sterile paper towel if a foot or knee pedal is not available.*	10	
Total Points		100	

CAAHEP Competencies Achieved
III. P (6)   Perform sterilization procedures

ABHES Competencies Achieved
9. (b) Apply principles of aseptic techniques and infection control

9. (o) 4. Perform sterilization techniques

PROCEDURE 44-3 Donning Sterile Gloves

Goal
To don sterile gloves without compromising the sterility of the gloves' outer surface.

OSHA Guidelines
This procedure does not involve exposure to blood, body fluids, or tissues.

Materials
Correctly sized, prepackaged, double-wrapped sterile gloves.

Method

Step Number	Procedure	Points Possible	Points Earned
1.	Obtain the correct size gloves.	4	
2.	Check the package for tears, and ensure that the expiration date has not passed.*	7	
3.	Perform a surgical scrub.	4	
4.	Peel the outer wrap from gloves, and place the inner wrapper on a clean surface above waist level.	4	
5.	Position gloves so the cuff end is closest to your body.	4	
6.	Touch only the flaps as you open the package.*	7	
7.	Use instructions provided on the inner package, if available.	4	
8.	Do not reach over the sterile inside of the inner package.	4	
9.	Follow these steps if there are no instructions:* **a.** Open the package so the first flap is opened away from you. **b.** Pinch the corner and pull to one side. **c.** Put your fingertips under the side flaps and gently pull until the package is completely open.	7	
10.	Use your nondominant hand to grasp the inside cuff of the opposite glove (the folded edge). Do not touch the outside of the glove. If you are right-handed, use your left hand to put on the right glove first, and vice versa.	4	
11.	Holding the glove at arm's length and waist level, insert the dominant hand into the glove, palm facing up. Do not let the outside of the glove touch any other surface.*	7	
12.	With your sterile gloved hand, slip the gloved fingers into the cuff of the other glove.	4	
13.	Pick up the other glove, touching only the outside. Do not touch any other surfaces.*	7	
14.	Pull the glove up and onto your hand, ensuring the sterile gloved hand does not touch your skin.*	7	
15.	Adjust your fingers as necessary, touching only glove to glove.	4	
16.	Do not adjust the cuffs because your forearms may contaminate the gloves.	4	
17.	Keep your hands in front of you, between your shoulders and waist. If you move your hands out of this area, they are considered contaminated.*	7	
18.	If contamination or the possibility of contamination occurs, change gloves.*	7	

(continued)

Step Number	Procedure	Points Possible	Points Earned
19.	Remove these gloves the same way you remove clean gloves, by touching only the inside.	4	
Total Points		100	

CAAHEP Competencies Achieved

III. P (3)   Select appropriate barrier/personal protective equipment (PPE) for potentially infectious situations

ABHES Competencies Achieved

9. (b) Apply principles of aseptic techniques and infection control

PROCEDURE 44-4 Wrapping and Labeling Instruments for Sterilization in the Autoclave

Goal
To enclose instruments and equipment to be sterilized in appropriate wrapping materials to ensure sterilization and to protect supplies from contamination after sterilization.

OSHA Guidelines

Materials
Dry, sanitized, and disinfected instruments and equipment; wrapping material (paper, muslin, gauze, bags, envelopes); sterilization indicators; autoclave tape; labels (if wrapping does not include space for labeling); and a waterproof pen.

Method

Step Number	Procedure	Points Possible	Points Earned
For Wrapping Instruments or Equipment in Pieces of Paper or Fabric			
1.	Wash your hands and don gloves before beginning to wrap the items to be sterilized.	5	
2.	Place a square of paper or muslin on the table with one point toward you. With muslin, use a double thickness. Ensure that the paper or fabric must be large enough to allow all four points to cover the instruments or equipment you will be wrapping and provide an overlap, which will be used as a handling flap.*	15	
3.	Place each item to be included in the pack in the center area of the paper or fabric "diamond." Items that will be used together should be wrapped together. Make sure, however, that surfaces of the items do not touch each other inside the pack so that steam can penetrate every surface of all instruments in the pack. Inspect each item to ensure it is operating correctly. Place hinged instruments in the pack in the open position. Wrap a small piece of paper, muslin, or gauze around delicate edges or points to protect against damage to other instruments or to the pack wrapping.*	15	
4	Place a sterilization indicator inside the pack with the instruments. Position the indicator correctly, following the manufacturer's guidelines.*	15	
5.	Fold the bottom point of the diamond up and over the instruments in to the center. Fold back a small portion of the point.	5	
6.	Fold the right point of the diamond in to the center. Again, fold back a small portion of the point to be used as a handle.	5	
7.	Fold the left point of the diamond in to the center, folding back a small portion to form a handle. The pack should now resemble an open envelope.	5	
8.	Grasp the covered instruments (the bottom of the envelope) and fold this portion up, toward the top point. Fold the top point down over the pack, making sure the pack is snug but not too tight.	5	

(continued)

Step Number	Procedure	Points Possible	Points Earned
9.	Secure the pack with autoclave tape. A "quick-opening tab" can be created by folding a small portion of the tape back onto itself. The pack must be snug enough to prevent instruments from slipping out of the wrapping or damaging each other inside the pack, but loose enough to allow adequate steam circulation through the pack.	5	
10.	Label the pack with your initials and the date. Then list the contents of the pack. If the pack contains syringes, be sure to identify the syringe size(s).*	15	
11.	Place the pack aside for loading into the autoclave.	5	
12.	Remove gloves, dispose of them in the appropriate waste container, and wash your hands.	5	
Total Points		100	
For Wrapping Instruments and Equipment in Bags or Envelopes			
1.	Wash your hands and put on gloves before beginning to wrap the items to be sterilized.	10	
2.	Insert the items into the bag or envelope as indicated by the manufacturer's directions. Hinged instruments should be opened before insertion into the package.*	20	
3.	Close and seal the pack. Make sure the sterilization indicator is not damaged or already exposed.*	20	
4.	Label the pack with your initials and the date. Then list the contents of the pack. The pens or pencils used to label the pack must be waterproof; otherwise, the contents of the pack and date of sterilization will be obliterated.*	20	
5.	Place the pack aside for loading into the autoclave.	15	
6.	Remove gloves, dispose of them in the appropriate waste container, and wash your hands.	15	
Total Points		100	

CAAHEP Competencies Achieved

III. P (5)   Prepare items for autoclaving

III. P (6)   Perform sterilization procedures

ABHES Competencies Achieved

9. (h) Wrap items for autoclaving

9. (p) 4. Perform sterilization techniques

PROCEDURE 44-5 Running a Load through the Autoclave

Goal
To run a load of instruments and equipment through an autoclave, ensuring sterilization of items by properly loading, drying, and unloading them.

OSHA Guidelines

Materials
Dry, sanitized, and disinfected instruments and equipment, both individual pieces and wrapped packs; oven mitts; sterile transfer forceps; and storage containers for individual items.

Method

Step Number	Procedure	Points Possible	Points Earned
1.	Wash your hands and don gloves before beginning to load items into the autoclave.	5	
2.	Rest packs on their edges, and place jars and containers on their sides.	5	
3.	Place lids for jars and containers with their sterile sides down.	5	
4.	If the load includes plastic items, make sure no other item leans against them.	5	
5.	If your load is mixed—containing both wrapped packs and individual instruments—place the tray containing the instruments below the tray containing the wrapped packs.*	8	
6.	Close the door and start the unit. For automatic autoclaves, choose the cycle based on the type of load you are running. Consult the manufacturer's recommendations before choosing the load type.*	8	
7.	For manual autoclaves, start the timer when the indicators show the recommended temperature and pressure.	5	
8.	Right after the end of the steam cycle and just before the start of the drying cycle, open the door to the autoclave slightly (between ¼ and ½ inch).*	8	
9.	Dry according to the manufacturer's recommendations. Packs and large items may require up to 45 minutes for complete drying.	5	
10.	Unload the autoclave after the drying cycle is finished. Do not unload any packs or instruments with wet wrappings, or the objects inside will be considered unsterile and must be processed again.*	8	
11.	Unload each package carefully. Wear oven mitts to protect yourself from burns when removing wrapped packs. Use sterile transfer forceps to unload unwrapped individual objects.	5	
12.	Inspect each package or item, looking for moisture on the wrapping, underexposed sterilization indicators, and tears or breaks in the wrapping. Consider the pack unsterile if any of these conditions is present.*	8	
13.	Place sterile packs aside for transfer to storage.	5	
14.	Place individual items that are not required to be sterile in clean containers.	5	

(continued)

Step Number	Procedure	Points Possible	Points Earned
15.	Place items that must remain sterile in sterile containers; close container covers tightly.	5	
16.	As you unload items, avoid placing them in an overly cool location; the cool temperature could cause condensation on the instruments or packs.	5	
17.	Remove gloves, dispose of them in the appropriate waste container, and wash your hands.	5	
Total Points		100	

CAAHEP Competencies Achieved

III. P (5)   Prepare items for autoclaving

III. P (6)   Perform sterilization procedures

ABHES Competencies Achieved

9. (h) Wrap items for autoclaving

9. (n) Assist physician with minor office surgical procedures

9. (o) 4. Perform sterilization techniques

PROCEDURE 44-6 Assisting as a Floater (Unsterile Assistant) during Minor Surgical Procedures

Goal
To provide assistance to the doctor during minor surgery while maintaining clean or sterile technique as appropriate.

OSHA Guidelines

Materials
Sterile towel, tray or Mayo stand, appropriate instrument pack(s), needles and syringes, anesthetic, antiseptic, sterile water or normal saline, small sterile bowl, sterile gauze squares or cotton balls, specimen containers half-filled with preservative, suture materials, sterile dressings, and tape.

Method

Step Number	Procedure	Points Possible	Points Earned
1.	Perform routine handwashing and don exam gloves.	10	
2.	Monitor the patient during the procedure; record the results in the patient's chart.	10	
3.	During the surgery, assist as needed.*	20	
4.	Add sterile items to the tray as necessary.	10	
5.	Pour sterile solution into a sterile bowl as needed.	10	
6.	Assist in administering additional anesthetic.* a. Check the medication vial two times. b. Clean the rubber stopper with an alcohol pad (write the date opened when using a new bottle); leave pad on top. c. Present the needle and syringe to the doctor. d. Remove the alcohol pad from the vial, and show the label to the doctor. e. Hold the vial upside down, and grasp the lower edge firmly; brace your wrist with your free hand. f. Allow the doctor to fill the syringe. g. Check the medication vial a final time.	20	
7.	Receive specimens for laboratory examination.* a. Uncap the specimen container; present it to the doctor for the specimen's introduction. b. Replace the cap and label the container. c. Treat all specimens as infectious. d. Place the specimen container in a transport bag or other container. e. Complete the requisition form to send the specimen to the laboratory.	20	
Total Points		100	

CAAHEP Competencies Achieved

    I. P (10)   Assist physician with patient care

    III. P (3)   Select appropriate barrier/personal protective equipment (PPE) for potentially infectious situations

ABHES Competencies Achieved

    9. (b) Apply principles of aseptic techniques and infection control

    9. (i) Prepare patient for examinations and treatments

    9. (n) Assist physician with minor office surgical procedures

PROCEDURE 44-7 Assisting as a Sterile Scrub Assistant during Minor Surgical Procedures

Goal
To provide assistance to the doctor during minor surgery while maintaining clean or sterile technique as appropriate.

OSHA Guidelines

Materials
Sterile towel, tray or Mayo stand, appropriate instrument pack(s), needles and syringes, anesthetic, antiseptic, sterile water or normal saline, small sterile bowl, sterile gauze squares or cotton balls, specimen containers half-filled with preservative, suture materials, sterile dressings, and tape.

Method

Step Number	Procedure	Points Possible	Points Earned
1.	Perform a surgical scrub and don sterile gloves. (Remember, remove the sterile towel covering the sterile field and instruments before gloving.)*	20	
2.	Close and arrange the surgical instruments on the tray.*	20	
3.	Prepare for swabbing by inserting gauze squares into the sterile dressing forceps.	12	
4.	Pass the instruments as necessary.	12	
5.	Swab the wound as requested.	12	
6.	Retract the wound as requested.	12	
7.	Cut the sutures as requested.	12	
Total Points		100	

CAAHEP Competencies Achieved

I. P (10)   Assist physician with patient care

III. P (3)   Select appropriate barrier/personal protective equipment (PPE) for potentially infectious situations

ABHES Competencies Achieved

9. (b) Apply principles of aseptic techniques and infection control

9. (i) Prepare patient for examinations and treatments

9. (n) Assist physician with minor office surgical procedures

PROCEDURE 44-8 Assisting after Minor Surgical Procedures

Goal
To provide assistance to the doctor during minor surgery while maintaining clean or sterile technique as appropriate.

OSHA Guidelines

Materials
Examination gloves, antiseptic, tray or Mayo stand, sterile dressings, and tape.

Method

Step Number	Procedure	Points Possible	Points Earned
1.	Monitor the patient.*	20	
2.	Don clean exam gloves, and clean the wound with antiseptic.	5	
3.	Dress the wound.*	20	
4.	Remove the gloves and wash your hands.	5	
5.	Give the patient oral postoperative instructions in addition to the release packet.*	20	
6.	Discharge the patient.	5	
7.	Put on clean exam gloves.	5	
8.	Properly dispose of used materials and disposable instruments.	5	
9.	Sanitize reusable instruments and prepare them for disinfection and/or sterilization as needed.	5	
10.	Clean equipment and the exam room according to OSHA guidelines.	5	
11.	Remove the gloves and wash your hands.	5	
Total Points		100	

CAAHEP Competencies Achieved

I. P (10)   Assist physician with patient care

III. P (3)   Select appropriate barrier/personal protective equipment (PPE) for potentially infectious situations

ABHES Competencies Achieved

9. (b) Apply principles of aseptic techniques and infection control

9. (n) Assist physician with minor office surgical procedures

PROCEDURE 44-9 Suture Removal

⟨ **WORK // DOC** ⟩

Goal

To remove sutures from a healing wound while maintaining sterile technique and protecting the integrity of the closed wound.

OSHA Guidelines

Materials

Tray or Mayo stand, suture removal pack (suture scissors and thumb forceps), sterile towel, antiseptic solution, hydrogen peroxide (3%), two small sterile bowls, sterile gauze squares, sterile strips or butterfly closures, sterile dressings, and tape.

Method

Step Number	Procedure	Points Possible	Points Earned
1.	Clean and disinfect the tray or Mayo stand.	2	
2.	Wash your hands and assemble the necessary materials.	2	
3.	Check the date and sterilization indicator on the suture removal pack.*	5	
4.	Unwrap the suture removal pack; place it on the tray or stand to create a sterile field.*	5	
5.	Unwrap the sterile bowls; add them to the sterile field.	2	
6.	Pour a small amount of antiseptic solution into one bowl, and a small amount of hydrogen peroxide into the other bowl.	2	
7.	Cover the tray with a sterile towel to protect the sterile field while you are out of the room.	2	
8.	Escort the patient to the exam room and explain the procedure.	2	
9.	Perform a routine hand wash, remove the towel from the tray, and don exam gloves.	2	
10.	Remove the old dressing.* a. Lift the tape toward the middle of the dressing to avoid pulling on the wound. b. If the dressing adheres to the wound, cover the dressing with gauze squares soaked in hydrogen peroxide. Leave the wet gauze in place for several seconds to loosen the dressing. c. Save the old dressing for the doctor to inspect.	5	
11.	Inspect the wound for signs of infection.	2	
12.	Clean the wound with gauze pads soaked in antiseptic; pat it dry with clean gauze pads.*	5	

(continued)

Step Number	Procedure	Points Possible	Points Earned
13.	Remove the gloves and wash your hands.	2	
14.	Notify the doctor that the wound is ready for examination.*	5	
15.	Once the doctor indicates the wound is sufficiently healed to proceed, don clean exam gloves.	2	
16.	Place a square of gauze next to the wound for collecting the sutures as they are removed.	2	
17.	Grasp the first suture knot with forceps.	2	
18.	Gently lift the knot away from the skin to allow room for the suture scissors.	2	
19.	Slide the suture scissors under the suture material, and cut the suture where it enters the skin.*	5	
20.	Gently lift the knot up and toward the wound to remove the suture without opening the wound.	2	
21.	Place the suture on the gauze pad; inspect to ensure the entire suture is present.*	5	
22.	Repeat the removal process until all sutures have been removed.	2	
23.	Count the sutures and compare the number with that indicated in the patient's record.*	5	
24.	Clean the wound with antiseptic; allow it to air-dry.*	5	
25.	Dress the wound as ordered, or notify the doctor if sterile strips or butterfly closures are to be applied.*	5	
26.	Observe the patient for signs of distress, like wincing or grimacing.	2	
27.	Properly dispose of used materials and disposable instruments.	2	
28.	Remove the gloves and wash your hands.	2	
29.	Instruct the patient on wound care.	2	
30.	In the patient's chart, record pertinent information, like the condition of the wound and the type of closures used, if any.	2	
31.	Escort the patient to the checkout area.	2	
32.	Don clean gloves.	2	
33.	Sanitize reusable instruments; prepare them for disinfection and/or sterilization as needed.	2	
34.	Clean the equipment and exam room according to OSHA guidelines.	2	
35.	Remove the gloves and wash your hands.	2	
Total Points		100	

CAAHEP Competencies Achieved

I. P (10) Assist physician with patient care

III. P (3) Select appropriate barrier/personal protective equipment (PPE) for potentially infectious situations

ABHES Competencies Achieved

9. (b) Apply principles of aseptic techniques and infection control

9. (h) Prepare patient for examinations and treatments

45

Orientation to the Lab

Name_____ Class_____ Date_____

R E V I E W

Vocabulary Review

Passage Completion

Study the key terms in the box. Use your textbook to find definitions of terms you do not understand.

centrifuge	optical microscope	quality assurance program
Certificate of Waiver tests	physician's office laboratory (POL)	reference laboratory
focus controls		

In the space provided, complete the following passage, using some of the terms from the box. You may change the form of a term to fit the meaning of the sentence.

Laboratory analysis plays an important role in any medical practice. Some physicians have all laboratory tests performed by a(n) (1)_____, which is owned and operated by an organization outside the practice. Other physicians do some laboratory work in the office, in the (2)_____. This allows quick turnaround of test results.

One piece of equipment used in the laboratory is a(n) (3)_____, which spins a specimen at high speed until it separates into its component parts. The laboratory equipment that is used most often in the POL, however, is the (4)_____. There are two (5)_____ on the optical microscope, coarse and fine.

A(n) (6)_____ is designed to monitor the quality of patient care that a medical laboratory provides. A laboratory can gain exemption from meeting certain federal standards if it performs only (7)_____.

1. _____
2. _____
3. _____
4. _____
5. _____
6. _____
7. _____

Matching

Match the key terms in the right column with the definitions in the left column by placing the letter of each correct answer in the space provided.

_____ 8. A foreign object visible through a microscope but unrelated to the specimen

_____ 9. A magnifying lens mounted on the nosepiece of a microscope

_____ 10. Something that measures the accuracy of test results and adherence to standard operating procedures

_____ 11. A laboratory owned and operated by an organization outside the practice

_____ 12. A device that spins a specimen at high speed until it separates into its component parts

_____ 13. A specimen with a known value that is used every time a patient sample is processed

_____ 14. The eyepiece of a microscope through which an image is viewed

_____ 15. A specimen with a known value that is used during calibration

_____ 16. A document that shows all procedures completed during the workday

_____ 17. Something that ensures accuracy in test results through careful monitoring of test procedures

a. proficiency testing program
b. centrifuge
c. artifact
d. reference laboratory
e. objective
f. standard
g. daily workload log
h. quality control program
i. control sample
j. ocular

True or False

Decide whether each statement is true or false. In the space at the left, write T for true or F for false. On the lines provided, rewrite the false statements to make them true.

_____ **18.** The objectives of the microscope are the eyepieces through which you view the image.

_____

_____ **19.** Placing the end of the oil-immersion objective in oil reduces the loss of light and produces a much sharper, brighter image.

_____

_____ **20.** The Supreme Court enacted the Clinical Laboratory Improvement Amendments of 1988, which established federal regulations for laboratories.

_____

_____ **21.** A hemocytometer is a slide that is calibrated to the exact measurements needed to count blood cells and sperm under a microscope.

_____

_____ **22.** Generally, positive and negative control samples are used with tests that yield a qualitative test response.

_____

Content Review

Multiple Choice

In the space provided, write the letter of the choice that best completes each statement or answers each question.

_____ **1.** Objectives are mounted on a swivel base called the
  a. Condenser
  b. Objective
  c. Stage
  d. Lens
  e. Nosepiece

_____ **2.** Chemicals or chemically treated substances used in testing procedures are known as
  a. Controls
  b. Standards
  c. Reagents
  d. Pipettes
  e. Objectives

_____ **3.** A specimen with a known value that is used to calibrate equipment is a
  a. Neutral reagent
  b. Standard
  c. Photometer
  d. Buffer
  e. Absolute

_____ 4. Which of the following is an instrument that measures light intensity?

    a. Artifact

    b. Hemocytometer

    c. Thermometer

    d. Photometer

    e. Pipette

_____ 5. Tests that measure the amount or concentration of a specific substance are known as

    a. Quantitative test results

    b. Moderate-complexity tests

    c. Reagent control tests

    d. Quality control tests

    e. Qualitative test results

Sentence Completion

In the space provided, write the word or phrase that best completes each sentence.

6. The iris of a microscope is used to _____ the amount of light illuminating the specimen.

7. When not in use, the microscope should be stored _____.

8. When transferring a blood specimen from a collection tube to another container, you should wear gloves and _____.

9. Using excessive lens cleaning products on the microscope lenses may loosen the lens by _____ the cement.

10. Tests that have been approved by the Food and Drug Administration (FDA) for use by patients at home are _____ tests.

11. CLIA '88 requires _____ _____ _____, which measure test result accuracy and adherence to standard operating procedures.

12. Specimens sent to another laboratory for testing should be recorded in the _____ _____ _____.

13. In a microscope, the _____ controls the amount of light on the specimen by opening and closing like a shutter.

14. Graduated flasks are used to measure large amounts of _____.

15. Treating patients with respect is part of the medical assistant's _____ skills.

6. _____

7. _____

8. _____

9. _____

10. _____

11. _____
_____
_____
_____

12. _____
_____
_____

13. _____

14. _____

15. _____

Short Answer
Write the answer to each question on the lines provided.

16. What three types of information does laboratory analysis of blood, urine, or other body fluids or substances provide about a patient?

_____

_____

_____

17. What record shows all procedures completed during the workday?

_____

_____

_____

18. As a medical assistant, what might your role be in the POL?

_____

_____

_____

19. Describe five steps you would take when troubleshooting equipment.

_____

_____

_____

20. Describe five steps you would take when troubleshooting a test kit.

_____

_____

_____

21. Describe the differences in a control sample and a standard.

_____

_____

_____

22. How are Certificate of Waiver tests defined? Give examples.

_____

_____

_____

23. Describe the records that must be kept as part of a quality control program in addition to the quality control log, the reagent control log, and the equipment maintenance log.

_____

_____

_____

24. Describe five laboratory housekeeping guidelines that must be taken to reduce the risk of infection and ensure good operating procedures.

_____

_____

_____

25. The following illustration shows the parts of a microscope. Write the name of each part on the line provided.

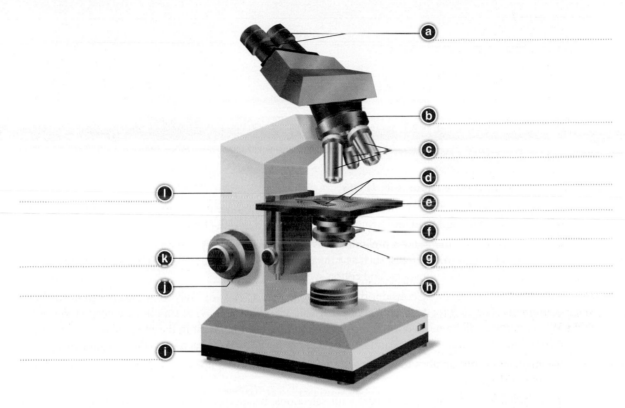

Critical Thinking
Write the answer to each question on the lines provided.

1. Why is it important to use a systematic approach when troubleshooting equipment problems?

_____

_____

_____

2. Why is it important to report an exposure incident even though you know the patient's HIV status is negative?

_____

_____

_____

3. Why should you change gloves every time you move from patient to patient when collecting specimens for testing?

_____

_____

_____

4. Why do you think mouth pipetting is prohibited at all times?

_____

_____

_____

5. Explain the meaning of the motto "If it is not written down, it was not done."

_____

_____

_____

A P P L I C A T I O N

Follow the directions for each application.

1. Equipping a Physician's Office Laboratory (POL)

Work with two partners. You are part of a team that is buying equipment for a new POL. Assume the POL will process routine tests involving blood and urine for a practice with two doctors.

a. You and your partners should make a preliminary list of all the laboratory equipment and supplies you think will be needed. Start with major items, such as a microscope. Then consider all the necessary support materials, such as coverslips, test tubes, dipsticks, and cotton swabs.

b. As you work with your partners, consider these questions: What tests are likely to be performed in the POL? What equipment is needed for each type of test that will be performed? What supplies are needed to run a POL? What supplies will be needed to care for and maintain the equipment in the POL? Make a list of all the possible tests the POL might perform and add the equipment needed for each procedure to your list.

c. Next, use medical supply catalogs to help you choose the laboratory equipment and supplies you would recommend for the POL.

d. Start an equipment inventory log and record your selections. Be specific about the type of equipment. Record model numbers, prices, and amounts. Use medical abbreviations as appropriate. Include illustrations as necessary.

e. Share your inventory log with another team and be prepared to justify your selections. Compare selections, prices, and amounts. Discuss items that are on one team's list but not the other. Check for completeness.

f. Then share your log with a different team.

g. On the basis of classmates' feedback, revise your inventory log to make it as complete as possible.

2. Setting Up a Microscope

The physician has asked you to set up the microscope so that she can do a wetprep examination. List the equipment and supplies you will need and how each is used.

3. Using a Microscope

Bring some items from home that you think would be interesting to view under the microscope. (Suggested items: newsprint, a feather, threads, dog or cat hair, sugar crystals.) Place each item under the microscope and view them using 10X and 40X objectives. Make drawings of each item under both magnifications. Write your observations about the materials underneath each drawing.

C A S E   S T U D I E S

Write your response to each case study on the lines provided.

Case 1

Your office is planning to close the POL and send all tests to a reference laboratory. The doctors say that the complexity and expense of meeting federal regulations is forcing them to take this action. In the past, your office has performed urinalyses, pregnancy tests, and blood glucose tests. Instead of closing the POL, what other option is available?

_____

_____

_____

Case 2

You have been put in charge of the care and maintenance of the microscope in the POL. Describe the procedure you would follow at the end of the workday.

_____

_____

_____

Case 3

You have been asked to train new laboratory personnel in the housekeeping duties essential in your lab. What information should you give new employees?

_____

_____

_____

Case 4

You are a medical assistant in a physician's office laboratory that performs Level II tests. Your employer has asked for your help in designing a quality assurance program. Describe the components the program must include.

_____

_____

_____

Case 5

A patient has arrived in the office for a scheduled blood test. Describe how you will communicate with her before, during, and after the test.

_____

_____

_____

Case 6

You are the supervisor in the POL at your medical office. You have a new employee starting in the lab this week. What information will you give this new employee regarding the subjects he or she will need to master in his or her role in the POL?

_____

_____

_____

PROCEDURE 45-1 Using a Microscope

Goal
To correctly focus the microscope using each of the three objectives for examination of a prepared specimen slide.

OSHA Guidelines

Materials
Microscope, lens paper, lens cleaner, prepared specimen slide, immersion oil, and tissues.

Method

Step Number	Procedure	Points Possible	Points Earned
1.	Wash your hands and don exam gloves.	3	
2.	Remove the protective cover from the microscope. Examine the microscope to make sure it is clean and that all parts are intact.	3	
3.	Plug in the microscope and make sure the light is working. If you need to replace the bulb, refer to the manufacturer's guidelines. Note bulb replacements in the microscope maintenance log. Turn the light off before cleaning the lenses.*	5	
4.	Clean the lenses and oculars with lens paper. Avoid touching the lenses with anything except lens paper. If a lens is particularly dirty, use a small amount of lens cleaner.	3	
5.	Place the specimen slide on the stage. Slide the edges of the slide under the slide clips to secure the slide to the stage.	3	
6.	Adjust the distance between the oculars to a position of comfort.	3	
7.	Adjust the objectives so the low-power (10X) objective points directly at the specimen slide. Before swiveling the objective assembly, be sure you have sufficient space for the objective. Recheck the distance between the oculars, making sure the field you see through the eyepieces is a merged field, not separate left and right fields. Raise the body tube by using the coarse adjustment control, and lower the stage as needed.*	5	
8.	Turn on the light and, using the iris controls, adjust the amount of light illuminating the specimen so the light fills the field but does not wash out the image.	3	
9.	Observe the microscope from one side, and slowly lower the body tube to move the objective closer to the stage and specimen slide, taking care not to strike the stage with the objective.*	5	
10.	Look through the oculars and use the coarse focus control to slowly adjust the image. If necessary, adjust the amount of light coming through the iris.*	5	
11.	Continue using the fine focus control to adjust the image.*	5	
12.	Switch to the high-power (40X) objective. Use the fine focus controls to view the specimen clearly.*	5	
13.	Rotate the objective assembly so that no objective points directly at the stage and specimen slide.	3	
14.	Apply a small drop of immersion oil to the specimen slide.*	5	

(continued)

Step Number	Procedure	Points Possible	Points Earned
15.	Gently swing the oil-immersion (100X) objective over the stage and specimen slide so it is surrounded by the immersion oil.	4	
16.	Examine the image and adjust the amount of light and focus as needed. Only use the fine focus adjustment with this objective. To eliminate air bubbles in the immersion oil, gently move the stage left and right.*	5	
17.	After you have examined the specimen as required by the testing procedure, lower the stage and raise the objectives.	3	
18.	Remove the slide. Dispose of it or store it as required by the testing procedure. If you must dispose of the slide, be sure to use the appropriate biohazardous waste container. If you must store the slide, remove the immersion oil with a tissue.*	5	
19.	Turn off the light. Unplug the microscope if that is your laboratory's standard operating procedure.	3	
20.	Clean the microscope stage, ocular lenses, and objectives. Be careful to remove all traces of immersion oil from the stage and oil-immersion objective. Clean the oil immersion lens last.*	5	
21.	Rotate the objective assembly so the low-power objective points toward the stage. Lower the objective so it comes close to but does not rest on the stage.	3	
22.	Cover the microscope with its protective cover. Check the work area to be sure you have cleaned everything correctly and disposed of all waste material.	3	
23.	Remove the gloves and wash your hands.	3	
Total Points		100	

CAAHEP Competencies Achieved

III. P (2)   Practice Standard Precautions

ABHES Competencies Achieved

9. (b) Apply principles of aseptic techniques and infection control

9. (i) Use standard precautions

10. (c) Dispose of Biohazardous materials

46

Microbiology and Disease

Name_____ Class_____ Date_____

R E V I E W

Vocabulary Review

Matching

Match the key terms in the right column with the definitions in the left column by placing the letter of each correct answer in the space provided.

_____ 1. An agent that kills or suppresses the growth of a microorganism

_____ 2. An organism that lives on or in another organism and that uses that other organism for its own nourishment or some other advantage, to the detriment of the host organism

_____ 3. A single-celled eukaryotic organism, generally much larger than bacteria and found in soil and water

_____ 4. A substance that contains all the nutrients a particular type of microorganism needs

_____ 5. A distinct group of organisms found on a culture plate

_____ 6. The result of a Gram stain in which the bacteria lose the purple color and pick up the red color of the safranin

_____ 7. A specimen spread thinly and evenly across a slide

_____ 8. Bacteria that appear blue after the Gram stain procedure

_____ 9. A procedure that involves culturing a specimen and then testing the isolated bacterium's susceptibility to certain antibiotics

_____ 10. A gelatin-like substance derived from seaweed that gives a medium its consistency

_____ 11. A preparation of a specimen in a liquid that allows organisms to remain alive and mobile while they are examined under a microscope

_____ 12. Fungi that grow mainly as single-celled organisms and reproduce by budding

_____ 13. A eukaryotic organism that has a rigid cell wall at some stage in the life cycle

_____ 14. A comma-shaped bacterium

_____ 15. A staining procedure for identifying bacteria that have a waxy cell wall

_____ 16. A solution of a dye or group of dyes that imparts a color to microorganisms

_____ 17. A spiral-shaped bacterium

_____ 18. A spherical, round, or ovoid bacterium

a. antimicrobial
b. coccus
c. acid-fast stain
d. yeast
e. spirillum
f. parasite
g. agar
h. vibrio
i. fungus
j. culture and sensitivity (C&S)
k. protozoan
l. colony
m. Gram-negative
n. smear
o. stain
p. wet mount
q. culture medium
r. Gram-positive

True or False

Decide whether each statement is true or false. In the space at the left, write T *for true or* F *for false. On the lines provided, rewrite the false statements to make them true.*

_____ **19.** Viruses are large, prokaryotic organisms.

_____

_____ **20.** Keratin is a tough, hard protein.

_____

_____ **21.** Eukaryotic microorganisms have a simple cell structure with no nucleus and no organelles in the cytoplasm.

_____

_____ **22.** Gonorrhea is a sexually transmitted infection caused by a Gram-negative, rod-shaped bacterium.

_____

_____ **23.** Gram stain is used to differentiate bacteria according to the chemical composition of their cell walls.

_____

_____ **24.** Aerobes are bacteria that grow best in the presence of oxygen.

_____

_____ **25.** Facultative organisms grow well whether oxygen is present or absent.

_____

_____ **26.** A protozoan is a multiple-celled eukaryotic organism that is generally smaller than a bacterium.

_____

_____ **27.** A mordant is a substance that can intensify or deepen the response of a specimen to a stain.

_____

_____ **28.** A parasite is an organism that lives on or in another organism and uses that other organism for its own nourishment.

_____

_____ **29.** Chlamydiae are bacteria that completely lack the rigid cell wall of other bacteria.

_____

_____ **30.** When performing a quantitative analysis of a urine specimen, mix the urine specimen well before taking the sample.

_____

_____ **31.** Trichinosis is an infection caused by *Trichinella spiralis*, a kind of virus.

_____

_____ **32.** An O&P specimen is a urine specimen that is examined for the presence of protozoans or parasites, including their eggs.

_____

_____ **33.** An etiologic agent is a living microorganism or its toxin that can cause human disease.

_____

_____ **34.** An ongoing system to evaluate the quality of medical care provided in a medical office is known as qualitative analysis.

_____

_____ **35.** A Gram stain result is referred to as Gram-positive when the bacteria appear red.

_____

Content Review

Multiple Choice

In the space provided, write the letter of the choice that best completes each statement or answers each question.

_____ **1.** A bacterium that grows best in the absence of oxygen is a(n)
   a. Protozoan
   b. Anaerobe
   c. Aerobe
   d. Vibrio
   e. Gram-positive

_____ **2.** A procedure to test a bacterium's susceptibility to certain antibiotics is
   a. A culture
   b. An antimicrobial
   c. A culture and sensitivity
   d. A qualitative analysis
   e. A quantitative analysis

_____ **3.** The label on a collection specimen container should include the patient's name and identification number, source of the specimen, doctor's name, your initials, and the
   a. Patient's insurance billing information
   b. Names of medications the patient is currently receiving
   c. Date and time of collection
   d. Doctor's presumptive diagnosis
   e. Doctor's DEA number

_____ **4.** A KOH mount is prepared with
   a. A 0.9% solution of sodium chloride
   b. A 10% solution of potassium hydroxide
   c. Iodine as a mordant
   d. Alcohol as a mordant
   e. Safranin as a stain

_____ **5.** A gelatin-like substance derived from seaweed that is used to give culture medium its consistency is known as
   a. Agar
   b. Smear
   c. Safranin
   d. Gentian violet
   e. Inoculum

Name_____ Class_____ Date_____

Sentence Completion

In the space provided, write the word or phrase that best completes each sentence.

6. Specific microorganisms are named with two words; the first word refers to the microorganism's _____, and the second word refers to its species.

7. Spherical, round, or ovoid bacteria are known as _____.

8. The medical term for head lice is _____.

9. To _____ a culture medium, you place a sample of a specimen in or on the medium.

10. Rod-shaped bacteria are known as _____.

11. A(n) _____ is an agent that kills microorganisms or suppresses their growth.

12. A _____ loop is a type of inoculating loop that measures a specific amount of fluid.

13. A fungus that grows mainly as a single-celled organism that reproduces by budding is referred to as a _____.

14. The most common type of culture medium used in the laboratory is _____, a nonselective medium.

15. Antimicrobial sensitivity tests are reported as sensitive (no growth), intermediate (little growth), or _____ (overgrown).

6. _____

7. _____

8. _____

9. _____

10. _____

11. _____

12. _____

13. _____

14. _____

15. _____

Short Answer

Write the answer to each question on the lines provided.

16. Clusters of cocci that appear Gram-positive typically suggest an infection with what microorganism?

_____

_____

_____

17. Compare and contrast prokaryotic and eukaryotic cells, and give examples of each.

_____

_____

_____

18. The four different bacterial shapes are shown here. On the lines provided, write the names of the bacteria that display these shapes.

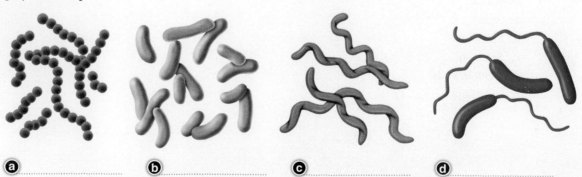

(a) _____ (b) _____ (c) _____ (d) _____

Copyright © 2014 by The McGraw-Hill Companies, Inc.

19. What are the six steps in diagnosing and treating an infection?

_____

_____

_____

_____

_____

20. Why is it important to process urine samples within 1 hour?

_____

_____

21. What are the three main objectives for collecting and transporting a microbiologic specimen to an outside laboratory?

_____

_____

_____

22. What is the procedure for preparing a KOH mount?

_____

_____

_____

23. Where should you label a culture plate? Why?

_____

_____

_____

24. Describe how you would prepare a microbiological specimen for transport by the U.S. Postal Service.

_____

_____

_____

25. What are the most common types of culture specimens?

_____

_____

_____

Critical Thinking

Write the answer to each question on the lines provided.

1. Why are cotton swabs no longer used for culture swabs?

_____

_____

_____

2. Why is it more difficult to grow and identify viruses than bacteria?

_____

_____

_____

3. Why is it important to follow the Gram staining procedure?

_____

_____

_____

4. Why is it important to develop an up-to-date laboratory procedures manual?

_____

_____

_____

5. Why are cultures collected from the human body usually incubated at 35° to 37°C?

_____

_____

_____

A P P L I C A T I O N

Follow the directions for the application.

Collecting a Specimen, Preparing a Specimen Smear, and Performing a Gram Stain

Working with a partner, you are to take a throat culture from him or her, prepare a smear of the specimen for staining, and perform a Gram stain. Your partner should serve as observer and evaluator.

a. Using a sterile swab, obtain a throat culture from your partner. Follow all safety precautions. Your partner should monitor the procedure while referring to Procedure 46-1 in the textbook and taking notes as needed for later discussion.

b. After you have obtained the specimen, prepare a specimen smear. Your partner should refer to the steps outlined in Procedure 46-3.

c. After you have prepared the smear, your partner should provide a critique of the procedure. Discuss any omissions or errors in the procedure.

d. Using the prepared smear, perform a Gram stain. Your partner should observe your technique while referring to Procedure 46-4 in the textbook and assess your performance on completion of the stain.

e. Exchange roles and allow your partner to collect a specimen, prepare a smear, and perform a Gram stain.

C A S E   S T U D I E S

Write your response to each case study on the lines provided.

Case 1

The doctor asks you to obtain a urine culture specimen from a patient. As you explain the procedure to the patient, he tells you that he is currently taking antibiotics that were prescribed by a doctor he visited for the same ailment while out of town on business. Should you have the patient collect the specimen? If not, what should you do?

_____

_____

_____

Case 2

You forgot to break the vial in the CULTURETTE before you sent it out to the lab. The lab rejected the specimen. Why?

_____

_____

_____

Case 3

While you are collecting a throat specimen, the patient gags and accidentally touches the swab with her tongue. What should you do? Why?

_____

_____

_____

Case 4

The physician takes scrapings from a patient's arm. He tells you he wants to perform a direct examination of the scrapings for the presence of fungus. What type of preparation should you do?

_____

_____

_____

PROCEDURE 46-1 Obtaining a Throat Culture Specimen

Goal
To isolate a pathogenic microorganism from the throat or to rule out strep throat.

OSHA Guidelines

Materials
Tongue depressor, sterile collection system, or sterile swab plus blood agar culture plate.

Method

Step Number	Procedure	Points Possible	Points Earned
1.	Identify the patient, introduce yourself, and explain the procedure.	5	
2.	Assemble the necessary supplies; label the culture plate if used.	5	
3.	Wash your hands and don examination gloves, goggles, and a mask or face shield.*	10	
4.	Have the patient assume a sitting position. (Having a small child lie down rather than sit may make the process easier. If the child refuses to open the mouth, gently squeeze the nostrils shut. The child will eventually open the mouth to breathe. Enlist the help of the parent to restrain the child's hands if necessary.)	5	
5.	Open the collection system or sterile swab package by peeling the wrapper halfway down; remove the swab with your dominant hand.	5	
6.	Ask the patient to tilt back her head and open her mouth as wide as possible.	5	
7.	With your other hand, depress the patient's tongue with the tongue depressor.	5	
8.	Ask the patient to say "Ah."	5	
9.	Insert the swab and quickly swab the back of the throat in the area of the tonsils, twirling the swab over representative areas on both sides of the throat. Avoid touching the uvula (the soft tissue hanging from the roof of the mouth), the cheeks, or the tongue.*	10	
10.	Remove the swab and then the tongue depressor from the patient's mouth.*	10	
11.	Discard the tongue depressor in a biohazardous waste container.	5	
To Transport the Specimen to a Reference Laboratory			
12.	Immediately insert the swab back into the plastic sleeve, being careful not to touch the outside of the sleeve with the swab.	5	
13.	Crush the vial of transport medium to moisten the tip of the swab.*	10	
14.	Label the collection system and arrange for transport to the laboratory.	5	
To Prepare the Specimen for Evaluation in the Physician's Office Laboratory		*or:*	
12.	Immediately inoculate the culture plate with the swab, using a back-and-forth motion.*	10	
13.	Discard the swab in a biohazardous waste container.	5	
14.	Place the culture plate in the incubator.	5	

(continued)

Step Number	Procedure	Points Possible	Points Earned
When Finished with All Specimens			
15.	Remove the gloves and wash your hands.	5	
16.	Document the procedure in the patient's chart.	5	
Total Points		100	

CAAHEP Competencies Achieved

III. P (7)   Obtain specimens for microbiological testing

III. P (8)   Perform CLIA-waived microbiology testing

ABHES Competencies Achieved

10. (b) Perform selected CLIA-waived tests that assist with diagnosis and treatment

5. Microbiology testing

10. (c) Dispose of Biohazardous materials

PROCEDURE 46-2 Performing a Quick Strep A Test on a Throat Swab Specimen

Goal
To determine the presence of Strep A antigen in a throat swab.

OSHA Guidelines

Materials
Strep A testing kit, throat swab specimen, and a timer or watch.

Method

Step Number	Procedure	Points Possible	Points Earned
1.	Review the laboratory requisition form and gather the supplies.*	10	
2.	Confirm the patient's identity, introduce yourself, and explain the procedure.	5	
3.	Wash your hands and don gloves, goggles, and a mask or face shield.	5	
4.	Open the Strep A testing kit and check the expiration date on the kit.	5	
5.	Obtain a throat specimen with a sterile swab, being careful not to touch the tongue, teeth, or cheeks.*	10	
6.	Complete the quality control tests provided with the testing kit.*	10	
7.	Put the required amount of the first reagent in the test tube or testing device provided in the kit.*	10	
8.	Place the swab into the test tube or testing device. Following the manufacturer's instructions, swirl the swab, and press it against the sides of the tube or device.*	10	
9.	Add the second reagent as directed.*	10	
10.	Read the results at the required time.*	10	
11.	Dispose of testing supplies in the appropriate waste container according to OSHA requirements.	5	
12.	Remove your gloves and wash your hands.	5	
13.	Document the results in the patient's chart.	5	
Total Points		100	

CAAHEP Competencies Achieved

   III. P (7)   Obtain specimens for microbiological testing

   III. P (8)   Perform CLIA-waived microbiology testing

ABHES Competencies Achieved

   10. (b) Perform selected CLIA-waived tests that assist with diagnosis and treatment

      (5) Microbiology testing

      (6) b. Kit testing: Quick strep

   10. (c) Dispose of Biohazardous materials

P R O C E D U R E 46-3 Preparing Microbiologic Specimens for Transport to an Outside Laboratory

Procedure Goal

To properly prepare a microbiologic specimen for transport to an outside laboratory.

OSHA Guidelines

Materials

Specimen-collection device, requisition form, secondary container or a zipper-type plastic bag.

Method

Step Number	Procedure	Points Possible	Points Earned
1.	Wash your hands and don examination gloves (and goggles and a mask or face shield if you are collecting a microbiologic throat culture specimen).	5	
2.	Obtain the microbiologic culture specimen.* a. Use the collection system specified by the outside laboratory for the test requested. b. Label the microbiologic specimen-collection device at the time of collection. c. Collect the microbiologic specimen according to the guidelines provided by the laboratory and office procedure.	15	
3.	Remove the gloves and wash your hands.	5	
4.	Complete the test requisition form.	5	
5.	Place the microbiologic specimen container in a secondary container or zipper-type plastic bag.	10	
6.	Attach the test requisition form to the outside of the secondary container or bag, per laboratory policy.	10	
7.	Log the microbiologic specimen in the list of outgoing specimens.	5	
8.	Store the microbiologic specimen according to guidelines provided by the laboratory for that type of specimen (for example, refrigerated, frozen, or 37°C).*	20	
9.	Call the laboratory for pickup of the microbiologic specimen, or hold it until the next scheduled pickup.*	15	
10.	At the time of pickup, ensure that the carrier takes all microbiologic specimens that are logged and scheduled to be picked up.	5	
11.	If you are ever unsure about collection or transportation details, call the laboratory.	5	
Total Points		100	

CAAHEP Competencies Achieved

    III. P (2)   Practice Standard Precautios

    III. P (7)   Obtain specimens for microbiological testing

ABHES Competencies Achieved

    9. (i) Use standard precautions

PROCEDURE 46-4 Preparing a Microbiologic Specimen Smear

Goal
To prepare a smear of a microbiologic specimen for staining.

OSHA Guidelines

Materials
Glass slide with frosted end, pencil, specimen swab, Bunsen burner, and forceps.

Method

Step Number	Procedure	Points Possible	Points Earned
1.	Wash your hands and don exam gloves.	10	
2.	Assemble all the necessary items.	10	
3.	Use a pencil to label the frosted end of the slide with the patient's name.	10	
4.	Roll the specimen swab evenly over the smooth part of the slide, making sure all areas of the swab touch the slide.	10	
5.	Discard the swab in a biohazardous waste container. (Retain the microbiologic specimen for culture as necessary or according to office policy.)	10	
6.	Allow the smear to air-dry. Do not wave the slide to dry it.	10	
7.	Heat-fix the slide by holding the frosted end with forceps and passing the clear part of the slide, with the smear side up, through the flame of a Bunsen burner three or four times. (Your office may use an alternate procedure for fixing the slide, such as flooding the smear with alcohol, allowing it to sit for a few minutes, and either pouring off the remaining liquid or allowing the smear to air-dry. Chlamydia slides come with their own fixative.)	10	
8.	Allow the slide to cool before the smear is stained.	10	
9.	Return the materials to their proper location.	10	
10.	Remove the gloves and wash your hands.	10	
Total Points		100	

CAAHEP Competencies Achieved

III. P. (7)   Obtain specimens for microbiological testing

ABHES Competencies Achieved

10. (b) Perform selected CLIA-waived tests that assist with diagnosis and treatment

   (5) Microbiology testing

10. (c) Dispose of Biohazardous materials

PROCEDURE 46-5 Performing a Gram Stain

Goal
To make bacteria present in a specimen smear visible for microscopic identification.

OSHA Guidelines

Materials
Heat-fixed smear, slide staining rack and tray, crystal violet dye, iodine solution, alcohol or acetone-alcohol decolorizer, safranin dye, wash bottle filled with water, forceps, and blotting paper or paper towels (optional).

Method

Step Number	Procedure	Points Possible	Points Earned
1.	Assemble all the necessary supplies.	4	
2.	Wash your hands and don examination gloves.	4	
3.	Place the heat-fixed smear on a level staining rack and tray, smear side up.	4	
4.	Completely cover the specimen area of the slide with the crystal violet stain.*	8	
5.	Allow the stain to sit for 1 minute; wash the slide thoroughly with water from the wash bottle.*	8	
6.	Use the forceps to hold the slide at the frosted end, tilting the slide to remove excess water.	4	
7.	Place the slide flat on the rack again, and completely cover the specimen area with iodine solution.*	8	
8.	Allow the iodine to remain for 1 minute; wash the slide thoroughly with water. *	8	
9.	Use the forceps to hold and tilt the slide to remove excess water.	4	
10.	While still tilting the slide, apply the alcohol or decolorizer drop by drop until no more purple color washes off. (This step usually takes 10 seconds to 30 seconds.)*	8	
11.	Wash the slide thoroughly with water; use the forceps to hold and tip the slide to remove excess water.*	8	
12.	Completely cover the specimen with safranin dye.*	8	
13.	Allow the safranin to remain for 1 minute; wash the slide thoroughly with water.*	8	
14.	Use the forceps to hold the stained smear by the frosted end, and carefully wipe the back of the slide to remove excess stain.	4	
15.	Place the smear in a vertical position and allow it to air-dry. (The smear may be blotted lightly between blotting paper or paper towels to hasten drying. Take care not to rub the slide, or the specimen may be damaged.)	4	
16.	Sanitize and disinfect the work area.	4	
17.	Remove the gloves and wash your hands.	4	
Total Points		100	

CAAHEP Competencies Achieved

III. P (7)   Obtain specimens for microbiological testing

ABHES Competencies Achieved

10. (b) Perform selected CLIA-waived tests that assist with diagnosis and treatment

(5) Microbiology testing

10. (c) Dispose of Biohazardous materials

Name_____ Class_____ Date_____

R E V I E W

Vocabulary Review

Matching
Match the key terms in the right column with the definitions in the left column by placing the letter of each correct answer in the space provided.

_____ 1. Excessive nighttime urination

_____ 2. Excess protein in urine

_____ 3. Excess glucose in urine

_____ 4. A tube used to collect urine specimens or instill medications

_____ 5. The presence of myoglobin in urine

_____ 6. A tube inserted in the ureter after plastic repair

_____ 7. A bile pigment formed from hemoglobin

_____ 8. A test to determine if there is hidden blood in the stool

_____ 9. A test for the presence of parasites and their eggs in a stool sample

_____ 10. Absence of urine production

_____ 11. A measure of the degree of acidity or alkalinity of urine

_____ 12. Insufficient production (or volume) of urine

_____ 13. Blood in urine

_____ 14. The presence of bilirubin in urine

_____ 15. A cylinder-shaped element that forms when protein accumulates in the kidney tubules and is washed into the urine

_____ 16. A test using antigens and antibodies conjugated to an enzyme

_____ 17. A naturally produced solid of definite form that is commonly found in urine specimens

_____ 18. The liquid portion of a centrifuged urine sample

_____ 19. A genetically inherited disorder in which the body cannot properly metabolize the nutrient phenylalanine

a. drainage catheter
b. nocturia
c. supernatant
d. anuria
e. enzyme immunoassay (EIA)
f. splinting catheter
g. bilirubin
h. proteinuria
i. crystal
j. cast
k. hematuria
l. bilirubinuria
m. phenylketonuria (PKU)
n. FOBT
o. oliguria
p. glycosuria
q. myoglobinuria
r. urinary pH
s. O&P

True or False

Decide whether each statement is true or false. In the space at the left, write T for true or F for false. On the lines provided, rewrite the false statements to make them true.

_____ **20.** When a timed urine specimen is obtained, only the first specimen and the last specimen are collected during a 2- to 24-hour period.

_____

_____ **21.** The normal water content of urine is about 50%.

_____

_____ **22.** Hyaline casts form as a result of increased urine flow.

_____

_____ **23.** A clean-catch midstream urine specimen is obtained after special cleansing of the external genitalia.

_____

_____ **24.** Hemoglobinuria is a rare condition in which free hemoglobin is present in urine.

_____

_____ **25.** Glomerular filtration occurs as blood moves through a tight ball of capillaries called the tubule.

_____

_____ **26.** A first morning urine specimen contains lesser concentrations of substances that collect over time than do specimens taken during the day.

_____

_____ **27.** Hemoglobin breaks down into urea in the intestines.

_____

_____ **28.** A random urine specimen is a single urine specimen that can be taken at any time of the day.

_____

_____ **29.** With adequate fluid intake, the average daily output volume of urine is 1250 mL.

_____

_____ **30.** A 24-hour urine specimen is used to complete a quantitative and qualitative analysis of one or more substances.

_____

_____ **31.** Yeast cells are often seen in the urine of patients with diabetes.

_____

Content Review

Multiple Choice

In the space provided, write the letter of the choice that best completes each statement or answers each question.

_____ **1.** The tube that carries urine from the bladder to the outside of the body is the
   a. Ureter
   b. Urethra
   c. Glomerulus
   d. Collecting tubule
   e. Renal tubule

_____ **2.** A single urine specimen taken at any time of the day is
    a. A clean-catch
    b. Timed
    c. Random
    d. 24-hour
    e. Quantitative

_____ **3.** Fresh urine specimens should be processed within
    a. 1 minute
    b. 1 hour
    c. 3 hours
    d. 1 day
    e. 1 week

_____ **4.** The first part of the urinalysis, a visual inspection of color, volume, odor, and specific gravity, is known as what type of test?
    a. Microscopic   **d.** Chemical
    b. Confirmatory   **e.** Metabolic
    c. Physical

_____ **5.** The normal pH range of freshly voided urine is
    a. 0–2.9   **d.** 4.5–8.0
    b. 2.4–4.8   **e.** 8.2–8.8
    c. 3.8–6.4

Sentence Completion

In the space provided, write the word or phrase that best completes each sentence.

6. The presence of _____ in the urine is one of the first signs of liver disease.

7. _____ is a yellow pigment that gives urine its color.

8. A(n) _____ catheter is designed to remain in place within the bladder.

9. Ketone bodies are intermediary products of fat and _____ metabolism.

10. Leukocyte _____ is a chemical seen when leukocytes are present in urine.

11. An increase in urine specific gravity indicates that the kidneys cannot properly _____ the urine.

12. A reagent strip can be used to test for _____, which suggests a bacterial infection of the urinary tract.

13. The three types of cells that are found in urine are epithelial cells, white blood cells, and _____.

14. Urine pregnancy tests determine the presence of the hormone _____.

15. A(n) _____ test should be done on a urine specimen before attempting to identify crystals in the specimen.

6. _____

7. _____

8. _____

9. _____

10. _____

11. _____

12. _____

13. _____

14. _____

15. _____

Short Answer

Write the answer to each question on the lines provided.

16. What conditions can cause hematuria?

_____

_____

_____

17. What should be done to refrigerated urine specimens before processing them?

_____

_____

_____

18. Why is it necessary to clean the external genitalia when collecting a clean-catch midstream urine specimen?

_____

_____

_____

19. Why is catheterization not routinely used for collecting urine specimens instead of the clean-catch midstream method?

_____

_____

_____

_____

20. What are the disadvantages of the nucleic acid amplification urine tests for STIs?

_____

_____

_____

21. What do changes in the color of a patient's urine generally indicate about changes in its specific gravity?

_____

_____

_____

22. What are the advantages of using a refractometer to measure urine specific gravity?

_____

_____

_____

23. Why might a doctor order the chemical testing of urine?

_____

_____

_____

24. After centrifugation, where should you pour the supernatant?

_____

_____

_____

25. What are three ways a patient can collect a stool specimen?

_____

_____

_____

Critical Thinking

Write the answer to each question on the lines provided.

1. During a microscopic urine exam, you find a higher than normal count of renal epithelial cells. What might this indicate?

_____

_____

_____

2. What is the purpose of taking the temperature of urine collected for a drug and alcohol analysis?

_____

_____

_____

3. Why should a glucose test be performed on a fresh urine specimen?

_____

_____

_____

4. Why is blood more commonly tested than urine for glucose?

_____

_____

_____

5. Will refrigeration cause a decrease or an increase in urine specific gravity? Explain.

_____

_____

_____

6. Why is it important to properly collect a stool sample so that it is not contaminated by water from the toilet or urine?

_____

_____

_____

A P P L I C A T I O N   WORK // DOC

Follow the directions for each application.

1. Collecting a Stool Specimen from an Elderly Patient

Working with two partners, conduct an interview with an elderly patient scheduled for a fecal occult blood test. One person should play the role of the elderly patient, one should take the role of the medical assistant conducting the interview, and the third should act as an observer and evaluator.

   a. Take a history of the patient, noting your questions and the patient's responses. On the basis of the responses, ask appropriate follow-up questions.

   b. Explain to the patient the procedure he is to follow. Allow the patient to interrupt at any time with questions, which you should answer to the best of your ability. Again, note your statements, the patient's questions, and your responses.

   c. Have the observer critique the interview. The critique should include the medical assistant's attitude, or approach, as well as the appropriateness and accuracy of the questions and responses to the elderly patient. The observer also should evaluate the order in which the assistant took the history and its completeness.

   d. As a team, discuss the observer's critique, noting the strengths and weaknesses of the interview.

2. Evaluating a Urine Specimen

Indicate whether each of the following results of a urinalysis is normal or abnormal by writing *normal* or *abnormal* in the space provided.

   a. Color: Red_____

   b. Turbidity: Clear_____

   c. Odor: Fruity_____

   d. Volume: 2200 mL/24 hours _____

   e. Specific gravity: 1.022 _____

   f. Ketones: Negative_____

   g. pH: 5.2_____

   h. Glucose: Positive_____

   i. Red blood cells: 8/high-power field _____

   j. Crystals: Negative_____

3. Completing a Laboratory Requisition Form

   a. Complete the sample reference laboratory requisition form, an example of which is found in the documentation section in the back of the book, using appropriate information from the following case.

   The physician has seen a young female patient in the office who has been complaining of vague abdominal pain, slight weight gain, fatigue, some nausea, and occasional fever. You have been asked to collect a urine specimen for this patient for a complete urinalysis and a qualitative urine pregnancy test. Your office does not perform any laboratory testing in-house.

   The patient's name is Mary Elizabeth Arnold, age 24. The physician's name is Dr. Travis Buffett; his UPIN number is 123456.

   The shaded areas must be completed, or the reference laboratory will reject the specimen. Remember that you must fill in the date and time of the collection even though those areas are not shaded in; use today's date and time. Do not forget to mark which tests are being requested. In addition, note the patient's unique control number, which the reference laboratory will use to track the specimen.

b. Complete the sample reference laboratory requisition form, an example of which is found in the documentation section in the back of the book, using appropriate information from the following case.

An elderly patient by the name of William Overtell has seen the physician in the office today. The physician suspects that this patient may be entering the early phases of kidney failure based on the patient's clinical picture. A key test in diagnosing a condition of this type can be a 24-hour urine specimen.

After measurement of the total volume of the 24-hour specimen, a small sample is prepared to forward to the reference laboratory for analysis. The physician's name is Dr. Felicia Mills, and her UPIN number is 98765443.

Because the patient has Medicare, the physician cannot bill the patient for the testing. The patient's Medicare number (112-33-5588B) must be provided in the appropriate block on the requisition form so that the laboratory can bill the insurance carrier directly. The total volume of the specimen was 980 mL. Identify the test number assigned to this test on the requisition form. Also, to ensure proper collection, detail the specific instructions that should be provided to the patient prior to the collection of the specimen.

CASE STUDIES

Write your response to each case study on the lines provided.

Case 1
A patient telephones and tells you she is concerned about not having a means at home of disinfecting a jar for a urine specimen. How would you respond to the patient?

_____
_____
_____

Case 2
You notice that the lid has been left off a urine specimen container that you are supposed to test for ketone bodies. Should you perform the test? Why or why not?

_____
_____
_____

Case 3
You open a fresh container of reagent test strips 5 months before the expiration date marked on the container. You note that the test strips are not discolored. What should your next step be?

_____
_____
_____

Case 4
Elizabeth comes to the office on a very hot day. She says she has been working outside all day and hasn't had much to drink. After you perform her urinalysis, you note that she has an abnormal urine specific gravity. Would you expect the urine specific gravity to be elevated or decreased? Why?

_____
_____
_____

Case 5

You have been asked to educate a mother about collecting a stool sample from her 1-year-old child. What tips can you give the mother about collecting the sample?

_____

_____

_____

PROCEDURE 47-1 Collecting a Clean-Catch Midstream Urine Specimen

WORK // DOC

Goal

To collect a urine specimen that is free from contamination.

OSHA Guidelines

Materials

Dry, sterile urine container with lid; label; written instructions (if the patient is to perform procedure independently); and antiseptic towelettes.

Method

Step Number	Procedure	Points Possible	Points Earned
1.	Confirm the patient's identity and be sure all forms are correctly completed.	8	
2.	Label the sterile urine specimen container with the patient's name, ID number, date of birth, the physician's name, the date and time of collection, and the initials of the person collecting the specimen.	8	
When the Patient Will Be Completing the Procedure Independently			
3.	Explain the procedure in detail. Provide the patient with written instructions, antiseptic towelettes, and the labeled sterile specimen container.	8	
4.	Confirm that the patient understands the instructions, especially not to touch the inside of the specimen container and to refrigerate the specimen until bringing it to the physician's office.	8	
When You Are Assisting a Patient			
3.	Explain the procedure and how you will be assisting in the collection.	8	
4.	Wash your hands and don exam gloves.	8	
When You Are Assisting in the Collection for Female Patients			
5.	Remove the lid from the specimen container, and place the lid upside down on a flat surface.	8	
6.	Use three antiseptic towelettes to clean the perineal area by spreading the labia and wiping from front to back. Wipe with the first towelette on one side and discard it. Wipe with the second towelette on the other side and discard it. Wipe with the third towelette down the middle and discard it. To remove soap residue that could cause a higher pH and affect chemical test results, rinse the area once from front to back with water.*	10	
7.	Keeping the patient's labia spread to avoid contamination, tell her to urinate into the toilet. After she has expressed a small amount of urine, instruct her to stop the flow.*	10	

(continued)

Step Number	Procedure	Points Possible	Points Earned
8.	Position the specimen container close to but not touching the patient.	8	
9.	Tell the patient to start urinating again. Collect the necessary amount of urine in the container. (If the patient cannot stop her urine flow, move the container into the urine flow and collect the specimen anyway.)	8	
10.	Allow the patient to finish urinating. Place the lid back on the collection container.	8	
11.	Remove the gloves and wash your hands.	8	
12.	Complete the test request slip, and record the collection in the patient's chart.	8	
When You Are Assisting in the Collection for Male Patients			
5.	Remove the lid from the specimen container, and place the lid upside down on a flat surface.	8	
6.	If the patient is circumcised, use an antiseptic towelette to clean the head of the penis. Wipe with a second towelette directly across the urethral opening. If the patient is uncircumcised, retract the foreskin before cleaning the penis. To remove soap residue that could cause a higher pH and affect chemical test results, rinse the area once from front to back with water.*	10	
7.	Keeping an uncircumcised patient's foreskin retracted, tell the patient to urinate into the toilet. After he has expressed a small amount of urine, instruct him to stop the flow.*	10	
8.	Position the specimen container close to but not touching the patient.	8	
9.	Tell the patient to start urinating again. Collect the necessary amount of urine in the container. (If the patient cannot stop his urine flow, move the container into the urine flow and collect the specimen anyway.)	8	
10.	Allow the patient to finish urinating. Place the lid back on the collection container.	8	
11.	Remove the gloves and wash your hands.	8	
12.	Complete the laboratory request form, and record the collection in the patient's chart.	8	
Total Points		100	

CAAHEP Competencies Achieved

    III. P (2)   Practice Standard Precautions

    III. A (1)   Display sensitivity to patient rights and feelings in collecting specimens

    III. A (2)   Explain the rationale for performance of a procedure to the patient

ABHES Competencies Achieved

    9. (i) Use standard precautions

    9. (q) Instruct patients with special needs

    10. (c) Dispose of Biohazardous materials

    10. (e) Instruct patients in the collection of a clean-catch mid-stream urine specimen

PROCEDURE 47-2 Collecting a 24-Hour Urine Specimen

WORK // DOC

Goal
To collect a urine specimen that is free from contaminants over a 24-hour period.

OSHA Guidelines

Materials
Urine collection container (disposable urinal or collection hat); sterile urine storage containers, and written instructions.

Method

Step Number	Procedure	Points Possible	Points Earned
1.	Review the laboratory requisition form and gather the supplies.	10	
2.	Confirm the patient's identity, introduce yourself, and check that all forms are completed correctly.	10	
3.	Label the sterile urine specimen storage containers with the patient's name, ID number, date of birth, and the physician's name.	10	
4.	Explain that the urine specimen storage container may have a preservative in it. Tell the patient what they should do if they get the preservative on their skin. (Usually flushing with cold water is sufficient; follow the manufacturer's provided instructions.)	10	
5.	Give the patient the following instructions: **a.** At the start of the observation period (usually early in the morning), void and discard the first urine specimen. This will start the collection period. Write the start date and time on the urine specimen storage containers. **b.** Do not discard the preservative in the urine specimen storage container. **c.** For the next 24 hours, each time the patient voids, collect the entire specimen in the provided specimen collection container. **d.** Carefully transfer the entire specimen in the urine storage container, being careful not to spill any urine. If the patient spills urine or accidentally urinates in the toilet, have them call to reschedule the test. **e.** Keep the specimen covered and in the refrigerator or in a cooler when not in use. **f.** 24 hours after you begin the test, void once more and transfer to the specimen storage container. Write the end date and time on the container. **g.** As quickly as possible, bring the specimen back to the office or deliver it to the laboratory if instructed to do so. Keep the specimen cool during transport.	20	

(continued)

Name_____ Date_____

Evaluated by_____ Score_____

Step Number	Procedure	Points Possible	Points Earned
6.	When the patient returns the urine specimen, wash your hands, don gloves, and then be sure to do the following:* a. Check that the container lid is secure. b. Clean the outside of the container with a tissue of gauze pad if necessary. c. Check that the start and end dates and times are recorded on the container. d. Note the volume of the collected specimen. e. Review the procedure with the patient to make sure the specimen was properly collected and stored during the collection period. f. Complete the necessary laboratory requisition forms. g. Notify the lab that the specimen is ready for transport. h. Keep the specimen cold until it is transported to the lab.	20	
7.	Remove the gloves and wash your hands.	10	
8.	Document the specimen collection, including volume, dates and times, and lab tests requested.	10	
Total Points		100	

CAAHEP Competencies Achieved

III. P. (2) Practice Standard Precautions

III. A (1) Display sensitivity to patient rights and feelings in collecting specimens

III. A (2) Explain the rationale for performance of a procedure to the patient

III. A (3) Show awareness of patients' concerns regarding their perceptions related to the procedure being performed

IV. P. (6) Prepare a patient for procedures and/or treatments

ABHES Competencies Achieved

9. (i) Use standard precautions

9. (q) Instruct patients with special needs

10. (c) Dispose of Biohazardous materials

P R O C E D U R E 47-3 Establishing Chain of Custody for a Urine Specimen

WORK // DOC

Goal
To collect a urine specimen for drug testing, maintaining a chain of custody.

OSHA Guidelines

Materials
Dry, sterile urine container with lid; chain of custody form (CCF); and two additional specimen containers.

Method

Step Number	Procedure	Points Possible	Points Earned
1.	Positively identify the patient. (Complete the top part of CCF with the drug testing laboratory's name and address, the requesting company's name and address, and the patient's Social Security number. Make a note on the form if the patient refuses to give her Social Security number.) Ensure the number on the printed label matches the number at the top of the form.*	10	
2.	Ensure the patient removes any outer clothing and empties her pockets, displaying all items.	4	
3.	Instruct the patient to wash and dry her hands.	4	
4.	Instruct the patient that no water is to be running while the specimen is being collected. Tape the faucet handles in the *off* position and add bluing agent to the toilet.*	10	
5.	Instruct the patient to provide the specimen as soon as it is collected so you may record the specimen's temperature.	4	
6.	Remain by the door of the restroom.	4	
7.	Measure and record the urine specimen's temperature within 4 minutes of collection. Make a note if its temperature is out of acceptable range.*	10	
8.	Examine the specimen for signs of adulteration (unusual color or odor).*	10	
9.	*In the presence of the patient,* check the "single specimen" or "split specimen" box. The patient should witness you transferring the specimen into the transport specimen bottle(s), capping the bottle(s), and affixing the label on the bottle(s).*	10	
10.	The patient should initial the specimen bottle label(s) *after* it is placed on the bottle(s).*	10	
11.	Complete any additional information requested on the form, including the authorization for drug screening. This information will include • Patient's daytime telephone number • Patient's evening telephone number • Test requested • Patient's name • Patient's signature • Date	4	

(continued)

Step Number	Procedure	Points Possible	Points Earned
12.	Sign the CCF; print your full name, and note the date and time of the collection and the name of the courier service.	4	
13.	Give the patient a copy of the CCF.	4	
14.	Place the specimen in a leakproof bag with the appropriate copy of the form.	4	
15.	Release the specimen to the courier service.	4	
16.	Distribute additional copies as required.	4	
Total Points		100	

CAAHEP Competencies Achieved

IX. P (7)   Document accurately in the patient record

IX. P (8)   Apply local, state, and federal health care legislation and regulation appropriate to the medical assisting practice

ABHES Competencies Achieved

3. (d) Recognize and identify acceptable medical abbreviations

9. (f) Screen and follow up patient test results

9. (q) Instruct patients with special needs

10. (e) Instruct patients in the collection of a clean-catch mid-stream urine specimen

PROCEDURE 47-4 Measuring Specific Gravity with a Refractometer

WORK // DOC

Goal
To measure the specific gravity of a urine specimen with a refractometer.

OSHA Guidelines

Materials
Urine specimen, refractometer, dropper, and laboratory report form.

Method

Step Number	Procedure	Points Possible	Points Earned
1.	Wash your hands and don exam gloves.	5	
2.	Check the specimen for proper labeling, and examine it to make sure there is no visible contamination and that no more than 1 hour has passed since collection (or since the specimen has been removed from the refrigerator and brought back to room temperature).*	10	
3.	Swirl the specimen.*	10	
4.	Confirm that the refractometer has been calibrated that day. If not, you must calibrate it with distilled water. You must also use two standard solutions as controls to check the refractometer's accuracy. Follow Steps 6 through 11, using each of the three samples in place of the specimen. Clean the refractometer and the dropper after each use, and record the calibration values in the quality control log.*	10	
5.	Open the hinged lid of the refractometer.	5	
6.	Draw up a small amount of the specimen into the dropper.	5	
7.	Place one drop of the specimen under the cover.	5	
8.	Close the lid.	5	
9.	Turn on the light, and look into the refractometer's eyepiece. As the light passes through the specimen, the refractometer measures the refraction of the light and displays the refractive index on a scale on the right with corresponding specific gravity values on the left.*	10	
10.	Read the specific gravity value at the line where light and dark meet.*	10	
11.	Record the value on the laboratory report form.	5	
12.	Sanitize and disinfect the refractometer and the dropper. Put them away when they are dry.	5	
13.	Clean and disinfect the work area.	5	
14.	Remove the gloves and wash your hands.	5	
15.	Record the value in the patient's chart.	5	
Total Points		100	

CAAHEP Competencies Achieved

I. P (14)   Perform CLIA-waived urinalysis

I. P (16)   Screen test results

ABHES Competencies Achieved

9. (f) Screen and follow up patient test results

10. (a) Practice quality control

10. (b) Perform selected CLIA-waived tests that assist with diagnosis and treatment

    1. Urinalysis

PROCEDURE 47-5 Performing a Reagent Strip Test

WORK // DOC

Goal

To perform chemical testing on urine specimens to screen for the presence of various elements, including leukocytes, nitrite, urobilinogen, protein, pH, blood, specific gravity, ketones, bilirubin, and glucose.

OSHA Guidelines

Materials

Urine specimen, laboratory report form, reagent strips, paper towel, and a timer.

Method

Step Number	Procedure	Points Possible	Points Earned
1.	Wash your hands and don personal protective equipment.	5	
2.	Check the specimen for proper labeling, and examine it to make sure there is no visible contamination. Perform the test as soon as possible after collection. Refrigerate the specimen if testing will take place more than 1 hour later. Bring the refrigerated specimen back to room temperature prior to testing.*	15	
3.	Check the expiration date on the reagent strip container and check the strip for damaged or discolored pads.*	15	
4.	Swirl the specimen.*	10	
5.	Dip a urine strip into the specimen, making sure each pad is completely covered. Briefly tap the strip sideways on a paper towel. *Do not blot* the test pads.*	15	
6.	Read each test pad against the chart on the bottle at the designated time. Note: It is important to read each pad at the appropriate time. Most reagent strip results are invalid after 2 minutes.*	15	
7.	Record the values on the laboratory report form.	5	
8.	Discard the used disposable supplies.	5	
9.	Clean and disinfect the work area.	5	
10.	Remove your gloves and wash your hands.	5	
11.	Record the result in the patient's chart.	5	
Total Points		100	

CAAHEP Competencies Achieved

    I. P (14)   Perform CLIA-waived urinalysis

    I. P (16)   Screen test results

ABHES Competencies Achieved

    3. (d) Recognize and identify acceptable medical abbreviations

    9. (f) Screen and follow up patient test results

  10. (a) Practice quality control

  10. (b) Perform selected CLIA-waived tests that assist with diagnosis and treatment

        1. Urinalysis

        6. Kit testing

    (c) Dip sticks

  10. (c) Dispose of Biohazardous materials

PROCEDURE 47-6 Pregnancy Testing Using the EIA Method

Goal

To perform the enzyme immunoassay in order to detect HCG in the urine (or serum) and to interpret results as positive or negative.

OSHA Guidelines

Materials

Gloves, urine specimen, timing device, surface disinfectant, pregnancy control solutions, and pregnancy test kits.

Method

Step Number	Procedure	Points Possible	Points Earned
1.	Wash your hands and don exam gloves.	10	
2.	Gather the necessary supplies and equipment.	10	
3.	If materials have been refrigerated, allow all materials to reach room temperature prior to conducting the testing.	10	
4.	Label the test chamber with the patient's name or identification number; label one test chamber for a negative and positive control.	10	
5.	Apply the urine (or serum) to the test chamber per the manufacturer's instructions.	10	
6.	At the appropriate time, read and interpret the results.	10	
7.	Document the patient's results in the chart; document the quality control results in the appropriate log book.	10	
8.	Dispose of used reagents in a biohazard container.	10	
9.	Clean the work area with a disinfectant solution.	10	
10.	Remove your gloves and wash your hands.	10	
Total Points		100	

CAAHEP Competencies Achieved

    I. P (16)   Screen test results

ABHES Competencies Achieved

    9. (f) Screen and follow up patient test results

    10. (a) Practice quality control

    10. (b) Perform selected CLIA-waived tests that assist with diagnosis and treatment

        6. Kit testing

    (a) Pregnancy

    10. (c) Dispose of Biohazardous materials

PROCEDURE 47-7 Processing a Urine Specimen for Microscopic Examination of Sediment

WORK // DOC

Goal
To prepare a slide for microscopic examination of urine sediment.

OSHA Guidelines

Materials
Fresh urine specimen, two glass or plastic test tubes, water, centrifuge, tapered pipette, glass slide with coverslip, microscope with light source, and laboratory report form.

Method

Step Number	Procedure	Points Possible	Points Earned
1.	Wash your hands and don exam gloves.	4	
2.	Check the specimen for proper labeling, and examine it to make sure there is no visible contamination and that no more than 1 hour has passed since collection (or since the specimen has been removed from the refrigerator and brought back to room temperature).*	8	
3.	Swirl the urine specimen.*	8	
4.	Pour approximately 10 mL of urine into one test tube and 10 mL of plain water into the balance tube.	4	
5.	Balance the centrifuge by placing the test tubes on either side.*	8	
6.	Make sure the lid is secure, and set the centrifuge timer for 5 to 10 minutes.*	8	
7.	Set the speed as prescribed by your office's protocol (usually 1500 to 2000 revolutions per minute) and start the centrifuge. Fill one test tube with approximately 10 mL of urine and the other with 10 mL of water.	4	
8.	After the centrifuge stops, lift out the tube containing the urine, and carefully pour most of the liquid portion—called the **supernatant**—down the sink drain.*	8	
9.	A few drops of urine should remain in the bottom of the test tube with any sediment. Mix the urine and sediment together by gently tapping the bottom of the tube on the palm of your hand.*	8	
10.	Use the tapered pipette to obtain a drop or two of urine sediment. Place the drops in the center of a clean glass slide.	4	
11.	Place the coverslip over the specimen, allow it to settle, and place it on the stage of the microscope.	3	

(continued)

Copyright © 2014 by The McGraw-Hill Companies, Inc.

Step Number	Procedure	Points Possible	Points Earned
12.	Correctly focus the microscope as directed in the *Microbiology and Disease* chapter. *Note:* Most medical assistants are trained to perform this procedure only up to this point. After this, the physician usually examines the specimen. You may, however, be asked to clean the items after the examination is completed. The remaining steps are provided for your information.	1	
13.	Use a dim light and view the slide under the low-power objective. Observe the slide for casts (found mainly around the coverslip's edges), and count the casts viewed.	1	
14.	Switch to the high-power objective. Identify the casts. Identify any epithelial cells, mucus, protozoa, yeasts, and crystals. Adjust the slide position so you can view and count the cells, protozoa, yeasts, and crystals from at least 10 different fields. Turn off the light after the examination is completed.	1	
15.	Record the observations on the laboratory report form.	5	
16.	Properly dispose of used disposable materials.	5	
17.	Sanitize and disinfect nondisposable items; put them away when they are dry.	5	
18.	Clean and disinfect the work area.	5	
19.	Remove the gloves and wash your hands.	5	
20.	Record the observations in the patient's chart.	5	
Total Points		100	

CAAHEP Competencies Achieved

I.P (14)   Perform CLIA-waived urinalysis

I. P (16)   Screen test results

ABHES Competencies Achieved

3. (d) Recognize and identify acceptable medical abbreviations

9. (f) Screen and follow up patient test results

10. (a) Practice quality control

10. (b) Perform selected CLIA-waived tests that assist with diagnosis and treatment

    1. Urinalysis

10. (c) Dispose of Biohazardous materials

PROCEDURE 47-8 Fecal Occult Blood Testing Using the Guaiac Testing Method   WORK // DOC

Goal
To test for the presence of blood in a fecal sample.

OSHA Guidelines

Materials
Fecal occult blood testing cards or slides, fecal collection spoon or other device, written patient instructions, and testing reagents.

Method

Step Number	Procedure	Points Possible	Points Earned
1.	Confirm the patient's identity, and ensure all forms are completed correctly.	10	
2.	Label the occult blood testing card or slide with the patient's name and date of birth. Give the patient the test card or slide and collecting spoon or applicator.	10	
3.	Give the patient pretest and collection instructions, including* **a.** Do not collect sample if you are menstruating or if visible blood is seen in the feces or toilet. **b.** For three days prior to collecting the sample, avoid red meats (beef, veal, and lamb), horseradish, vitamin C supplements, some fruits and vegetables, aspirin or other nonsteroidal anti-inflammatory drugs, and other medications including corticosteroids. (Consult the specific test instructions for dietary and medication restrictions as these may vary from test to test.) **c.** Collect the samples (depending on the specific test) on two or three different days. **d.** Collect the specimen before it comes into contact with the toilet water. (The patient may use a clean container or a specimen collection hat.) **e.** Place a small amount of fecal material on each slide or test card window with the applicator. The sample should be thinly smeared in the sample area. Close the card window or place the slide in the provided container, and write the collection date on the card or slide. **f.** Return the card or slide to the office.	15	
Processing the Test			
4.	Wash your hands and don gloves.	10	
5.	Open the back of the card. Add the recommended amount of developing reagent directly over the smeared area on the back side of the paper and over the positive and negative controls, if present on the card.*	15	

(continued)

Step Number	Procedure	Points Possible	Points Earned
6.	Read the test results at the appropriate time according to the manufacturer's instructions (usually within 60 seconds). There will be a blue color on the guaiac paper if blood is present.	10	
7.	Dispose of the testing card according to OSHA regulations.	10	
8.	Remove your gloves and wash your hands.	10	
9.	Document the results in the patient's chart.	10	
Total Points		100	

CAAHEP Competencies Achieved

I. P (16)   Screen test results

ABHES Competencies Achieved

3. (d) Recognize and identify acceptable medical abbreviations

9. (f) Screen and follow up patient test results

10. (a) Practice quality control

10. (f) Instruct patients in the collection of a fecal specimen

Collecting, Processing, and Testing Blood Specimens

Name_____ Class_____ Date_____

R E V I E W

Vocabulary Review

Matching

Match the key terms in the right column with the definitions in the left column by placing the letter of each correct answer in the space provided.

_____ 1. The liquid part of blood in which other components are suspended

_____ 2. The process of blood clotting

_____ 3. The study of the shape or form of objects

_____ 4. The portion of blood volume that includes red blood cells, white blood cells, and platelets

_____ 5. The insertion of a needle into a vein for the purpose of withdrawing blood

_____ 6. Granular leukocytes that capture invading bacteria and antigen/antibody complexes

_____ 7. The rupturing of blood cells

_____ 8. A white blood cell

_____ 9. The fever-producing substance released by a neutrophil

_____ 10. A white blood cell with a solid nucleus and clear cytoplasm

_____ 11. A winged infusion set

_____ 12. Clear, yellow liquid that remains after a blood clot forms

_____ 13. The area of a spun sample of blood that contains the white blood cells and platelets

_____ 14. A nongranular leukocyte that regulates immunologic response

_____ 15. The heaviest part of whole blood, which moves to one end of a microhematocrit tube after being spun in a centrifuge

_____ 16. A blood collection device that includes a double-pointed needle, a plastic needle holder, and collection tubes

_____ 17. A flat, broad length of vinyl or rubber used during venipuncture procedures

_____ 18. The puncture of a vein

a. agranular leukocyte
b. phlebotomy
c. eosinophils
d. serum
e. morphology
f. pyrogen
g. formed elements
h. buffy coat
i. plasma
j. evacuation system
k. venipuncture
l. packed red blood cells
m. coagulation
n. butterfly system
o. leukocyte
p. T lymphocyte
q. tourniquet
r. hemolysis

True or False

Decide whether each statement is true or false. In the space at the left, write T *for true or* F *for false. On the lines provided, rewrite the false statements to make them true.*

_____ **19.** Hemoglobin is found in red blood cells.

_____

_____ **20.** The last step in preparing to draw blood for testing is to review the written testing request.

_____

_____ **21.** Morphologic tests are done to monitor therapeutic levels of drugs like Coumadin.

_____

_____ **22.** An erythrocyte sedimentation rate is performed on freshly collected, anticoagulated blood.

_____

_____ **23.** Blood chemistry tests routinely conducted in the POL include blood glucose monitoring.

_____

_____ **24.** Hemoglobin A1c may be tested after a patient has eaten.

_____

_____ **25.** A small, calibrated glass tube that holds a small, precise volume of fluid is a hematocrit.

_____

_____ **26.** When counting RBCs and WBCs, you use a concentrated blood sample and a hemocytometer.

_____

_____ **27.** Hemoglobin is released during hemolysis, the rupturing of red blood cells.

_____

_____ **28.** Capillary puncture requires a superficial puncture of the skin with a sharp point.

_____

_____ **29.** Neutrophils have a light green nucleus and pale pink cytoplasm, which contains fine pink or lavender granules.

_____

_____ **30.** Through hematocrit determination, you can identify how much of the volume of a sample of blood is made up of red blood cells after the sample has been spun in a centrifuge.

_____

_____ **31.** In a tube of blood that has been spun in a centrifuge, the packed red blood cells are separated from the white blood cells by the buffy coat.

_____

_____ **32.** A complete blood count is a type of serologic test.

_____

_____ **33.** An erythrocyte sedimentation rate (ESR) test measures the rate at which red blood cells settle to the bottom of a blood sample.

_____

_____ **34.** A hematocrit is a test that measures the percentage of white blood cells in a blood sample.

_____

Content Review

Multiple Choice

In the space provided, write the letter of the choice that best completes each statement or answers each question.

_____ 1. Blood is transported throughout the body by the
   a. Circulatory system
   b. Plasma
   c. Hemoglobin
   d. Transrespiratory system
   e. Lungs

_____ 2. Which of the following gives red blood cells their color?
   a. Hemoglobin
   b. Hemolysis
   c. Oxygen
   d. B lymphocytes
   e. Transferrin

_____ 3. The study of blood is known as
   a. Morphology
   b. Cytology
   c. Histology
   d. Hematology
   e. Cardiology

_____ 4. Other than assembling the equipment and supplies necessary, the first step in preparing to draw blood is reviewing the
   a. Patient's blood type
   b. Procedure with the patient
   c. Written request for the test
   d. Health of the patient
   e. Patient's insurance plan

_____ 5. A small, disposable instrument with a sharp point used to puncture the skin and make a small incision is a
   a. Micropipette
   b. Lancet
   c. Syringe
   d. Tourniquet
   e. Butterfly device

_____ 6. Fragments of megakaryocytes are known as
   a. Neutrophils
   b. Basophils
   c. Red blood cells.
   d. Monocytes
   e. Thrombocytes

_____ 7. Which of the following methods of blood collection would be best to use with patients who have small or fragile veins?

    a. Evacuation system

    b. VACUTAINER system

    c. Butterfly system

    d. Venipuncture

    e. Syringe

_____ 8. Lancets are used

    a. When the amount of blood required for a procedure is not large

    b. When the amount of blood required for a procedure is large

    c. For infants only

    d. For adults only

    e. Only for chemistry tests

_____ 9. A test used to monitor the health of a patient with diabetes is a

    a. Complete blood count

    b. Hemoglobin A1c

    c. Creatine kinase

    d. ESR

    e. Differential count

Sentence Completion

In the space provided, write the word or phrase that best completes each sentence.

10. When drawing a patient's blood, you should make no more than _____ attempts.

11. The most common patient question you will encounter when drawing blood is, _____.

12. Probably the greatest fear of patients undergoing blood tests is contracting _____.

13. The additive in a lavender topped tube is _____.

14. _____ form a gel-like barrier between serum and the clot in a coagulated blood sample.

15. Blood cell destruction is called _____.

16. The normal range for a total carbon dioxide blood test is _____.

17. _____ are the first line of defense during a phlebotomy procedure.

10. _____

11. _____

12. _____

13. _____

14. _____

15. _____

16. _____

17. _____

Short Answer

Write the answer to each question on the lines provided.

18. Why might you need to wear a mask during a phlebotomy procedure?

_____

_____

_____

19. What two goals are met by wearing personal protective equipment during phlebotomy procedures?

_____

_____

_____

20. Describe three advantages of an evacuation system of blood drawing.

_____

_____

_____

21. How can you prevent infections caused by phlebotomy?

_____

_____

_____

22. Describe the biggest challenge in blood drawing that children present.

_____

_____

_____

23. Describe how you would determine the concentration of hemoglobin in a blood sample.

_____

_____

_____

24. Describe two desired characteristics of engineered safety devices.

_____

_____

_____

25. Describe the staining characteristics of each of the following white blood cells.

    a. Neutrophils _____

    b. Basophils _____

    c. Eosinophils _____

    d. Lymphocytes _____

    e. Monocytes _____

Critical Thinking

Write the answer to each question on the lines provided.

    1. Why is it important to dispose of sharps promptly, using approved sharps containers?

_____

_____

_____

2. What should you do if you suffer a needlestick injury?

_____

_____

_____

3. Why is it important to be absolutely sure of the meaning of any abbreviations used in laboratory work?

_____

_____

_____

4. Why is it important to identify the patient correctly before drawing blood?

_____

_____

_____

5. What are the advantages of pen-like capillary puncture devices?

_____

_____

_____

A P P L I C A T I O N   WORK // DOC

Follow the directions for each application.

1. Identifying Blood Test Collection Tubes

For each test listed, name the color and additive of the collection tube used to perform the test.

a. Creatine kinase _____

b. Bilirubin _____

c. Leukocyte count _____

d. Fasting glucose _____

e. Phenylalanine _____

f. Prothrombin _____

g. Thyroid stimulating hormone _____

h. Complete blood count _____

2. Collecting Blood Specimens

Practice each of the following techniques or role-play each of the following situations with a partner. Critique each other by using the space provided to note pointers and suggestions that you think will help the other person perform the technique better. For situations in which you draw blood, use a mannequin arm. If a mannequin arm is not available, attach a piece of rubber tubing to a rolled piece of fabric. Then tape over a portion of the tubing to simulate skin.

a. Venipuncture with a needle and syringe

b. Preparing a smear slide

c. Capillary puncture with an automatic puncturing device

d. Preparing patients for blood drawing

e. Handling a patient who faints during blood drawing

3. Completing a Laboratory Requisition Form

a. Complete the sample reference laboratory requisition form, found at the end of the workbook, using appropriate information from the following case.

A female patient was seen in the physician's office today. After examining the patient and reviewing her history, the physician has requested that blood be drawn for the following tests: thyroid profile II, basic chemistry, and total glycohemoglobin.

The patient's name is Janice Jondahl, age 56. The physician's name is Dr. Rebecca Adamson; her UPIN number is 97644521.

Remember to use today's date and time for the specimen date and time and do not omit any of the shaded areas. After completing the form, name the type of specimen and tube type that are required according to the requisition form. In addition, note the test numbers assigned to each of the tests requested by the physician.

b. Complete the sample reference laboratory requisition form, found at the end of the workbook, using appropriate information from the following case.

Charles Riffe, age 83, has seen Dr. Domingo Krishnan in the office today for a follow-up for high blood cholesterol, which has been an ongoing problem for him. The physician has placed the patient on a cholesterol-reducing medication for 6 weeks now and has asked that this patient return the next morning without eating to have the following blood tests drawn: lipid profile I to include a lipoprotein analysis, glucose, and a liver profile A (to rule out liver damage from the prescribed medication).

The patient has Medicare, which means that the physician cannot bill the patient for the service. The patient's Medicare number, 678-35-0022B, must be provided to the reference laboratory in order for the laboratory to bill the insurance carrier directly.

Remember to use today's date and time for the specimen collection date and time. After completing the form, answer the following questions:

1. Why would the physician request that the patient return the next day without having eaten?

2. What are the specimen requirements for the tests requested?

3. Is there any information missing from this scenario that you must have before sending the specimen to the reference laboratory?

C A S E   S T U D I E S

Write your response to each case study on the lines provided.

Case 1

While you are preparing a patient for a blood test, she asks whether her symptoms are signs of rheumatoid arthritis. How should you respond?

_____

_____

_____

Case 2

A patient arrived in the office for a blood test. What steps should you follow, from this moment to the time you draw the blood?

_____

_____

_____

Case 3

As you are assembling the equipment for drawing blood from a patient, you notice her eyeing the needle and tubes nervously. She then asks, "Will this hurt?" As you draw the blood, the patient comments, "I guess this test is pretty common, right? I mean, do you usually need so many tubes of blood?" How should you respond to her concerns?

_____

_____

_____

Case 4

While performing a capillary puncture, you notice the patient's hands are very cold. What should you do?

_____

_____

_____

Case 5

You have been asked to prepare a blood sample for transport to an outside lab. How should you do this?

_____

_____

_____

PROCEDURE 48-1 Quality Control Procedures for Blood Specimen Collection

[WORK // DOC]

Goal
To follow proper quality control procedures when taking a blood specimen.

OSHA Guidelines

Materials
Necessary sterile equipment, specimen-collection container, paperwork related to the type of blood test the specimen is being drawn for, requisition form, marker, and proper packing materials for transport.

Method

Step Number	Procedure	Points Possible	Points Earned
1.	Review the request form for the test ordered, verify the procedure, prepare the necessary equipment and paperwork, and prepare the work area.	8	
2.	Identify the patient and explain the procedure. Confirm the patient's identification. Ask the patient to spell her name. Make sure the patient understands the procedure to be performed, even if she has had it done before.	8	
3.	Confirm the patient has followed any pretest preparation requirements such as fasting, taking any necessary medication, or stopping a medication. For example, if a fasting specimen is being taken, the patient should not have eaten anything after midnight of the day before. Some doctors' offices will let the patient drink water or black coffee, however. It often depends on the type of specimen being taken.*	15	
4.	Collect the specimen properly. Collect it at the right time intervals if that applies. Use sterile equipment and proper technique.	8	
5.	Use the correct specimen-collection containers and the right preservatives, if required.*	15	
6.	Immediately label the specimens. The label should include the patient's name, the date and time of collection, the test's name, and the name of the person collecting the specimen. Do not label the containers before collecting the specimen.*	15	
7.	Follow correct procedures for disposing of hazardous specimen waste and decontaminating the work area. Used needles, for instance, should immediately be placed in a biohazard sharps container.	8	
8.	Thank the patient. Keep the patient in the office if any follow-up observation is necessary.	8	

(continued)

Step Number	Procedure	Points Possible	Points Earned
9.	If the specimen is to be transported to an outside laboratory, prepare it for transport in the proper container for that type of specimen, according to OSHA regulations. Place the container in a clear plastic bag with a zip closure and dual pockets with the international biohazard label imprinted in red or orange. The requisition form should be placed in the bag's outside pocket. This ensures protection from contamination if the specimen leaks. Have a courier pick up the specimen and place it in an appropriate carrier (like an insulated cooler) with the biohazard label. Place specimens to be sent by mail in appropriate plastic containers, and then place the containers inside a heavy duty plastic container with a screw-down, nonleaking lid. Then place this container in either a heavy-duty cardboard box or nylon bag. The words *Human Specimen* or *Body Fluids* should be imprinted on the box or bag. Seal with a strong tape strip.*	15	
Total Points		100	

CAAHEP Competencies Achieved

I. P (2)   Perform Venipuncture

ABHES Competencies Achieved

10. (a) Practice quality control

10. (c) Dispose of Biohazardous materials

10. (d) Collect, label, and process specimens

1. Perform venipuncture

2. Perform capillary puncture

PROCEDURE 48-2 Performing Venipuncture Using an Evacuation System

WORK//DOC

Goal
To collect a venous blood sample using an evacuation system.

OSHA Guidelines

Materials
VACUTAINER components (safety needle, needle holder/adapter, collection tubes), antiseptic and cotton balls or antiseptic wipes, tourniquet, sterile gauze squares, and sterile adhesive bandages.

Method

Step Number	Procedure	Points Possible	Points Earned
1.	Review the laboratory request form, and make sure you have the necessary supplies.	2	
2.	Greet the patient, confirm the patient's identity, and introduce yourself.	2	
3.	Explain the purpose of the procedure, and confirm that the patient has followed the pretest instructions.*	10	
4.	Make sure the patient is sitting in a venipuncture chair or is lying down.	2	
5.	Wash your hands. Don exam gloves.	2	
6.	Prepare the safety needle holder/adapter assembly by inserting the threaded side of the needle into the adapter and twisting the adapter in a clockwise direction. Push the first collection tube into the other end of the needle holder/adapter until the outer edge of the collection tube stopper meets the guideline.*	10	
7.	Ask the patient whether one arm is better than the other for the venipuncture. The chosen arm should be positioned slightly downward.	2	
8.	Properly apply the tourniquet to the patient's upper arm midway between the elbow and the shoulder.*	10	
9.	Palpate the proposed site, and use your index finger to locate the vein. Do not draw blood from an artery. If you cannot locate the vein within 1 minute, release the tourniquet and allow blood to flow freely for 1 to 2 minutes. Then reapply the tourniquet and try again to locate the vein.	2	
10.	After locating the vein, clean the area with a cotton ball moistened with antiseptic or an antiseptic wipe. Use a circular motion to clean the area, starting at the center and working outward. Allow the site to air-dry.*	10	

(continued)

Step Number	Procedure	Points Possible	Points Earned
11.	Remove the plastic cap from the outer point of the needle cover, and ask the patient to tighten the fist. Hold the patient's skin taut below the insertion site.*	10	
12.	With a steady and quick motion, insert the needle—held at a 15-degree angle, bevel side up, and aligned parallel to the vein—into the vein. You will feel a slight resistance as the needle tip penetrates the vein wall. Penetrate to a depth of ¼ to ½ inch. Grasp the holder/adapter between your index and great (middle) fingers. Using your thumb, seat the collection tube firmly into place over the needle point, puncturing the rubber stopper. Blood will begin to flow into the collection tube.	2	
13.	Fill each tube until the blood stops running to ensure the correct proportion of blood to additives. Switch tubes as needed by pulling one tube out of the adapter and inserting the next in a smooth and steady motion.	2	
14.	Once blood is flowing steadily, ask the patient to release the fist, and untie the tourniquet by pulling the end of the tucked-in loop. The tourniquet should, in general, be left on no longer than 1 minute. You must remove the tourniquet before you withdraw the needle from the vein.*	10	
15.	As you withdraw the needle in a smooth and steady motion, place a sterile gauze square over the insertion site. Immediately activate the safety device on the needle if it is not self-activating. Properly dispose of the needle immediately. Instruct the patient to hold the gauze pad in place with slight pressure. The patient should keep the arm straight and slightly elevated for several minutes.	2	
16.	If the collection tubes contain additives, you will need to invert them slowly several times.*	10	
17.	Label specimens and complete the paperwork.	2	
18.	Check the patient's condition and the puncture site for bleeding. Replace the sterile gauze square with a sterile adhesive bandage.	2	
19.	Properly dispose of used supplies and disposable instruments, and disinfect the work area.	2	
20.	Remove the gloves and wash your hands.	2	
21.	Instruct the patient about care of the puncture site.	2	
22.	Document the procedure in the patient's chart.	2	
Total Points		100	

CAAHEP Competencies Achieved

  I. P (2)   Perform venipuncture

ABHES Competencies Achieved

   3. (d) Recognize and identify acceptable medical abbreviations

   9. (f) Screen and follow up patient test results

  10. (c) Dispose of Biohazardous materials

  10. (d) Collect, label, and process specimens

       1. Perform venipuncture

PROCEDURE 48-3 Performing Capillary Puncture WORK // DOC

Goal
To collect a capillary blood sample using the finger puncture method.

OSHA Guidelines

Materials
Capillary puncture device (safety lancet or automatic puncture device like an Autolet or Glucolet), antiseptic and cotton balls or antiseptic wipes, sterile gauze squares, sterile adhesive bandages, reagent strips, micropipettes, and smear slides.

Method

Step Number	Procedure	Points Possible	Points Earned
1.	Review the laboratory request form, and make sure you have the necessary supplies.	2	
2.	Greet the patient, confirm the patient's identity, and introduce yourself.	2	
3.	Explain the purpose of the procedure, and confirm that the patient has followed the pretest instructions, if indicated.*	10	
4.	Make sure the patient is sitting in the venipuncture chair or is lying down.*	10	
5.	Wash your hands. Don exam gloves.	2	
6.	Examine the patient's hands to determine which finger to use for the procedure. Avoid fingers that are swollen, bruised, scarred, or calloused. Generally, the ring and great (middle) fingers are the best choices. If you notice the patient's hands are cold, you may want to warm them between your own, have the patient put them in a warm basin of water or under warm running water, or wrap them in a warm cloth.*	10	
7.	Prepare the patient's finger with a gentle "massaging" or rubbing motion toward the fingertip. Keep the patient's hand below heart level so that gravity helps the blood flow.	2	
8.	Clean the area with a cotton ball moistened with antiseptic or an antiseptic wipe. Allow the site to air-dry.*	10	
9.	Hold the patient's finger between your thumb and forefinger. Hold the safety lancet or automatic puncture device at a right angle to the patient's fingerprint. Puncture the skin on the pad of the fingertip with a quick, sharp motion. The depth to which you puncture the skin is generally determined by the length of the lancet point. Most automatic puncturing devices are designed to penetrate to the correct depth.*	10	

(continued)

Copyright © 2014 by The McGraw-Hill Companies, Inc.

Step Number	Procedure	Points Possible	Points Earned
10.	Allow a drop of blood to form at the end of the patient's finger. If the blood droplet is slow in forming, apply steady pressure. Avoid milking the patient's finger.*	10	
11.	Wipe away the first droplet of blood. Then fill the collection devices, as described.* *Micropipettes:* Hold the tip of the tube just to the edge of the blood droplet. The tube will fill through capillary action. If you are preparing microhematocrit tubes, you need to seal one end of each tube with clay sealant. *Reagent strips:* With some reagent strips (dipsticks), you must touch the strip to the blood drop but not smear it; with other strips, you must smear it. Follow the manufacturer's guidelines. *Smear slides:* Gently touch the blood droplet to the smear slide and process the slide as described in Procedure 48-4.	10	
12.	After you have collected the required samples, dispose of the lancet immediately. Then wipe the patient's finger with a sterile gauze square. Instruct the patient to apply pressure to stop the bleeding.	2	
13.	Label specimens and complete the paperwork. Some tests, such as glucose monitoring, must be completed immediately.*	10	
14.	Check the puncture site for bleeding. If necessary, replace the sterile gauze square with a sterile adhesive bandage.	2	
15.	Properly dispose of used supplies and disposable instruments, and disinfect the work area.	2	
16.	Remove the gloves and wash your hands.	2	
17.	Instruct the patient about care of the puncture site.	2	
18.	Document the procedure in the patient's chart. (If the test has been completed, include the results.)	2	
Total Points		100	

CAAHEP Competencies Achieved

I. P (2) Perform capillary puncture

ABHES Competencies Achieved

3. (d) Recognize and identify acceptable medical abbreviations

10. (c) Dispose of Biohazardous materials

10. (d) Collect, label, and process specimens

   2. Perform capillary puncture

PROCEDURE 48-4 Preparing a Blood Smear Slide

Goal
To prepare a blood specimen to be used in a morphologic or other study.

OSHA Guidelines

Materials
Blood specimen (either from a capillary puncture or a specimen tube containing anticoagulated blood), capillary tubes, sterile gauze squares, slide with frosted end, and wooden applicator sticks.

Method

Step Number	Procedure	Points Possible	Points Earned
1.	Wash your hands and don exam gloves.	7	
2.	If using blood from a capillary puncture, follow the steps in Procedure 48-3 to express a drop of blood from the patient's finger. If using a venous sample, check the specimen for proper labeling, carefully uncap the specimen tube, and use wooden applicator sticks to remove any coagulated blood from the inside rim of the tube. You may use a special safety transfer device if available.*	10	
3.	Touch the tip of the capillary tube to the blood specimen either from the patient's finger or the specimen tube. The tube will take up the correct amount through capillary action.	8	
4.	Pull the capillary tube away from the sample, holding it carefully to prevent spillage. Wipe the outside of the capillary tube with a sterile gauze square.	8	
5.	With the slide on the work surface, hold the capillary tube in one hand and the frosted end of the slide against the work surface with the other.	8	
6.	Apply a drop of blood to the slide, about ¾ inch from the frosted end. Place the capillary tube in the sharps container.*	10	
7.	Pick up the spreader slide with your dominant hand. Hold the slide at approximately a 30- to 35-degree angle. Place the edge of the spreader slide on the smear slide close to the unfrosted end. Pull the spreader slide toward the frosted end until the spreader slide touches the blood drop. Capillary action will spread the droplet along the edge of the spreader slide.*	10	
8.	As soon as the drop spreads out to cover most of the spreader slide edge, push the spreader slide back toward the unfrosted end of the smear slide, pulling the sample across the slide behind it. Maintain the 30- to 35-degree angle.*	10	

(continued)

Step Number	Procedure	Points Possible	Points Earned
9.	Continue pushing the spreader until you come off the end, still maintaining the angle. The resulting smear should be approximately 1½ inches long, preferably with a margin of empty slide on all sides.*	10	
10.	Properly label the slide, allow it to dry, and follow the manufacturer's directions for staining it for the required tests.	7	
11.	Properly dispose of used supplies and disinfect the work area.	6	
12.	Remove the gloves and wash your hands.	6	
Total Points		100	

CAAHEP Competencies Achieved

I. P (12)   Perform CLIA-waived hematology testing

ABHES Competencies Achieved

10. (c) Dispose of Biohazardous materials

10. (d) Collect, label, and process specimens

PROCEDURE 48-5 Measuring Hematocrit Percentage WORK//DOC After Centrifuge

Goal

To identify the percentage of a blood specimen represented by RBCs after the sample has been spun in a centrifuge.

OSHA Guidelines

Materials

Blood specimen (either from a capillary puncture or a specimen tube containing anticoagulated blood), microhematocrit tube, sealant tray containing sealing clay, centrifuge, hematocrit gauge, wooden applicator sticks, and gauze squares.

Method

Step Number	Procedure	Points Possible	Points Earned
1.	Wash your hands and don exam gloves.	5	
2.	If using blood from a capillary puncture, follow the steps in Procedure 48-3 to express a drop of blood from the patient's finger. If using a venous blood sample, check the specimen for proper labeling, carefully uncap the specimen tube, and use wooden applicator sticks to remove any coagulated blood from the inside rim of the tube. Alternately, use a special safety transfer device if available.*	10	
3.	Touch the tip of one of the microhematocrit tubes to the blood sample. The tube will take up the correct amount through capillary action.	5	
4.	Pull the microhematocrit tube away from the sample, holding it carefully to prevent spillage. Wipe the outside of the microhematocrit tube with a gauze square.*	10	
5.	Hold the microhematocrit tube in one hand with a gloved finger over one end to prevent leakage, and press the other end of the tube gently into the clay in the sealant tray. The clay plug must completely seal the end of the tube.*	10	
6.	Repeat the process to fill another microhematocrit tube. Tubes must be processed in pairs.*	10	
7.	Place the tubes in the centrifuge, with the sealed ends pointing outward. If you are processing more than one sample, record the position identification number in the patient's chart to track the sample.	5	
8.	Seal the centrifuge chamber.	5	
9.	Run the centrifuge for the required time, usually between 3 and 5 minutes. Allow the centrifuge to come to a complete stop before unsealing it.	5	

(continued)

Step Number	Procedure	Points Possible	Points Earned
10.	Determine the hematocrit percentage by comparing the column of packed RBCs in the microhematocrit tubes with the hematocrit gauge. Position each tube so the boundary between sealing clay and RBCs is at zero on the gauge. Some centrifuges are equipped with gauges, but others require separate handheld gauges.*	10	
11.	Record the percentage value on the gauge that corresponds to the top of the column of RBCs for each tube. Compare the two results. They should not vary by more than 2%. If you record a greater variance, at least one of the tubes was filled incorrectly, and you must repeat the test.	5	
12.	Calculate the average result by adding the two tube figures and dividing that number by 2.	5	
13.	Properly dispose of used supplies, and clean and disinfect the equipment and the area.	5	
14.	Remove the gloves and wash your hands.	5	
15.	Record the test result in the patient's chart. Be sure to identify abnormal results.	5	
Total Points		100	

CAAHEP Competencies Achieved

I. P (12)   Perform CLIA-waived hematology testing

ABHES Competencies Achieved

3. (d) Recognize and identify acceptable medical abbreviations

9. (f) Screen and follow up patient test results

10. (b) Perform selected CLIA-waived tests that assist with diagnosis and treatment

      2. Hematology testing

10. (c) Dispose of Biohazardous materials

10. (d) Collect, label, and process specimens

PROCEDURE 48-6 Measuring Blood Glucose Using a Handheld Glucometer

WORK // DOC

Goal
To measure the amount of glucose present in a blood sample.

OSHA Guidelines

Materials
Safety engineered capillary puncture device (automatic puncture device or other safety lancet), antiseptic and cotton balls or antiseptic wipes, sterile gauze squares, sterile adhesive bandages, handheld glucometer, and reagent strips appropriate for the device.

Method

Step Number	Procedure	Points Possible	Points Earned
1.	Wash your hands and don exam gloves.	5	
2.	Review the manufacturer's instructions for the specific device used.	5	
3.	Check the expiration date on the reagent strips.*	10	
4.	Code the meter to the reagent strips if required.*	10	
5.	Turn the device on according to the manufacturer's instructions.	5	
6.	Perform the required quality control procedures.*	10	
7.	Insert the strip into the meter following the manufacturer's instructions.	5	
8.	Perform a capillary puncture following the steps outlined in Procedure 48-3.	5	
9.	Touch the drop of blood to the reagent strip, allowing it to be taken up by the strip.*	10	
10.	Read the digital result after the required amount of time.*	10	
11.	Discard the reagent strip and used supplies according to OSHA standards.	5	
12.	Record the time of the test and the result on the laboratory slip.	5	
13.	Disinfect the equipment and area.	5	
14.	Remove the gloves and wash your hands.	5	
15.	Document the test results in the patient's chart. Record the quality control tests in the laboratory control log.	5	
Total Points		100	

CAAHEP Competencies Achieved

    I. P (12)   Perform CLIA-waived chemistry testing

ABHES Competencies Achieved

    9. (f) Screen and follow up patient test results

  10. (a) Practice quality control

  10. (b) Perform selected CLIA-waived tests that assist with diagnosis and treatment

        3. Chemistry testing

  10. (c) Dispose of Biohazardous materials

  10. (d) Collect, label, and process specimens

PROCEDURE 48-7 Rapid Infectious Mononucleosis Test   [WORK // DOC]

Goal

To determine the presence of antibodies associated with infectious mononucleosis using whole blood, serum, or plasma.

OSHA Guidelines

Materials

Infectious mononucleosis test kit, patient blood sample, and a watch or timer.

Method

Step Number	Procedure	Points Possible	Points Earned
1.	Review the laboratory request form and gather the necessary supplies.	5	
2.	Greet the patient, confirm the patient's identity, and introduce yourself.	5	
3.	Explain the procedure.	5	
4.	Wash your hands and don required PPE.	5	
5.	Obtain a sample of the patient's blood using appropriate venipuncture technique.*	10	
6.	Process the blood sample to obtain whole blood, plasma, or serum as required by the testing procedure.	5	
7.	Open the test kit and check the expiration date.	5	
8.	Run the recommended controls according to manufacturer's instructions.*	10	
9.	Place the required amount of blood, serum, or plasma onto the testing device, following manufacturer's instructions.	5	
10.	Add testing reagent or reagents to the testing device, according to manufacturer's instructions.*	10	
11.	Wait the required amount of time. Do not go over the recommended time.*	10	
12.	Read the results and record them in the patient's chart.	5	
13.	Discard the testing supplies according to OSHA regulations.	5	
14.	Disinfect the work area.	5	
15.	Remove your PPE and wash your hands.	5	
16.	Document the results in the patient's chart.	5	
Total Points		100	

CAAHEP Competencies Achieved

I. P. (15)   Perform CLIA waived immunology testing

ABHES Competencies Achieved

9. (f) Screen and follow up patient test results

10. (a) Practice quality control

10. (b) Perform selected CLIA-waived tests that assist with diagnosis and treatment

   3. Chemistry testing

10. (c) Dispose of Biohazardous materials

10. (d) Collect, label, and process specimens

Electrocardiography and Pulmonary Function Testing

Name_____ Class_____ Date_____

R E V I E W

Vocabulary Review

Matching
Match the key terms in the right column with the definitions in the left column by placing the letter of each correct answer in the space provided.

_____ 1. The condition of having two separate poles, one of which is positive and the other negative

_____ 2. An electrical impulse that initiates a chain reaction, resulting in a contraction of the heart muscle

_____ 3. A period of electrical recovery during which polarity is restored

4. An instrument that measures and displays the electrical impulses responsible for the cardiac cycle

_____ 5. A wave recorded on an electrocardiogram that is produced by the electrical impulses responsible for the cardiac cycle

_____ 6. An erroneous mark or defect on an ECG tracing

_____ 7. An irregularity in heart rhythm

_____ 8. An instrument that measures the activity of the heart in a 24-hour period

_____ 9. The greatest volume of air that a person can expel when performing rapid, forced expiration

_____ 10. A standardized measuring instrument used to calibrate a spirometer

a. calibration syringe
b. forced vital capacity
c. Holter monitor
d. polarity
e. depolarization
f. arrhythmia
g. repolarization
h. artifact
i. electrocardiogram
j. deflection

True or False
Decide whether each statement is true or false. In the space at the left, write T for true or F for false. On the lines provided, rewrite the false statements to make them true.

_____ 11. Spirometry measures the air taken in by and expelled from the lungs.

_____

_____ 12. A spirometer or peak flow meter is used to measure breathing capacity.

_____

_____ 13. A heart attack is referred to as a myocardial infarction.

_____

_____ 14. A lead is attached to the patient's skin during electrocardiography.

_____

_____ **15.** A pen-like instrument that records movement on ECG paper is called a stylus.

_____ **16.** An instrument that measures and displays the electrical impulses responsible for the cardiac cycle is referred to as an electrocardiography.

_____ **17.** An electrolyte is a substance that decreases transmission of electrical impulses.

_____ **18.** The atrioventricular node is a mass of specialized conducting cells located at the bottom of the right atrium that delays transmission of electrical impulses so the atria can completely contract.

_____ **19.** The bundle of His is an area of specialized conductive tissue in the heart that sends impulses through a series of bundle branches.

_____ **20.** The sequence of contraction and relaxation is referred to as a pulmonary cycle.

_____ **21.** A procedure that measures and evaluates a patient's lung capacity and volume is referred to as a pulmonary function test.

_____ **22.** The process by which a graphic pattern is created from the electrical impulses generated within the heart as it pumps is called repolarization.

Content Review

Multiple Choice

In the space provided, write the letter of the choice that best completes each statement or answers each question.

_____ **1.** When performing routine electrocardiography, you place electrodes on the
  a. Right arm, left arm, right leg, left leg, and six on the chest
  b. Right arm, left arm, right temple, left temple, and six on the chest
  c. Right arm, right leg, and five on the chest
  d. Right arm, left arm, and one on the chest, which is moved to six different positions
  e. Right leg, left leg, right hip, left hip, and three on the chest

_____ **2.** Augmented leads monitor
  a. Bipolar leads
  b. One electrode and a point within the heart
  c. One limb electrode and a point midway between two other limb electrodes
  d. Electrical activity between two limb electrodes
  e. All leads at once

_____ **3.** A flat line on the ECG tracing of one of the leads is typically caused by
  a. Switching two of the wires
  b. A loose or disconnected wire
  c. A loose or disconnected patient cable
  d. Cardiac arrest
  e. None of the above

_____ 4. A patient who is to wear a Holter monitor should be instructed
   a. To take baths rather than showers
   b. To avoid excessive or unusual exercise
   c. In how to remove the electrodes before going to bed and how to replace them in the morning
   d. To keep a written record of activities, emotional upsets, physical symptoms, and medications
   e. To stop the recording while eating

_____ 5. When administering spirometry,
   a. Emergency resuscitation equipment should always be in the room
   b. Explain the procedure, but once the test begins, avoid coaching patients on their performance
   c. Position the patient with the chin slightly elevated and the neck slightly extended
   d. Position the patient with the chin bent slightly toward the chest and the back straight
   e. Have the patient recline in the chair during the procedure

_____ 6. Electrocardiography records the transmission, _____, and duration of the various electrical impulses of the heart.
   a. Heart rate   d. Blood pressure
   b. Magnitude   c. Strength
   c. Amplification

_____ 7. A single-channel electrocardiograph records the electrical activity of one lead, whereas a(n) _____ electrocardiograph records more than one lead at a time.
   a. Deflection   d. Electronic
   b. Pulse oximeter   e. Rhythm strip
   c. Multichannel

_____ 8. To ensure the conductivity of electrical impulses from the skin, you must apply _____ to each electrode before placing it on the patient's body.
   a. Alcohol   d. Lotion
   b. Soap and water   e. An electrolyte
   c. Talcum powder

_____ 9. On an electrocardiograph, the _____ is used to adjust the position of the stylus.
   a. Sensitivity selector
   b. Amplifier
   c. Centering control
   d. Default switch
   e. Interpretative mode

_____ 10. Exercise electrocardiography typically continues until the patient reaches a(n) _____, has chest pain or fatigue, or develops complications.
   a. Arrhythmia
   b. Target heart rate
   c. Personal best peak expiratory flow rate
   d. Exhaustion rate
   e. Specified amount of time

_____ 11. Why is it important for a medical assistant to recognize abnormal heart rhythms?
   a. To effectively triage a medical emergency
   b. To alert the physician or nurse that the patient has an irregular ECG
   c. To take control of the medical emergency
   d. Both a and b
   e. Both a and c

_____ **12.** The cardiac arrhythmia that resembles a "saw tooth" is

    a. A bundle branch block

    b. Ventricular fibrillation

    c. Atrial tachycardia

    d. Bradycardia

    e. Sinus tachycardia

_____ **13.** The green zone on the peak flow zone chart indicates

    a. Good asthma control

    b. That airways are beginning to narrow

    c. That airways are constricted

    d. Low oxygen saturation

    e. 70% of the highest peak flow rate

_____ **14.** Patient symptoms that include wheezing, shortness of breath, and difficulty talking and/or walking indicate patients in the _____ zone.

    a. Green

    b. Red

    c. Yellow

    d. Black

    e. Safe

_____ **15.** The noninvasive procedure that measures oxygen saturation in blood is

    a. Peak flow

    b. Arterial blood gases

    c. Pulse oximetry

    d. ECG

    e. Forced vital capacity

Short Answer

Write the answer to each question on the lines provided.

16. Briefly describe the heart's process of conduction.

_____

_____

_____

17. Examine the following ECG tracings. Then follow the directions.

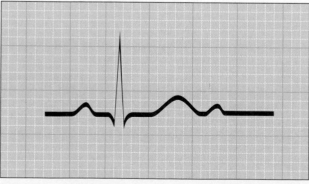

(a)

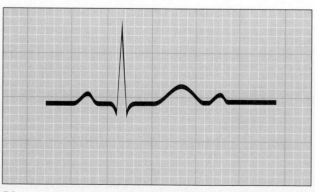

(b)

Source: Courtesy of Cardiac Science Corporation, Milton, Wisconsin.

a. Circle and label the QRS complex on part (a).

b. Label the R wave on part (a).

c. Label the T wave on part (a).

d. Label the P wave on part (a).

e. On part (b), draw lines and label the tracing to show when atrial relaxation occurs.

f. On part (b), draw an arrow and label the tracing to show when atrial contraction takes place.

g. On part (b), draw an arrow and label the tracing to show when repolarization takes place.

18. Review the abnormal ECG tracings and label each cardiac arrhythmia.

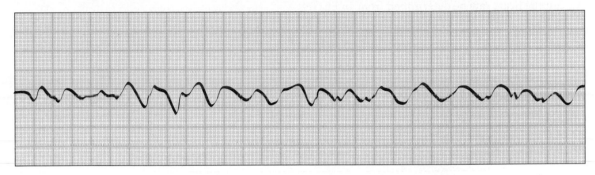

a

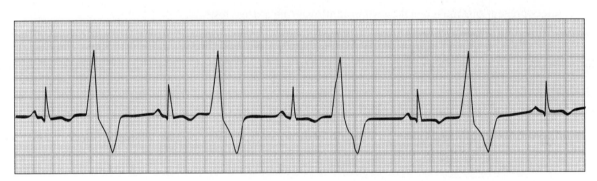

b

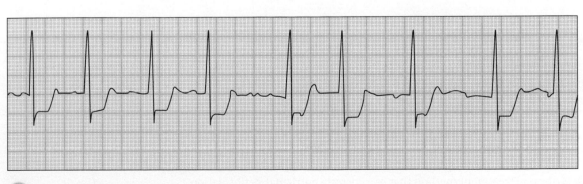

c

Source: Courtesy of Cardiac Science Corporation, Milton, Wisconsin.

19. What are four possible causes of mechanical problems that can result in a wandering baseline?

_____

_____

_____

20. How do muscles cause somatic interference that shows up as artifacts on ECG tracings?

_____

_____

_____

21. How can the heart rate be determined from an ECG?

_____

_____

_____

22. While calibrating the spirometer, you notice that the reading is getting progressively less each time you calibrate. What could be the cause? What should you do?

_____

_____

_____

23. What safety precautions must be taken when administering a stress test?

_____

_____

_____

24. What are four conditions and activities that can affect the outcome of a spirometry test?

_____

_____

_____

25. An acceptable maneuver on a spirometer must have what five features?

_____

_____

_____

26. Describe what occurs during a premature ventricular contraction.

_____

_____

_____

27. Describe one treatment method that can correct ventricular defibrillation.

_____

_____

_____

28. List three causes of atrial fibrillation.

_____

_____

_____

29. What should a patient do if his or her peak expiratory flow is in the red zone?

_____

_____

_____

30. What is the normal range for the peak expiratory flow rate?

_____

_____

_____

Critical Thinking

Write the answer to each question on the lines provided.

1. What may happen if you fail to allow the electrocardiograph to warm up properly?

_____

_____

_____

2. Why might a physician order a series of ECGs for a patient after he has changed her medication?

_____

_____

_____

3. In what situation might it be better to position the electrodes on the upper arms and the thighs rather than lower on the arms and legs?

_____

_____

_____

4. A patient has complained of periodic arrhythmias, but repeated ECGs have not shown any evidence of them. Why might the doctor order a Holter monitor to be used by the patient?

_____

_____

_____

5. What is the purpose of coaching the patient to improve performance during spirometry?

_____

_____

_____

6. Why is averaging the readings of the peak expiratory flow rate not recommended?

_____

_____

_____

7. While observing a pulse oximetry, you notice the reading states 89%. What should you do and why?

_____

_____

_____

A P P L I C A T I O N

Follow the directions for the application.

Preparing a Patient for Electrocardiography

Working with two partners, prepare a patient for electrocardiography. One partner should play the role of the patient, one should take the role of the medical assistant preparing the patient for the procedure, and the third should act as an observer and evaluator. The patient is elderly and is anxious about the procedure.

a. The medical assistant should introduce herself and explain the procedure to the patient. The patient should ask questions and express concerns about what will happen and what he will experience. The medical assistant should answer all questions to the best of her ability and provide help in allaying the patient's anxieties.

b. The medical assistant should help the patient get into position for the procedure, helping him find the position that is most comfortable.

c. Following the preparation, the observer should critique what the medical assistant did. The critique should include the assistant's skill in communicating with the patient, the accuracy of her descriptions of the procedure, her responses to the patient's questions, how well the medical assistant succeeded in allaying the patient's concerns, and the effectiveness of the assistant's positioning of the patient.

d. As a team, discuss the observer's critique, noting the strengths and weaknesses of preparation of the patient for the procedure.

e. Exchange roles and repeat the preparation for another procedure, such as spirometry, peak flow, or providing a patient with a Holter monitor. The new observer should choose the type of procedure.

f. Exchange roles one final time so that each team member plays all three roles once.

C A S E   S T U D I E S

Write your response to each case study on the lines provided.

Case 1

After completing an ECG on a patient, you examine the tracing and find the wave peaks are very low, making it difficult to clearly read the tracing. What should you do?

_____

_____

_____

Case 2

While performing an ECG on a 55-year-old female patient, you note that all of the limb electrodes are coming off. What might cause the electrodes to come off of the patient's arms and legs? What action should you take?

_____

_____

_____

Case 3

Sam Smith is recovering from a heart attack. While you are preparing him for a stress test to determine how his heart is functioning, Mr. Smith expresses his fears. He is afraid the test will cause another heart attack. What do you tell him?

_____

_____

_____

Case 4

You are administering spirometry to a patient. She has been very cooperative but is having difficulty achieving the three acceptable maneuvers that are required. After several attempts, she complains of dizziness. You check her pulse and blood pressure and find that both are significantly elevated. What should you do?

_____

_____

_____

Case 5

You are working in an outpatient surgical clinic in the preoperative holding area. Each patient is monitored with a pulse oximeter. You check Mrs. O'Shaughnessy's fingers and notice that they are cold to the touch and have poor blood return. What should you do?

_____

_____

_____

PROCEDURE 49-1 Obtaining an ECG   WORK // DOC

Goal
To obtain a graphic representation of the electrical activity of a patient's heart.

OSHA Guidelines

Materials
Electrocardiograph, ECG paper, electrodes, electrolyte preparation, wires, patient gown, drape, blanket, pillows, gauze pads, alcohol, moist towel, and scissors for trimming hair (if needed).

Method

Step Number	Procedure	Points Possible	Points Earned
1.	Turn on the electrocardiograph and, if necessary, allow the stylus to heat up.	3	
2.	Identify the patient, introduce yourself, and explain the procedure.	3	
3.	Wash your hands.	3	
4.	Ask the patient to disrobe from the waist up and remove jewelry, socks or stockings, bra, and shoes. If the electrodes will be placed on the patient's legs, have the patient roll up his or her pant legs. Sometimes the electrodes are placed on the sides of the lower abdomen—check the manufacturer's instructions. Provide a gown if the patient is female, and instruct her to wear the gown with the opening in front.	3	
5.	Assist the patient onto the table and into a supine position. Cover the patient with a drape (and a blanket if the room is cool). If the patient experiences difficulty breathing or cannot tolerate lying flat, use a Fowler's or semi-Fowler's position, adjusting with pillows under the head and knees for comfort if needed.	3	
6.	Tell the patient to rest quietly and breathe normally. Explain the importance of lying still to prevent false readings.	3	
7.	Wash the patient's skin, using gauze pads moistened with alcohol. If needed, rub it vigorously with dry gauze pads to promote better contact of the electrodes.*	6	
8.	If the patient's leg or chest hair is dense, use a small pair of scissors to closely trim the hair where you will attach the electrode. (Shaving is not recommended because of the risk of bleeding and infection.)	3	
9.	Apply electrodes to fleshy portions of the limbs, making sure the electrodes on one arm and leg are placed similarly to those on the other arm and leg. Attach electrodes to areas that are not bony or muscular. The arm lead tabs on the electrode point downward and the electrode tabs for the leg leads point upward. Peel off the backings of the disposable electrodes and press them into place.*	6	
10.	Apply the precordial electrodes at specified locations on the chest. Precordial electrode tabs point downward.*	6	
11.	Attach wires and cables, making sure all wire tips follow the patient's body contours.*	6	

(continued)

Step Number	Procedure	Points Possible	Points Earned
12.	Check all electrodes and wires for proper placement and connection; drape wires over the patient to avoid creating tension on the electrodes that could result in artifacts *	6	
13.	Enter the patient data into the electrocardiograph. Press the on, run, or record button. Standardize the machine, if necessary, by following these steps: a. Set the paper speed to 25 mm per second or as instructed. b. Set the sensitivity setting to 1 or as instructed. c. Turn the lead selector to standardization mode. d. Adjust the stylus so the baseline is centered. e. Press the standardization button. The stylus should move upward above the baseline 10 mm (two large squares).	3	
14.	Run the ECG.* a. If the machine has an automatic feature, set the lead selector to automatic. b. For manual tracings, turn the lead selector to standby mode. Select the first lead (I), and record the tracing. Switch the machine to standby, and then repeat the procedure for all 12 leads.	6	
15.	Check tracings for artifacts.	3	
16.	Correct problems and repeat any tracings that are not clear.	3	
17.	Disconnect the patient from the machine.	3	
18.	Remove the tracing from the machine, and label it with the patient's name, the date, and your initials.	3	
19.	Disconnect the wires from the electrodes, and remove the electrodes from the patient.	3	
20.	Clean the patient's skin with a moist towel.	3	
21.	Assist the patient into a sitting position.	3	
22.	Allow a moment for rest, and then assist the patient from the table.	4	
23.	Assist the patient in dressing if necessary, or allow the patient privacy to dress.	3	
24.	Wash your hands.	3	
25.	Record the procedure in the patient's chart.	3	
26.	Properly dispose of used materials and disposable electrodes.	3	
27.	Clean and disinfect the equipment and the room according to OSHA guidelines.	3	
Total Points		100	

CAAHEP Competencies Achieved

I. P (5)   Perform electrocardiography

ABHES Competencies Achieved

2. (c) Assist the physician with the regimen of diagnostic and treatment modalities as they relate to each body system

9. (o) Perform:

1. Electrocardiograms

PROCEDURE 49-2 Holter Monitoring

WORK // DOC

Goal
To monitor the electrical activity of a patient's heart over a 24-hour period to detect cardiac abnormalities that may go undetected during routine electrocardiography or stress testing.

OSHA Guidelines

Materials
Holter monitor, battery, cassette tape, patient diary or log, alcohol, gauze pads, disposable shaving supplies, disposable electrodes, hypoallergenic tape, drape, and electrocardiograph.

Method

Step Number	Procedure	Points Possible	Points Earned
1.	Identify the patient, introduce yourself, and explain the procedure.	5	
2.	Ask the patient to remove clothing from the waist up; provide a drape if necessary.	4	
3.	Wash your hands and assemble the equipment.	4	
4.	Assist the patient into a comfortable position (sitting or supine).	3	
5.	If the patient's body hair is particularly dense, don examination gloves and trim the areas where the electrodes will be attached.	4	
6.	Clean the electrode sites with alcohol and gauze.*	7	
7.	Rub each electrode site vigorously with a dry gauze square.	5	
8.	Attach wires to the electrodes, and peel off the paper backing on the electrodes. Apply electrodes, pressing firmly to ensure that each electrode is securely attached and is making good contact with the skin.*	7	
9.	Attach the patient cable.*	7	
10.	Insert a fresh battery, and position the unit.*	7	
11.	Tape wires, cable, and electrodes as necessary to avoid tension on the wires as the patient moves.*	7	
12.	Insert the cassette tape if applicable, and turn on the unit .*	7	
13.	If the unit uses a cassette tape, confirm that the tape or other recording device is actually running. Indicate the start time in the patient's chart.*	7	
14.	Instruct the patient on proper use of the monitor and how to enter information in the diary. Caution the patient not to alter any diary entries; it is crucial to know what the patient is doing at all times.*	7	
15.	Schedule the patient's return visit for the same time on the following day.	5	
16.	On the following day, remove the electrodes, discard them, and clean the electrode sites.	5	
17.	Wash your hands.	4	

(continued)

Step Number	Procedure	Points Possible	Points Earned
18.	Remove the cassette tape and obtain a printout of the tracing OR transfer the data from the monitor to patient's electronic chart according to office procedure and the manufacturer's directions. Document all parts of the procedure.	5	
Total Points		100	

CAAHEP Competencies Achieved

I. P (5)   Perform electrocardiography

ABHES Competencies Achieved

2. (c) Assist the physician with the regimen of diagnostic and treatment modalities as they relate to each body system

9. (o) Perform:

1. Electrocardiograms

PROCEDURE 49-3 Measuring Forced Vital Capacity Using Spirometry [WORK//DOC]

Goal
To determine a patient's forced vital capacity using a volume-displacing spirometer.

OSHA Guidelines

Materials
Adult scale with height bar, spirometer, patient tubing (tubing that runs from the mouthpiece to the machine), mouthpiece, nose clip, and disinfectant.

Method

Step Number	Procedure	Points Possible	Points Earned
1.	Prepare the equipment. Ensure the paper supply in the machine is adequate.	5	
2.	Calibrate the machine as necessary.*	6	
3.	Identify the patient and introduce yourself.	3	
4.	Check the patient's chart to see whether there are special instructions to follow.	3	
5.	Ask whether the patient has followed instructions.	3	
6.	Wash your hands and don examination gloves.	5	
7.	Measure and record the patient's height and weight.*	6	
8.	Explain the proper positioning.*	6	
9.	Explain the procedure.	5	
10.	Demonstrate the procedure.*	6	
11.	Turn on the spirometer, and enter applicable patient data and the number of tests to be performed.	5	
12.	Ensure the patient has loosened any tight clothing, is comfortable, and is in the proper position. Apply the nose clip.*	6	
13.	Have the patient perform the first maneuver, coaching when necessary.*	6	
14.	Determine whether the maneuver is acceptable.	5	
15.	Offer feedback to the patient and recommendations for improvement if necessary.*	6	
16.	Have the patient perform additional maneuvers until three acceptable maneuvers are obtained.	5	
17.	Record the procedure in the patient's chart, and place the chart and the test results on the physician's desk for interpretation.	5	
18.	Ask the patient to remain until the physician reviews the results.	5	
19.	Properly dispose of used materials and disposable instruments.	3	

(continued)

Step Number	Procedure	Points Possible	Points Earned
20.	Sanitize and disinfect patient tubing, reusable mouthpiece, and nose clip.	3	
21.	Clean and disinfect the equipment and room according to OSHA guidelines.	3	
Total Points		100	

CAAHEP Competencies Achieved

I. P (4)   Perform pulmonary function testing

ABHES Competencies Achieved

2. (c) Assist the physician with the regimen of diagnostic and treatment modalities as they relate to each body system

9. (o) Perform:

2. Respiratory testing

PROCEDURE 49-4 Obtaining a Peak Expiratory Flow Rate

WORK // DOC

Goal
To determine a patient's peak expiratory flow rate.

OSHA Guidelines

Materials
Peak flow meter and a disposable mouthpiece.

Method

Step Number	Procedure	Points Possible	Points Earned
1.	Assemble all necessary equipment and supplies for the test.	4	
2.	Wash your hands and identify the patient.	4	
3.	Explain and demonstrate the procedure to the patient *	10	
4.	Position the patient in a sitting or standing position with good posture. Make sure any chewing gum or food is removed from the patient's mouth.*	10	
5.	Set the indicator to zero.*	10	
6.	Ensure the disposable mouthpiece is securely placed onto the peak flow meter.	4	
7.	Hold the peak flow meter with the gauge uppermost, and ensure your fingers are away from the gauge.	4	
8.	Instruct the patient to take as deep a breath as possible.*	10	
9.	Instruct the patient to place the mouthpiece into his mouth and close his lips tightly around the mouthpiece, sealing his lips around it.	4	
10.	Instruct the patient to blow out as fast and as hard as possible.*	10	
11.	Observe the reading where the arrowhead is on the indicator.	4	
12.	Reset the indicator to zero and repeat the procedure two times, for a total of three readings. You will know the technique is correct if the reading results are close. If coughing occurs during the procedures, repeat the step.	4	
13.	Document the readings into the patient's chart. The highest reading will be the peak flow rate.*	10	
14.	Dispose of the mouthpiece in a biohazardous waste container.	4	
15.	Disinfect or dispose of the peak flow meter per office policy.	4	
16.	Wash your hands.	4	
Total Points		100	

CAAHEP Competencies Achieved

I. P (4)   Perform pulmonary function testing

ABHES Competencies Achieved

2. (c) Assist the physician with the regimen of diagnostic and treatment modalities as they relate to each body system

9. (o) Perform:

   2. Respiratory testing

PROCEDURE 49-5 Obtaining a Pulse Oximetry Reading

WORK // DOC

Goal
To obtain a pulse oximetry reading.

OSHA Guidelines

Materials
Pulse oximeter.

Method

Step Number	Procedure	Points Possible	Points Earned
1.	Assemble all the necessary equipment and supplies.	5	
2.	Wash your hands and correctly identify the patient.	5	
3.	Select the appropriate site to apply the sensor to by assessing capillary refill in the patient's toe or finger.*	15	
4.	Prepare the selected site, removing nail polish or earrings if necessary. Wipe the selected site with alcohol and allow it to air dry.*	15	
5.	Attach the sensor to the site (if a finger is used, place in the clip).*	15	
6.	Instruct the patient to breathe normally.	10	
7.	Attach the sensor cable to the oximeter. Turn on the oximeter and listen to the tone.	5	
8.	Set the alarm limits for high and low oxygen saturations and high and low pulse rates, as directed by the physician's order, and turn on the oximeter.	10	
9.	Read the saturation level and document it in the patient's chart. Report to the physician readings that are less than 95%. Manually check the patient's pulse and compare it to the pulse oximeter. Document all the readings and the application site in the patient's medical chart.	10	
10.	Wash your hands.	5	
11.	Rotate the patient's finger sites every four hours if using a pulse oximeter long-term.	5	
Total Points		100	

CAAHEP Competencies Achieved

I. P (4)   Perform pulmonary function testing

ABHES Competencies Achieved

2. (c) Assist the physician with the regimen of diagnostic and treatment modalities as they relate to each body system

9. (o) Perform:

   2. Respiratory testing

50

Diagnostic Imaging

Name_____ Class_____ Date_____

R E V I E W

Vocabulary Review

Matching

Match the key terms in the right column with the definitions in the left column by placing the letter of each correct answer in the space provided.

_____ **1.** Contrast medium is injected through a urethral catheter to evaluate the function of the ureters, bladder, and urethra

_____ **2.** A type of radiation therapy that allows deep penetration of tissue to treat deep tumors

_____ **3.** The use of radionuclides or radioisotopes to evaluate the bone, brain, lungs, kidneys, liver, pancreas, thyroid, or spleen

_____ **4.** A nuclear medicine procedure used to locate and determine the extent of brain damage from a stroke

_____ **5.** An X-ray exam of the internal breast tissues

_____ **6.** An X-ray of the abdomen used to assess the urinary organs, evaluate urinary system diseases or disorders, and detect kidney stones

_____ **7.** A series of X-rays taken while an IV contrast medium travels through the kidneys, ureters, and bladder

_____ **8.** A type of radiation therapy that uses radioactive implants close to or directly in cancerous tissue to treat the tumor

_____ **9.** A test used to detect gallstones and other abnormalities of the gallbladder

_____ **10.** An X-ray procedure in which barium sulfate is instilled through the anus into the rectum and then into the colon to help diagnose abnormalities of the colon or rectum

_____ **11.** An invasive procedure that requires the insertion of a catheter, wire, or other testing device into a patient's blood vessel to obtain an image of the vessel

_____ **12.** The use of X-ray technology for diagnostic purposes

_____ **13.** The use of special ultrasound technology to study blood flow through vessels

a. angiography
b. barium enema
c. brachytherapy
d. cholecystography
e. doppler echocardiography
f. intravenous pyelogram
g. diagnostic radiology
h. KUB radiography
i. mammography
j. nuclear medicine
k. SPECT
l. teletherapy
m. retrograde pyelography

True or False

Decide whether each statement is true or false. In the space at the left, write T for true or F for false. On the lines provided, rewrite the false statements to make them true.

_____ **14.** A contrast medium makes internal organs denser and blocks the passage of X-rays to the photographic film.

_____

_____ 15. Standard X-rays and ultrasound, which do not require inserting devices or breaking the skin, are types of invasive procedures.

_____

_____ 16. A MUGA scan is a type of nuclear medicine test used to evaluate the condition of the heart's myocardium.

_____

_____ 17. For patients with poor kidney function, doctors often use an IVP to evaluate the function of the ureters, bladder, and urethra.

_____

_____ 18. Myelography is a type of fluoroscopy of the abdomen.

_____

_____ 19. A dosimeter is a radiation exposure badge that contains a sensitized piece of film.

_____

_____ 20. In PET, special isotopes emit positrons, which are processed by computer and viewed to diagnose brain-related conditions.

_____

_____ 21. In ultrasound, low-frequency sound waves directed through the skin produce echoes that are converted by computer into an image on a screen.

_____

_____ 22. 4-D ultrasound provides live-action images for observation of fetal movement.

_____

_____ 23. Radiation therapy is used to treat cancer by promoting cellular reproduction.

_____

_____ 24. A roentgen ray is another name for an X-ray.

_____

_____ 25. Hysterosalpingography is a radiological exam of a vagina.

_____

Content Review

Multiple Choice

In the space provided, write the letter of the choice that best completes each statement or answers each question.

_____ 1. An X-ray is a type of electromagnetic wave that has a
   a. Low energy level and an extremely long wavelength
   b. Low energy level and an extremely short wavelength
   c. High energy level and an extremely short wavelength
   d. High energy level and an extremely long wavelength
   e. Low energy level and a variable wavelength

_____ 2. A test that utilizes a contrast medium and fluoroscopy to help diagnose abnormalities or injuries in the cartilage, tendons, or ligaments of the joints is called
   a. Arthrography   d. Angiography
   b. Cholangiography   e. Tomography
   c. Thermography

_____ 3. Which of the following duties in connection with diagnostic radiology are medical assistants most likely to perform?

   a. Operating X-ray equipment

   b. Assisting a radiologist with X-ray procedures

   c. Assisting a radiologic technologist with X-ray procedures

   d. Providing preprocedure and postprocedure patient care

   e. Repairing X-ray equipment

_____ 4. Angiography requires insertion of a catheter into a patient's

   a. Knee or shoulder

   b. Pancreatic duct

   c. Urethra

   d. Common bile duct

   e. Blood vessel

_____ 5. During which of the following procedures does the patient eat a specially prepared fatty meal?

   a. Cholecystography

   b. Cholangiography

   c. A barium swallow

   d. An intravenous pyelogram

   e. A MUGA scan

_____ 6. The test that uses nonionizing radiation and a strong magnetic field is known as

   a. SPECT

   b. CT

   c. PET

   d. MRI

   e. CAT

_____ 7. Myelography is a fluoroscopic exam of the

   a. Heart

   b. Spinal cord

   c. Bone marrow

   d. Gallbladder

   e. Liver

_____ 8. The digital storage area where digital images are sent and stored for diagnostic viewing and electronic image storage and distribution is known as

   a. DICOM

   b. IHE

   c. PAC

   d. EHR

   e. CMS

_____ 9. Stereotaxis is an example of

   a. Magnetic resonance imaging

   b. Nuclear medicine

   c. Stereoscopy

   d. Teletherapy

   e. Echocardiography

Sentence Completion

In the space provided, write the word or phrase that best completes each sentence.

10. _____ is a type of ultrasound test used to study the structure and function of the heart.

11. Before an MRI, it is important to determine whether the patient has any internal _____ materials.

12. In a double-contrast barium enema, _____ is forced into the colon to distend the tissue.

13. During an IVP, a radiologist injects a contrast medium into a patient's _____.

14. A test used to help diagnose and evaluate obstructions, ulcers, polyps, diverticulosis, tumors, or motility problems of the esophagus, stomach, duodenum, and small intestine is a _____ swallow.

15. A type of teletherapy that uses CT or MRI scanning in conjunction with radiation to treat brain tumors, acoustic neuromas, and arteriovenous malformations is _____ radiosurgery.

16. The _____ dense areas of an X-ray are the lightest on the film.

17. Prior to having a mammogram, a patient should not use _____, powders, or perfumes.

10. _____

11. _____

12. _____

13. _____

14. _____

15. _____

16. _____

17. _____

Short Answer

Write the answer to each question on the lines provided.

18. What are four general duties that medical assistants may perform for patients who will undergo radiologic testing?

_____

_____

_____

19. Why are contrast media used in some diagnostic radiologic tests? List three ways that contrast media can be administered.

_____

_____

_____

20. Describe the mechanics of the diagnostic procedure fluoroscopy.

_____

_____

_____

21. Why do some radiologic diagnostic procedures require patients to be admitted to a hospital or same-day surgical facility? Give one example of such a procedure.

_____

_____

_____

22. How are conventional tomography and computed tomography similar? How are they different?

_____

_____

_____

23. Describe three ways for medical assistants to protect themselves against excessive radiation exposure.

_____

_____

_____

24. What four items of information about a patient's X-rays should be documented in the patient report card or record book?

_____

_____

_____

25. How might a cardiologist use electronic medicine to monitor a patient from afar?

_____

_____

_____

26. For what conditions do radiologists assess when performing a hysterosalpingography?

_____

_____

_____

27. What is the difference between PAC and DICOM?

_____

_____

_____

28. What are three advantages of digital radiography?

_____

_____

_____

Critical Thinking

Write the answer to each question on the lines provided.

1. Why is it important to take an X-ray only within 10 days of the last menstrual period for women of childbearing age?

_____

_____

_____

2. How might a patient undergoing an invasive radiologic diagnostic procedure be at greater risk than a patient undergoing a noninvasive procedure?

_____

_____

_____

3. Why is preprocedure care especially important for patients who are scheduled to undergo an MRI?

_____

_____

_____

4. Why is it important for the patient to remain still during an X-ray exam?

_____

_____

_____

5. How could a radiologist use electronic medicine to interpret and report on a tomogram produced in another country?

_____

_____

_____

6. Why is it important to ask a patient if they have had a previous mammogram when assisting a patient with setting up an appointment for a mammogram?

_____

_____

_____

A P P L I C A T I O N

Follow the directions for each application.

1. Preparing a Patient for a Radiologic Diagnostic Test

Work with two partners. One student should take the role of a patient scheduled for a radiologic diagnostic procedure in a few days. The second student should assume the role of medical assistant in a radiology facility or medical office. The third student should act as an observer and evaluator.

a. Choose one of the following procedures: arthrography, barium enema, barium swallow, cholecystography, CT scan with contrast medium, or IVP. Review the description of the chosen procedure and the preprocedure care steps.

b. The medical assistant should schedule a time for the procedure with the patient, taking into account such factors as whether the patient's digestive tract must be empty and whether the patient will want to sleep through the procedure to avoid experiencing hunger.

c. The medical assistant should describe the procedure to the patient according to the guidelines presented in the student textbook. The patient should ask questions about the procedure, which the medical assistant should answer clearly and completely.

d. The medical assistant should explain the preparation instructions. The patient should ask questions about the instructions. The medical assistant may want to have the patient repeat the instructions to ensure that the patient understands them.

e. After the instructions have been given and the patient's questions have been answered, the observer should provide a critique of the medical assistant's preprocedure care. Comments should include positive feedback and suggestions for improvement.

f. Change roles and repeat the exercise, using a different diagnostic test. Then change roles again so that each student has a turn at each role and all students become familiar with various procedures for different tests.

2. Develop an office policy and procedure plan for the proper storage and handling of X-ray film. Present your plan to the class.

C A S E   S T U D I E S

Write your response to each case study on the lines provided.

Case 1

A patient arrives in the office for a diagnostic test that will involve the use of a contrast medium that contains iodine. In your preprocedure interview with the patient a week ago, she reported no known allergies to iodine or shellfish. As you are preparing the patient for the procedure, she informs you that 2 days ago, after eating boiled shrimp at a party, she awoke in the middle of the night with nausea and joint pain. She says these symptoms subsided after 24 hours. You suspect the woman had a mild case of food poisoning from eating the shrimp. What should you do and why?

_____

_____

_____

Case 2

An elderly patient has just been examined by the physician, who has momentarily stepped out of the exam room. You are in the room with the patient and his son. The patient has just learned that he must undergo a barium enema in 2 days. When he asks you to explain this procedure, his son tells him that he is better off not knowing because it will only make him anxious. What, if anything, do you say to the patient?

_____

_____

_____

Case 3

A patient's mammogram indicates a small nodule in one breast. Without further testing, the physician cannot know whether the nodule is benign or malignant. He asks you to call the patient to schedule an ultrasound exam of the breast. When you call the patient to make the appointment, she tells you that she has never had an ultrasound and fears additional exposure to radiation. What can you say to the patient to reassure her?

_____

_____

_____

Case 4

You are interviewing a patient before his cholecystography procedure. When you ask if he was able to take the contrast media tablets the night before, he states that he did take them, but he thinks he might have dropped one of the pills. What should you do?

_____

_____

_____

PROCEDURE 50-1 Assisting with an X-ray Examination

WORK // DOC

Goal
To assist with a radiologic procedure under the supervision of a radiologic technologist.

OSHA Guidelines
This procedure does not involve exposure to blood, body fluids, or tissue. You must wear a radiation exposure badge (dosimeter), however, and will be required to wear a garment containing a lead or approved nonlead shield if you remain in the room during the operation of X-ray equipment.

Materials
X-ray examination order, X-ray machine, X-ray film and holder, X-ray film developer, drape, and patient shield.

Method

Step Number	Procedure	Points Possible	Points Earned
1.	Check the X-ray examination order and equipment needed.	20	
2.	Identify the patient and introduce yourself.	20	
3.	Determine whether the patient has complied with the preprocedure instructions. Do not depend on the patient to inform you, but ask the patient if and how they prepped for the procedure.	20	
4.	Explain the procedure and the purpose of the examination to the patient.	20	
5.	Instruct the patient to remove clothing and all metals (including jewelry) as needed, according to the body area to be examined, and to put on a gown. Explain that metals may interfere with the image. Ask whether the patient has any surgical metal or a pacemaker, and report this information to the radiologic technologist. Leave the room to ensure patient privacy.	20	
Total Points		100	
	Note: Steps 6 through 11 are nearly always performed by a radiologic technologist and are not scored. They are left here for reference only.		
6.	Position the patient according to the X-ray view ordered.		
7.	Drape the patient and place the patient shield appropriately.		
8.	Instruct the patient about the need to remain still and to hold the breath when requested.		
9.	Leave the room or stand behind a lead shield during the exposure.		
10.	Ask the patient to assume a comfortable position while the films are developed. Explain that X-rays sometimes must be repeated.		
11.	Develop the films.		
12.	Determine if the X-ray films are satisfactory by allowing the radiologist to review the films.		
13.	Instruct the patient to dress and tell the patient when to contact the physician's office for the results.		

(continued)

Step Number	Procedure	Points Possible	Points Earned
14.	Label the dry, finished X-ray films, place them in a properly labeled envelope, and file them according to your office's policies.		
15.	Record the X-ray examination, along with the final written findings, in the patient's chart.		

CAAHEP Competencies Achieved

IV. P (6)   Prepare a patient for procedures and/or treatments

III. A (2)   Explain the rationale for performance of a procedure to the patient

III. A (3)   Show awareness of patient's concerns regarding their perceptions related to the procedure being performed

ABHES Competencies Achieved

2. (c) Assist the physician with the regimen of diagnostic and treatment modalities as they relate to each body system

9. (m) Assist physician with routine and specialty examinations and treatments

PROCEDURE 50-2 Documentation and Filing Techniques for X-rays

WORK // DOC

Goal
To document X-ray information and file X-ray films properly.

OSHA Guidelines
This procedure does not involve exposure to blood, body fluids, or tissues.

Materials
X-ray film(s), patient X-ray record card or book, label, film-filing envelopes, film-filing cabinet, inserts, and a marking pen.

Method

Step Number	Procedure	Points Possible	Points Earned
1.	Document the patient's X-ray information on the patient record card or in the record book. Include the patient's name, the date, the type of X-ray, and the number of X-rays taken.	25	
2.	Verify that the film is properly labeled with the referring doctor's name, the date, and the patient's name. To note corrections or unusual positions or to identify a film that does not include labeling, attach the appropriate label and complete the necessary information. Some facilities also record the name of the radiologist who interpreted the X-ray.	25	
3.	Place the processed film in a film-filing envelope. File the envelope alphabetically or chronologically (or according to your office's protocol) in the filing cabinet.	25	
4.	If you remove an envelope for any reason, put an insert or an "out card" in its place until it is returned to the cabinet.	25	
Total Points		100	

CAAHEP Competencies Achieved

IV. P (3)   Use medical terminology, pronouncing medical terms correctly, to communicate information, patient history, data, and observation

IV. P (8)   Document Patient Care

ABHES Competencies Achieved

8. (jj) Perform fundamental writing skills including correct grammar, spelling, and formatting techniques when writing prescriptions, documenting medical records, etc.

8. (ll) Apply electronic technology

51

Principles of Pharmacology

Name_____ Class_____ Date_____

R E V I E W

Vocabulary Review

Matching
Match the key terms in the right column with the definitions in the left column by placing the letter of each correct answer in the space provided.

_____ 1. A drug's official name

_____ 2. The study of what drugs do to the body

_____ 3. A drug that is categorized as potentially dangerous or addictive

_____ 4. The use of magnets of various shapes and sizes to relieve pain or treat disease

_____ 5. Distribute a drug to a patient who is to use it

_____ 6. The science or study of drugs

_____ 7. A statement of the forms of a drug and its approved indications

_____ 8. A prescription that is entered electronically and transmitted directly to a pharmacy

_____ 9. Produces opium-like effects

_____ 10. Absorption, distribution, metabolism, and excretion

_____ 11. Government term for opioid

_____ 12. The act of ordering a drug for a patient from a pharmacy

_____ 13. Also called clinical pharmacology

_____ 14. Study of the characteristics of natural drugs and their sources

_____ 15. The study of poisons or poisonous effects of drugs

_____ 16. To give a drug by any route that introduces the drug into a patient's body

_____ 17. A drug's brand or proprietary name

_____ 18. The therapeutic value of a drug

_____ 19. Description of a drug, its purpose and effects, indications, contraindications, warnings, precautions, adverse reactions, and other information

_____ 20. The purpose or reason for using a drug

a. toxicology
b. dispense
c. pharmacodynamics
d. e prescribing
e. indication
f. administer
g. labeling
h. efficacy
i. opioid
j. trade name
k. controlled substance
l. generic name
m. magnetic therapy
n. pharmacology
o. package insert
p. pharmacokinetics
q. pharmacotherapeutics
r. pharmacognosy
s. prescribe
t. narcotic

True or False

Decide whether each statement is true or false. In the space at the left, write T for true or F for false. On the lines provided, rewrite the false statements to make them true.

_____ **21.** Pharmacology is the study of the characteristics of natural drugs and their sources.

_____

_____ **22.** The study of what the body does to drugs is known as pharmacokinesis.

_____

_____ **23.** Pharmacotherapeutics is the study of the chemical properties of drugs.

_____

_____ **24.** A physician prescribes a drug by giving a patient a prescription to be filled by a pharmacy.

_____

_____ **25.** Drugs are eliminated from the body through absorption.

_____

_____ **26.** Labeling for a drug includes the purpose or reason for using the drug and the form of the drug.

_____

_____ **27.** Metabolism is the process of transporting a drug from its administration site to its site of action.

_____

_____ **28.** Prescription drugs are medications that can be used only by order of a physician.

_____

_____ **29.** An opioid is a Schedule I substance.

_____

_____ **30.** Narcotics such as codeine, morphine, and meperidine have a lower abuse potential than Schedule IV drugs.

_____

Content Review

Multiple Choice

In the space provided, write the letter of the choice that best completes each statement or answers each question.

_____ **1.** Bacteria and fungi are simple organisms used to make
    a. Antiserums and antitoxins   **d.** Nucleic acids
    b. Antibiotics   **e.** Ointments
    c. Enzymes

_____ **2.** Which of the following is the generic name for a medication that lowers cholesterol?
    a. Raloxifene   **d.** Digoxin
    b. Toprol XL   **e.** Atorvastatin
    c. Tramadol

_____ **3.** Administering morphine to reduce the accompanying pain of cancer is an example of
    a. Maintenance drug therapy   **d.** Supplemental drug therapy
    b. Curative drug therapy   **e.** Prophylactic drug therapy
    c. Palliative drug therapy

_____ 4. The government agency that regulates the manufacture and distribution of all drugs in the United States is the
   a. Drug Enforcement Agency
   b. Federal Bureau of Investigation
   c. Occupational Safety and Health Administration
   d. Food and Drug Administration
   e. Centers for Disease Control and Prevention

_____ 5. The study of adverse reactions or drug interactions is known as
   a. Epidemiology
   b. Pharmacology
   c. Toxicology
   d. Virology
   e. Pathology

_____ 6. Which types of drugs cannot be renewed without a written order or prescription?
   a. Schedule I
   b. Schedule II
   c. Schedule III
   d. Schedule IV
   e. Schedule V

_____ 7. A physician who needs Schedule II drugs for her practice must order them using
   a. DEA form 222
   b. DEA form 214
   c. DEA form 224
   d. DEA form 41
   e. DEA forms 41 and 224

_____ 8. Which of the following is the generic name for a medication that controls seizures?
   a. Zolpidem
   b. Cetirizine
   c. Fluconazole
   d. Promethazine
   e. Clonazepam

_____ 9. According to the Controlled Substances Act of 1970, physicians are not allowed to prescribe drugs in which of the following schedules?
   a. Schedule I
   b. Schedule II
   c. Schedule III
   d. Schedule IV
   e. Schedule V

_____ 10. Which of the following generic medications is used to relieve diarrhea?
   a. Quinapril
   b. Valacyclovir
   c. Naproxen
   d. Bismuth subsalicylate
   e. Diphenhydramine HCl

_____ 11. Which of the following drugs is given to treat asthma?
   a. Advair Diskus®
   b. Fosamax®
   c. Lidoderm®
   d. Norvasc®
   e. Prevacid®

_____ 12. What is the most likely reason someone would take the medication Zetia®?
   a. To reduce blood pressure
   b. To reduce cholesterol
   c. To treat depression
   d. To replace a hormone
   e. To treat an allergy

Sentence Completion

In the space provided, write the word or phrase that best completes each sentence.

13. Antiserums and antitoxins for vaccines are examples of _____ substances used as drugs.

14. Tablets and capsules are absorbed through the stomach or intestines into the _____.

15. Drug metabolism usually takes place in the _____.

16. Distribution can pertain to the length of time between dosing and _____ in the bloodstream.

17. Pharmacotherapeutics is sometimes called _____.

18. A drug's trade name is selected by, is copyrighted by, and is the property of its _____.

19. A nonprescription, or _____, drug is one that the FDA has approved for use without the supervision of a licensed practitioner.

20. A physician's written order that authorizes the dispensing and administering of drugs to a patient is called a(n) _____.

21. The official name of a drug is its _____ name.

22. The purpose or reason for using a drug is called the _____.

23. A popular drug reference book used by physician practices that is published annually is the _____.

24. A drug that is potentially dangerous and addictive is referred to as a(n) _____ substance.

25. A preparation made from microorganisms that is used to prevent a specific disease in children and adults is a(n) _____.

13. _____

14. _____

15. _____

16. _____

17. _____

18. _____

19. _____

20. _____

21. _____

22. _____

23. _____

24. _____

25. _____

Short Answer

Write the answer to each question on the lines provided.

26. What are the regulatory functions of the Food and Drug Administration (FDA) with regard to drugs?

_____

_____

_____

27. What are the four processes of pharmacokinetics?

_____

_____

_____

28. In what ways are drugs excreted?

_____

_____

_____

29. What is off-label prescribing?

_____

_____

_____

30. What factors determine the safety of a drug?

_____

_____

_____

31. List four main sources of drug information, and describe the contents of each.

    a. _____

_____

    b. _____

_____

    c. _____

_____

    d. _____

_____

32. How does regulation of the use of an OTC drug differ from that of a prescription drug?

_____

_____

_____

33. Compare how the five schedules of drugs described in the Controlled Substances Act of 1970 differ according to degree of potential abuse or nontherapeutic effects of the drugs in each schedule.

_____

_____

_____

_____

_____

_____

_____

34. What requirements does the CSA place on physicians who administer, dispense, or prescribe any controlled substance?

_____

_____

_____

35. Explain how controlled substances are identified on their labels.

_____

_____

_____

36. How does the ordering of Schedule II drugs differ from the ordering of drugs from Schedules III, IV, and V?

_____

_____

_____

37. List in order the four parts of a prescription and explain what information is contained in each part.

a. _____

_____

b. _____

_____

c. _____

_____

d. _____

_____

38. Complete the following chart.

Action of Drug	Drug Category	EXAMPLE	
		Generic Name	Trade Name
a. Counteracts effects of histamine and relieves allergic symptoms		Cetirizine	
b. Dilates blood vessels, decreases blood pressure		Nitroglycerin	
c. Increases urine output, reduces blood pressure and cardiac output		Furosemide	
d. Kills microorganisms or inhibits or prevents their growth		Azithromycin	
e. Normalizes heartbeat in cases of certain cardiac arrhythmias		Propafenone HCl	
f. Prevents blood from clotting		Warfarin sodium	
g. Prevents or relieves nausea and vomiting		Prochlorperazine	
h. Prevents sensation of pain (generally, locally, or topically)		Lidocaine HCl	
i. Reduces blood pressure		Quinapril	
j. Reduces fever		Acetaminophen	
k. Reduces inflammation		Triamcinolone	
l. Relieves depression		Escitalopram	
m. Relieves diarrhea		Loperamide HCl	
n. Relieves mild to severe pain		Oxycodone HCl	
o. Relieves or controls convulsions		Divalproex	
p. Reduces blood sugar		Metformin	

39. Identify the purpose of each part of the package insert template pictured here.

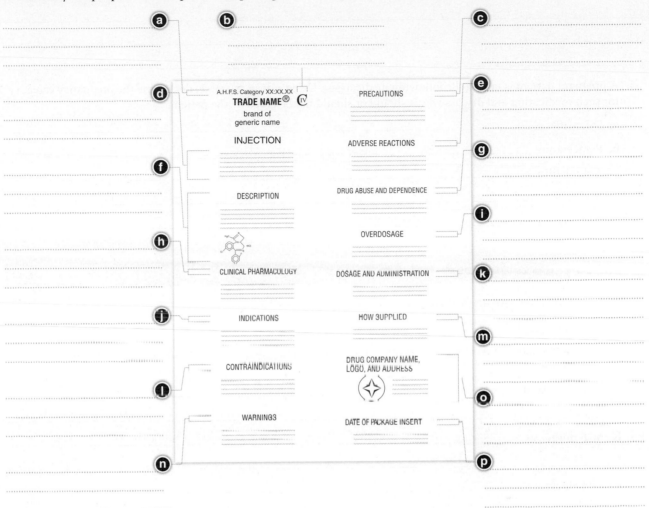

Critical Thinking

Write the answer to each question on the lines provided.

1. Why do clinical studies include both healthy individuals and patients?

_____
_____
_____

2. Why is it important that patients inform their pharmacist of all prescription and OTC drugs they are currently taking when medication is prescribed for them?

_____
_____
_____

3. Why is it important that the patient chart be consulted before a prescription refill is authorized?

_____
_____
_____

4. What is the first thing a medical assistant does if a patient requests drug samples?

_____

_____

_____

5. A pregnant patient is taking the following medications. Using a drug resource, determine the pregnancy category for each medication and discuss why it should or should not be taken by the patient.

   a. Dilantin® _____

   b. Paracetamol _____

   c. Amoxicillin _____

   d. Accutane® _____

   e. Codeine _____

A P P L I C A T I O N

WORK // DOC

Follow the directions for each application.

1. Antihypertensives

What are the actions and differences of the following types of antihypertensives? Use the *PDR* or another credible drug reference.

   a. Calcium channel blockers _____

_____

   b. ACE inhibitors _____

_____

   c. Beta blockers _____

_____

   d. Diuretics _____

_____

2. Interpreting Prescriptions

The physician has written the following prescriptions. Interpret each prescription on the lines provided.

   a. Proloprim® 200 mg 10 caps
      Sig 1 cap po daily. 10 d

_____

_____

   b. Nasalide® 25 mL nasal sol
      Sig II sprays t.i.d. PRN

_____

_____

   c. Furosemide oral sol (10 mg/mL)
      Sig 1 tsp po b.i.d.

_____

_____

    d. Nitro-Dur® 0.3 mg transdermal nitroglycerin infusion system
       Sig 1 patch daily

_____

_____

    e. Cylert® 18.75 mg 14 tabs
       Sig II tabs po qam 7 d

_____

_____

3. Conducting an Inventory of Dispensed Controlled Drugs

On a separate sheet of paper, write an office procedural plan for conducting a controlled drug inventory. The procedure should include the following information:

- How often the inventory is to be conducted
- Information you must have about each drug
- Where this information is obtained for Schedule II drugs
- Where this information is obtained for Schedules III, IV, and V drugs
- How the information for each drug is processed
- What records must be included in the inventory
- How the inventory is maintained
- How long the inventory is retained

4. Charting Prescription Refills on a Progress Note

Read each of the following cases and chart the information on the progress note. An example form for progress notes is provided in the back of the workbook.

    a. A patient calls to request a refill for Lexapro 10 mg. She takes 1 tablet per day. Her pharmacy number is 216-444-0000. She states that she has no known drug allergies. The physician authorized 4 refills.

    b. The pharmacy calls for a refill for Mr. Smith. He would like his Ativan® 1 gr refilled. He has not been seen in the office in 6 months, and the physician does not authorize the refill.

    c. Ms. Thompson calls to confirm the correct dosage and dosing schedule for her prescription of Zithromax that she received that morning.

    d. A patient calls to request a refill for Zocor 40 mg, 1 tablet per day. The physician authorized 3 refills.

C A S E   S T U D I E S

Write your response to each case study on the lines provided.

Case 1

You are interviewing a new patient who has arrived with her 1-month-old child. The patient tells you that the over-the-counter medication she has been taking for allergies does not seem to be working. She thinks she may need a prescription drug for her allergies. What are two important questions you should ask this patient in case the doctor prescribes medication?

_____

_____

_____

Case 2

Your workplace has been burglarized. Schedules III, IV, and V drugs were stolen. (Your workplace does not administer or dispense Schedule II drugs.) What should you do?

_____

_____

_____

Case 3

The physician has written a prescription for Achromycin, 250-mg capsules. After checking a drug reference, you find that Achromycin is a trade name for tetracycline HCl, a generic drug that is available in 250-mg capsules at a lower cost than Achromycin. Returning to the prescription, you note that the physician has failed to check the "Generic Equivalent OK" box on the prescription form. What should you do?

_____

_____

_____

PROCEDURE 51-1 Helping the Physician Comply with the Controlled Substances Act of 1970

WORK // DOC

Goal
To comply with the Controlled Substances Act of 1970.

OSHA Guidelines
This procedure does not involve exposure to blood, body fluids, or tissues.

Materials
DEA Form 224, DEA Form 222, DEA Form 41, computer or pen.

Method

Step Number	Procedure	Points Possible	Points Earned
1.	Use DEA Form 224 to register the physician with the Drug Enforcement Administration. Renew all registrations every 3 years using DEA Form 224a.	10	
2.	Order Schedule II drugs using DEA Form 222, as instructed by the physician. (Stocks of these drugs should be kept to a minimum.)	25	
3.	Include the physician's DEA registration number on every prescription for a drug in Schedules II through V.*	25	
4.	Complete an inventory of all drugs in Schedules II through V every 2 years (as permitted in your state; this task may be reserved for other healthcare professionals).	5	
5.	Store all drugs in Schedules II through V in a secure, locked safe or cabinet (as permitted in your state).*	25	
6.	Keep accurate dispensing and inventory records for at least 2 years.	5	
7.	Dispose of expired or unused drugs according to the DEA regulations. Always complete DEA Form 41 when disposing of controlled drugs.	5	
Total Points		100	

CAAHEP Competencies Achieved

IX. C (13)   Discuss all levels of governmental legislation and regulation as they apply to medical assisting practice, including FDA and DEA regulations

ABHES Competencies Achieved

6. (e) Comply with federal, state, and local health laws and regulations

PROCEDURE 51-2 Interpreting a Prescription

`WORK//DOC`

Goal
To read and accurately interpret a prescription.

OSHA Guidelines
This procedure does not involve exposure to blood, body fluids, or tissues.

Materials
Prescription, Table 51-4 Abbreviations Used in Prescriptions in textbook, method of recording (pen or electronic).

Method

Step Number	Procedure	Points Possible	Points Earned
1.	Verify the prescriber information. This is especially important in a multiphysician practice or electronic health record.*	15	
2.	Ensure that patient information is accurate, including correct spelling of name, date of birth, and address. For written prescriptions, check legibility.*	15	
3.	Confirm the date of the prescription.	10	
4.	Check the medication name and double-check spelling.ˣ	25	
5.	Verify that instructions to the pharmacist are complete and include refill authorization and generic substitution.	10	
6.	Translate the instructions to the patient using Table 51–4.	10	
7.	Make sure that the prescription is signed in ink for handwritten prescriptions and digitally for electronic prescriptions.*	15	
Total Points		100	

CAAHEP Competencies Achieved

II. C (6) Identify both abbreviations and symbols used in calculating medication dosages

IV. P (3) Use medical terminology, pronouncing medical terms correctly, to communicate information, patient history, data, and observations

ABHES Competencies Achieved

6. (c) Identify and define common abbreviations that are accepted in prescription writing

6. (d) Understand legal aspects of writing prescriptions, including federal and state laws

8. (jj) Perform fundamental writing skills, including correct grammar, spelling, and formatting techniques when writing prescriptions, documenting medical records, etc.

52

Dosage Calculations

Name_____ Class_____ Date_____

R E V I E W

Vocabulary Review

Matching

Match the key terms in the right column with the definitions in the left column by placing the letter of each correct answer in the space provided.

_____ 1. A measurement system that includes units such as drops and teaspoons

_____ 2. Quantity of the dose on hand

_____ 3. Calculating dosages by setting up equivalent measures and cross multiplying

_____ 4. An older measurement system that includes units such as fluid drams and grains

_____ 5. The total surface area of the body

_____ 6. A measurement system based on multiples of 10

_____ 7. The amount of medication in each unit of a drug

_____ 8. A set of scales arranged so that a ruler aligned with two values shows the corresponding value on a third scale

_____ 9. The amount of medication the physician has ordered the patient to take

_____ 10. The amount of space a drug occupies

_____ 11. Calculating dosages by substituting values into a standard equation

_____ 12. The heaviness of a drug

a. proportion method
b. weight
c. apothecary system
d. desired dose
e. nomogram
f. dosage unit
g. metric system
h. formula method
i. BSA
j. volume
k. dose on hand
l. household system

True or False

Decide whether each statement is true or false. In the space at the left, write T for true or F for false. On the lines provided, rewrite the false statements to make them true.

_____ 13. The apothecary system of measurement is based on multiples of 10.

_____

_____ 14. The preferred abbreviation for milliliters is ml.

_____

_____ 15. When a number has no whole-number part, you should write a zero to the left of the decimal point.

_____

_____ 16. In the metric system, 1 kg equals 1000 mg.

_____

_____ **17.** An ounce in the apothecary system of measurement is equal to an ounce in the household system of measurement.

_____

_____ **18.** The basic formula for dosage calculations is D/H ÷ Q.

_____

_____ **19.** Drug doses for pediatric patients are often determined on the basis of body surface area.

_____

_____ **20.** To find a person's BSA, you can use a complex formula or a pyelogram.

_____

Content Review

Multiple Choice

In the space provided, write the letter of the choice that best completes each statement or answers each question.

_____ **1.** How many milliliters are in 1 liter?

    a. 0.001

    b. 0.1

    c. 10

    d. 100

    e. 1000

_____ **2.** How many grams are in 1 milligram?

    a. 0.001

    b. 0.1

    c. 10

    d. 100

    e. 1000

_____ **3.** How many micrograms are in 1 milligram?

    a. 0.001

    b. 0.1

    c. 10

    d. 100

    e. 1000

_____ **4.** What is 5.48645 rounded to the nearest hundredth?

    a. 5.486

    b. 5.48

    c. 5.49

    d. 5.4

    e. 5.5

_____ **5.** What is 1.59654 rounded to the nearest thousandth?

    a. 1.596

    b. 1.597

    c. 1.5965

    d. 1.5964

    e. 1.59654

_____ 6. The label on a bottle of Depakote® tablets shows that each tablet contains 125 mg. How many grams is this?

    a. 125 grams

    b. 12.5 grams

    c. 1.25 grams

    d. 0.125 grams

    e. 0.0125 grams

_____ 7. The physician has ordered Erythromycin 0.5 g. On hand are 250 mg Erythromycin tablets. How many tablets will you give?

    a. 0.5 tablet

    b. 1 tablet

    c. 1.5 tablet

    d. 2 tablet

    e. 2.5 tablet

_____ 8. The physician tells a patient to take 2 tbsp of Robitussin cough syrup twice daily. What system of measurement is the physician using?

    a. Apothecary

    b. Household

    c. Universal

    d. Metric

    e. International

_____ 9. A medication order specifies 800 mcg Nitrostat® sublingually as needed for chest pain. On hand are 0.4 mg Nitrostat® sublingual tablets. What is the desired dose in milligrams?

    a. 0.04 mg

    b. 0.4 mg

    c. 4.0 mg

    d. 8.0 mg

    e. 0.8 mg

_____ 10. The physician has ordered Atacand 16 mg po bid, and on hand are Atacand 8 mg tablets. What is the dosage unit for this medication order?

    a. Tablet

    b. 2 mg

    c. 5 mg

    d. 16 mg

    e. 2.5 tablets

_____ 11. Tranxene 7.5 mg po at bedtime has been ordered. On hand are Tranxene 3.75 mg tablets. How many tablets do you need to give?

    a. 3.75 tablets

    b. 2 tablets

    c. 1.5 tablets

    d. 1 tablet

    e. 0.5 tablet

_____ 12. Vistaril suspension 50 mg po qid has been ordered. On hand is Vistaril suspension 100 mg per 5 mL. How many milliliters must be given to deliver the ordered dose?

    a. 1 mL

    b. 2 mL

    c. 2.5 mL

    d. 5 mL

    e. 10 mL

_____ 13. The physician has ordered 100 mg Docusate and on hand is Docusate sodium elixir 150 mg/15 mL. What is the dosage unit?

    a. 100 mg

    b. 150 mg

    c. 15 mL

    d. 1 mL

    e. 0.6 mL

_____ 14. The physician has ordered 1 mg of B-12 (cyanocobalamin) by subcutaneous injection (subcut). The following label shows the available form of the drug. What is the desired dose?

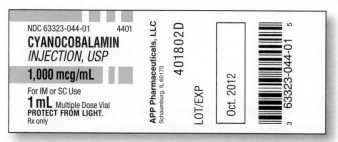

Source: Reprinted with permission of APP Pharmaceuticals, LLC.

    a. 10 mcg   **d.** 1 mg

    b. 1000 mcg   **e.** 1 mcg

    c. 1 mL

_____ 15. Clarithromycin 500 mg has been ordered. The following label shows the available form of the drug. What amount should the patient take?

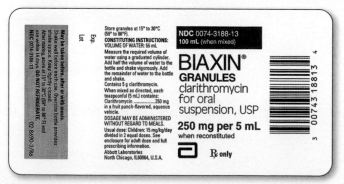

Source: Kathryn A. Booth et al., MATH & DOSAGE CALCULATIONS FOR HEALTHCARE PROFESSIONALS, 4/e. © 2012 McGraw Hill Companies, Inc. Reprinted with permission. Medication label copyright © Abbott Pharmaceuticals Division. Reproduced with permission.

    a. 5 mL   **d.** 1 tbsp

    b. 1 tsp   **e.** 2.5 mL

    c. 10 mL

_____ **16.** The physician has ordered Zithromax 50 mg PO every 8 hours. The following label shows the available form of the drug. What is the dose on hand?

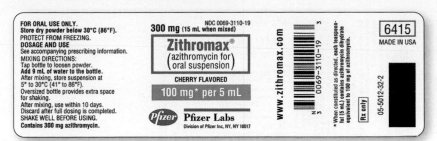

Source: Kathryn A. Booth et al., MATH & DOSAGE CALCULATIONS FOR HEALTHCARE PROFESSIONALS, 4/e. © 2012 McGraw Hill Companies, Inc. Reprinted with permission. Medication label copyright Pfizer Inc. Reproduced with permission.

a. 100 mg/5 mL	**d.** 2.5 mL
b. 50 mg/5 mL	**e.** 1 tablet
c. 5 mL	

_____ **17.** The physician has ordered Amoxicillin 300 mg PO every 12 hours and on hand is Amoxicillin suspension labeled 50 mg/mL. How much Amoxicillin should be administered in 1 dose?

a. 1 mL

b. 3 mL

c. 6 mL

d. 30 mL

e. 50 mL

_____ **18.** The physician has ordered Erythromycin 100 mg po 3 times daily. The following label shows the available form of the drug. What is the desired dose?

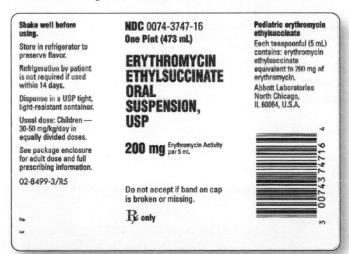

Source: Kathryn A. Booth et al., MATH & DOSAGE CALCULATIONS FOR HEALTHCARE PROFESSIONALS, 4/e. © 2012 McGraw Hill Companies, Inc. Reprinted with permission. Medication label copyright © Abbott Pharmaceuticals Division. Reproduced with permission.

a. 5 mL	**d.** 100 mg
b. 200 mg	**e.** 300 mg
c. 2.5 mL	

_____ **19.** The physician has ordered Amoxicillin 500 mg 4 times daily. The following label shows the available form of the drug. How much Amoxicillin should be administered in 1 dose?

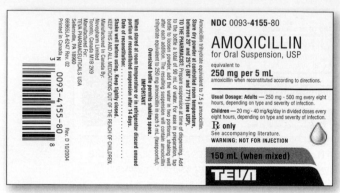

Source: Label reproduced with permission from Teva Pharmaceuticals. This label is a representation only and should not be used for any official purposes.

   a. 5 mL

   b. 10 mL

   c. 2.5 mL

   d. 500 mg

   e. 250 mg

_____ **20.** The physician has ordered a 5 mcg dose of Hepatitis B vaccine be given to a newborn infant. The following label shows the available form of the drug. What is the amount to administer?

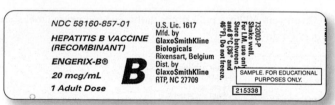

   a. 20 mcg

   b. 1 mL

   c. 0.5 mL

   d. 25 mcg

   e. 0.25 mL

Short Answer

Write the answer to each question on the lines provided.

21. What question should you ask yourself every time you perform a dosage calculation?

_____

_____

_____

22. Name the three systems of measurement that are used in the United States. Which is the most widely used?

_____

_____

_____

23. Briefly describe the process for rounding decimals.

_____

_____

_____

24. List the two rules for converting between measurements within the metric system.

_____

_____

_____

25. Why are pediatric dosages often calculated by BSA or weight?

_____

_____

_____

Critical Thinking

Write the answer to each question on the lines provided.

1. What is the difference between the formula method and the proportion method of dosage calculation?

_____

_____

_____

2. A patient with recurrent angina (chest pain) is given the medication shown in the label below. The patient is instructed to take the medication under his tongue at the first sign of angina and may repeat the dose every 5 minutes up to 15 minutes before seeking medical attention. How many total tablets can he take before contacting medical attention? The patient takes two tablets and his pain subsides. How many mcg of medication did he take?

_____

_____

_____

Copyright © 2014 by The McGraw-Hill Companies, Inc.

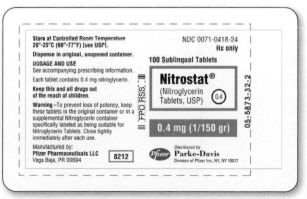

Source: Kathryn A. Booth et al., MATH & DOSAGE CALCULATIONS FOR HEALTHCARE PROFESSIONALS, 4/e. © 2012 McGraw Hill Companies, Inc. Reprinted with permission. Medication label copyright Pfizer Inc. Reproduced with permission.

A P P L I C A T I O N

Follow the directions for each application.

1. Dosage Based on BSA

The following figure is a nomogram that has been used to calculate a patient's body surface area. Refer to the nomogram to answer each of the following questions. Round your answers to the nearest tic mark on the nomogram.

a. What is this patient's current weight in pounds? _____

b. What is the patient's height in centimeters? _____

c. What is the patient's body surface area? _____

d. If the patient were the same height but weighed 20 kilograms, what would the patient's body surface area be?

_____

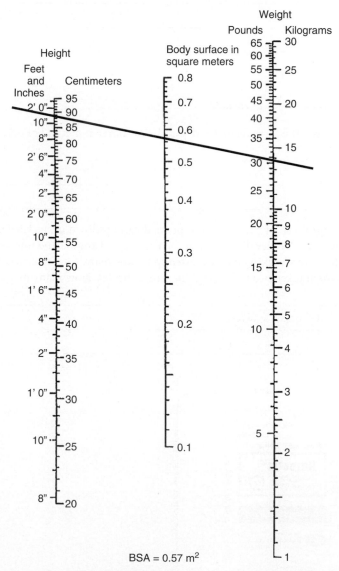

BSA = 0.57 m²

Source: Kathryn A. Booth and James Whaley, MATH AND DOSAGE CALCULATIONS FOR MEDICAL CAREERS, 2/e, © 2007 McGraw-Hill Companies, Inc. Reprinted with permission.

2. Dosage Based on Weight

For a child who weighs 55 pounds, the physician has ordered Amoxicillin 30 mg/kg/day po every 8 hours. The following label shows the available form of the drug. On the basis of this information, perform the necessary calculations to answer the following questions.

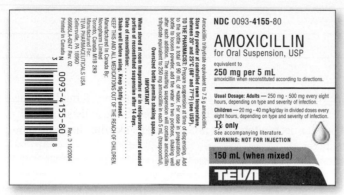

Source: Label reproduced with permission from Teva Pharmaceuticals. This label is a representation only and should not be used for any official purposes.

a. What is the child's weight in kilograms? _____

b. What is the desired dose for 24 hours? _____

c. What is the desired dose for 1 dose? _____

d. What is the amount to administer in each dose? (Round your answer to the nearest tenth.) _____

CASE STUDIES

Write your response to each case study on the lines provided.

Case 1

Frances Underwood is a 52-year-old female who is suffering from abnormal uterine bleeding. The physician orders Provera 5 mg for 10 days beginning on the 16th day of her menstrual cycle. Francis is given the medication shown in the label below. How many tablets will she take per day? How many total tablets will she be given to fill the prescription? Her menstrual period started on January 20th, so what day should she take her first dose of Provera?

_____

_____

_____

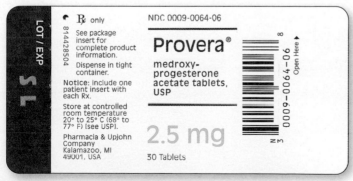

Source: Kathryn A. Booth et al., MATH & DOSAGE CALCULATIONS FOR HEALTHCARE PROFESSIONALS, 4/e. © 2012 McGraw Hill Companies, Inc. Reprinted with permission. Medication label copyright Pfizer Inc. Reproduced with permission.

Case 2

A patient in an agitated state is brought to the emergency department. The physician verbally orders 2 mL IM (intramuscular) of Vistaril. The healthcare professional draws up 2 mL from a vial labeled 50 mg/mL. Then she notices another vial of Vistaril labeled 25 mg/mL. What should she do?

_____

_____

_____

Case 3

A patient is brought to the physician's office with severe vomiting. The physician orders Compazine™ 5 mg IM to be given now. The healthcare professional obtains a vial of Compazine™ labeled 5 mg/mL. The label also lists the total quantity of medication as 5 mL. The healthcare professional injects a total of 5 mL. What mistake did the healthcare professional make? How could he have avoided this mistake?

_____

_____

_____

53

Medication Administration

Name_____ Class_____ Date_____

R E V I E W

Vocabulary Review

Matching

Match the key terms in the right column with the definitions in the left column by placing the letter of each correct answer in the space provided.

_____ 1. Liquid used to dissolve and dilute a drug

_____ 2. Beneath the skin

_____ 3. Indented line in a tablet along which the tablet can be broken

_____ 4. A technique of IM injection that prevents a drug from leaking into the subcutaneous tissue and causing irritation

_____ 5. Between the cheek and gum

_____ 6. Within the upper layers of the skin

_____ 7. The way a drug is introduced into the body

_____ 8. Under the tongue

_____ 9. Slow drip

_____ 10. Salve

_____ 11. Through the skin

_____ 12. Vaginal irrigation

_____ 13. Within a muscle

_____ 14. A homogeneous mixture of solid, liquid, or gaseous substance in a liquid

_____ 15. Directly into a vein

a. solution
b. intramuscular (IM)
c. Z-track method
d. buccal
e. intravenous (IV)
f. infusion
g. score
h. intradermal (ID)
i. transdermal
j. douche
k. ointment
l. route
m. diluent
n. sublingual
o. subcutaneous (subcut)

True or False

Decide whether each statement is true or false. In the space at the left, write T for true or F for false. On the lines provided, rewrite the false statements to make them true.

_____ 16. Patients should sign a consent form before receiving a vaccine.

_____

_____ 17. Medical assistants document drug administration immediately before administering the drug.

_____

_____ 18. If you make a medication error but the patient has no ill effects, you do not need to report the error.

_____

_____ 19. Tablets that are to be given sublingually are placed between the patient's gum and cheek.

_____ 20. Oral administration is contraindicated in patients who have severe nausea.

_____ 21. Intermuscular injections are a form of parenteral administration.

_____ 22. An 18-gauge needle is larger than a 16-gauge needle.

_____ 23. Two needles and syringe sets are needed to draw and administer medication from an ampule.

_____ 24. The vastus lateralis is a good injection site for an infant.

_____ 25. A douche may be used to administer a medication by the rectal route.

Content Review

Multiple Choice

In the space provided, write the letter of the choice that best completes each statement or answers each question.

_____ 1. Inhalation therapy can be administered through the nose or
   a. Ear
   b. Eye
   c. Skin
   d. Rectum
   e. Mouth

_____ 2. Which of the following forms of drugs is administered by the transdermal route?
   a. Capsule
   b. Pill
   c. Spray
   d. Patch
   e. Suppository

_____ 3. The office sharps container should be properly disposed of when it is
   a. One-third full
   b. Half full
   c. Two-thirds full
   d. Three-quarters full
   e. Full

_____ 4. What information must you ask a patient every time before administering an injection?
   a. Blood pressure results
   b. Age
   c. Route preference
   d. Any known drug allergies
   e. Weight

_____ 5. What is the best site for administering an intramuscular injection to a pediatric patient?
   a. Vastus lateralis
   b. Dorsogluteal
   c. Biceps
   d. Triceps
   e. Deltoid

_____ 6. You are administering a sublingual medication. Which education statement would be correct?
   a. Place the medication between your cheek and gum until it dissolves
   b. Place the medication under your tongue and then take a drink of water
   c. Take a drink of water, then swallow this pill with your second drink of water
   d. Inhale the medication, holding your breath for 30 seconds after each inhalation
   e. Place the medication under your tongue until it dissolves

_____ 7. Why should you wear gloves during the administration of a transdermal patch?
   a. To prevent contamination of the patch
   b. To prevent the medication from getting on your skin
   c. To keep the patch sterile until it is administered
   d. To prevent infection
   e. To prevent patient discomfort

_____ 8. You have just finished administering a drug intramuscularly. How long will it take the drug to be absorbed?
   a. 7 to 20 seconds   d. 20 to 30 minutes
   b. 15 to 30 seconds   e. 2 to 3 hours
   c. 3 to 5 minutes

_____ 9. A patient was given her antibiotic tablet before breakfast, but the instructions indicate that the drug should be taken after meals. Which right of administration does this violate?
   a. Right drug   d. Right time
   b. Right technique   e. Right route
   c. Right reason

_____ 10. Which of the following is *not* a contraindication for an injection site?
   a. Mole   d. Birthmark
   b. Hair   e. Edema
   c. Scar

Sentence Completion

In the space provided, write the word or phrase that best completes each sentence.

11. Topical administration is the direct application of a drug on the _____.

12. Drugs that produce systemic effects are administered by routes that allow the drugs to be absorbed and distributed in the _____ throughout the body.

13. Parenteral administration of a drug generally applies to giving drugs by _____.

14. The _____ of a needle is a measure of its inside diameter.

15. Skin tests are usually administered by _____ injection.

16. Physicians usually prescribe vaginal drugs to treat local bacterial or _____ infections.

17. Before administering a medication, you should always check the medication _____ times.

18. Failing to report a medication error is _____ and sometimes illegal.

19. You may break a tablet to provide a smaller dose only if the tablet is _____.

20. After using a needle, you should engage the safety mechanism and immediately place the needle in a(n) _____.

11. _____

12. _____

13. _____

14. _____

15. _____

16. _____

17. _____

18. _____

19. _____

20. _____

Short Answer

Write the answer to each question on the lines provided.

21. To ensure accuracy, when should you read the label of a drug you are about to administer?

_____

_____

_____

22. Why do drugs that are administered buccally and sublingually produce therapeutic effects more quickly than do orally administered drugs?

_____

_____

_____

23. Why is the tip of an injection needle beveled?

_____

_____

_____

24. Why does parenteral administration of a drug pose more safety risks for patients than administration by other routes?

_____

_____

_____

25. Why do you inject aspirated air from the syringe into the vial of diluent when you are reconstituting a drug for injection?

_____

_____

_____

26. After cleansing the site of an intradermal injection with an alcohol swab, why should you let the skin dry before giving the injection?

_____

_____

_____

27. When administering a subcutaneous injection, why would you avoid an injection site that is hardened or fatty?

_____

_____

_____

28. What is the function of the small amount of air you draw into the syringe when you administer an intramuscular injection?

_____

_____

_____

29. How does a drug-drug interaction differ from the adverse effects of a drug?

_____

_____

30. The following illustration shows a standard syringe. Write the name of each part of the instrument on the lines provided.

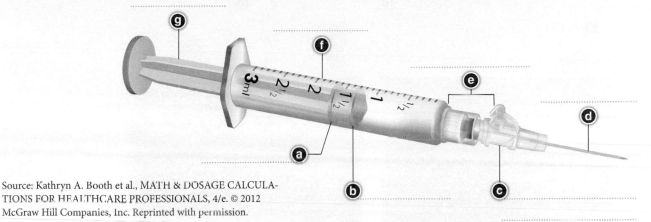

31. Why is it important to ask patients about drug allergies every time they come into the office?

_____

_____

_____

32. What is the purpose of having a patient sign a consent form before administering a medication?

_____

_____

_____

33. What are some methods to ensure a smooth procedure when administering a pediatric injection?

_____

_____

_____

_____

_____

34. Why is the vastus lateralis the best site for administering an injection to a pediatric patient?

_____

_____

_____

35. Why is accurate charting essential in a medical facility?

_____

_____

_____

36. What information is documented after giving an injection to a patient?

_____

_____

_____

37. On the following figure, label the type of injection that is being given on the basis of the location of the needle.

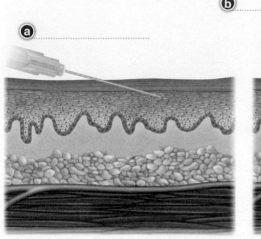 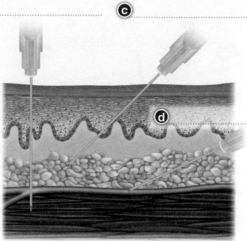

Critical Thinking

Write the answer to each question on the lines provided.

1. Why do you place a 2 × 2 gauze or cotton ball over the injection site when you withdraw the needle during an intramuscular or subcutaneous injection?

_____

_____

_____

2. The doctor has asked you to administer eye ointment and eyedrops to a patient. In what order should you administer the drugs to the patient? Why?

_____

_____

_____

3. When charting medications in the patient chart, why is it important to refrain from using statements such as "appears" or "seems like"?

_____

_____

_____

4. Why is it important to include the expiration date, lot number, and manufacturer when charting medications?

_____

_____

_____

A P P L I C A T I O N

Follow the directions for each application.

1. **Demonstrating Proper Medication Administration for Medications Given Orally, Sublingually, and Buccally**

   Using Procedures 53-1, Administering Oral Drugs, and 53-2, Administering Buccal or Sublingual Drugs, review and practice administering medications orally, sublingually, and buccally. Use the following circumstances during your practice:

   a. Working with a partner, role-play giving the proper instructions for each type of medication.

   b. Chart the following medications as being administered in the sample progress note provided in the back of the workbook. Make certain your charting is complete, including patient reactions and any patient education in the patient's chart. (To make the charting complete, create any information not provided as follows.)
      - 650 mg acetaminophen PO
      - Nitroglycerin gr 1/100 SL
      - Methyltestosterone 10 mg buccal

2. **Demonstrating Proper Medication Preparation for Medications Given by Injection**

   Using Procedures 53-3, Drawing a Drug from an Ampule, and 53-4, Reconstituting and Drawing a Drug for Injection, practice preparing medications for administration.

3. **Demonstrating Proper Medication Administration for Medications Given by Injection**

   Using Procedures 53-5, Giving an Intradermal Injection; 53-6, Giving a Subcutaneous Injection; and 53-7, Giving an Intramuscular Injection, practice administering injections. Use the following circumstances during your practice:

   a. Working with a partner and a manikin, role-play giving the injections while providing the proper communication to the patient for each type of injection.

   b. Chart the following injections as being administered in the sample progress note or medication flow sheet provided. Make certain your charting is complete, including the date, time, drug name, dosage, expiration date, lot number, manufacturer, route, site, significant patient reactions, and any patient education in the patient's chart. (To make charting complete, create any information not provided as follows.)
      - Tigan 200 mg intramuscularly
      - Humulin R 20 units subcutaneously
      - Mantoux TB test intradermally

4. **Demonstrating Proper Medication Administration for Medications Given by Various Routes**

   Using Procedures 53-8, Administering Inhalation Therapy; 53-9, Administering and Removing a Transdermal Patch and Providing Patient Instruction; 53-10, Assisting with Administration of a Urethral Drug; 53-11, Administering a Vaginal Medication; and 53-12, Administering a Rectal Medication, practice administering medications through various routes. Use the following circumstances in your practice.

   a. Research names of medications that would be administered by the various routes, or obtain medication names from your instructor.

   b. Working with a partner and a manikin, when necessary, role-play giving the proper instructions for each procedure performed. Take turns with a partner and review any steps in your instruction you have missed.

   c. Chart each medication you have researched and/or procedure performed in the sample **progress note** provided. Make certain your charting is complete by creating information based on your practice session.

C A S E   S T U D I E S

Write your response to each case study on the lines provided.

Case 1

A patient received from the pharmacy a prescription for hyoscyamine sulfate tablets for buccal administration. She telephones the office and asks you if it would be all right to take the medication while having her second cup of coffee in the morning. What do you tell her? Why?

_____

_____

_____

Case 2

Heparin 1.5 mL subcut has been ordered for a patient. What volume syringe and needle (gauge and length) should you prepare?

_____

_____

_____

Case 3

The doctor has written an order for you to administer two 250-mg tablets of Trimox® (amoxicillin) to a patient who has an infection. The patient reluctantly takes the first tablet but spits out the second. What do you do?

_____

_____

_____

Case 4

You had just administered a drug to a child, and within 5 minutes the child vomited. Should you readminister the drug?

_____

_____

_____

Case 5

You are explaining the dosage instructions to a mother, and the medication is ordered in tablet form. The mother tells you that the child has difficulty swallowing tablets. What should you do?

_____

_____

_____

PROCEDURE 53-1 Administering Oral Drugs   〔WORK//DOC〕

Goal
To safely administer an oral drug to a patient.

OSHA Guidelines
This procedure does not involve exposure to blood, body fluids, or tissues.

Materials
Drug order (in patient chart), container of oral drug, small paper cup (for tablets, capsules, or caplets) or plastic calibrated medicine cup (for liquids), glass of water or juice, straw (optional), package insert or drug information sheet.

Method

Step Number	Procedure	Points Possible	Points Earned
1.	Identify the patient and wash your hands.	4	
2.	Select the ordered drug (tablet, capsule, or liquid).	4	
3.	Check the rights, comparing information against the drug order.*	8	
4.	If you are unfamiliar with the drug, check a drug reference, read the package insert, or speak with the physician. Determine whether the drug may be taken with or followed by water or juice.	4	
5.	Ask the patient about any drug or food allergies. If the patient is not allergic to the ordered drug or other ingredients used to prepare it, proceed.*	8	
6.	Perform any calculations needed to provide the prescribed dose. If you are unsure of your calculations, check them with a coworker or the physician.	4	
If You Are Giving Tablets or Capsules			
7.	Open the container and tap the correct number into the cap. Do not touch the inside of the cap because it is sterile. If you pour out too many tablets or capsules and you have not touched them, tap the excess back into the container.	8	
8.	Tap the tablets or capsules from the cap into the paper cup.	4	
9.	Recap the container immediately.*	8	
10.	Give the patient the cup along with a glass of water or juice. If the patient finds it easier to drink with a straw, unwrap the straw and place it in the fluid. If patients have difficulty swallowing pills, have them drink some water or juice before putting the pills in the mouth.*	8	
If You Are Giving a Liquid Drug			
11.	If the liquid is a suspension, shake it well.	4	
12.	Locate the mark on the medicine cup for the prescribed dose. Keeping your thumbnail on the mark, hold the cup at eye level and pour the correct amount of the drug. Keep the label side of the bottle on top as you pour or put your palm over it.*	8	
13.	After pouring the drug, place the cup on a flat surface, and check the drug level again. If you poured out too much, discard it.*	8	
14.	Give the medicine cup to the patient with instructions to drink the liquid. If indicated, offer a glass of water or juice to wash down the drug.	4	

(continued)

Step Number	Procedure	Points Possible	Points Earned
After You Have Given an Oral Drug			
15.	Wash your hands.	4	
16.	Give the patient an information sheet about the drug. Discuss the information with the patient and answer any questions she may have. If the patient has questions you cannot answer, refer her to the physician.	4	
17.	Document the drug administration with the date, time, drug name, dosage, expiration date, lot number, manufacturer, route, site, significant patient reactions, and any patient education in the patient's chart.*	8	
Total Points		100	

CAAHEP Competencies Achieved

I. P (8)   Administer oral medications

II. P (1)   Prepare proper dosages of medication for administration

II. A (1)   Verify ordered doses/dosages prior to administration

ABHES Competencies Achieved

9. (j) Prepare and administer oral and parenteral medications as directed by physicians

PROCEDURE 53-2 Administering Buccal or Sublingual Drugs

WORK // DOC

Goal

To safely administer a buccal or sublingual drug to a patient.

OSHA Guidelines

This procedure does not involve exposure to blood, body fluids, or tissues.

Materials

Drug order (in patient chart), container of buccal or sublingual drug, small paper cup, package insert or drug information sheet.

Method

Step Number	Procedure	Points Possible	Points Earned
1.	Identify the patient and wash your hands.	4	
2.	Select the ordered drug.	4	
3.	Check the rights, comparing information against the drug order.*	10	
4.	If you are unfamiliar with the drug, check the *PDR* or other creditable drug reference, read the package insert, or speak with the physician.	4	
5.	Ask the patient about any drug or food allergies. If the patient is not allergic to the ordered drug or other ingredients used to prepare it, proceed.*	10	
6.	Perform any calculations needed to provide the prescribed dose. If you are unsure of your calculations, check them with a coworker or the physician.	6	
7.	Open the container and tap the correct number into the cap. Do not touch the inside of the cap because it is sterile. If you pour out too many tablets or capsules and you have not touched them, tap the excess back into the container.	6	
8.	Tap the tablets or capsules from the cap into the paper cup.	4	
9.	Recap the container immediately.*	10	
If You Are Giving Buccal Medication			
10.	For a buccal drug, provide patient instruction, including • Tell the patient not to chew or swallow the tablet. • Place the medication between the cheek and gum until it dissolves.* • Instruct the patient not to eat, drink, or smoke until the tablet is completely dissolved.*	10	
If You Are Giving a Sublingual Drug			
11.	For a *sublingual* drug, provide patient instruction including • Tell the patient not to chew or swallow the tablet. • Place the medication under the tongue until it dissolves.* • Instruct the patient not to eat, drink, or smoke until the tablet is completely dissolved.*	10	

(continued)

Step Number	Procedure	Points Possible	Points Earned
After You Have Given a Buccal or Sublingual Medication			
12.	Remain with the patient until the tablet dissolves to monitor for possible adverse reaction and to ensure that the patient has allowed the tablet to dissolve in the mouth instead of chewing or swallowing it.	4	
13.	Wash your hands.	4	
14.	Give the patient an information sheet about the drug. Discuss the information with the patient and answer any questions she may have. If the patient has questions you cannot answer, refer her to the physician.	4	
15.	Document the drug administration with the date, time, drug name, dosage, expiration date, lot number, manufacturer, route, site, significant patient reactions, and any patient education in the patient's chart.*	10	
Total Points		100	

CAAHEP Competencies Achieved

I. P (7) Select proper sites for administering parenteral medication

I. P (9) Administer parenteral (excluding IV) medications

II. P (1) Prepare proper dosages of medication for administration

II. A (1) Verify ordered doses/dosages prior to administration

ABHES Competencies Achieved

9. (j) Prepare and administer oral and parenteral medications as directed by physicians

Name_____ Date_____

Evaluated by_____ Score_____

PROCEDURE 53-3 Drawing a Drug from an Ampule

Goal
To safely open an ampule and draw a drug, using sterile technique.

OSHA Guidelines

Materials
Ampule of drug, alcohol swab, 2 × 2 gauze square, small file (provided by the drug manufacturer), sterile filtered needle, sterile needle, and a syringe of the appropriate size.

Method

Step Number	Procedure	Points Possible	Points Earned
1.	Wash your hands and put on exam gloves.	12	
2.	Gently tap the top of the ampule with your forefinger to settle the liquid to the bottom of the ampule.	12	
3.	Wipe the ampule's neck with an alcohol swab.	12	
4.	Wrap the 2 × 2 gauze square around the ampule's neck. Then snap the neck away from you. If it does not snap easily, score the neck with the small file and snap it again.	12	
5.	Insert the filtered needle into the ampule without touching the side of the ampule.*	25	
6.	Pull back on the plunger to aspirate (remove by vacuum or suction) the liquid completely into the syringe.	12	
7.	Replace with the regular needle and push the plunger on the syringe until the medication just reaches the tip of the needle. The drug is now ready for injection.	15	
Total Points		100	

CAAHEP Competencies Achieved

II. P (1)   Prepare proper dosages of medication for administration

II. A (1)   Verify ordered doses/dosages prior to administration

ABHES Competencies Achieved

9. (j) Prepare and administer oral and parenteral medications as directed by physicians

PROCEDURE 53-4 Reconstituting and Drawing a Drug for Injection

Goal
To reconstitute and draw a drug for injection, using sterile technique.

OSHA Guidelines

Materials
Vial of drug, vial of diluent, alcohol swabs, two disposable sterile needle and syringe sets of appropriate size, sharps container.

Method

Step Number	Procedure	Points Possible	Points Earned
1.	Wash your hands and put on exam gloves.	8	
2.	Place the drug vial and diluent vial on the countertop. Wipe each rubber diaphragm with a fresh alcohol swab.	8	
3.	Remove the cap from the needle and the guard from the syringe. Pull the plunger back to the mark that equals the amount of diluent needed to reconstitute the drug ordered.*	18	
4.	Puncture the diaphragm of the vial of diluent with the needle, and inject the air into the diluent.*	18	
5.	Invert the vial and aspirate the diluent.	8	
6.	Remove the needle from the diluent vial, inject the diluent into the drug vial, and withdraw the needle. Properly dispose of this needle and syringe.	8	
7.	Roll the vial between your hands to mix the drug and diluent thoroughly. Do not shake the vial unless so directed on the drug label.	8	
8.	Remove the cap and guard from the second needle and syringe.	8	
9.	Pull back the plunger to the mark that reflects the amount of drug ordered. Inject the air into the drug vial.	8	
10.	Invert the vial and aspirate the proper amount of the drug into the syringe. The drug is now ready for injection.	8	
Total Points		100	

CAAHEP Competencies Achieved

II. P (1)   Prepare proper dosages of medication for administration

II. A (1)   Verify ordered doses/dosages prior to administration

ABHES Competencies Achieved

9. (j) Prepare and administer oral and parenteral medications as directed by physicians

PROCEDURE 53-5 Giving an Intradermal Injection WORK // DOC

Goal
To administer an intradermal injection safely and effectively, using sterile technique.

OSHA Guidelines

Materials
Drug order (in patient chart), alcohol swab, disposable needle and syringe of the appropriate size filled with the ordered dose of drug, sharps container.

Method

Step Number	Procedure	Points Possible	Points Earned
1.	Identify the patient. Wash your hands and put on exam gloves.	6	
2.	Check the rights, comparing information against the drug order.*	15	
3.	Identify the injection site on the patient's forearm. To do so, rest the patient's arm on a table with the palm up. Measure 2 to 3 finger-widths below the antecubital space and a hand-width above the wrist. The space between is available for the injection.	6	
4.	Prepare the skin with the alcohol swab, moving in a circle from the center out.	6	
5.	Let the skin dry before giving the injection.*	15	
6.	Hold the patient's forearm, and stretch the skin taut with one hand.	6	
7.	With the other hand, place the needle—bevel up—almost flat against the patient's skin. Press the needle against the skin and insert it.	6	
8.	Inject the drug slowly and gently. You should see the needle through the skin and feel resistance. As the drug enters the upper layer of skin, a wheal (raised area of the skin) will form.	6	
9.	After the full dose of the drug has been injected, withdraw the needle. Properly dispose of used materials and the needle and syringe immediately.	6	
10.	Remove the gloves and wash your hands.	7	
11.	Stay with the patient to monitor for unexpected reactions.	6	
12.	Document the injection with the date, time, drug name, dosage, expiration date, lot number, manufacturer, route, site, significant patient reactions, and any patient education in the patient's chart.*	15	
Total Points		100	

CAAHEP Competencies Achieved

    I. P (7)   Select proper sites for administering parenteral medication

    I. P (9)   Administer parenteral (excluding IV) medications

    II. P (1)   Prepare proper dosages of medication for administration

    II. A (1)   Verify ordered doses/dosages prior to administration

ABHES Competencies Achieved

   9. (j) Prepare and administer oral and parenteral medications as directed by physicians

PROCEDURE 53-6 Giving a Subcutaneous Injection [WORK // DOC]

Goal
To administer a subcutaneous injection safely and effectively, using sterile technique.

OSHA Guidelines

Materials
Drug order (in patient's chart), alcohol swabs, sterile 2 × 2 gauze or cotton ball, container of the ordered drug, disposable needle and syringe of the appropriate size, sharps container.

Method

Step Number	Procedure	Points Possible	Points Earned
1.	Identify the patient. Wash your hands and put on exam gloves.	6	
2.	Check the rights, comparing information against the drug order.*	10	
3.	Prepare the drug and draw it up to the mark on the syringe that matches the ordered dose.	6	
4.	Choose a site and clean it with an alcohol swab, moving in a circle from the center out. Let the area dry.	6	
5.	Pinch the skin firmly to lift the subcutaneous tissue.	6	
6.	Position the needle—bevel up—at a 45- to 90-degree angle to the skin.*	10	
7.	Insert the needle in one quick motion. Then release the skin and inject the drug slowly. With some medications, you will check the placement of the needle by pulling back on the plunger before injecting. If blood is seen in the hub, you should withdraw the needle and start with a fresh needle and syringe. If no blood is seen, inject the medication slowly.	6	
8.	After the full dose of the drug has been injected, place a 2 × 2 gauze over the site, and withdraw the needle at the same angle you inserted it.	6	
9.	Apply pressure at the puncture site with the gauze or cotton ball.	6	
10.	Massage the site gently to help distribute the drug, if indicated. Do not massage insulin, heparin, or other anticoagulant medications.*	10	
11.	Properly dispose of the used materials and the needle and syringe.	6	
12.	Remove the gloves and wash your hands.	6	
13.	Stay with the patient to monitor for unexpected reactions.	6	
14.	Document the injection with the date, time, drug name, dosage, expiration date, lot number, manufacturer, route, site, significant patient reactions, and any patient education in the patient's chart.*	10	
Total Points		100	

Copyright © 2014 by The McGraw-Hill Companies, Inc.

Name_____ Date_____

Evaluated by_____ Score_____

CAAHEP Competencies Achieved

    I. P (7)   Select proper sites for administering parenteral medication

    I. P (9)   Administer parenteral (excluding IV) medications

    II. P (1)   Prepare proper dosages of medication for administration

    II. A (1)   Verify ordered doses/dosages prior to administration

ABHES Competencies Achieved

    9. (j) Prepare and administer oral and parenteral medications as directed by physicians

PROCEDURE 53-7 Giving an Intramuscular Injection [WORK//DOC]

Goal
To administer an intramuscular injection safely and effectively, using sterile technique.

OSHA Guidelines

Materials
Drug order (in patient's chart), alcohol swabs, sterile 2 × 2 gauze or cotton ball, container of the ordered drug, disposable needle and syringe of the appropriate size, sharps container.

Method

Step Number	Procedure	Points Possible	Points Earned
1.	Identify the patient. Wash your hands and put on exam gloves.	6	
2.	Check the rights, comparing information against the drug order.*	10	
3.	Prepare the drug and draw it up to the mark on the syringe that matches the ordered dose.	6	
4.	Choose a site and gently tap it. Tapping stimulates the nerve endings and reduces pain caused by the needle insertion.	6	
5.	Clean the site with an alcohol swab, moving in a circle from the center out. Let the site dry.	6	
6.	Stretch the skin taut over the injection site.	6	
7.	Hold the needle and syringe at a 90-degree angle to the skin. Then insert the needle with a quick, dart-like thrust.*	10	
8.	Release the skin and aspirate by pulling back slightly on the plunger to check the needle placement. If pulling back on the plunger produces blood, placement is incorrect and you must begin again with a fresh needle and syringe. If pulling back on the plunger produces no blood, placement is correct. Inject the drug slowly.*	10	
9.	After the full dose of the drug has been injected, place a 2 × 2 gauze over the site. Then quickly remove the needle at a 90-degree angle.	6	
10.	Use the 2 × 2 gauze to apply pressure to the site and massage it, if indicated.	6	
11.	Properly dispose of used materials and the needle and syringe.	6	
12.	Remove the gloves and wash your hands.	6	
13.	Stay with the patient to monitor for unexpected reactions.	6	
14.	Document the injection with the date, time, drug name, dosage, expiration date, lot number, manufacturer, route, site, significant patient reactions, and any patient education in the patient's chart.*	10	
Total Points		100	

CAAHEP Competencies Achieved

I. P (7)   Select proper sites for administering parenteral medication

I. P (9)   Administer parenteral (excluding IV) medications

II. P (1)   Prepare proper dosages of medication for administration

II. A (1)   Verify ordered doses/dosages prior to administration

ABHES Competencies Achieved

9. (j) Prepare and administer oral and parenteral medications as directed by physicians

PROCEDURE 53-8 Administering Inhalation Therapy WORK // DOC

Goal
To administer inhalation therapy safely and effectively.

OSHA Guidelines
This procedure does not involve exposure to blood, body fluids, or tissues.

Materials
Drug order (in patient's chart), container of the ordered drug, tissues, package insert or patient education sheet about medication.

Method

Step Number	Procedure	Points Possible	Points Earned
1.	Identify the patient. Wash your hands.	7	
2.	Check the rights, comparing information against the drug order. Make sure you have the correct type of inhaler based upon the order (oral or nasal).*	14	
3.	Prepare the container of medication as directed. Use the package insert and show the directions to the patient.	7	
4.	Shake the container as directed and stress this step to the patient.*	7	
For a Nasal Inhaler			
5.	Instruct the patient to complete the following steps: • Have the patient blow the nose to clear the nostrils. • Tilt the head back, and with one hand, place the inhaler tip about ½ inch into the nostril. • Point the tip straight up toward the inner corner of the eye.* • Use the opposite hand to block the other nostril. • Inhale gently while quickly and firmly squeezing the inhaler. • Remove the inhaler tip and exhale through the mouth. • Shake the inhaler and repeat the process in the other nostril. • If indicated in the package insert, instruct patients to keep the head tilted back and not to blow their nose for several minutes.	14	
For an Oral Inhaler			
6.	Instruct the patient to complete the following steps: • Warm the canister by rolling it between the palms of your hands. • Uncap the mouthpiece and assemble the inhaler as directed on the package insert. • Hold the mouth open and place the canister in the mouth or about 1 inch from the mouth. Check the package insert for the proper placement. • Exhale normally and inhale through the canister as he or she depresses it. The medication must be inhaled. • Breathe in until the lungs are full and hold the breath for 10 seconds • Breathe out normally.	9	
After You Have Given an Inhalation Medication			
7.	Remain with the patient to monitor for changes and possible adverse reaction.	7	
8.	Recap and secure the medication container. Instruct the patient in this procedure.	7	
9.	Wash your hands.	7	

(continued)

Step Number	Procedure	Points Possible	Points Earned
10.	Give the patient an information sheet about the drug. Discuss the information with the patient and answer any questions she may have. If the patient has questions you cannot answer, refer her to the physician.	7	
11.	Document the drug administration with the date, time, drug name, dosage, expiration date, lot number, manufacturer, route, site, significant patient reactions, and any patient education in the patient's chart.*	14	
Total Points		100	

CAAHEP Competencies Achieved

I. P (7)   Select proper sites for administering parenteral medication

I. P (9)   Administer parenteral (excluding IV) medications

II. P (1)   Prepare proper dosages of medication for administration

II. A (1)   Verify ordered doses/dosages prior to administration

ABHES Competencies Achieved

9. (j) Prepare and administer oral and parenteral medications as directed by physicians

PROCEDURE 53-9 Administering and Removing a Transdermal Patch and Providing Patient Instruction

WORK // DOC

Goal
To safely administer and remove a transdermal patch drug to a patient.

OSHA Guidelines
This procedure does not involve exposure to blood, body fluids, or tissues.

Materials
Drug order (in patient chart), transdermal patch medication, gloves, package insert or drug information sheet, patient chart.

Method

Step Number	Procedure	Points Possible	Points Earned
1.	Identify the patient, wash your hands, and put on gloves.*	9	
2.	Select the ordered transdermal patch and check the rights, comparing information against the drug order.*	9	
3.	Ask the patient about any drug or food allergies. If the patient is not allergic to the ordered drug or other ingredients used to prepare it, proceed.*	9	
4.	If you are unfamiliar with the drug, check the *PDR* or other credible drug reference, read the package insert, or speak with the physician.	5	
5.	Perform any calculations needed to provide the prescribed dose. If you are unsure of your calculations, check them with a coworker or the physician.	5	
Applying the Transdermal Medication			
6.	Remove the patch from its pouch. The plastic backing is easily peeled off once the patch is removed from the pouch. For patches without a protective pouch, bend the sides of the transdermal unit back and forth until the clear plastic backing snaps down the middle.	5	
7.	For either type of patch, demonstrate how to peel off the clear plastic backing to expose the sticky side of the patch.	5	
8.	Apply the patch to a reasonably hair-free site, such as the abdomen. Note that estrogen patches are usually placed on the hip.	5	
9.	Instruct the patient on how to apply the patch. Advise the patient to avoid using the extremities below the knee or elbow, skin folds, scar tissue, or burned or irritated areas.*	9	
Removing the Transdermal Patch			
10.	Gently lift and slowly peel the patch back from the skin. Wash the area with soap and dry it with a towel. Instruct the patient on this technique.	5	
11.	Explain to the patient that the skin may appear red and warm, which is normal. Reassure the patient that the redness will disappear. In some cases, lotion may be applied to the skin if it feels dry.	5	

(continued)

Step Number	Procedure	Points Possible	Points Earned
12.	Instruct the patient to notify the doctor if the redness does not disappear in several days or if a rash develops.	5	
13.	*Never* apply a new patch to the site just used. It is best to allow each site to rest between applications. Some transdermal systems call for waiting 7 days before using a site again. Be sure to check the package directions regarding site rotation.	5	
After You Have Applied and/or Removed the Transdermal Patch			
14.	Wash your hands and instruct the patient to do the same after applying or removing a transdermal system at home.	5	
15.	Give the patient an information sheet about the drug. Discuss the information with the patient and answer any questions she may have. If the patient has questions you cannot answer, refer her to the physician.	5	
16.	Document the drug administration with the date, time, drug name, dosage, expiration date, lot number, manufacturer, route, site, significant patient reactions, and any patient education in the patient's chart.*	9	
Total Points		100	

CAAHEP Competencies Achieved

I. P (7)   Select proper sites for administering parenteral medication

I. P (9)   Administer parenteral (excluding IV) medications

II. P (1)   Prepare proper dosages of medication for administration

II. A (1)   Verify ordered doses/dosages prior to administration

ABHES Competencies Achieved

9. (j) Prepare and administer oral and parenteral medications as directed by physicians

PROCEDURE 53-10 Assisting with Administration of a Urethral Drug

WORK // DOC

Goal
To assist with a urethral administration.

OSHA Guidelines

Materials
Urinary catheter kit, either a syringe without a needle or tubing and a bag (depending on the amount of drug to be administered), sterile gloves, the prescribed drug, a drape, and a bedsaver pad.

Method

Step Number	Procedure	Points Possible	Points Earned
1.	Wash your hands and use sterile technique to assemble the equipment.	7	
2.	Check the rights, comparing information against the drug order, and explain the procedure and the drug order to the patient.*	15	
3.	Assist the patient into the lithotomy position and drape her to preserve her modesty while exposing the vulva.	6	
4.	Place a bedsaver pad under the buttocks.	6	
5.	Open the catheter kit.	6	
6.	Put on sterile gloves.	6	
7.	Cleanse the vulva as you would to perform catheterization, using the materials in the kit. As you sweep down with the antiseptic swab, watch for the urethral opening to "wink."*	15	
8.	The physician or nurse will insert the lubricated catheter. Tell the patient that she should feel pressure, not pain, and that the physician or nurse is going to attach the syringe to the catheter and insert the drug (or attach the tubing and bag to the catheter and let the drug run in by gravity).	6	
9.	After instilling the drug, the physician or nurse will clamp the catheter and leave the drug in place for the ordered amount of time.	6	
10.	Stay with the patient not only to ensure that she remains still but also to reassure her that the full feeling in the bladder is normal. She may also say she feels the need to urinate. Advise her that this feeling, too, is normal and is caused by the catheter.	6	
11.	When the time is up, unclamp the catheter, gently remove it, and allow the patient to urinate. Assist the patient as needed.	6	
12.	While the patient is dressing, immediately document the drug instillation with date, time, drug, dose, route, and any significant patient reactions.*	15	
Total Points		100	

CAAHEP Competencies Achieved

I. P (7)   Select proper sites for administering parenteral medication

I. P (9)   Administer parenteral (excluding IV) medications

II. P (1)   Prepare proper dosages of medication for administration

II. A (1)   Verify ordered doses/dosages prior to administration

ABHES Competencies Achieved

9. (j) Prepare and administer oral and parenteral medications as directed by physicians

Copyright © 2014 by The McGraw-Hill Companies, Inc.

PROCEDURE 53-11 Administering a Vaginal Medication

WORK // DOC

Goal

To safely administer a vaginal medication with patient instruction.

OSHA Guidelines

Materials

Prescription or drug order in the patient's chart, a cloth or paper drape, a bedsaver pad, gloves, cotton balls, water-soluble lubricant, and the prescribed drug.

Method

Step Number	Procedure	Points Possible	Points Earned
1.	Wash your hands.	5	
2.	Check the rights, comparing information against the drug order, and explain the procedure and the drug order to the patient.*	14	
3.	Give the patient the opportunity to empty her bladder before beginning.	5	
4.	Assist the patient into the lithotomy position and drape her.*	13	
5.	Place a bedsaver pad under the buttocks.	5	
6.	Put on gloves.	5	
7.	Cleanse the perineum with soap and water, using one cotton ball per stroke, and cleanse the center last, while spreading the labia.*	14	
8.	Lubricate the vaginal suppository applicator in lubricant spread on a paper towel. For vaginal drugs in the forms of creams, ointments, gels, and tablets, use the appropriate applicator, preparing it according to the package insert.	5	
9.	While spreading the labia with one hand, insert the applicator with the other (the applicator should be about 2 inches into the vagina and angled toward the sacrum).	5	
10.	Release the labia and push the applicator's plunger to release the suppository into the vagina.	5	
11.	Remove the applicator, and wipe any excess lubricant off the patient.	5	
12.	Help her to a sitting position, and assist with dressing if needed.	5	
13.	Document the administration with date, time, drug, dose, route, and any significant patient reactions.*	14	
Total Points		100	

Name_____ Date_____

Evaluated by_____ Score_____

CAAHEP Competencies Achieved

  I. P (7)   Select proper sites for administering parenteral medication

  I. P (9)   Administer parenteral (excluding IV) medications

  II. P (1)   Prepare proper dosages of medication for administration

  II. A (1)   Verify ordered doses/dosages prior to administration

ABHES Competencies Achieved

  9. (j) Prepare and administer oral and parenteral medications as directed by physicians

PROCEDURE 53-12 Administering a Rectal Medication

`WORK//DOC`

Goal
To safely administer a rectal medication.

OSHA Guidelines

Materials
Prescription or drug order in the patient's chart, a cloth or paper drape, a bedsaver pad, gloves, water-soluble lubricant, and the prescribed drug.

Method

Step Number	Procedure	Points Possible	Points Earned
1.	Check the rights, comparing information against the drug order.*	11	
2.	Explain the procedure and the drug order to the patient.	4	
3.	Give the patient the opportunity to empty the bladder before beginning.	4	
4.	With the patient in a gown, help the patient into Sims' position and use a drape to prevent exposing the patient. Place a bedsaver pad under the patient.	4	
5.	Lift the patient's gown to expose the anus.	4	
6.	Wash your hands, put on gloves, and prepare the medication.	4	
When Administering a Suppository			
7.	Lubricate the tapered end of the suppository with about 1 tsp of lubricant.	4	
8.	While spreading the patient's buttocks with one hand, insert the suppository—tapered end first—into the anus with the other hand.	4	
9.	Gently advance the suppository past the sphincter with your index finger. Before it passes the sphincter, the suppository may feel as if it is being pushed back out the anus. When it passes the sphincter, it seems to disappear.	4	
10.	Use tissues to remove excess lubricant from the area.	4	
11.	Remove your gloves and ask the patient to lie quietly and retain the suppository for at least 20 minutes. When the treatment is completed, help the patient to a sitting, then standing, position.*	11	
When Administering a Retention Enema			
12.	Place the tip of a syringe into a rectal tube. Let a little rectal solution flow through the syringe and tube. While holding the tip up, clamp the tubing.	4	
13.	Lubricate the end of the tube and spread the patient's buttocks, and slide the tube into the rectum about 4 inches.	4	
14.	Slowly pour the rectal solution into the syringe, release the clamp, and let gravity move the solution into the patient. When you have administered the ordered amount of solution, clamp the tube and then remove it.	4	

(continued)

Step Number	Procedure	Points Possible	Points Earned
15.	Using tissues, apply pressure over the anus for 20 seconds to stifle the patient's urge to defecate, and then wipe any excess lubricant or solution from the area. Encourage the patient to retain the enema for the time ordered.*	11	
16.	When the time has passed, help the patient use a bedpan or direct the patient to a toilet to expel the solution.	4	
After the Administration Is Complete			
17.	Remove your gloves and wash your hands.	4	
18.	Immediately document the drug administration with date, time, drug, dose, route, and any significant patient reactions.*	11	
Total Points		100	

CAAHEP Competencies Achieved

I. P (7)   Select proper sites for administering parenteral medication

I. P (9)   Administer parenteral (excluding IV) medications

II. P (1)   Prepare proper dosages of medication for administration

II. A (1)   Verify ordered doses/dosages prior to administration

ABHES Competencies Achieved

9. (j) Prepare and administer oral and parenteral medications as directed by physicians

54

Physical Therapy and Rehabilitation

Name_____ Class_____ Date_____

R E V I E W

Vocabulary Review

Matching
Match the key terms in the right column with the definitions in the left column by placing the letter of each correct answer in the space provided.

_____ 1. Applying cold to a patient's body for therapeutic reasons

_____ 2. A protractor device that measures the range of motion in degrees

_____ 3. Body position or alignment

_____ 4. Applying heat to a patient's body for therapeutic reasons

_____ 5. Redness of the skin

_____ 6. A type of heat therapy in which a machine produces high-frequency waves

_____ 7. A device designed to improve a patient's ability to move

a. cryotherapy
b. diathermy
c. erythema
d. goniometer
e. mobility aid
f. posture
g. thermotherapy

True or False
Decide whether each statement is true or false. In the space at the left, write T for true or F for false. On the lines provided, rewrite the false statements to make them true.

_____ 8. Art therapy provides treatment of musculoskeletal, nervous, and cardiovascular disorders.

_____

_____ 9. The most common form of diathermy is a hot pack.

_____

_____ 10. Cryotherapy causes blood vessels to constrict.

_____

_____ 11. Applying heat for therapeutic reasons is known as hydrotherapy.

_____

_____ 12. The degree to which a joint is able to move is known as gait.

_____

_____ 13. Posture is your body position and alignment.

_____

_____ 14. During ROM exercises, the patient builds muscle strength.

_____

_____ 15. Ultraviolet lamps are used to treat psoriasis.

_____

Content Review

Multiple Choice

In the space provided, write the letter of the choice that best completes each statement or answers each question.

_____ 1. Which of the following is a mobility aid?
- **a.** Traction
- **b.** Cane
- **c.** ROM
- **d.** Diathermy
- **e.** Massage

_____ 2. Fluid accumulation in tissues is known as
- **a.** Constriction
- **b.** Erythema
- **c.** Edema
- **d.** Inflammation
- **e.** Hematoma

_____ 3. When using the three-point gait with crutches, the patient moves both the crutches and the affected leg forward from the tripod position and then
- **a.** Moves the unaffected leg forward while weight is balanced on both crutches
- **b.** Moves the left crutch and the right foot forward at the same time
- **c.** Moves the right foot forward to level with the left crutch
- **d.** Swings both legs forward together ahead of the crutches
- **e.** Swings both legs forward together even with the crutches

_____ 4. Redness of the skin is known as
- **a.** Cyanosis
- **b.** Edema
- **c.** Diathermy
- **d.** Erythema
- **e.** ROM

_____ 5. A treatment that uses heated wax and mineral oil is known as
- **a.** A paraffin bath
- **b.** Diathermy
- **c.** Fluidotherapy
- **d.** A hot pack
- **e.** Neuromuscular massage

Sentence Completion

In the space provided, write the word or phrase that best completes each sentence.

6. Cold compresses and ice massages are types of _____ _____ applications used in cryotherapy.

7. Static traction is also called _____ traction.

8. _____ _____ exercises are self-directed exercises that the patient does without help.

9. During _____ traction, a physical therapist pulls gently on a patient's limb or head.

10. During _____ _____ exercises, the physical therapist moves a patient's body part.

11. _____ _____ stimulate muscles by delivering controlled amounts of low-voltage electric current to motor and sensory nerves.

6. _____

7. _____

8. _____

9. _____

10. _____

11. _____

Short Answer

Write the answer to each question on the lines provided.

12. What are four benefits of physical therapy?

_____

_____

_____

13. Why is it important to ask a patient how a hot pack feels?

_____

_____

14. What are four beneficial results that can be achieved through cryotherapy?

_____

_____

15. What is the process by which thermotherapy promotes healing?

_____

_____

16. What are two types of dry heat therapy?

_____

_____

17. What are two benefits of manual traction?

_____

_____

18. What is the difference between active and passive mobility exercises?

_____

_____

19. To make sure that crutches fit a patient properly, what conditions should you check before the patient leaves the office?

_____

_____

20. What factors determine the type of mobility aid chosen for a patient?

_____

_____

_____

21. Describe the following Swedish massage strokes: (a) pétrissage, (b) effleurage, (c) tapotement.

_____

_____

_____

Critical Thinking

Write the answer to each question on the lines provided.

1. Why is it important to check a chemical cold pack for leaks before applying the pack to the patient?

_____

_____

_____

2. How might a reduction in a patient's ROM affect the type of mobility device the patient should be using?

_____

_____

_____

3. Why is it important that a patient not lie on a heating pad?

_____

_____

_____

4. Why is it important to ensure that a patient knows how to perform exercises correctly?

_____

_____

_____

5. Why might a doctor prescribe cryotherapy, thermotherapy, or some other type of therapy in addition to exercise therapy for a patient with a sports injury?

_____

_____

_____

6. What should you do if a patient who uses a walker tells you there are steps in his house?

_____

_____

_____

A P P L I C A T I O N

Follow the directions for each application.

1. **Teaching a Patient How to Use a Walker**

   Work with two partners to teach a patient how to use a mobility aid. One partner should take the role of the patient, one should take the role of a medical assistant who is teaching the patient how to use a mobility aid, and the third should serve as observer and evaluator.

   a. Role-play teaching a patient to use a walker. The medical assistant should assist the patient in stepping into the walker and explain how to grip the sides of the walker. The assistant should then instruct the patient in how to position his feet and to walk securely. The patient should ask questions during the instruction. The observer should refer to the steps outlined in Procedure 54-4 while observing the teaching.

   b. The medical assistant should next explain how to maneuver the walker for sitting down in a chair or on a bed.

   c. The medical assistant should then teach the patient how to ascend and descend stairs.

   d. Following the teaching, the observer should critique the session, pointing out any errors or omissions in the instruction. The three partners should then discuss the session and the evaluator's comments.

   e. Team members should exchange roles and review the use of another mobility aid. The new observer should evaluate the session, and all three partners should discuss the session.

   f. Team members should exchange roles one more time and go through the use of a third mobility aid. Each student should have the opportunity to play each role.

2. **Learning Crutch Walking and Preparing an Educational Brochure**

   Workings in pairs, teach each other various gaits:

   a. Two-point gait

   b. Three-point gait

   c. Four-point gait

   d. Swing-to gait

   e. Swing-through gait

   Follow these steps:

   1. First review text Procedure 54-5.

   2. Discuss the steps necessary to perform each type of gait. Write a list of the steps to use for each gait while performing the instruction.

   3. Practice teaching and performing the various gaits.

   4. Practice getting up and sitting down.

   5. Practice ascending and descending stairs.

   6. After you have mastered the gaits, create a patient teaching brochure for each of the types of gaits.

C A S E   S T U D I E S

Write your response to each case study on the lines provided.

Case 1

The doctor has prescribed use of a chemical ice pack for a 62-year-old patient with a sprained ankle. After the ice pack has been on the ankle for 15 minutes, the patient complains of increased pain in the ankle. What should you do?

_____

_____

_____

Case 2

While applying a moist heat pack, you notice that the patient is shivering. What should you do?

_____

_____

_____

Case 3

After a few minutes, the patient from Case 2 complains of being uncomfortably hot. What should you do?

_____

_____

_____

Case 4

A patient with paraplegia needs crutches. What type of crutches will most likely be prescribed? Why?

_____

_____

_____

Case 5

A patient who is having difficulty recovering from a leg injury sustained in an automobile accident is considering dance therapy. What will you tell her?

_____

_____

_____

Case 6

The doctor prescribed massage therapy for a patient with neck and back spasms. The patient doesn't think it will help him. What can you tell him about the benefits of massage therapy?

_____

_____

_____

PROCEDURE 54-1 Administering Cryotherapy

WORK//DOC

Goal
To reduce pain and swelling by safely and effectively administering cryotherapy.

OSHA Guidelines

Materials
Gloves, cold application materials required as ordered: ice bag, ice collar, chemical cold pack, washcloth or gauze squares, or ice.

Method

Step Number	Procedure	Points Possible	Points Earned
1.	Double-check the physician's order. Be sure you know where to apply therapy and how long it should remain in place.	5	
2.	Identify the patient, and explain the procedure and its purpose. Ask if the patient has any questions.	5	
3.	Have the patient undress and put on a gown, if required; provide privacy or assistance as needed.	5	
4.	Wash your hands and don gloves.	5	
5.	Position the patient comfortably and drape appropriately.*	10	

6.	Prepare the therapy as ordered.*
	• Ice bag or collar
	  a. Prior to use, check the ice bag or collar for leaks.
	  b. Fill the ice bag or collar two-thirds full with ice chips or small ice cubes. Compress the container to expel any air and then close it.
	  c. Dry the bag or collar completely and cover it with a towel. This will absorb moisture and provide comfort.
	• Chemical ice pack
	  a. Check the pack for leaks.
	  b. Shake or squeeze the pack to activate the chemicals, or use a cold chemical pack taken from a refrigerator or freezer.
	  c. Cover the pack with a towel.
	• Cold compress
	  a. Place the washcloth or gauze squares under a stream of running water.
	  b. Wring them out.
	  c. Rewet at frequent intervals.
		10	

7.	Place the device on the patient's affected body part. If you are using a compress, place an ice bag on it, if desired, to keep it colder longer.*	10	
8.	Ask the patient how the device feels.*	10	
9.	Explain the cold is of great benefit, although it may be somewhat uncomfortable.	5	

(continued)

Step Number	Procedure	Points Possible	Points Earned
10.	Leave the device in place for the length of time ordered by the physician. Periodically check the skin for color, feeling, and pain. If the area becomes excessively pale or blue, numb, or painful, remove the device and have the physician examine the area. For cold application using ice, limit application time to 20 minutes.*	10	
11.	Remove the application and observe the area for reduced swelling, redness, and pain. If the patient has a dressing, replace it at this time.	5	
12.	Help the patient dress, if needed.	5	
13.	Remove equipment and supplies, properly discarding used disposable materials; sanitize, disinfect, and/or sterilize reusable equipment and materials as needed.	5	
14.	Remove the gloves and wash your hands.	5	
15.	Document the treatment and your observation in the patient's chart. If you teach the patient or the patient's family how to use the device, document your instructions.	5	
Total Points		100	

CAAHEP Competencies Achieved

IV. P (6)   Prepare a patient for procedures and/or treatments

ABHES Competencies Achieved

2. (c) Assist the physician with the regimen of diagnostic and treatment modalities as they relate to each body system

PROCEDURE 54-2 Administering Thermotherapy WORK//DOC

Goal
To administer thermotherapy safely and effectively.

OSHA Guidelines

Materials
Gloves, towels, blanket, heat application materials required for order: chemical hot pack, heating pad, hot-water bottle, heat lamp, container and medication for hot soak, and container and gauze for hot compress.

Method

Step Number	Procedure	Points Possible	Points Earned
1.	Double-check the physician's order. Be sure you know where to apply therapy, the proper temperature for the application, and how long it should remain in place.	5	
2.	Identify the patient and explain the procedure and its purpose. Ask if the patient has any questions.	5	
3.	Have the patient undress and put on a gown, if required; provide privacy or assistance as needed.	5	
4.	Wash your hands and don gloves.	5	
5.	Position the patient comfortably and drape appropriately.*	8	
6.	If the patient has a dressing, check the dressing for blood and change as necessary. Alert the physician and ask if treatment should continue.*	8	
7.	Check the temperature by touch and look for the presence of adverse skin conditions (excessive redness, blistering, or irritation) on all applications before and during the treatment.*	8	
8.	As necessary, reheat devices or solutions to provide therapeutic temperatures and then reapply them.	5	

9.	Prepare the therapy as ordered.*
	• Chemical hot pack
	  a. Check the pack for leaks.
	  b. Activate the pack. (Check manufacturer's directions.)
	  c. Cover the pack with a towel.
	• Heating pad
	  a. Turn the heating pad on, selecting the appropriate temperature setting.
	  b. Cover the pad with a towel or pillowcase.
	  c. Make sure the patient's skin is dry, and do not allow the patient to lie on top of the heating pad.
		8	

(continued)

Step Number	Procedure	Points Possible	Points Earned

	• Hot-water bottle
	  a. Fill the bottle one-half full with hot water of the correct temperature—usually 110°F to 115°F. Use a thermometer. The physician can provide information on the ideal temperature of water that should be used, which will depend on the area being treated.
	  b. Expel the air and close the bottle.
	  c. Cover the bottle with a towel or pillowcase.
	• Heat lamp
	  a. Place the lamp 2 feet to 4 feet away from the treatment area. (Check manufacturer's directions.)
	  b. Follow the treatment time as ordered.
	• Hot soak
	  a. Select a container of the appropriate size for the area to be treated.
	  b. Fill the container with hot water that is no more than 110°F. Use a thermometer. Add medication to the container if ordered.
	• Hot compress
	  a. Soak a washcloth or gauze in hot water. Wring it out.
	  b. Frequently rewarm the compress to maintain the temperature.		

10.	Place the device on the patient's affected body part, or place the affected body part in the container. If you are using a compress, place a hot-water bottle on top, if desired, to keep it warm longer.	5	
11.	Ask the patient how the device feels. During any heat therapy, remember, dilated blood vessels cause heat loss from the skin and this heat loss may make the patient feel chilled. Be prepared to cover the patient with sheets or blankets.	5	
12.	Leave the device in place for the length of time ordered by the physician. Periodically check the skin for redness, blistering, or irritation. If the area becomes excessively red or develops blisters, remove the patient from the heat source and have the physician examine the area.*	8	
13.	Remove the application and observe the area for inflammation and swelling. Replace the patient's dressing if necessary.	5	
14.	Help the patient dress, if needed.	5	
15.	Remove equipment and supplies, properly discarding used disposable materials, and sanitize, disinfect, and/or sterilize reusable equipment and materials as needed.	5	
16.	Remove the gloves and wash your hands.	5	
17.	Document the treatment and your observation in the patient's chart. If you teach the patient or the patient's family how to use the device, document your instructions.	5	
Total Points		100	

CAAHEP Competencies Achieved

IV. P (6)   Prepare a patient for procedures and/or treatments

ABHES Competencies Achieved

2. (c) Assist the physician with the regimen of diagnostic and treatment modalities as they relate to each body system

PROCEDURE 54-3 Teaching a Patient How to Use a Cane

Goal
To teach a patient how to use a cane safely.

OSHA Guidelines
This procedure does not involve exposure to blood, body fluids, or tissues.

Materials
A cane suited to the patient's needs.

Method

Step Number	Procedure	Points Possible	Points Earned
Standing from a Sitting Position			
1.	Instruct the patient to slide his buttocks to the edge of the chair.	5	
2.	Tell the patient to place his right foot slightly behind and inside the right front leg of the chair and his left foot slightly behind and inside the left front leg of the chair. (This provides him with a wide, stable stance.)*	7	
3.	Instruct the patient to lean forward and use the armrests or seat of the chair to push upward. Caution the patient not to lean on the cane.*	7	
4.	Have the patient position the cane for support on the uninjured or strong side of his body, as indicated	5	
Walking			
1.	Teach the patient to hold the cane on the uninjured or strong side of her body with the tip(s) of the cane 4 to 6 inches from the side and in front of her strong foot. Remind the patient to make sure the tip is flat on the ground.	5	
2.	Have the patient move the cane forward approximately 8 inches and then move her affected foot forward, parallel to the cane.*	7	
3.	Next, have the patient move her strong leg forward past the cane and her weak leg.*	7	
4.	Observe as the patient repeats this process.	5	
Ascending Stairs			
1.	Instruct the patient to always start with his uninjured or strong leg when going up stairs.	5	
2.	Advise the patient to keep the cane on the uninjured or strong side of his body and to use the wall or rail, if available, for support on the weak side. If a rail is not available, the patient may need assistance for safety.*	7	
3.	After the patient steps on the strong leg, instruct him to bring up his weak leg and then the cane.*	7	
4.	Remind the patient not to rush.	5	
Descending Stairs			
1.	Instruct the patient to always start with her weak leg when going down stairs.	5	
2.	Advise the patient to keep the cane on the uninjured or strong side of her body and to use the wall or rail, if available, for support on the weak side. If a rail is not available, the patient may need assistance for safety.*	7	

(continued)

Step Number	Procedure	Points Possible	Points Earned
3.	Have the patient use the uninjured or strong leg and wall or rail to support her body, put the cane on the next step, and bend the strong leg as she lowers the weak leg to the next step.*	7	
4.	Instruct the patient to step down with the strong leg.	5	
Walking on Snow or Ice			
1.	Suggest the patient try a metal ice-gripping cane or a ski pole. These can be dug into the snow or ice to prevent slipping. Instruct the patient to avoid walking on ice unless absolutely necessary.	4	
Total Points		100	

CAAHEP Competencies Achieved

XI. C (10)   Identify principles of body mechanics and ergonomics

ABHES Competencies Achieved

5. (b) Identify and respond appropriately when working/caring for patients with special needs

9. (q) Instruct patients with special needs

PROCEDURE 54-4 Teaching a Patient How to Use a Walker

Goal
To teach a patient how to use a walker safely.

OSHA Guidelines
This procedure does not involve exposure to blood, body fluids, or tissues.

Materials
A walker suited to the patient's needs.

Method

Step Number	Procedure	Points Possible	Points Earned
Walking			
1.	Instruct the patient to step into the walker.*	10	
2.	Tell the patient to place her hands on the handgrips on the sides of the walker.*	10	
3.	Make sure the patient's feet are far enough apart so she feels balanced.*	10	
4.	Instruct the patient to pick up the walker and move it forward about 6 inches.*	10	
5.	Have the patient move one foot forward and then the other foot.*	10	
6.	Instruct the patient to pick up the walker again and move it forward. If the patient is strong enough, explain that she may advance the walker after moving each leg rather than waiting until she has moved both legs.*	10	
Sitting			
1.	Teach the patient to turn his back to the chair or bed.	5	
2.	Instruct the patient to take small, careful steps and to back up until he feels the chair or bed at the back of his legs.*	10	
3.	Instruct the patient to keep the walker in front of himself, let go of the walker, and place both his hands on the arms or seat of the chair or on the bed.*	10	
4.	Teach the patient to balance himself on his arms while lowering himself slowly to the chair or bed.	5	
5.	If the patient has an injured or affected leg, he should keep it forward while bending his unaffected leg and lowering his body to the chair or bed.*	10	
Total Points		100	

CAAHEP Competencies Achieved

XI. C (10) Identify principles of body mechanics and ergonomics

ABHES Competencies Achieved

5. (b) Identify and respond appropriately when working/caring for patients with special needs

9. (q) Instruct patients with special needs

Name_____ Date_____

Evaluated by_____ Score_____

PROCEDURE 54-5 Teaching a Patient How to Use Crutches

Goal
To teach a patient how to use crutches safely.

OSHA Guidelines
This procedure does not involve exposure to blood, body fluids, or tissues.

Materials
A pair of crutches suited to the patient's needs.

Method

Step Number	Procedure	Points Possible	Points Earned
1.	Verify the physician's order for the type of crutches and gait to be used.	8	
2.	Wash your hands, identify the patient, and explain the procedure.	8	
3.	Elderly patients or patients with muscle weakness should be taught muscle strength exercises for their arms	8	
4.	Have the patient stand erect and look straight ahead.	8	
5.	Tell the patient to place the crutch tips 2 to 4 inches in front of and 4 to 6 inches to the side of each foot.	8	
6.	When instructing a patient to use an axillary crutch, make sure the patient has a 2-inch gap between the axilla and the axillary bar and that each elbow is flexed 25 degrees to 30 degrees.*	10	
7.	Teach the patient how to get up from a chair:* **a.** Instruct the patient to hold both crutches on his affected or weaker side. **b.** Have the patient slide to the edge of the chair. **c.** Tell the patient to push down on the arm or seat of the chair on his stronger side and use his strong leg to push up. If indicated, keep the affected leg forward. **d.** Advise the patient to put the crutches under his arms and press down on the hand grips with his hands.	10	
8.	Teach the patient the required gait. Which gait the patient will use depends on the patient's muscle strength and coordination. It also depends on the type of crutches, the injury, and the patient's condition. Check the physician's orders, and see Figures 54-11 and 54-12 for examples.*	10	
9.	Teach the patient how to ascend stairs:* **a.** Start the patient close to the bottom step, and tell him to push down with his hands. **b.** Instruct the patient to step up on the first step with his good foot. **c.** Tell the patient to lift the crutches to the same step and then lift his other foot. Advise the patient to keep his crutches with his affected limb. **d.** Remind the patient to check his balance before he proceeds to the next step.	10	

(continued)

Step Number	Procedure	Points Possible	Points Earned
10.	Teach the patient how to descend stairs:* a. Have the patient start at the edge of the steps. b. Instruct the patient to bring his crutches and then the affected foot down first. Advise the patient to bend at the hips and knees to prevent leaning forward, which could cause him to fall. c. Tell the patient to bring his unaffected foot to the same step. d. Remind the patient to check his balance before he proceeds. In some cases, a handrail may be easier and can be used with both crutches in one hand.	10	
11.	Give the patient the following general information related to the use of crutches:* a. Do not lean on crutches. b. Report to the physician any tingling or numbness in the arms, hands, or shoulders. c. Support body weight with the hands. d. Always stand erect to prevent muscle strain. e. Look straight ahead when walking. f. Generally, move the crutches not more than 6 inches at a time to maintain good balance. g. Check the crutch tips regularly for wear; replace the tips as needed. h. Check the crutch tips for wetness; dry the tips if they are wet. i. Check all wing nuts and bolts for tightness. j. Wear flat, well-fitting, nonskid shoes. k. Remove throw rugs and other unsecured articles from traffic areas. l. Report any unusual pain in the affected leg.	10	
Total Points		100	

CAAHEP Competencies Achieved

XI. C (10)   Identify principles of body mechanics and ergonomics

ABHES Competencies Achieved

5. (b) Identify and respond appropriately when working/caring for patients with special needs

9. (q) Instruct patients with special needs

55

Nutrition and Health

Name_____ Class_____ Date_____

REVIEW

Vocabulary Review

Matching

Match the key terms in the right column with the definitions in the left column by placing the letter of each correct answer in the space provided.

_____ 1. The phase of metabolism in which a complex substance is broken into simpler substances and converted to energy

_____ 2. A fat-related substance produced by the liver that can also be obtained through dietary sources

_____ 3. A condition in which people get too little water or lose too much water due to vomiting, diarrhea, and similar causes

_____ 4. Natural, inorganic substances the body needs to carry on life functions

_____ 5. Weight loss technique aimed at changing patterns that lead to overeating

_____ 6. A unit of food that provides the same amounts of protein, fat, and carbohydrate as all other units in a food category

_____ 7. Injecting nutrients directly into a patient's veins

_____ 8. An eating disorder in which people starve themselves

_____ 9. Fats that are usually solid at room temperature

_____ 10. A chemical agent that fights free radicals

_____ 11. A protein substance found in wheat, rye, and barley

_____ 12. Fats that are usually liquid at room temperature

_____ 13. A long chain of sugar units

_____ 14. The amount of energy needed to raise the temperature of 1 kg of water by 1°C

_____ 15. A type of complex carbohydrate that is not absorbed by the body

_____ 16. An eating disorder in which people binge and then attempt to counter the effects by vomiting, exercising, or using laxatives

_____ 17. The phase of metabolism in which nutrients are changed into more complex substances and used to build body tissues

_____ 18. Natural organic compounds found in plant and animal foods

_____ 19. An essential nutrient for building and repairing cells and tissue

_____ 20. Organic substances that are essential for normal body growth and maintenance

a. anorexia nervosa
b. behavior modification
c. calorie
d. cholesterol
e. antioxidant
f. complex carbohydrate
g. dehydration
h. amino acids
i. fiber
j. vitamins
k. catabolism
l. food exchange
m. gluten
n. protein
o. saturated fat
p. anabolism
q. bulimia
r. minerals
s. unsaturated fat
t. parenteral nutrition

True or False

Decide whether each statement is true or false. In the space at the left, write T for true or F for false. On the lines provided, rewrite the false statements to make them true.

_____ **21.** Antigens are chemical agents that fight cell-destroying free radicals.

_____

_____ **22.** The body uses amino acids to create proteins.

_____

_____ **23.** Fiber can help lower blood cholesterol levels.

_____

_____ **24.** Incomplete carbohydrates lack one or more of the essential amino acids.

_____

_____ **25.** Starch is the tough, stringy part of vegetables and fruits that is not absorbed by the body but aids in a variety of bodily functions.

_____

_____ **26.** Lipids are carried through the bloodstream by soluble fiber.

_____

_____ **27.** Each gram of protein contains 4 calories.

_____

_____ **28.** Complete proteins are also known as polysaccharides.

_____

_____ **29.** Saturated fats are derived from animal sources.

_____

_____ **30.** Triglycerides are simple lipids that consist of glycerol and three fatty acids.

_____

Content Review

Multiple Choice

In the space provided, write the letter of the choice that best completes each statement or answers each question.

_____ **1.** Which of the following nutrients can help prevent diverticular disease, constipation, and irritable bowel syndrome?

  a. Lipids   **d.** Fiber

  b. Calcium   **e.** Complete proteins

  c. Electrolytes

_____ **2.** An increased risk of heart disease, stroke, and peripheral vascular disease has been linked with high levels of

  a. Folate   **d.** Lipoproteins and unsaturated fats

  b. Vitamins A and K   **e.** Iron and fluoride

  c. Triglycerides and cholesterol

_____ 3. Which of the following is *not* a function of water in the human body?

    a. Aiding in digestion   **d.** Flushing out wastes

    b. Regulating body temperature   **e.** Promoting the healing of wounds

    c. Lubricating the body's moving parts

_____ 4. Which of the following statements about diet therapy is *false*?

    a. Diet therapy sometimes involves restricting certain foods

    b. Diet therapy always involves lowering the daily caloric intake

    c. Diet therapy may involve changing the number of meals per day

    d. Physicians and dietitians cooperate to determine which diet therapy is best for a patient

    e. Diet therapy sometimes involves changing or specifying the texture of foods

_____ 5. The optimal percentage of body fat for women younger than age 50 is

    a. 10% to 14%   **d.** 16% to 25%

    b. 12% to 19%   **e.** 18% to 30%

    c. 14% to 23%

_____ 6. Dietary guidelines that aim to reduce the risk of heart attack recommend choosing a diet that is

    a. Low in saturated fats and cholesterol   **d.** High in salt

    b. Low in fiber   **e.** Supplemented by vitamins

    c. Moderate in sugars

_____ 7. What is the chief difference between a full-liquid diet and a clear-liquid diet?

    a. A full-liquid diet is higher in carbohydrates

    b. A full-liquid diet includes strained cooked cereals and soups

    c. A clear-liquid diet contains large amounts of fiber

    d. A clear-liquid diet is higher in proteins

    e. A clear-liquid diet allows citrus juices

_____ 8. The term *reduced cholesterol* on a food label means that the food has

    a. Less than or equal to 2 mg of cholesterol per serving

    b. Less than or equal to 20 mg of cholesterol per serving

    c. At least 25% less cholesterol per serving than the food it replaces

    d. At least 50% less cholesterol per serving than the food it replaces

    e. At least 75% less cholesterol per serving than the food it replaces

_____ 9. A sign of bulimia is

    a. Mood swings

    b. Self-starvation

    c. Cessation of menstruation

    d. Weight gain

    e. Malnourishment

_____ 10. The 2010 USDA Dietary Guidelines encourage people to do all of the following *except*

    a. Increase vegetable and fruit intake

    b. Maintain appropriate calorie balance during each stage of life

    c. Decrease intake of fat-free or low-fat milk products

    d. Promote a healthy weight by improving physical activity

    e. Control total calorie intake to manage body weight

Sentence Completion

In the space provided, write the word or phrase that best completes each sentence.

11. A physician or _____ prescribes a diet for a patient after determining the patient's nutritional status.

12. _____ fiber, found in the bran in whole wheat bread and brown rice, promotes regular bowel movements by contributing to stool bulk.

13. The Recommended Daily Allowance of vitamin C for an adult female is _____.

14. Trans fatty acids form through a process known as _____, which turns liquid oils into solid fats.

15. Iron deficiency can cause _____, a blood disorder that can leave a person fatigued, weak, and mentally impaired.

16. The 2011 guidelines of the _____ recommend that people be as lean as possible throughout life without being underweight.

17. Wheat, milk, eggs, and chocolate are some of the most common food _____.

18. Patients with diabetes should not miss a meal because skipping meals disturbs the balance of _____ and metabolism.

19. You can learn about a packaged food's caloric, fat, and sodium content per serving by reading the _____ label.

20. Managed care and other health insurance providers require documentation of _____ about nutrition.

11. _____

12. _____

13. _____

14. _____

15. _____

16. _____

17. _____

18. _____

19. _____

20. _____

Short Answer

Write the answer to each question on the lines provided.

21. What are the three major ways in which the human body uses nutrients?

_____

_____

_____

22. What are RDAs? Why do you need to know about them?

_____

_____

_____

23. What is the purpose of the USDA Dietary Guidelines for Americans?

_____

_____

_____

24. Under what circumstances might a physician be likely to prescribe a diet to help a patient gain weight?

_____

_____

_____

25. Describe five guidelines that you can follow when discussing diets with a patient.

_____

_____

_____

_____

_____

26. Describe MyPlate and label the parts on the following figure.

_____

_____

_____

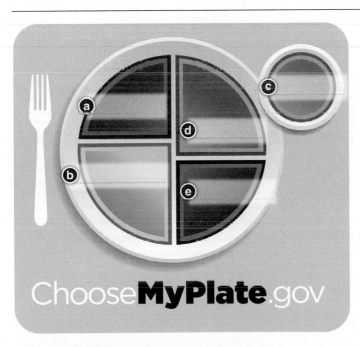

Source: www.choosemyplate.gov.

27. What are the four basic recommendations from the American Cancer Society to prevent cancer?

_____

_____

_____

_____

28. What is BMI, and how is it used?

_____

_____

_____

29. List the recommended foods for each of the following patients.

    a. 1½-year-old child _____

_____

    b. 10-month-old infant _____

_____

    c. 3-month-old infant _____

_____

Critical Thinking

Write the answer to each question on the lines provided.

1. Cities that host marathons often provide a spaghetti dinner for participants who want to "carbo-load" the night before the race. Why would marathon runners want to eat a lot of carbohydrates?

_____

_____

_____

2. What is the difference between trans fats and saturated fats?

_____

_____

_____

3. Why is behavior modification generally more successful than fad dieting when it comes to long-term weight loss?

_____

_____

_____

4. Why is it important to take a patient's culture and religion into account when planning the patient's diet?

_____

_____

_____

A P P L I C A T I O N
WORK // DOC

Follow the directions for each application.

1. Modifying Diets

Using the Internet, research diabetic diet exchanges and prepare a travel diet for a diabetic patient. Suggestions for research include the American Diabetes Association and the American Dietetic Association.

2. Preparing Patient Education Materials

In teams of three or four, choose a disease or condition for each team to research, such as hyperlipidemia, hypertension, food allergies, or another condition. Each team should design a poster or informational booklet describing the disease and associated diet restrictions. Each team should present their findings to the class for discussion.

3. **Educating patients**

Role-play educating a patient about his or her daily water food allergies, how to read food labels, and a special diet. Use the sample progress note form at the back of this workbook to document your patient education.

CASE STUDIES

Write your response to each case study on the lines provided.

Case 1

You hear Joe, another medical assistant in your office, talking to a patient about the diet the doctor has prescribed. Joe says, "Well, if you really like red meat, go ahead and eat it. Just try to cut back your fat intake from other foods." What, if anything, has Joe done wrong?

_____

_____

_____

Case 2

"Why is the doctor telling me to cut back on beer?" complains Mr. Kowalski, who is being treated for hypertension. "I've heard that beer can be good for you!" How should you respond?

_____

_____

_____

Case 3

The physician has just prescribed a low-cholesterol diet for Mrs. Ryan. "But how am I supposed to know how much cholesterol my food has?" she asks you. How could you help Mrs. Ryan?

_____

_____

_____

PROCEDURE 55-1 Teaching Patients How to Read Food Labels

Goal
To explain how patients can use food labels to plan or follow a diet.

OSHA Guidelines
This procedure does not involve exposure to blood, body fluids, or tissues.

Materials
Food labels from products.

Method

Step Number	Procedure	Points Possible	Points Earned
1.	Identify the patient and introduce yourself.	10	
2.	Explain that food labels can be used as a valuable source of information when planning or implementing a prescribed diet.	10	
3.	Using a label from a food package, point out the Nutrition Facts section.	10	
4.	Describe the various elements on the label—in this case the ice-cream label: • Serving size is the basis for the nutrition information provided.* • Calories and calories from fat show the proportion of fat calories in the product. • The % Daily Value section shows how many grams (g) or milligrams (mg) of a variety of nutrients are contained in one serving. Then the label shows the percentage (%) of the recommended daily intake of each given nutrient (assuming a diet of 2000 calories a day). • Recommendations for total amounts of various nutrients for both a 2000-calorie and a 2500-calorie diet are shown in chart form near the bottom of the label. These numbers provide the basis for the daily value percentages. • Ingredients are listed in order from largest quantity to smallest quantity.	30	
5.	Inform the patient that a variety of similar products with significantly different nutritional values are often available. Explain that patients can use nutrition labels to evaluate and compare such similar products. Patients must consider what a product contributes to their diets, not simply what it lacks. To do this, patients must read the entire label.	10	
6.	Ask the patient to compare two other similar products and determine which would fit in better as part of a healthy, nutritious diet that meets that patient's individual needs.	10	
7.	Document the patient education session in the patient's chart, indicate the patient's understanding, and initial the entry.*	20	
Total Points		100	

CAAHEP Competencies Achieved

IV. P (5) Instruct patients according to their needs to promote health maintenance and disease prevention

ABHES Competencies Achieved

9. (r) Teach patients methods of health promotion and disease prevention

PROCEDURE 55-2 Alerting Patients with Food Allergies to the Dangers of Common Foods

WORK // DOC

Goal
To explain how patients can eliminate allergy-causing foods from their diets.

OSHA Guidelines
This procedure does not involve exposure to blood, body fluids, or tissues.

Materials
Results of the patient's allergy tests, patient's chart, pen, patient education materials.

Method

Step Number	Procedure	Points Possible	Points Earned
1.	Identify the patient and introduce yourself.	8	
2.	Discuss the results of the patient's allergy tests (if available), reinforcing the physician's instructions. Provide the patient with a checklist of the foods that the patient has been found to be allergic to and review this list with the patient.	8	
3.	Discuss with the patient the possible allergic reactions those foods can cause.*	17	
4.	Discuss with the patient the need to avoid or eliminate those foods from the diet. Point out that the patient needs to be alert to avoid the allergy-causing foods not only in their basic forms but also as ingredients in prepared dishes and packaged foods. (Patients allergic to peanuts, for example, should avoid products containing peanut oil as well as peanuts.)	8	
5.	Tell the patient to read labels carefully and to inquire at restaurants about the use of those ingredients in dishes listed on the menu.	8	
6.	With the physician's or dietitian's consent, talk with the patient about the possibility of finding adequate substitutes for the foods if they are among the patient's favorites. Also discuss, if necessary, how the patient can obtain the nutrients in those foods from other sources (for example, the need for extra calcium sources if the patient is allergic to dairy products). Provide these explanations to the patient in writing, if appropriate, along with supplementary materials such as recipe pamphlets, a list of resources for obtaining food substitutes, and so on.	8	
7.	Discuss with the patient the procedures to follow if the allergy-causing foods are accidentally ingested.*	18	
8.	Answer the patient's questions and remind the patient that you and the rest of the medical team are available if any questions or problems arise later on.	8	
9.	Document the patient education session or interchange in the patient's chart, indicate the patient's understanding, and initial the entry.*	17	
Total Points		100	

CAAHEP Competencies Achieved

    IV. P (5)   Instruct patients according to their needs to promote health maintenance and disease prevention

ABHES Competencies Achieved

    9. (r) Teach patients methods of health promotion and disease prevention

56

Practice Management

Name_____ Class_____ Date_____

R E V I E W

Vocabulary Review

Matching
Match the key terms in the right column with the definitions in the left column by placing the letter of each correct answer in the space provided.

_____ 1. How unemployment taxes are filed by employers

_____ 2. PAs and NPs for example

_____ 3. Defines the hierarchy of an organization

_____ 4. Bank account that holds taxes to be paid

_____ 5. Facilitates communication in nonadversarial manner

_____ 6. List of meeting topics

_____ 7. Form required when there is potential liability for event

_____ 8. Reporting to a direct supervisor

_____ 9. Withholding allowance certificate

_____ 10. Trial period of usually 90 days

_____ 11. Issues between employees and management

_____ 12. Prediction of revenue and expenses

_____ 13. Synopsis of HR policies and procedures

_____ 14. Wage and Tax Statement

_____ 15. Unwelcome conduct of sexual nature

_____ 16. Verification of employment eligibility

_____ 17. Gross pay minus taxes and withholdings

_____ 18. Process when employee feels unfairly treated

_____ 19. Rules for office and guidelines for procedures

_____ 20. Unemployment contributions at the state level

a. agenda
b. budget
c. chain of command
d. employee handbook
e. Form I-9
f. FUTA
g. grievance process
h. incident report
i. labor relations
j. mediation
k. midlevel provider
l. net earnings
m. organizational chart
n. policies and procedures (P&Ps)
o. probationary period
p. sexual harassment
q. SUTA
r. tax liability account
s. W-2 tax form
t. W-4 tax form

True or False

Decide whether each statement is true or false. In the space at the left, write T for true or F for false. On the lines provided, rewrite the false statements to make them true.

_____ **21.** The medical director is in charge of the physician assistants and nurse practitioners.

_____

_____ **22.** Since medical assistants work closely with the physicians, it is appropriate to ask the physician for time off from work.

_____

_____ **23.** It is not anticipated that the practice manager will have communication or interaction with bankers and lawyers.

_____

_____ **24.** If the medical practice is renting office space, the practice manager has no responsibility for the facility safety.

_____

_____ **25.** The human resources department is very likely the only department in the medical office that does not involve the patient.

_____

_____ **26.** Under FMLA regulations, an employer is required to pay the employee's salary up to 12 weeks when he or she is on an approved leave from work.

_____

_____ **27.** In order for sexual harassment to have taken place, the victim must prove there was a physical encounter with the accused person.

_____

_____ **28.** The practice manager is usually responsible for ensuring that the budgeted expenses and revenues are met.

_____

_____ **29.** When using the problem-solving model to resolve a quality assurance issue, it is important to "close the loop."

_____

_____ **30.** To calculate an employee's take-home paycheck, subtract all taxes and other withholdings from the employee's net earnings.

_____

_____ **31.** The W4 form should be completed upon the employee's hire and updated annually.

_____

_____ **32.** FUTA taxes help fund the Social Security program.

_____

_____ **33.** In the policies and procedures manual, the procedures outline the intent or goal of the practice, and the policy outlines the steps to achieve that goal.

_____

_____ **34.** Federal taxes for the office may be filed biweekly, monthly or quarterly depending on the office size and schedule.

_____

_____ **35.** All states require that SUTA taxes be filed in addition to FUTA taxes.

_____

Content Review

Multiple Choice
In the space provided, write the letter of the choice that best completes each statement or answers each question.

_____ **1.** Which of the following duties is not usually performed by the practice manager?
    a. Evaluating employees
    b. Taking vital signs
    c. Hiring an administrative medical assistant
    d. Ensuring that employees are trained
    e. Terminating a medical assistant

_____ **2.** In a typical organizational structure of a physician-owned practice, the
    a. Medical assistant directly reports to the physician at all times
    b. Office manager reports to the medical assistants
    c. Physician is solely responsible for all office activities
    d. Practice manager reports to the corporate board of directors
    e. Medical assistant reports to the practice manager

_____ **3.** If you are following the chain of command for your organization, when a problem arises, you should initially report to your
    a. Receptionist
    b. Supervisor
    c. Physician
    d. Coworker
    e. Practice manager

_____ **4.** A medical practice budget could be negatively affected by
    a. Increased patient payments
    b. Decreased use of office supplies
    c. Increased patient load
    d. Decreased revenue
    e. New contractual agreements for annual sports physicals

_____ **5.** At least 1 week prior to a staff meeting, the office manager should
    a. Decide where to hold the meeting
    b. Put out a call for agenda items
    c. Send around a sign-in sheet
    d. Determine when the subsequent meetings will be held
    e. Notify the physician of the meeting

_____ **6.** Mediating appropriate issues between staff members is the responsibility of the
    a. Human resources department   **d.** Recruiting staff
    b. Risk management department   **e.** Quality assurance team
    c. Staff and employees

_____ 7. The qualifications and requirements for the medical assistant position are found
   a. In the policies and procedure manual
   b. In the job description
   c. In the MSDS binder
   d. In a QA manual
   e. On the organizational chart

_____ 8. In a company-owned medical practice, the person who has ultimate responsibility is the
   a. Administrative medical assistant
   b. Office manager
   c. Chief executive officer
   d. Physician
   e. Physician's designee

_____ 9. Maintaining an entryway free of ice and other hazards is considered what area of management?
   a. Human resources
   b. Quality assurance
   c. Health and safety
   d. Legal and business
   e. Organizational

_____ 10. If a patient slips and falls on a slippery floor in the medical office, this accident falls under
   a. Human resources
   b. Quality assurance
   c. Health and safety
   d. Legal and business
   e. Risk management

_____ 11. If a patient falls on a slippery floor, the type of form that must be initiated is a/n
   a. I-9
   b. W-2
   c. Grievance
   d. Incident report
   e. W-4

_____ 12. An effective practice manager should possess all the following attributes except
   a. Fairness
   b. Firmness
   c. Judgmental attitude
   d. Tact
   e. Open-mindedness.

_____ 13. Which of the following topics would be covered in the benefits section of an employee handbook?
   a. A leave of absence from work
   b. Payroll amounts
   c. ADA policy
   d. Safety and security
   e. 401(K) plan

_____ **14.** A newly hired employee is required to complete a Form I-9, which is used to

    a. State the number of deductions the employee wishes to claim for income tax

    b. Certify citizenship or other legal status to work in the United States

    c. Arrange for direct deposit of payroll checks into a bank account

    d. Assign a beneficiary for the life insurance policy provided by the employer

    e. Identify the person to contact in case of emergency

_____ **15.** Which of the following is an accurate statement regarding the human relations department of a medical practice?

    a. It is often the only department that does not involve the patient

    b. The human relations department deals with people services

    c. This department assists the employer with the hiring process

    d. HR also is known as the *personnel department*

    e. All of the above

_____ **16.** According to the FMLA requirements, how many weeks is an employee allowed to take leave from work without pay?

    a. 6 weeks

    b. 8 weeks

    c. 10 weeks

    d. 12 weeks

    e. 15 weeks

_____ **17.** Components of a typical job description include

    a. Requirements and qualifications

    b. The number of holidays that are included as paid time off

    c. The criteria for enrolling in the 401(k) plan

    d. Instructions for handling emergencies and incidents

    e. A copy of the organizational chart for the practice

_____ **18.** When a medical practice has a probationary period to evaluate a new employee, the customary time period is

    a. 120 days

    b. 90 days

    c. 60 days

    d. 30 days

    e. 2 weeks

_____ **19.** An employee who feels unjustly treated should

    a. Contact an attorney

    b. Write a letter to the board of directors

    c. Bring up the topic at the next staff meeting

    d. Follow the steps of the grievance process

    e. File a complaint with the EEOC

_____ **20.** An incident report should never include

    a. The identification of the injured party

    b. Assumptions

    c. The medical treatment provided

    d. Statements

    e. Names of witnesses

Sentence Completion

In the space provided, write the word that best completes the sentence or phrase.

21. The organizational design and/or _____ shows the structure and relationship between different functions and positions within the medical practice.

22. When the medical assistant has a complaint, it is not appropriate to go outside the _____ with the complaint, even if the complaint is about your supervisor.

23. The role of the practice manager is to ensure that all communication is _____, _____, _____, and HIPAA-compliant.

24. Other names for the human relations department are personnel _____, personnel _____, or people _____.

25. Three laws that prevent discrimination in hiring are _____, _____, and _____.

26. When an adverse event occurs in the medical practice, a/an _____ is completed.

27. The medical practice must comply with the health and safety regulations established by _____.

28. Most states require that, when a medical assistant is involved in a clinical aspect of patient care, he or she must be supervised by a _____.

29. In order for the practice and its healthcare providers to legally provide care, all _____, _____, and _____ must be up-to-date.

30. To pay for small office expenses, the _____ fund is often used.

21. _____

22. _____

23. _____

_____

_____

24. _____

_____

25. _____

_____

_____

26. _____

27. _____

28. _____

29. _____

_____

_____

30. _____

Short Answer

Write the answer to each question on the lines provided.

31. Provide at least six items that are the responsibility of the practice manager.

_____

_____

_____

_____

_____

_____

32. Explain the difference between risk management and quality assurance.

_____

_____

_____

_____

33. Explain the purpose of a probationary period for a new employee.

_____

_____

34. List at least five items that are included in a job description.

_____

_____

_____

_____

_____

35. Explain the Fair Labor Standards Act.

_____

_____

_____

36. Explain the purpose of the payroll register and the information it contains.

_____

_____

Critical Thinking

Write the answer to each question on the lines provided.

1. Anna and Stephanie are both medical assistants who have worked at the same medical clinic for over 5 years. A new employee, Greg, has been hired to work in the back office as a lab assistant. During a lunch break in the employee lounge, Greg, Anna, and Stephanie engage in a conversation about dating since all three are single. Greg begins to make inappropriate comments about couples dating. These comments make Anna and Stephanie uncomfortable. They try to change the subject, but Greg continues to make inappropriate sexual comments about couples dating. Anna and Stephanie leave the employee lounge, and as they leave, Greg says, "What's the matter, girls? Can't you lighten up and have fun?"

   a. What is the main problem with Greg's behavior?

   _____

   _____

   _____

   b. How should situations like this be avoided in the workplace?

   _____

   _____

   _____

2. Marilyn's annual employee performance review is due next week. Her supervisor asks her to complete the Employee Review Input form. This is Marilyn's opportunity to provide her input about her job performance over the past year. She is asked to list her areas of weakness and her strengths. The employee is also asked to list continuing education that was completed over the past year. Marilyn realizes that she did not do any continuing education even though her employer requires at least 5 hours a year.

a. How should Marilyn respond to the continuing education section of the review?

_____

_____

_____

b. Why do employers require medical personnel to participate in annual continuing education?

_____

_____

_____

3. Using the problem-solving model in the chapter, explain how to go about creating a solution to the problem of only one microwave in the staff kitchen and the backup this causes at lunchtime (1 hour).

_____

_____

_____

APPLICATION

WORK // DOC

Follow the directions for each application.

1. Creating an Agenda

Malik has asked you to assist him in creating the agenda for the staff meeting planned for November 15, 20xx. The following items will be included: Information to be presented at the meeting includes the following list of items. Organize the topics appropriately to develop the agenda. Produce the agenda in the appropriate format using word processing software.

- Announce new physician assistant starting at the clinic, James Thomas, PA.
- Approve prior minutes and agenda.
- Update the status of the building renovation.
- Announce that CPR class will be held next month for new employees.
- Discuss the office hours during holiday as well as the holiday party.
- Provide an update on EHR software implementation.

2. Payroll

Below is a partially completed payroll register. Calculate the total gross earnings and then the net earnings for each employee with the information provided

Name	Rate	Reg Hrs	OT Hrs	OT Earned	Total Gross	FICA W/H	State W/H	Health Ins	Life/ Disbl	Net
George, T	15.25	40	4			101.05	37.00	35.00	6.75	
Vega, M	14.50	35				85.17	22.85	35.00	4.18	
Knight, A	17.10	37.5				92.62	33.48	22.49	8.10	
Moran, J	13.75	40	8			105.63	41.97	52.00	9.52	

3. Incident Report

While walking into the break room this morning at 10:15 a.m., your coworker Juanita Small slipped on a small amount of water that had been spilled on the floor and fell to her knees. You witnessed the accident and have been asked to help her complete the incident report, even though she says she is not hurt. Using an incident form blank such as Figure 56-10, assist Juanita with completing this form for submission to Malik Katahri, the office manager.

PROCEDURE 56-1 Preparing a Travel Expense Report ⬚WORK//DOC⬚

(Imagine that you attended the latest AAMA or AMT annual conference. Research the price of airfare from your locale to the city of the conference. Determine registration and other costs. Use these figures to perform the procedure.)

Goal
To obtain reimbursement or account for preapproved travel funds; to provide documentation of expenses for the medical office.

OSHA Guidelines
This procedure does not involve exposure to blood, body fluids, or tissues.

Materials
Travel expense form (Figure 56-6), pen, receipts, conference Web information, calculator.

Method

Step Number	Procedure	Points Possible	Points Earned
1.	Ensure your travel was prior approved.	10	
2.	Save receipts from the event.	10	
3.	Complete the personal identifying information on the form.	10	
4.	Insert the purpose of the travel, the location, dates, and number of days.	10	
5.	Place the amounts as labeled in the expense table.	10	
6.	Total the amounts.	10	
7.	Check the appropriate box to indicate if you missed work and the dates and total number of days.	10	
8.	Sign and date the form.	10	
9.	Attach receipts (generally, original receipts are submitted; keep copies for your own records).	10	
10.	Submit completed form and receipts.	10	
Total Points		100	

CAAHEP Competencies Achieved

None

ABHES Competencies Achieved

None

PROCEDURE 56-2 Preparing an Agenda

Goal
To facilitate a meeting's organization and focus by providing a list of meeting topics, the name of the person reporting, and the order in which each topic will be addressed.

OSHA Guidelines
This procedure does not involve exposure to blood, body fluids, or tissues.

Materials
Paper and pen or computer, copy machine, minutes from last meeting.

Method

Step Number	Procedure	Points Possible	Points Earned
1.	Approximately one week before the meeting, e-mail or post a memo to staff offering them an opportunity to add items to the agenda. This is referred to as a *Call for Agenda Items*.	10	
2.	Place the following on top of the form used to create the agenda: • Name of the practice • Site name, if the practice has more than one location • Title: *Staff Meeting Agenda* • Date and time the meeting is scheduled to begin and end	10	
3.	Many offices have standing topics which go on the agenda every month; examples are • Introduction of new staff members • Approval of minutes if formal minutes are kept • Staff news (promotions, birthdays, weddings, births, etc.) • Quality assurance report • Policy and procedure updates • Committee reports • Report from individuals who may have attended a conference	10	
4.	Review the minutes from the previous meeting to determine any topics that required action with the person responsible. List these on the agenda under *Old Business*.	10	
5.	Add topics obtained from the *Call for Agenda Items* and any new topics the manager wishes to discuss. List these under *New Business*.	10	
6.	Add *Other* on the agenda to allow announcements or other brief information.	10	
7.	Place the date and time of the next meeting at the end of the agenda.	10	
8.	At least one week prior to the meeting, inform and verify persons on the agenda who will present a topic at the meeting.	10	
9.	Send agenda to staff members prior to the meeting.	10	
10.	Make copies available at the staff meeting.	10	
Total Points		100	

CAAHEP Competencies Achieved

V. A (2)   Implement time management principles to maintain effective office function

ABHES Competencies Achieved

8. (dd) Serve as liaison between physician and others

PROCEDURE 56-3 Completing an Incident Report   [WORK // DOC]

Goal
To provide documentation of an adverse occurrence or potential risk to facilitate investigation, correction, and aid in the avoidance of future occurrences.

OSHA Guidelines
This procedure does not involve exposure to blood, body fluids, or tissues.

Materials
A paper and pen, an incident report (Figure 56-9 may be used)

Method

Step Number	Procedure	Points Possible	Points Earned
1.	Make sure appropriate initial first aid and appropriate assistive steps are taken to help the injured person	15	
2.	Interview the person to whom the incident occurred, gathering the required facts as needed for the incident report, including contact information.	15	
3.	Interview witnesses, gathering the required facts as needed for the incident report, including contact information.	14	
4.	Ensure information is complete.	14	
5.	Transfer the information to the incident report form.	14	
6.	Review the form for accuracy and clarity.	14	
7.	Submit the form to the appropriate supervisor.	14	
Total Points		100	

CAAHEP Competencies Achieved

IX. P (6)   Complete an incident report

ABHES Competencies Achieved

8. (jj) Perform fundamental writing skills including correct grammar, spelling, and formatting techniques when writing prescriptions, documenting medical records, etc.

PROCEDURE 56-4 Generating Payroll
WORK // DOC

Goal
To handle the practice's payroll as efficiently and accurately as possible for each pay period.

OSHA Guidelines
This procedure does not involve exposure to blood, body fluids, or tissues.

Materials
Employees' time cards, employees' earnings records, payroll register, IRS tax tables, check register.

Method

Step Number	Procedure	Points Possible	Points Earned
1.	Calculate the total regular and overtime hours worked, based on the employee's time card. Enter those totals under the appropriate headings on the payroll register.	9	
2.	Check the pay rate on the employee earnings record. Multiply the hours worked (including any paid vacation or paid holidays, if applicable) by the rates for regular time and overtime (time and a half or double time). This yields gross earnings.	9	
3.	Enter the gross earnings under the appropriate heading on the payroll register. Subtract any nontaxable benefits, such as healthcare or retirement programs.	10	
4.	Using IRS tax tables and data on the employee earnings record, determine the amount of federal income tax to withhold based on the employee's marital status and number of exemptions. Also compute the amount of FICA tax to withhold for Social Security (6.2%) and Medicare (1.45%).	9	
5.	Following state and local procedures, determine the amount of state and local income taxes (if any) to withhold based on the employee's marital status and number of exemptions	9	
6.	Calculate the employer's contributions to FUTA and to the state unemployment fund, if any. Post these amounts to the employer's account.	9	
7.	Enter any other required or voluntary deductions, such as health insurance or contributions to a 401(k) fund.	9	
8.	Subtract all deductions from the gross earnings to get the employee's net earnings.	9	
9.	Enter the total amount withheld from all employees for FICA under the headings for Social Security and Medicare. Remember that the employer must match these amounts. Enter other employer contributions, such as for federal and state unemployment taxes, under the appropriate headings.	9	
10.	Fill out the check stub, including the employee's name, date, pay period, gross earnings, all deductions, and net earnings. Make out the paycheck for the net earnings.	9	
11.	Deposit each deduction in a tax liability account.	9	
Total Points		100	

CAAHEP Competencies Achieved

None

ABHES Competencies Achieved

8. (j) Perform accounts payable procedures

Emergency Preparedness

Name_____ Class_____ Date_____

R E V I E W

Vocabulary Review

Matching

Match the key terms in the right column with the definitions in the left column by placing the letter of each correct answer in the space provided.

_____ 1. A condition resulting from massive, widespread infection that affects the ability of the blood vessels to circulate blood

_____ 2. The vomiting of blood

_____ 3. Low blood sugar

_____ 4. A condition that results from insufficient blood volume in the circulatory system

_____ 5. A jarring injury to the brain

_____ 6. A muscle injury that results from overexertion

_____ 7. A swelling caused by blood under the skin

_____ 8. A brain attack caused by impaired blood supply to the brain

_____ 9. Unusually rapid, strong, or irregular pulsations of the heart

_____ 10. A nosebleed

a. strain
b. hematemesis
c. palpitations
d. hypoglycemia
e. epistaxis
f. hematoma
g. hypovolemic shock
h. concussion
i. septic shock
j. stroke

True or False

Decide whether each statement is true or false. In the space at the left, write T for true or F for false. On the lines provided, rewrite the false statements to make them true.

_____ 11. A splint is used to bandage a laceration or an incision.

_____

_____ 12. A cast is a rigid, external dressing that is molded to the contours of the body part to which it is applied.

_____

_____ 13. The displacement of a bone end from the joint is a sprain.

_____

_____ 14. Botulism is a life-threatening allergic reaction.

_____

_____ 15. When caring for a person who has a poisonous snakebite, it is important to apply ice to the bite.

_____

_____ **16.** A contusion is a type of closed wound.

_____

_____ **17.** A person having a seizure should be positioned on the floor with his head turned toward the side.

_____

_____ **18.** Ventricular fibrillation is an unusually rapid, strong, or irregular pulsation of the heart.

_____

_____ **19.** The first priority for medical assistants in an emergency is a victim's airway.

_____

_____ **20.** When assisting in a disaster, you should accept an assignment that is appropriate to your age.

_____

_____ **21.** Hyperglycemia is a lack of adequate water in the body.

_____

_____ **22.** The lower extension of the breastbone is the xiphoid process.

_____

_____ **23.** Establishing a chain of custody is important in cases of rape and when testing for illicit drug use.

_____

_____ **24.** An automated external defibrillator (AED) is used during a cardiac emergency to correct abnormal rhythms such as ventricular fibrillation (VF).

_____

_____ **25.** A person is placed in the recovery position when a fracture, dislocation, sprain, or strain is suspected.

_____

_____ **26.** When treating a bee sting, use tweezers to remove the stinger.

_____

_____ **27.** Bioterrorism is the intentional release of a chemical agent with the intent to harm individuals.

_____

Content Review

Multiple Choice

In the space provided, write the letter of the choice that best completes each statement or answers each question.

_____ **1.** Dry mouth, intense thirst, muscle weakness, and blurred vision are symptoms of
   a. Hypoglycemia   **d.** Hyperthermia
   b. Dehydration   **e.** Epilepsy
   c. Hyperglycemia

_____ **2.** Which of the following is the main symptom of a choking emergency?
   a. A fearful look   **d.** Unconsciousness
   b. The inability to speak **e.** Pallor
   c. Coughing

_____ **3.** Which of the following is a type of head injury?
   a. A contusion   **d.** Epistaxis
   b. A dislocation   **e.** An avulsion
   c. Viral encephalitis

Name_____ Class_____ Date_____

4. The most common abnormal rhythm that occurs during cardiac arrest is
 a. Tachycardia
 b. Ventricular fibrillation
 c. Palpitations
 d. CVA
 e. Myocardial infarction

5. Asthma is a common disorder caused by
 a. Wheezing and coughing
 b. Electrolyte imbalances
 c. Diabetes
 d. Narrowing of the bronchi
 e. Head injury

6. An insufficient blood volume in the circulatory system causes
 a. Insulin shock
 b. Ventricular fibrillation
 c. Septic shock
 d. Myocardial infarction
 e. Hypovolemic shock

7. A series of violent and involuntary contractions of the muscles is known as
 a. Epilepsy
 b. Stroke
 c. Strain
 d. Concussion
 e. Cramps

8. A symptom specific to toxic shock syndrome is
 a. High fever
 b. Vomiting
 c. A decreased level of consciousness
 d. A red rash on the hands and feet
 e. Seizures

9. A life-threatening allergic reaction is known as
 a. Asthma
 b. Botulism
 c. Anaphylaxis
 d. Sepsis
 e. Urticaria

10. Which of the following is an electrical device that shocks the heart to restore normal beating?
 a. CVA
 b. MI
 c. AED
 d. PPE
 e. EMT

Sentence Completion

In the space provided, write the word or phrase that best completes each sentence.

11. An important ally in providing emergency care is your local _____ system.

12. An electrical burn is caused by exposure to electrical currents or _____.

13. A scalp hematoma can be reduced by applying _____ immediately after the injury.

14. If you suspect bioterrorism, your facility should first contact _____.

15. Acute abdominal pain in the right upper quadrant may signal _____.

16. A _____ is a rolling cart of emergency supplies and equipment.

17. A severe condition that is the end result of severe hyperglycemia is known as _____.

11. _____
12. _____
13. _____
14. _____
15. _____
16. _____
17. _____

Chapter 57: Emergency Preparedness **795**

Name_____ Class_____ Date_____

Short Answer
Write the answer to each question on the lines provided.

18. What are four ways in which first aid can benefit victims of accidents or sudden illness?

_____

_____

_____

_____

19. How should you position a person who is having a seizure?

_____

_____

_____

20. Name and describe the types of wounds that are depicted in the following illustrations.

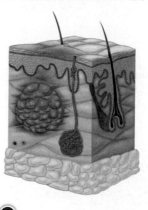
a ....

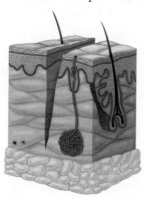
b ....

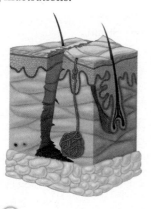
c ....

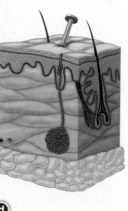
d ....

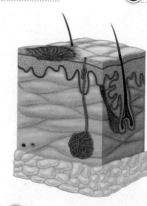
e ....

21. Describe four steps to follow when treating a patient who has swallowed poison but who is alert and not having convulsions.

_____

_____

_____

_____

22. What are the five symptoms of dehydration?

_____

_____

_____

23. What are the symptoms of a sprain?

_____

_____

_____

24. What actions are medical personnel required to take when treating a victim of rape?

_____

_____

_____

25. Briefly describe the process of triage during a disaster.

_____

_____

_____

Critical Thinking

Write the answer to each question on the lines provided.

1. Your neighbor has been cutting down trees today. He comes to your door and says that a tree limb slid by his head and amputated his ear. What should you do?

_____

_____

_____

2. Three patients arrive in the office of a general practitioner at about the same time. One is suffering from a second-degree burn on her hand, another has been bitten by a spider, and the third is experiencing chest pain. In what order should these patients be treated? Why?

_____

_____

_____

3. Why should you look for additional symptoms when a patient complains of headache, dizziness, or vomiting?

_____

_____

_____

4. A patient arrives at your office feeling restless and confused. She has a rapid pulse; shallow respirations; hunger; profuse sweating; pale, cool, clammy skin; double vision; and tremors. She states that she took her regular dose of insulin this morning but was not able to eat breakfast. What could be wrong with this patient? What should you do?

_____

_____

_____

5. When performing an emergency assessment, why should you check for a medical identification card, necklace, or bracelet?

_____

_____

_____

A P P L I C A T I O N

Follow the directions for each application.

1. **Performing Emergency Procedures**

   Each of the following descriptions of emergency procedures contains at least one error. On the lines provided, rewrite the procedures to make them correct.

   a. When treating a dog bite that has caused a puncture wound, wash the area with antiseptic soap and water and use pressure to stop the bleeding.

   _____

   _____

   b. When treating a spider bite, wash the area thoroughly with soap and water and apply a hot pack to the area to reduce swelling and pain.

   _____

   _____

   c. When treating a first-degree burn, immerse the affected area in cold water. Then pat the area dry and apply petroleum jelly or ointment.

   _____

   _____

   d. When treating a scalp laceration, apply indirect pressure, wash the area with soap and water, and apply a moist, sterile dressing over the area.

   _____

   _____

2. **Choosing Personal Protective Equipment for Emergencies**

   For each emergency described as follows, list personal protective equipment that should be worn.

   a. Vomiting _____.

   _____

   b. Childbirth _____.

   _____

   c. Heart attack _____.

   _____

   d. Eye injury _____.

   _____

   e. Bleeding _____.

   _____

3. **Developing a Safety Plan for Patients and Employees**

   Create a safety plan including

   a. A first aid kit checklist

   b. Household emergency evacuation plan

   c. List of emergency contacts

C A S E   S T U D I E S

Write your response to each case study on the lines provided.

Case 1

While eating dinner in a restaurant, you hear a commotion across the dining room. A man appears to be choking. A woman is slapping him on the back. What, if anything, should you do?

_____

_____

_____

Case 2

While walking at the local park, you see a woman stumble and fall. You notice that she catches herself with her arms extended. As you reach the victim, you notice that her right wrist looks swollen and she is complaining of severe pain in her arm. What should you do?

_____

_____

_____

Case 3

A patient who has been sitting in the waiting room comes to the reception desk and asks you for a glass of water. She seems disoriented and short of breath, and her skin appears flushed. When you lean forward to ask the patient whether she is all right, you notice that her breath has a sweet odor. What might be happening, and how should you handle the situation?

_____

_____

Case 4

An infant comes in your office with a high fever. While her mother is talking to you, the infant begins to have a seizure. What should you do?

_____

_____

_____

Case 5

Your neighbor, Jane Chung, has been working in her garage for most of the morning, spray-painting some patio furniture. You notice that she has had the door closed while she was working. You decide to check on her and find her sitting down, holding her chest. She says that she feels dizzy and nauseated and has a headache. What could be wrong with Jane? What should you do?

_____

_____

_____

PROCEDURE 57-1 Stocking the Crash Cart

Goal
To ensure the crash cart includes all appropriate drugs, supplies, and equipment needed for emergencies.

OSHA Guidelines
This procedure does not involve exposure to blood, body fluids, or tissues.

Materials
Protocol for or list of crash cart items, and crash cart.

Method

Step Number	Procedure	Points Possible	Points Earned
1.	Review the office protocol for or list of items that should be on the crash cart.	20	
2.	Verify each drug on the crash cart, and check the amount against the office protocol or list. Restock those that were used, and replace those that have passed their expiration date.	20	
3.	Check the supplies on the crash cart against the list. Restock items that were used, and make sure the packaging of supplies on the cart has not been opened.	20	
4.	Check the equipment on the crash cart against the list, and examine it to make sure it is in working order. Restock missing or broken equipment.	20	
5.	Check miscellaneous items on the crash cart against the list, and restock as needed.	20	
Total Points		100	

CAAHEP Competencies Achieved

XI. P (3)   Develop a personal (patient and employee) safety plan

ABHES Competencies Achieved

None

Name_____ Date_____

Evaluated by_____ Score_____

PROCEDURE 57-2 Performing an Emergency Assessment

Goal

To assess a medical emergency quickly and accurately.

OSHA Guidelines

Materials

Patient's chart, pen, gloves, and other PPE appropriate to the situation.

Method

Step Number	Procedure	Points Possible	Points Earned
1.	Put on gloves.	2	
2.	Form a general impression of the patient, including his level of responsiveness, level of distress, facial expressions, age, ability to talk, and skin color.	10	
3.	If the patient can communicate clearly, ask what happened. If not, ask someone who observed the accident or injury.	3	
4.	Assess an unresponsive patient by tapping on his shoulder and asking, "Are you OK?" If there is no response, proceed to the next step.*	15	
5.	Assess the patient's circulation, airway, and breathing. Perform CPR as needed.	15	
6.	Is there any serious external bleeding? Control any significant bleeding.	15	
7.	If all life-threatening problems have been identified and treated, perform a focused exam. Start at the head and perform the following steps rapidly, taking about 90 seconds.* **a.** Head: Check for deformities, bruises, open wounds, tenderness, depressions, and swelling. Check the ears, nose, and mouth for fluid, blood, or foreign bodies. **b.** Eyes: Open the eyes and compare the pupils. They should be the same size. **c.** Neck: Look and feel for deformities, bruises, depressions, open wounds, tenderness, and swelling. Check for a medical alert bracelet or necklace. **d.** Chest: Look and feel for deformities, bruises, open wounds, tenderness, depressions, and swelling. **e.** Abdomen: Look and feel for deformities, bruises, open wounds, tenderness, depressions, and swelling. **f.** Pelvis: Look and feel for deformities, bruises, open wounds, tenderness, depressions, and swelling. **g.** Arms: Look and feel for deformities, bruises, open wounds, depressions, tenderness, and swelling. Compare the arms for any differences in size, color, or temperature.	15	

(continued)

Step Number	Procedure	Points Possible	Points Earned
	h. Legs: Look and feel for deformities, bruises, open wounds, depressions, tenderness, and swelling. Compare the legs for any differences in size, color, or temperature. i. Back: Look and feel for deformities, bruises, open wounds, depressions, tenderness, and swelling. Feel under the patient for pools of blood.		
8.	Check vital signs and observe the patient for pallor (paleness) or cyanosis (a bluish tint). If the patient is dark-skinned, observe for pallor or cyanosis on the inside of the lips and mouth.	10	
9.	Document your findings and report them to the doctor or emergency medical technician (EMT).	5	
10.	Assist the doctor or EMT as requested.	2	
11.	Dispose of biohazardous waste according to OSHA guidelines.	5	
12.	Remove your gloves and wash your hands.	3	
Total Points		100	

CAAHEP Competencies Achieved

XI. P (10)   Perform first aid procedures

ABHES Competencies Achieved

9. (e) Recognize emergencies and treatments and minor office surgical procedures

9. (o) 5) First aid and CPR

PROCEDURE 57-3 Foreign Body Airway Obstruction in a Responsive Adult or Child

Goal

To correctly relieve a foreign body from the airway of an adult or child.

OSHA Guidelines

This procedure does not involve exposure to blood, body fluids, or tissues.

Materials

Choking adult or child patient.

Caution: Never perform this procedure on someone who is not choking.

Method

Step Number	Procedure	Points Possible	Points Earned
1.	Ask, "Are you choking?" If the answer is "Yes," indicated by a nod of the head or some other sign, tell the patient you can help. A choking person cannot speak, cough, or breathe, and exhibits the universal sign of choking. If the patient is coughing, observe him closely to see if he clears the object. If he is not coughing or stops coughing, use abdominal thrusts.*	15	
2.	Position yourself behind the patient. Place your fist against the abdomen just above the navel and below the xiphoid process.	10	
3.	Grasp your fist with your other hand, and provide quick inward and upward thrusts into the patient's abdomen. Note: If a pregnant or obese person is choking, you will need to place your arms around the chest and perform thrusts over the center of the breastbone.*	15	
4.	Continue the thrusts until the object is expelled or the patient becomes unresponsive.	10	
5.	If the patient becomes unresponsive, call EMS and position the patient on his back and begin chest compressions without a pulse check.*	15	
6.	Use the head tilt-chin lift to open the patient's airway.	10	
7.	Look into the mouth. If you see the foreign body, remove it using your index finger. **Do not perform any blind finger sweeps**.	10	
8.	Open the airway. If the patient is not breathing, attempt a rescue breath. Observe the chest. If it does not rise with the breath, reposition the airway and administer another rescue breath. If the chest does not rise after the second attempt, assume the airway is still blocked and continue CPR.*	15	
Total Points		100	

CAAHEP Competencies Achieved

XI. P (9)   Maintain provider/professional level CPR certification.

XI. P (10) Perform first aid procedures

ABHES Competencies Achieved

9. (e) Recognize emergencies and treatments and minor office surgical procedures

9. (o) 5) First aid and CPR

PROCEDURE 57-4 Foreign Body Airway Obstruction in a Responsive Infant

Goal
To correctly relieve a foreign body from the airway of an infant.

OSHA Guidelines
This procedure does not involve exposure to blood, body fluids, or tissues.

Materials
Choking infant.

Caution: Never perform this procedure on an infant who is not choking.

Method

Step Number	Procedure	Points Possible	Points Earned
1.	Assess the infant for signs of severe or complete airway obstruction, which include* **a.** Sudden onset of difficulty in breathing. **b.** Inability to speak, make sounds, or cry. **c.** A high-pitched, noisy, wheezing sound, or no sounds while inhaling. **d.** Weak, ineffective coughs. **e.** Blue lips or skin.	10	
2.	Hold the infant with his head down, supporting the body with your forearm. His legs should straddle your forearm and you should support his jaw and head with your hand and fingers. This is best done in a sitting or kneeling position.	8	
3.	Give up to five back blows with the heel of your free hand. Strike the infant's back forcefully between the shoulder blades. At any point, if the object is expelled, discontinue the back blows.*	10	
4.	If the obstruction is not cleared, turn the infant over as a unit, supporting the head with your hands and the body between your forearms.	8	
5.	Keep the head lower than the chest and perform five chest thrusts. Place two fingers over the breastbone (sternum), above the xiphoid. Give five quick chest thrusts about ½ to 1 inch deep. Stop the compressions if the object is expelled.*	10	
6.	Alternate five back blows and five chest thrusts until the object is expelled or until the infant becomes unconscious. If the infant becomes unconscious, call EMS or have someone do it for you.*	10	
7.	Open the infant's mouth by grasping both the tongue and the lower jaw between the thumb and fingers, and pull up the lower jawbone. *If you see the object, remove it using your smallest finger.* **Do not use blind finger sweeps on an infant**.	8	
8.	Open the airway and attempt to provide rescue breaths. If the chest does not rise, reposition the airway (both head and chin) and try to provide another rescue breath.*	10	
9.	If the rescue breaths are unsuccessful, begin CPR.*	10	

(continued)

Step Number	Procedure	Points Possible	Points Earned
10.	Open the infant's mouth and look for the foreign object. If you see an object, remove it with your smallest finger.	8	
11.	Open the airway and attempt to provide rescue breaths. If the chest does not rise, continue CPR until the doctor or EMS arrives.	8	
Total Points		100	

CAAHEP Competencies Achieved

XI. P (9)   Maintain provider/professional level CPR certification

XI. P (10)   Perform first aid procedures

ABHES Competencies Achieved

9. (e) Recognize emergencies and treatments and minor office surgical procedures

9 (o) 5) First aid and CPR

PROCEDURE 57-5 Controlling Bleeding   WORK//DOC

Goal

To control bleeding and minimize blood loss.

OSHA Guidelines

Materials

Clean or sterile dressings.

Method

Step Number	Procedure	Points Possible	Points Earned
1.	If you have time, wash your hands and don exam gloves, face protection, and a gown.	10	
2.	Using a clean or sterile dressing, apply direct pressure over the wound.*	15	
3.	If blood soaks through the dressing, do not remove it. Apply an additional dressing over the original one.*	15	
4.	If possible, elevate the bleeding body part.	10	
5.	If direct pressure and elevation do not stop the bleeding, apply pressure over the nearest pressure point between the bleeding and the heart. For example, if the wound is on the lower arm, apply pressure on the brachial artery. For a lower-leg wound, apply pressure on the femoral artery in the groin.*	15	
6.	When the doctor or EMT arrives, assist as requested.	5	
7.	After the patient has been transferred to a hospital, properly dispose of contaminated materials.	10	
8.	Remove the gloves and wash your hands.	10	
9.	Document your care in the patient's chart.	10	
Total Points		100	

CAAHEP Competencies Achieved

XI. P (10)   Perform first aid procedures

ABHES Competencies Achieved

9. (e) Recognize emergencies and treatments and minor office surgical procedures

9. (o) 5) First aid and CPR

PROCEDURE 57-6 Cleaning Minor Wounds WORK // DOC

Goal
To clean and dress minor wounds.

OSHA Guidelines

Materials
Sterile gauze squares, basin, antiseptic soap, warm water, and sterile dressing.

Method

Step Number	Procedure	Points Possible	Points Earned
1.	Wash your hands and don exam gloves.	10	
2.	Dip several gauze squares in a basin of warm, soapy water.	5	
3.	Wash the wound from the center outward, using a new gauze square for each cleansing motion.*	15	
4.	As you wash, remove debris that could cause infection.	10	
5.	Rinse the area thoroughly, preferably by placing the wound under warm, running water.*	15	
6.	Pat the wound dry with sterile gauze squares.	5	
7.	Cover the wound with a dry, sterile dressing. Bandage the dressing in place.	10	
8.	Properly dispose of contaminated materials and decontaminate surfaces potentially exposed to blood or body fluid.	10	
9.	Remove the gloves and wash your hands.	10	
10.	Instruct the patient on wound care.	5	
11.	Record the procedure in the patient's chart.	5	
Total Points		100	

CAAHEP Competencies Achieved

XI. P (10)   Perform first aid procedures

ABHES Competencies Achieved

9. (e) Recognize emergencies and treatments and minor office surgical procedures

9. (o) 5) First aid and CPR

PROCEDURE 57-7 Caring for a Patient Who Is Vomiting

Goal
To increase comfort and minimize complications, such as aspiration, for a patient who is vomiting.

OSHA Guidelines

Materials
Emesis basin; cool compress; cup of cool water; paper tissues or a towel; and (if ordered) intravenous fluids, electrolytes, and an antinausea drug.

Method

Step Number	Procedure	Points Possible	Points Earned
1.	Wash your hands and don exam gloves and other PPE.	10	
2.	Ask the patient when and how the vomiting started and how frequently it occurs. Find out whether she is nauseated or in pain.*	15	
3.	Give the patient an emesis basin to collect vomit. Observe and document its amount, color, odor, and consistency. Particularly note blood, bile, undigested food, or feces in the vomit.*	15	
4.	Place a cool compress on the patient's forehead to make her more comfortable. Offer water and paper tissues or a towel to clean her mouth.	10	
5.	Monitor for signs of dehydration, like confusion, irritability, and flushed, dry skin. Also monitor for signs of electrolyte imbalances, like leg cramps or an irregular pulse.*	15	
6.	If requested, assist by laying out supplies and equipment for the physician to use in administering intravenous fluids and electrolytes. Administer an antinausea drug if prescribed.*	15	
7.	Prepare the patient for diagnostic tests if instructed.	10	
8.	Remove the gloves and wash your hands.	10	
Total Points		100	

CAAHEP Competencies Achieved
XI. P (10)   Perform first aid procedures

ABHES Competencies Achieved
9. (e) Recognize emergencies and treatments and minor office surgical procedures

9. (o) 5) First aid and CPR

9. (q) Instruct patients with special needs

PROCEDURE 57-8 Performing Triage in a Disaster

Goal
To prioritize disaster victims.

OSHA Guidelines

Materials
Disaster tag and a pen.

Method

Step Number	Procedure	Points Possible	Points Earned
1.	Wash your hands and don exam gloves and other PPE if available.	5	
2.	Quickly assess each victim.	5	
3.	Sort victims by type of injury and need for care, classifying them as emergent, urgent, nonurgent, or dead.	10	
4.	Label the emergent patients no. 1, and send them to appropriate treatment stations immediately. Emergent patients, such as those who are in shock or who are hemorrhaging, need immediate care.*	20	
5.	Label the urgent patients no. 2, and send them to basic first-aid stations. Urgent patients need care within the next several hours. Such patients may have lacerations that can be dressed quickly to stop the bleeding but can wait for suturing.*	20	
6.	Label nonurgent patients no. 3, and send them to volunteers who will be empathic and provide refreshments. Nonurgent patients are those for whom timing of treatment is not critical, like patients who have no physical injuries but are emotionally upset.*	20	
7.	Label patients who are dead no. 4. Ensure the bodies are moved to an area where they will be safe until they can be identified and proper action can be taken.*	20	
Total Points		100	

CAAHEP Competencies Achieved

XI. P (6)   Participate in a mock environmental exposure event with documentation of steps taken

ABHES Competencies Achieved

2. (c) Assist the physician with the regimen of diagnostic and treatment modalities as they relate to each body system

9 (e) Recognize emergencies and treatments and minor office surgical procedures

Preparing for the World of Work

Name_____ Class_____ Date_____

Vocabulary Review

Matching

Match the key terms in the right column with the definitions in the left column by placing the letter of each correct answer in the space provided.

_____ 1. A résumé format that is used when an individual does not have relevant job experience

_____ 2. The person who organizes and assigns your applied training experience

_____ 3. A document that outlines the expectations of the academic institution and the medical facility

_____ 4. A résumé that highlights specialty areas of accomplishments and strengths

_____ 5. A résumé for individuals who have a strong work history

_____ 6. Making contacts with relatives, friends, and acquaintances who may have information about how to find a job in your field

_____ 7. A type of critique that is aimed at giving an individual feedback about his or her performance in order to improve

_____ 8. A recommendation for employment from a clinical preceptor or medical facility

_____ 9. A collection of an applicant's résumé, reference letter, and other documents of interest to show to a potential employer

a. affiliation agreement
b. chronological résumé
c. applied training coordinator
d. constructive criticism
e. functional résumé
f. networking
g. portfolio
h. reference
i. targeted résumé

Content Review

Sentence Completion

In the space provided, write the word or phrase that best completes each sentence.

1. _____ is the opportunity to work within a medical facility to gain the on-the-job training that is essential for beginning your new career.

2. Educational institutions in which applied training is mandatory are accredited by _____ and _____.

3. The minimum number of hours required for applied training by an accredited institution is _____.

4. _____ should be turned off during working hours.

1. _____

2. _____

3. _____

4. _____

5. The two major credentialing agencies for medical assisting are _____ and _____.

6. Medical facilities expect the applied training student to appear as a _____.

7. Accepting all assignments with enthusiasm and looking for extra work when idle is an example of showing _____.

5. _____

6. _____

7. _____

Short Answer
Write the answer to each question on the lines provided.

8. What are three ways you might learn about open positions in your field?

_____

_____

_____

9. Describe how to prepare for an interview.

_____

_____

_____

10. What types of questions are you not required to answer at a job interview?

_____

_____

_____

11. What is expected of a medical assisting student in his or her applied training at a medical facility?

_____

_____

_____

12. When may you take the CMA exam?

_____

_____

_____

13. Name five reasons an employer might not hire a job candidate.

_____

_____

_____

14. What types of documents should be in a portfolio?

_____

_____

_____

15. What is important to remember when filling out a job application?

_____

_____

_____

Critical Thinking

Write the answer to each question on the lines provided.

1. Should a job candidate send résumés to employers whose ads state qualifications that are higher or different from the candidate's experience or education? Why or why not?

_____

_____

_____

2. What might a site ask of a medical assisting applied training student prior to beginning his clinical rotation?

_____

_____

_____

3. What two things should you know before preparing for a national certification exam?

_____

_____

_____

4. In choosing a résumé, what style might be the best strategy for you?

_____

_____

_____

5. List the five steps for applying for a national certification exam.

_____

_____

_____

A P P L I C A T I O N

Follow the directions for each application.

1. Preparing for the Certification Exam

Develop a strategy for studying for a national certification exam. First, identify areas you need to study more by taking a practice test. Once you have done this, set up a study calendar. Make sure you assess your knowledge along the way, taking practice tests at various intervals.

2. Interview Practice

Work in groups of three to four students. Assign three or four interview questions each and write responses to the questions. Practice interviewing each other and then compile a list of the best responses. Share your group's responses with the class by holding a mock interview with someone in your group. Type an official copy of the findings and pass it out to the class. Refer to the text chapter for interview questions and research additional questions on the Internet.

3. Employment Interview

Working in teams of three or four, contact local temporary employment agencies to come to your class and conduct mock interviews with your class. To begin this process, use the following steps:

a. Assign each team member a duty or role.

b. Contact local employment agencies and speak with a recruiter.

c. Follow up your call with a letter that recaps what was discussed and an invitation to participate in mock interviews on an established date and time. Mail the letter using campus letterhead.

d. Working in teams, use the information in the text about proper interviewing skills to establish a critique form for the interviewer to use during the interview.

e. The day of the mock interviews, supply a light snack for the interviewers.

f. Wear professional interview apparel.

g. Share critiques with the class.

C A S E   S T U D I E S

Write your response to each case study on the lines provided.

Case 1

During a job interview, a prospective employer asks you if you are a single mother. Explain whether the question is appropriate and how you might respond to such a question.

_____

_____

_____

Case 2

You are interviewing with a popular, busy surgeon's office. As the interview is wrapping up, the physician tells you that all applicants will be notified either way regarding the candidate selection. Should you phone the physician to follow up? Do you think it will appear that you are motivated to obtain the position if you call often?

_____

_____

_____

Case 3

A fellow student tells you he is afraid to take the national certification test and he is not sure it will help him anyway. What can you tell him about the advantages of becoming certified? What tips can you give him to help him with a study plan?

_____

_____

_____

PROCEDURE 58-1 Résumé Writing

Goal
To develop a résumé that defines your career objective and highlights your skills.

OSHA Guidelines
This procedure does not involve exposure to blood, body fluids, or tissues.

Materials
Paper, pen, dictionary, thesaurus, and a computer.

Method

Step Number	Procedure	Points Possible	Points Earned
1.	Type your full name, address (temporary and permanent, if you have both), telephone number with area code, and email address (if you have one).*	15	
2.	List your general career objective. You may also choose to summarize your skills. If you want to phrase your objective to fit a specific position, you should include that information in a cover letter to accompany the résumé.	5	
3.	List the highest level of education or the most recently obtained degree first. Include the school name, degree earned, and date of graduation. Be sure to list any special projects, courses, or participation in overseas study programs.	10	
4.	Summarize your work experience. List your most recent or most relevant employment first. Describe your responsibilities and list job titles, company names, and dates of employment. Summer employment, volunteer work, and student applied training may also be included. Use short sentences with strong action words such as *directed, designed, developed,* and *organized.* For example, condense a responsibility into "Handled insurance and billing" or "Drafted correspondence as requested."*	15	
5.	List any memberships and affiliations with professional organizations alphabetically or by order of importance.*	15	
6.	Do not list references on your résumé.	10	
7.	Do not list the salary you wish to receive in a medical assisting position. Salary requirements should not be discussed until a job offer is received. If the ad you are answering requests that you include a required salary, it is best to state a range (no broader than $5,000 from lowest to highest point in the range for an annual salary).*	15	
8.	Print your résumé on an 8½-by-11-inch sheet of high-quality white or off-white bond paper. Carefully check your résumé for spelling, punctuation, and grammatical errors. Have someone else double-check your résumé whenever possible.	15	
Total Points		100	

CAAHEP Competencies Achieved

None

ABHES Competencies Achieved

11. (a) Perform the essential requirements for employment such as résumé writing, effective interviewing, dressing professionally, and following up appropriately

PROCEDURE 58-2 Writing Thank-You Notes

Goal
To develop an appropriate, professional thank-you note after an interview or applied training.

OSHA Guidelines
This procedure does not involve exposure to blood, body fluids, or tissues.

Materials
Paper, pen, dictionary, thesaurus, computer, a #10 business envelope.

Method

Step Number	Procedure	Points Possible	Points Earned
1.	Complete the letter within two days of the interview or completion of the applied training. Begin by typing the date at the top of the letter.*	15	
2.	Type the name of the person who interviewed you (or who was your mentor in the applied training). Include credentials and title, such as Dr. or Director of Client Services. Include the complete address of the office or organization.	15	
3.	Start the letter with "Dear Dr., Mr., Mrs., Miss, or Ms."	10	
4.	In the first paragraph, thank the interviewer for his time and for granting the interview. Discuss some specific impressions, for example, "I found the interview and tour of the facilities an enjoyable experience. I would welcome the opportunity to work in such a state-of-the-art medical setting." If you are writing to thank your mentor for her time during your applied training and for allowing you to perform your applied training at her office, practice, or clinic, discuss the knowledge and experience you gained during the applied training.*	15	
5.	In the second paragraph, mention the aspects of the job or applied training that you found most interesting or challenging. For a job interview thank-you note, state how your skills and qualifications will make you an asset to the staff. When preparing an applied training thank-you letter, mention interest in any future positions.*	15	
6.	In the last paragraph, thank the interviewer for considering you for the position. Ask to be contacted at his earliest convenience regarding his employment decision.*	15	
7.	Close the letter with "Sincerely," and type your name. Leave enough space—usually 4 spaces—above your typewritten name to sign your name.	5	
8.	Type your return address in the upper left corner of the #10 business envelope. Then type the interviewer's name and address in the envelope's center, apply the proper postage, and mail the letter. You can also email your thank-you letter. Proper letter format and professional tone and appearance still apply. Send the thank-you letter as an attachment.	10	
Total Points		100	

CAAHEP Competencies Achieved

None

ABHES Competencies Achieved

11. (a) Perform the essential requirements for employment such as resume writing, effective interviewing, dressing professionally, and following up appropriately

Work Documentation: Administrative

Use these documents when performing application activities and procedures that include a work document icon.

WORK // DOC

LIST OF WORK DOCUMENTS

WORK DOCUMENTS BY CHAPTER

The documents needed to complete the application activities and procedures for each chapter are listed as follows. Notice that some of the documents are used in more than one chapter. Only one copy of each document is included in this workbook, so you will need to make enough additional copies to complete all of the application activities or procedures identified.

Name_____ Date_____

AGE ANALYSIS WORKSHEET

Accounts Receivable–Age Analysis   Date: _____

Patient	Balance	Date of Charges	Most Recent Payment	30 days	60 days	90 days	120 days	Remarks

APPOINTMENT CARD

BWW

BWW Medical Associates, PC
305 Main Street
Port Snead, YZ 12345-9876

Patient Name: _____

Date: _____
Month   Day   Year

Time: _____ A.M.   P.M.

Appointment with: _____

APPOINTMENT RECORD

APPOINTMENT RECORD

12 November Tuesday			**13** November Wednesday	
		DOCTOR		
		AM		
		8:00		
		8:15		
		8:30		
		8:45		
		9:00		
		9:15		
		9:30		
		9:45		
		10:00		
		10:15		
		10:30		
		10:45		
		11:00		
		11:15		
		11:30		
		11:45		
		12:00		
		12:15		
		12:30		
		12:45		
		PM		
		1:00		
		1:15		
		1:30		
		1:45		
		2:00		
		2:15		
		2:30		
		2:45		
		3:00		
		3:15		
		3:30		
		3:45		
		4:00		
		4:15		
		4:30		
		4:45		
		5:00		
		5:15		
		5:30		
		5:45		

REMARKS & NOTES _____

This document will be used multiple times. Make photocopies before writing on this document, or download it from the Online Learning Center at www.mhhe.com/BoothMA5e for any future uses.

AUTHORIZATION TO RELEASE INFORMATION

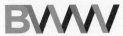

BWW Medical Associates, PC
305 Main Street, Port Snead YZ 12345-9876
Tel: 555-654-3210, Fax: 555-987-6543
Web: BWWAssociates.com

Paul F. Buckwalter, MD
Alexis N. Whalen, MD
Elizabeth H. Williams, MD

Authorization to Release Health Information

I, _____ residing at

_____ and DOB of

_____ give permission to (name of practice) _____

to release to _____ of BWW Medical Associates, PC the

following information: _____

_____

_____

Reason for the request: _____

_____

Signature of Patient or Legal Guardian _____

Printed Name of Patient or Legal Guardian _____

If Guardian, relationship to Patient _____

This authorization will expire on: _____

YOU MAY REFUSE TO SIGN THIS AUTHORIZATION. You may revoke this authorization at any time by notifying BWW Medical Associates, PC in writing. Revocation will have no effect on actions taken prior to receipt of any revocation. Any disclosure of information carries the potential for unauthorized redisclosure and the information may not be protected by federal confidentiality rules.

BANK DEPOSIT SLIP

DEPOSIT TICKET

BWW Medical Associates, PC

305 Main St.
Port Snead, YZ 12345-9876

DATE _____ 20 _____
DEPOSITS MAY NOT BE AVAILABLE FOR IMMEDIATE WITHDRAWAL

_____

CASH	CURRENCY		
	COIN		
LIST CHECKS SINGLY			
	TOTAL		
	LESS CASH RECEIVED		
	NET DEPOSIT		

89-852
622

→

BE SURE EACH ITEM IS
PROPERLY ENDORSED

FIRST NATIONAL BANK
CLINTON BRANCH

⑆062208525⑆ 526 6612 ⑈ 0789

CHECKS AND OTHER ITEMS ARE RECEIVED FOR DEPOSIT SUBJECT TO THE PROVISIONS OF THE UNIFORM COMMERCIAL CODE OR ANY APPLICABLE COLLECTION AGREEMENT

CHECKS LIST SINGLY	DOLLARS	CENTS
1		
2		
3		
4		
5		
6		
7		
8		
9		
10		
11		
12		
13		
14		
15		
TOTAL		

ENTER TOTAL ON THE FRONT SIDE OF THIS TICKET

Name_____ Date_____

BANK RECONCILIATION FORM

BANK RECONCILIATION

CLIENT NAME: _____ MONTH OF: _____

BANK: _____ ACCOUNT NO. : _____

GENERAL LEDGER		BALANCE PER BANK STATEMENT	
ACCOUNT BALANCE............................		AS OF:	
ADD DEBITS:		ADD DEPOSITS IN TRANSIT:	

TOTAL DR.............

TOTAL..

TOTAL IN TRANSIT

TOTAL.......................................

LESS CREDITS:

Checks

Auto Withdrawals

Bank Fees

LESS CHECKS OUTSTANDING:

  (SEE LIST BELOW)

TOTAL CR..............

  BANK BAL PER GENERAL LEDGER..

TOTAL.................

  BANK BALANCE PER REC.................

CHECKS:

NUMBER	AMOUNT	NUMBER	NUMBER	NUMBER	AMOUNT
					TOTAL
					GRAND TOTAL
TOTAL		TOTAL			

BWW LETTERHEAD

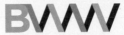

BWW Medical Associates, PC
305 Main Street, Port Snead YZ 12345-9876
Tel: 555-654-3210, Fax: 555-987-6543
Web: BWWAssociates.com

Paul F. Buckwalter, MD
Alexis N. Whalen, MD
Elizabeth H. Williams, MD

This document will be used multiple times. Make photocopies before writing on this document, or download it from the Online Learning Center at www.mhhe.com/BoothMA5e for any future uses.

CMS 1500

1500

HEALTH INSURANCE CLAIM FORM

APPROVED BY NATIONAL UNIFORM CLAIM COMMITTEE 08/05

□□□ PICA

PICA □□□

CARRIER →

| 1. MEDICARE ☐ (Medicare #) | MEDICAID ☐ (Medicaid #) | TRICARE CHAMPUS ☐ (Sponsor's SSN) | CHAMPVA ☐ (Member ID#) | GROUP HEALTH PLAN ☐ (SSN or ID) | FECA BLK LUNG ☐ (SSN) | OTHER ☐ (ID) | 1a. INSURED'S I.D. NUMBER (For Program in Item 1) |

| 2. PATIENT'S NAME (Last Name, First Name, Middle Initial) | 3. PATIENT'S BIRTH DATE MM DD YY SEX M ☐ F ☐ | 4. INSURED'S NAME (Last Name, First Name, Middle Initial) |

| 5. PATIENT'S ADDRESS (No., Street) | 6. PATIENT RELATIONSHIP TO INSURED Self ☐ Spouse ☐ Child ☐ Other ☐ | 7. INSURED'S ADDRESS (No., Street) |

| CITY | STATE | 8. PATIENT STATUS Single ☐ Married ☐ Other ☐ | CITY | STATE |

| ZIP CODE | TELEPHONE (Include Area Code) ( ) | Employed ☐ Full-Time Student ☐ Part-Time Student ☐ | ZIP CODE | TELEPHONE (Include Area Code) ( ) |

| 9. OTHER INSURED'S NAME (Last Name, First Name, Middle Initial) | 10. IS PATIENT'S CONDITION RELATED TO: | 11. INSURED'S POLICY GROUP OR FECA NUMBER |

| a. OTHER INSURED'S POLICY OR GROUP NUMBER | a. EMPLOYMENT? (Current or Previous) YES ☐ NO ☐ | a. INSURED'S DATE OF BIRTH MM DD YY SEX M ☐ F ☐ |

| b. OTHER INSURED'S DATE OF BIRTH MM DD YY SEX M ☐ F ☐ | b. AUTO ACCIDENT? PLACE (State) YES ☐ NO ☐ | b. EMPLOYER'S NAME OR SCHOOL NAME |

| c. EMPLOYER'S NAME OR SCHOOL NAME | c. OTHER ACCIDENT? YES ☐ NO ☐ | c. INSURANCE PLAN NAME OR PROGRAM NAME |

| d. INSURANCE PLAN NAME OR PROGRAM NAME | 10d. RESERVED FOR LOCAL USE | d. IS THERE ANOTHER HEALTH BENEFIT PLAN? YES ☐ NO ☐ If yes, return to and complete item 9 a-d. |

PATIENT AND INSURED INFORMATION →

READ BACK OF FORM BEFORE COMPLETING & SIGNING THIS FORM.

12. PATIENT'S OR AUTHORIZED PERSON'S SIGNATURE. I authorize the release of any medical or other information necessary to process this claim. I also request payment of government benefits either to myself or to the party who accepts assignment below.

SIGNED _____ DATE _____

13. INSURED'S OR AUTHORIZED PERSON'S SIGNATURE I authorize payment of medical benefits to the undersigned physician or supplier for services described below.

SIGNED _____

| 14. DATE OF CURRENT: MM DD YY ◄ ILLNESS (First symptom) OR INJURY (Accident) OR PREGNANCY(LMP) | 15. IF PATIENT HAS HAD SAME OR SIMILAR ILLNESS. GIVE FIRST DATE MM DD YY | 16. DATES PATIENT UNABLE TO WORK IN CURRENT OCCUPATION MM DD YY MM DD YY FROM TO |

| 17. NAME OF REFERRING PROVIDER OR OTHER SOURCE | 17a. _____ 17b. NPI _____ | 18. HOSPITALIZATION DATES RELATED TO CURRENT SERVICES MM DD YY MM DD YY FROM TO |

| 19. RESERVED FOR LOCAL USE | | 20. OUTSIDE LAB? YES ☐ NO ☐ $ CHARGES |

| 21. DIAGNOSIS OR NATURE OF ILLNESS OR INJURY (Relate Items 1, 2, 3 or 4 to Item 24E by Line) 1. ____.____ 3. ____.____ 2. ____.____ 4. ____.____ | 22. MEDICAID RESUBMISSION CODE ORIGINAL REF. NO. 23. PRIOR AUTHORIZATION NUMBER |

24. A. DATE(S) OF SERVICE		B. PLACE OF SERVICE	C. EMG	D. PROCEDURES, SERVICES, OR SUPPLIES (Explain Unusual Circumstances)		E. DIAGNOSIS POINTER	F. $ CHARGES	G. DAYS OR UNITS	H. EPSDT Family Plan	I. ID. QUAL.	J. RENDERING PROVIDER ID. #
From MM DD YY	To MM DD YY			CPT/HCPCS	MODIFIER						
1										NPI	
2										NPI	
3										NPI	
4										NPI	
5										NPI	
6										NPI	

| 25. FEDERAL TAX I.D. NUMBER SSN EIN ☐ ☐ | 26. PATIENT'S ACCOUNT NO. | 27. ACCEPT ASSIGNMENT? (For govt. claims, see back) YES ☐ NO ☐ | 28. TOTAL CHARGE $ | 29. AMOUNT PAID $ | 30. BALANCE DUE $ |

| 31. SIGNATURE OF PHYSICIAN OR SUPPLIER INCLUDING DEGREES OR CREDENTIALS (I certify that the statements on the reverse apply to this bill and are made a part thereof.) SIGNED _____ DATE _____ | 32. SERVICE FACILITY LOCATION INFORMATION a. NPI b. | 33. BILLING PROVIDER INFO & PH # ( ) a. NPI b. |

PHYSICIAN OR SUPPLIER INFORMATION →

NUCC Instruction Manual available at: www.nucc.org

APPROVED OMB-0938-0999 FORM CMS-1500 (08/05)

This document will be used multiple times. Make photocopies before writing on this document, or download it from the Online Learning Center at www.mhhe.com/BoothMA5e for any future uses.

Name_____ Date_____

DAILY CHECKLIST FOR CLOSING THE OFFICE

Daily Checklist for Closing BWW Medical Associates, PC				W/E _____		
	M	**T**	**W**	**Th**	**F**	**S**
1. Computers are logged off and shut down						
2. Contaminated supplies/equipment are properly disposed of or tagged for cleaning/sterilization						
3. Areas are restocked						
4. Patient charts are pulled/reviewed for next day and all test results are available						
5. Laboratory specimens are in pick-up receptacle						
6. All office equipment is turned off (including kitchen)						
7. Reception area is neat and organized						
8. Calls are forwarded to voicemail/answering machine						
9. Medical records are secured						
10. All doors and windows are locked						
11. Security system is armed						

Name_____ Date_____

DAILY CHECKLIST FOR OPENING THE OFFICE

Daily Checklist for Opening BWW Medical Associates, PC	M	T	W	Th	F	S
1. Security system is disarmed						
2. Voicemail/answering service messages are retrieved						
3. Messages are routed and ready for callback						
4. Fax machine is checked						
5. Computers are turned on						
6. Appointments and insurance rosters are checked						
7. Charts are pulled and paperwork is attached						
8. Equipment is working properly						
9. Rooms are supplied and ready						
10. Refrigerator temperature is checked						
11. Emergency supplies, including O_2, are checked						
12. Reception area is in order and patient education material is available						
13. Lab specimens from the day before were picked up						

W/E _____

Name_____ Date_____

DAILY LOG

Date: Today						
Patient	**Services**	**Charge**	**Payment**	**Adj**	**Cur. Bal.**	**Prev. Bal.**
TOTALS						

DISBURSEMENTS JOURNAL

Record of Office Disbursements
20XX

DATE	PAYEE	CK. NO.	TOTAL AMOUNT	RENT	UTILITIES	POSTAGE	LAE/ X-RAY	MEDICAL SUPPLIES	OFFICE SUPPLIES	WAGES	INSURANCE	TAXES	TRAVEL	MISC.

Name_____ Date_____

EMPLOYEES EARNING RECORD

Name _____   Soc. Sec. No. _____   Dependents _____   Year _____

Address _____   Birth Date _____   Deductions _____

_____   Job Title _____   Pay Rate

Spouse _____   Employed on _____   Record of

Phone _____   Terminated on _____   Changes

Reason _____

Date	Rate

Check Number	Period Number	Earnings			Deductions					Net Pay	Cumulative FICA
		Regular	OT	Total	FICA	Fed. Tax	State	SUI	SDI		
1st Quarter Total											
2nd Quarter Total											
3rd Quarter Total											
4th Quarter Total											

This document will be used multiple times. Make photocopies before writing on this document, or download it from the Online Learning Center at www.mhhe.com/BoothMA5e for any future uses.

Employees Earning Record   **853**

FAX COVER SHEET

BWW

BWW Medical Associates, PC
305 Main Street, Port Snead YZ 12345-9876
Tel: 555-654-3210, Fax: 555-987-6543
Web: BWWAssociates.com

Paul F. Buckwalter, MD
Alexis N. Whalen, MD
Elizabeth H. Williams, MD

FACSIMILE COVER SHEET

Date: _____

To: _____   From: _____

Fax #: _____   Fax #: _____

# of pages (including this cover sheet): _____

Message:

_____

_____

_____

_____

_____

_____

_____

INCIDENT REPORT

BWW

BWW Medical Associates, PC
305 Main Street, Port Snead YZ 12345-9876
Tel: 555-654-3210, Fax: 555-987-6543
Web: BWWAssociates.com

Paul F. Buckwalter, MD
Alexis N. Whalen, MD
Elizabeth H. Williams, MD

Incident Report
(Only for Internal Use)

Date/time of incident: _____ Location: _____

Name of injured or at risk party: _____

Circle one: Patient   Staff Member   Other (complete blank) _____

Address of above party: _____

Phone numbers of above party: home _____ cell _____

Describe the incident (use back of sheet if additional space needed): _____

_____

_____

Describe action(s) taken and by whom: _____

_____

_____

Name(s)/contact information of witnesses: _____

_____

_____

Name(s)/time of parties notified: _____

_____

Name of person completing report: _____ Date/time: _____

Report submitted to: _____ Date/time: _____

(Submit form to immediate supervisor of area where the incident occurred)

This document will be used multiple times. Make photocopies before writing on this document, or download it from the Online Learning Center at www.mhhe.com/BoothMA5e for any future uses.

INSURANCE CLAIMS REGISTER

| Patient Name | Insurance Company | Claim Filing | | Insurance Response Pd, Denied, Rejct, Suspd, Info Req | Date Resubmitted | Payment | | Patient Balance | Date Patient Billed |
		Date	Amount	Date		Date	Amount		

LEDGER CARD

BWW

BWW Medical Associates, PC
305 Main Street, Port Snead YZ 12345-9876
Tel: 555-654-3210, Fax: 555-987-6543
Web: BWWAssociates.com

Paul F. Buckwalter, MD
Alexis N. Whalen, MD
Elizabeth H. Williams, MD

Patient's Name _____

Home Phone _____ Work Phone _____

Social Security No. _____

Employer _____

Insurance _____

Policy # _____

Person Responsible for Charges (if Different from Patient) _____

Address

Date	Reference	Description	Charge	Credits		Current Balance
				Payments	Adj.	

Please Pay Last Amount in This Column

OV—Office Visit   C—Consultation   EX—Examination
X—X-ray   NC—No Charge   INS—Insurance
ROA—Received on Account MA—Missed Appointment

PATIENT MEDICAL HISTORY FORM

BWW

BWW Medical Associates, PC
305 Main Street, Port Snead YZ 12345-9876
Tel: 555-654-3210, Fax: 555-987-6543
Web: BWWAssociates.com

Paul F. Buckwalter, MD
Alexis N. Whalen, MD
Elizabeth H. Williams, MD

Patient Medical History

Name: _____ Age: _____ Sex: _____ MS: S M W D

Address: _____

Occupation: _____

Reason for visit: _____

History of present illness: _____

Allergies: _____

Current medications: _____

Cigarettes _____ Alcohol _____ Drugs _____

Past medical history:
Surgeries and dates: _____

Illnesses/Immunizations:

Chickenpox _____ Measles _____ Rubella _____ Mumps_____ DTP _____ TD _____ Polio ___ Whooping _____

cough _____ Flu_____ Pneumonia _____ Hepatitis B _____

Other_____

Females: Age first period _____ LMP _____ # pregnancies _____ # children _____

Family history:

Relationship	Age if Alive	Medical Issues	Age at Death	Cause of Death
Mother				
Father				
Brothers				
Sisters				

Have you or an immediate family member (mother, father, sister, brother, grandparent) been diagnosed with:

Cancer _____ Location _____ Whom _____ Hypertension _____

Thyroid disorder _____ Heart disease _____ GI disorder _____ Blood disorder _____

Depression _____ Nervous disorder _____ Asthma _____ Migraines _____

This document will be used multiple times. Make photocopies before writing on this document, or download it from the Online Learning Center at www.mhhe.com/BoothMA5e for any future uses.

Name_____ Date_____

PATIENT PHYSICAL EXAMINATION FORM

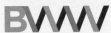

BWW Medical Associates, PC
305 Main Street, Port Snead YZ 12345-9876
Tel: 555-654-3210, Fax: 555-987-6543
Web: BWWAssociates.com

Paul F. Buckwalter, MD
Alexis N. Whalen, MD
Elizabeth H. Williams, MD

Review of Systems and Physical Examination
ROS

HEENT:_____

CV_____

Resp_____

GI_____

GU_____

MS_____

Integ_____

Neuro_____

Psych_____

Endo_____

Allergic/Immuno_____

Physical Examination

T_____ P_____ BP_____ R_____ HT_____ WT_____

Appearance_____ Skin_____ Mucus membrane_____

Eyes_____ Vision_____ Pupils_____ Fundus_____

Ears_____ Nose_____ Throat_____

Chest_____ Breasts_____

Heart_____

Lungs_____

Abdomen_____

Genitalia_____

Rectum_____

Pelvic_____

Extremities_____ Pulses_____

Lymph nodes_____ Neck_____ Axilla_____ Inguinal_____ Abd_____

Neuro_____

This document will be used multiple times. Make photocopies before writing on this document, or download it from the Online Learning Center at www.mhhe.com/BoothMA5e for any future uses.

PATIENT REGISTRATION FORM

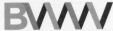

BWW Medical Associates, PC
305 Main Street, Port Snead YZ 12345-9876
Tel: 555-654-3210, Fax: 555-987-6543
Web: BWWAssociates.com

Paul F. Buckwalter, MD
Alexis N. Whalen, MD
Elizabeth H. Williams, MD

Patient Registration

Patient Information

Name: _____   Today's date: _____

Address: _____

City: _____   State: _____   Zip code: _____

Telephone (home): _____   (Work): _____   (Cell): _____

Birthdate: _____   Age: _____   Sex: M   F   Marital status: M   S   W   D

Social security number: _____   Employer: _____   Occupation: _____

Primary physician: _____

Referred by: _____

Person to contact in emergency: _____

Emergency telephone: _____

Special needs: _____

Responsible Party

Party responsible for payment: Self   Spouse   Parent   Other

Name (If other than self): _____

Address: _____

City: _____   State: _____   Zip code: _____

Primary Insurance

Primary medical insurance: _____

Insured party: Self   Spouse   Parent   Other

ID#/Social security no.: _____   Group/Plan no.: _____

Name (If other than self): _____

Address: _____

City: _____   State: _____   Zip code: _____

Secondary Insurance

Secondary medical insurance: _____

Insured party: Self   Spouse   Parent   Other

ID#/Social security no.: _____   Group/Plan no.: _____

Name (If other than self): _____

Address: _____

City: _____   State: _____   Zip code: _____

This document will be used multiple times. Make photocopies before writing on this document, or download it from the Online Learning Center at www.mhhe.com/BoothMA5e for any future uses.

PAYROLL REGISTER

Pay Period _____

Emp. No.	Name	Earnings to date	Hrly. Rate	Reg. Hrs.	OT Hrs.	OT Earnings	TOTAL GROSS	Earnings Subject to Unemp.	Earnings Subject to FICA	Social Security (FICA)	Medicare	Federal W/H	State W/H	Health Ins.	Net pay	Check No.

This document will be used multiple times. Make photocopies before writing on this document, or download it from the Online Learning Center at www.mhhe.com/BoothMA5e for any future uses.

PRIVACY VIOLATION COMPLAINT FORM

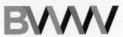

BWW Medical Associates, PC
305 Main Street, Port Snead YZ 12345-9876
Tel: 555-654-3210, Fax: 555-987-6543
Web: BWWAssociates.com

Paul F. Buckwalter, MD
Alexis N. Whalen, MD
Elizabeth H. Williams, MD

Privacy Violation Complaint

As per our Privacy Policies and Procedures, we are providing this form for individuals who feel they have a complaint regarding how their protected health information was handled by our office. You have the right to make a complaint and we may take no retaliatory actions against you because of it. We will respond to this complaint within 30 days of its receipt.

Patient Name: _____

Address: _____

DOB: _____ Date of Complaint: _____

Phone: Home _____ Cell _____ Work _____

Best time to reach you: _____

Reason for the complaint (Please be as specific as possible, attaching additional documentation as necessary): _____
_____
_____
_____
_____

_____   _____
Signature   Date

Office Use Only

Received by: _____ Date _____

Follow-up Started on (date): _____

PROGRESS NOTE

BWW

BWW Medical Associates, PC
305 Main Street, Port Snead YZ 12345-9876
Tel: 555-654-3210, Fax: 555-987-6543
Web: BWWAssociates.com

Paul F. Buckwalter, MD
Alexis N. Whalen, MD
Elizabeth H. Williams, MD

PROGRESS NOTES

Name _____ Chart #_____

DATE	

This document will be used multiple times. Make photocopies before writing on this document, or download it from the Online Learning Center at www.mhhe.com/BoothMA5e for any future uses.

RECEIPT OF PRIVACY PRACTICES

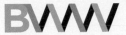

BWW Medical Associates, PC
305 Main Street, Port Snead YZ 12345-9876
Tel: 555-654-3210, Fax: 555-987-6543
Web: BWWAssociates.com

Paul F. Buckwalter, MD
Alexis N. Whalen, MD
Elizabeth H. Williams, MD

Notice of Privacy Practices

I understand that BWW Medical Associates, PC creates and maintains medical records describing my health history, symptoms, examinations, test results, diagnoses, treatments, and plans for my future care and/or treatment. I further understand that this information may be used for any of the following:

1. Plan and document my care and treatment
2. Communicate with health professionals involved in my care and treatment
3. Verify insurance coverage for planned procedures and/or treatments for the applicable diagnoses
4. Application of any medical or surgical procedures and diagnoses (codes) to my medical insurance claim forms as application for payment of services rendered
5. Assessment of quality of care and utilization review of the health care professionals providing my care

Additionally, it has been explained to me that:

1. A complete description of the use and disclosure of this information is included in the *Notice of Information of Privacy Practices* which has been provided to me
2. I have had a right to review this information prior to signing this consent
3. BWW Medical Associates, PC has the right to change this notice and their practices
4. Any revision of this notice will be mailed to me at the address I provided to them prior to its implementation
5. I may object to the use of my health information for specific purposes
6. I may request restrictions as to the manner my information may be used or disclosed in order to carry out treatment, payment, or health information
7. I understand that it is not required that my requested restrictions be honored
8. I may revoke this consent in writing, except for those disclosures which may have taken place prior to the receipt of my revocation

At the time of the document signing, I request the following restrictions to disclosure or use of my health information: _____

_____

_____   _____
Printed Name of Patient or Legal Guardian   Signature of Parent or Legal Guardian

_____   _____
Printed Name of Witness/Title   Signature of Witness/Title

Date: _____

Name_____ Date_____

SELF-EVALUATION OF PROFESSIONAL BEHAVIORS

Behavior	Example(s)	Rate Yourself (5 = Best)					Improvements Needed
		1	2	3	4	5	
Integrity	Consistently honest; able to be trusted with the property of others; can be trusted with confidential information; completes tasks accurately.						
Appearance	Clothing and uniform appropriate for circumstance; neat, clean, and well-kept appearance; good personal hygiene and grooming.						
Teamwork	Places the success of the team above self-interest; does not undermine the team; helps and supports other team members; shows respect to all team members; remains flexible and open to change; communicates with others to help resolve problems.						
Self-confidence	Demonstrates the ability to trust personal judgment; demonstrates an awareness of strengths and limitations; exercises good personal judgment.						
Communication	Speaks clearly; writes legibly; listens actively; adjusts communication strategies to various situations.						
Commitment to diversity	Consistently demonstrates respect for varied cultural backgrounds, ethnicities, religions, sexual orientations, social classes, abilities, political beliefs, and disabilities.						
Punctuality and attendance	Arrives at class and work on the appointed day and time.						
Acceptance of criticism	Listens when constructive criticism is given; does not become defensive with criticism; appreciates constructive criticism and incorporates suggestions into behavior as appropriate.						
Organization	Coordinates more than one task at a time; keeps work area neat and orderly; anticipates future work; works efficiently and systematically.						
Knowledge and comprehension	Learns new things easily; retains new information; associates theory with practice.						

STANDARDIZED PRIOR AUTHORIZATION FORM

Standardized Prior Authorization Request Form

COMPLETE ALL INFORMATION ON THE "STANDARDIZED PRIOR AUTHORIZATION FORM".
INCOMPLETE SUBMISSIONS MAY BE RETURNED UNPROCESSED.

Please direct any questions regarding this form to the *plan* to which you submit your request for claim review.

The Standardized Prior Authorization Form is not intended to replace payer specific prior authorization procedures, policies and documentation requirements. For payer specific policies, please reference the payer specific websites.

Health Plan:	Health Plan Fax #:	*Date Form Completed and Faxed:

Service Type Requiring Authorization[1, 2, 3] (Check all that apply)

Ambulatory/Outpatient Services
- ☐ Surgery/Procedure (SDC)
- ☐ Infusion or Oncology Drugs

Ancillary
- ☐ Acupuncture
- ☐ Chiropractic
- ☐ IVF/ART
- ☐ Non-Participating Specialist

Dental
- ☐ Adjunctive Dental Services
- ☐ Endodontics
- ☐ Maxilliofacial Prosthetics
- ☐ Oral Surgery
- ☐ Restorative

Durable Medical Equipment
- ☐ Prosthetic Device
- ☐ Purchase
- ☐ Renal Supplies
- ☐ Rental

Home Health/Hospice
- ☐ Home Health (Please circle: SN, PT, OT, ST, HHA, MSW)
- ☐ Hospice
- ☐ Infusion Therapy
- ☐ Respite Care

Inpatient Care/Observation
- ☐ Acute Medical/Surgical
- ☐ Long Term Acute Care
- ☐ Acute Rehab
- ☐ Skilled Nursing Facility
- ☐ Observation

Nutrition/Counseling
- ☐ Counseling
- ☐ Enteral Nutrition
- ☐ Infant Formula
- ☐ Total Parental Nutrition

Outpatient Therapy
- ☐ Occupational Therapy
- ☐ Physical Therapy
- ☐ Pulmonary/Cardiac Rehab
- ☐ Speech Therapy

Transportation
- ☐ Non-emergent Ground
- ☐ Non-emergent Air

☐ Other—please specify:

Provider Information (*Denotes required field)

*Requesting Provider Name and NPI#:	*Phone:	Fax:
*Servicing Provider Name and NPI# (and Tax ID if required): ☐ Same as Requesting Provider	*Phone:	Fax:
*Servicing Facility Name and NPI#: ☐ Same as Requesting Provider	*Phone:	Fax:
*Contact Person:	*Phone:	Fax:

Member Information (*Denotes required field)

*Patient Name:	*☐ Male ☐ Female	*DOB:
*Health Insurance ID#: If other insurance, please specify:	*Patient Account/Control Number:	
Address:	Phone:	

Diagnosis/Planned Procedure Information (*Denotes required field)

*Principal Diagnosis Description:	*Principal Planned Procedure (Description and CPT/HCPCS Code):
ICD-9 Codes:	# of Units Being Requested: ☐ Hours ☐ Days ☐ Months ☐ Visits ☐ Dosage
Secondary Diagnosis Description:	Secondary Planned Procedure (Description and CPT/HCPCS Code):
ICD-9 Codes:	# of Units Being Requested: ☐ Hours ☐ Days ☐ Months ☐ Visits ☐ Dosage
*Service Start Date:	*Service End Date:

[1] Please attach plan specific templates that are required for supporting clinical documentation.
[2] Not all services listed will be covered by the benefits in a member's health plan product.
[3] This form does not replace payer specific prior authorization requirements.

Clear Form

Massachusetts Administrative Simplification Collaborative–Standardized Prior Authorization Request Form V1.1   May 2012

This document will be used multiple times. Make photocopies before writing on this document, or download it from the Online Learning Center at www.mhhe.com/BoothMA5e for any future uses.

SUPERBILL

BWW Medical Associates, PC
305 Main Street, Port Snead YZ 12345-9876, Tel: 555-654-3210, Fax: 555-987-6543

☐ PRIVATE ☐ BLUECROSS ☐ IND. ☐ MEDICARE ☐ MEDI-CAL ☐ HMO ☐ PPO

PATIENT'S LAST NAME	FIRST	ACCOUNT #	BIRTHDATE / /	SEX ☐ MALE ☐ FEMALE	TODAY'S DATE / /
INSURANCE COMPANY	SUBSCRIBER		PLAN #	SUB. #	GROUP

ASSIGNMENT: I hereby assign my insurance benefits to be paid directly to the undersigned physician. I am financially responsible for non-covered services.
SIGNED: (Patient, or Parent, if Minor)　　　DATE: / /

RELEASE: I hereby authorize the physician to release to my insurance carrers any information required to process this claim.
SIGNED: (Patient, or Parent, if Minor)　　　DATE: / /

✔	DESCRIPTION	M/Care CPT/Mod	DxRe	FEE	✔	DESCRIPTION	M/Care CPT/Mod	DxRe	FEE	✔	DESCRIPTION	M/Care	CPT/Mod	DxRe	FEE
	OFFICE CARE					PROCEDURES					INJECTIONS/IMMUNIZATIONS				
	NEW PATIENT					Tread Mill (In Office)	93015				Tetanus/Diphtheria		90718		
	Brief	99201				24 Hour Holter	93224				MMR		90707		
	Limited	99202				If Medicare (Set up Fee)	93225				Pneumococcal		90732		
	Intermediate	99203				Physician Interpret	93227				Influenza		90656		
	Extended	99204				EKG w/Interpretation	93000				TB Skin Test (PPD)		86580		
	Comprehensive	99205				EKG (tracing only)	93005				Antigen Injection-Single		95115		
						Sigmoidoscopy	45300				Multiple		95117		
	ESTABLISHED PATIENT					Sigmoidoscopy, Flexible	45330				B12 Injection	J3420	90782		
	Minimal	99211				Sigmoidos. , Flex. w/Bx.	45331				Injection, IM		90782		
	Brief	99212				Spirometry, FEV/FVC	94010				Compazine	J0780	90782		
	Limited	00213				Spirometry, Post Dilator	94060				Demerol	J2175	00782		
	Intermediate	99214									Vistaril	J3410	90782		
	Extended	99215				LABORATORY					Susphrine	J0170	90782		
	Comprehensive	99215				Blood Draw Fee	36415				Decadron	J0890	90782		
						Urinalysis, Chemical	81000				Estradiol	J1000	90782		
	CONSULTATION-OFFICE					Throat Culture	87081				Testosterone	J1080	90782		
	Focused	99241				Occult Blood	82270				Lidocaine	J2000	90782		
	Expanded	99242				Pap Handling Charge	99000				Solumedrol	J2920	90782		
	Detailed	99243				Pap Life Guard	88150-90				Solucortef	J1720	90782		
	Comprehensive 1	99244				Gram Stain	87205				Hydeltra	J1690	90782		
	Comprehensive 2	99245				Hanging Drop	87210								
	MCR Pts - use E/M codes					Urine Drug Screen	80100				INJECTIONS - JOINT/BURSA				
	Case Management	98900									Small Joints		20600		
											Intermediate		20605		
	Post-op Exam	99024									Large Joints		20610		
						SUPPLIES					Trigger Point		20552		
											MISCELLANEOUS				

	DIAGNOSIS:	ICD-9												
	Abdominal Pain	709.0	__ Gout	274.0	__ C.V.A. - Acute	436.	__ Electrolyte Dis.	276.9	__ Herpes Simplex	054.9
	Abscess (Site)	682.9	__ Asthma	493.90	__ Cere. Vas. Accid. (Old)	438	__ Fatigue	780.7	__ Herpes Zoster	053.9
	Adverse Drug Rx	995.2	__ Asthmatic Bronchitis	493.90	__ Cerumen	380.4	__ Fibrocys. Br. Dis	610.1	__ Hydrocele	603.9
	Alcohol Detox	291.8	__ Atrial Fib.	427.31	__ Chestwall Pain	786.59	__ Fracture (Site)	829.0	__ Hyperlipidemia	272.4
	Alcoholism	303.90	__ Atrial Tachi.	427.0	__ Cholecystitis	575.0	__ Open/Close		__ Hypertension	401.9
	Allergic Rhinitis	477	__ Bowel Obstruct.	560.9	__ Cholelithiasis	574.00	__ Fungal Infect. (Site)	110.8	__ Hyperthyroidism	242.9
	Allergy	995.3	__ Breast Mass	611.72	__ COPD	492.8	__ Gastric Ulcer	531.90	__ Hypothyroidism	244.9
	Alzheimer's Dis.	290.1	__ Bronchitis	490	__ Cirrhosis	571.5	__ Gastritis	535.0	__ Labyrinthitis	386.30
	Anemia	285.9	__ Bursitis	727.3	__ Cong. Heart Fail.	428.9	__ Gastroenteritis	558.9	__ Lipoma (Site)	214.9
	Anemia - Pernicious	281.0	__ Cancer, Breast (Site)	174.9	__ Conjunctivitis	372.30	__ G.I. Bleeding	578.9	__ Lymphoma	202.8
	Angina	413.9	__ Metastatic (Site)	199.1	__ Contusion (Site)	924.9	__ Glomerulonephritis	583.9	__ Mit. Valve Prolapse	424.0
	Anxiety Synd.	300.00	__ Colon	153.9	__ Costochondritis	733.99	__ Headache	784.0	__ Myocard. Infarction (Area)	410.9
	Appendicitis	541	__ Cancer, Rectal	154.1	__ Depression	311.	__ Headache, Tension	307.81	__ M.I., Old	412
	Arterioscl. H.D.	414.0	__ Lung (Site)	162.9	__ Dermatitis	692.9	__ Migraine (Type)	346.9	__ Myositis	729.1
	Arthritis, Osteo.	715.90	__ Skin (Site)	173.9	__ Diabetes Mellitus	250.00	__ Hemorrhoids	455.6	__ Nausea/Vomiting	787.0
	Rheumatoid	714.0	__ Card. Arrhythmia (Type)	427.9	__ Diabetic Ketosis	250.1	__ Hernia, Hiatal	553.3	__ Neuralgia	729.2
	Arthritis, Osteo.		__ Cardiomyopathy	425.4	__ Diverticulitis	562.11	__ Inguinal	550.9	__ Nevus (Site)	216.9
	Lupus	710.0	__ Cellulitis (Site)	682.9	__ Diverticulosis	562.10	__ Hepatitis	573.3	__ Obesity	278.0

DIAGNOSIS: (IF NOT CHECKED ABOVE)

SERVICES PERFORMED AT: ☐ Office ☐ E.R. ☐ CLAIM CONTAINS NO ORDERED REFERRING SERVICE

REFERRING PHYSICIAN & I.D. NUMBER

RETURN APPOINTMENT INFORMATION:	NEXT APPOINTMENT		ACCEPT ASSIGNMENT?	DOCTOR'S SIGNATURE
5 - 10 - 15 - 20 - 30 - 40 - 60	M - T - W - TH - F - S		☐ YES	
[DAYS] [WKS.] [MOS.] [PRN]	DATE / / TIME:	AM / PM	☐ NO	

INSTRUCTIONS TO PATIENT FOR FILING INSURANCE CLAIMS:

1. Complete upper portion of this form, sign and date.
2. Attach this form to your own insurance company's form for direct reimbursement.

MEDICARE PATIENTS - DO NOT SEND THIS TO MEDICARE. WE WILL SUBMIT THE CLAIM FOR YOU.

☐ CASH
☐ CHECK #_____
☐ VISA
☐ MC
☐ CO-PAY

TOTAL TODAY'S FEE	
OLD BALANCE	
TOTAL DUE	
AMOUNT REC'D. TODAY	

SURGICAL GUIDELINES (SAMPLE)

BVVV

BWW Medical Associates, PC
305 Main Street, Port Snead YZ 12345-9876
Tel: 555-654-3210, Fax: 555-987-6543
Web: BWWAssociates.com

Paul F. Buckwalter, MD
Alexis N. Whalen, MD
Elizabeth H. Williams, MD

Pre-Operative Instructions for Surgery
Use the following guidelines to prepare for your upcoming surgery.

Medications:
1. If you take anticoagulants such as aspirin, warfarin, Coumadin, Plavix, Heparin, Ticlid, or Lovenox, you may need to stop taking the medication before the surgery.
2. STOP all herbal medications, vitamin E, diet pills, multivitamins, and NSAIDS such as ibuprofen, Advil, Nuprin, Aleve, Naprosyn, or Naproxen 7 to 10 days prior to surgery.
3. STOP all cholesterol lowering medications, such as Lipitor, Zocor, or Pravachol, 48 HOURS PRIOR to surgery.
4. DO NOT TAKE ANY diuretics or water pills the morning of surgery.
5. DO NOT TAKE these medications the morning of surgery. BENAZEPRIL, CAPTOPRIL, ALAPRIL, QUINAPRIL.
6. DO TAKE any HEART MEDICATIONS or BLOOD PRESSURE MEDICATIONS the morning of surgery with a sip of water, unless otherwise indicated.
7. You MAY USE PRESCRIBED INHALERS AND you MUST BRING THEM WITH YOU the day of surgery.
8. If you are a diabetic, DO NOT TAKE ANY DIABETIC PILLS OR INSULIN the morning of surgery. Your blood sugar will be checked at the hospital prior to surgery and will be taken care of as needed.

Skin Preparation:
BEFORE surgery, your body must be thoroughly cleaned with a special soap to decrease the amount of germs on the skin. Dial antibacterial soap may be used for this purpose. Using this soap will help reduce the chance of getting a wound infection after surgery.

Follow these instructions for proper skin preparation:
DO NOT shave the day of surgery. Shaving can cause small abrasions or nicks in the skin, which allow germs to enter. If you want to shave, it must be done the night before surgery.

DO NOT use any creams, lotions, powders, or underarm deodorant in the area where your surgery will take place. These items interfere with the solution used to prepare your skin in the operating room.

The evening before surgery:
Take a shower and wash your entire body with antibacterial soap. Work the soap up into lather. Wash your body, especially the surgical area, with a clean, fresh washcloth. Rinse thoroughly because soap can leave a film, which may interfere with the antiseptics used to clean the skin in the operating room. Dry your body with a clean, fresh towel. Wear clean, fresh pajamas to bed.

(continued)

SURGICAL GUIDELINES (SAMPLE) *(concluded)*

BWW

BWW Medical Associates, PC
305 Main Street, Port Snead YZ 12345-9876
Tel: 555-654-3210, Fax: 555-987-6543
Web: BWWAssociates.com

Paul F. Buckwalter, MD
Alexis N. Whalen, MD
Elizabeth H. Williams, MD

The morning of surgery:

Take a shower or wash the surgical area again with antibacterial soap. Work into lather and clean your body or the surgical site with a clean, fresh washcloth. Again, rinse thoroughly. Dry your body with a clean, fresh towel, and put on clean, fresh clothes.

Additional Instructions:

1. DO NOT eat or drink anything after midnight the day before surgery, or the morning of surgery (except for certain morning medications). This includes candy, mints, coffee, water, gum, and cigarettes.

2. DO NOT wear any jewelry, makeup, nail polish, hair clips, or contact lenses the day of surgery. Bring your contact lens case and cleaning solution to the hospital if you wear contacts.

3. DO NOT bring any valuables with you to the hospital or they will have to be placed with security or left with the accompanying person.

4. It is recommended that you wear loose, comfortable clothing to the hospital the day of surgery. Wear something that is loose enough to fit over the operated site, which may have a bandage over it, especially if you are going home the same day.

5. Plan to arrive at the hospital 2 hours prior to your surgery time as told by your doctor's office.

6. If you are having OUTPATIENT SURGERY, it is REQUIRED that you have a responsible person provide you with transportation after surgery, and someone must be able to stay with you 24 hours following surgery. You cannot take the bus or a taxicab home alone.

7. If you are staying overnight after your surgery, you will be transported to your room after a short stay in the recovery room.

8. ALL patients for ALL surgeries REQUIRE pre-testing unless otherwise told by your surgeon. Additional pre-testing information will be given to you.

9. Please call our office if you have any further questions or concerns.

TELEPHONE MESSAGE SHEET

BVVW

BWW Medical Associates, PC

TELEPHONE MESSAGE

For:_____

_____

_____

_____

_____

_____

_____

Name of Caller: _____

Name of Patient (if not caller): _____

Date/Time Called:_____

Message Taken by:_____

This document will be used multiple times. Make photocopies before writing on this document, or download it from the Online Learning Center at www.mhhe.com/BoothMA5e for any future uses.

TRAVEL EXPENSE REPORT

BWW

BWW Medical Associates, PC
305 Main Street, Port Snead YZ 12345-9876
Tel: 555-654-3210, Fax: 555-987-6543
Web: BWWAssociates.com

Paul F. Buckwalter, MD
Alexis N. Whalen, MD
Elizabeth H. Williams, MD

TRAVEL EXPENSE REPORT
(Travel with estimated expenses must be approved prior to the event)

Applicant's name: _____ Date: _____

Applicant's address: _____

Applicant's cell phone and home phone: _____

Name of activity and type (example: professional meeting, conference; attach Web or brochure

information): _____

Purpose of travel: _____

Location of activity: _____

Dates: _____ Number of days: _____

Registration fee	$
Transportation: *indicate major mode of travel	$
Airport shuttle or parking	$
Taxi	$
Lodging (daily rate _____ × _____ number of days)	$
Meals ($30 per day × _____ number of days)	$
Other (explain)	$
Total	$

Did you miss work days: [ ] NO [ ] YES (If "YES" include dates and number of days)

Dates: _____ Number of days: _____

Signature: _____

*If using your own vehicle, mileage is reimbursed at the current rate. Check with your supervisor prior to travel.

This form must be submitted with receipts in 10 working days upon return. Noncompliance may result in denial of reimbursement or if funds were previously awarded, payroll deduction may occur to recover the amount.

For Management Use Only

[ ] Not approved   [ ] Approved   Amount: _____

Name (print): _____ Date: _____

Signature: _____

Work Documentation: Clinical

Use these documents while performing application activities and procedures that include a work document icon.

WORK // DOC

LIST OF WORK DOCUMENTS

WORK DOCUMENTS BY CHAPTER

The blank documents needed to complete the application activities and procedures for each chapter are listed below. Notice that some of the documents are used in more than one chapter. Only one copy of each blank document is included in this workbook, so you will need to make enough additional copies to complete all of the application activities or procedures identified.

CHAPTER 3

CHAPTER 5

AUTHORIZATION TO RELEASE INFORMATION

BWW

BWW Medical Associates, PC
305 Main Street, Port Snead YZ 12345-9876
Tel: 555-654-3210, Fax: 555-987-6543
Web: BWWAssociates.com

Paul F. Buckwalter, MD
Alexis N. Whalen, MD
Elizabeth H. Williams, MD

Authorization to Release Health Information

I, _____ residing at

_____ and DOB of

_____ give permission to (name of practice) _____

to release to _____ of BWW Medical Associates, PC the

following information: _____

_____

_____

Reason for the request: _____

_____

Signature of Patient or Legal Guardian _____

Printed Name of Patient or Legal Guardian _____

If Guardian, relationship to Patient _____

This authorization will expire on: _____

YOU MAY REFUSE TO SIGN THIS AUTHORIZATION. You may revoke this authorization at any time by notifying BWW Medical Associates, PC in writing. Revocation will have no effect on actions taken prior to receipt of any revocation. Any disclosure of information carries the potential for unauthorized redisclosure and the information may not be protected by federal confidentiality rules.

BODY MASS INDEX (BMI) CHART

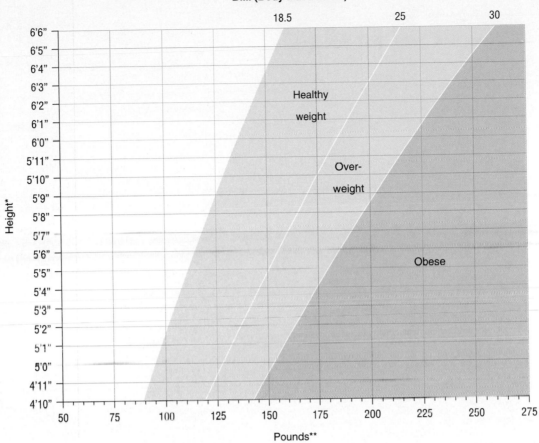

BMI (Body Mass Index)

BWW LETTERHEAD

BWW Medical Associates, PC
305 Main Street, Port Snead YZ 12345-9876
Tel: 555-654-3210, Fax: 555-987-6543
Web: BWWAssociates.com

Paul F. Buckwalter, MD
Alexis N. Whalen, MD
Elizabeth H. Williams, MD

This document will be used multiple times. Make photocopies before writing on this document, or download it from the Online Learning Center at www.mhhe.com/BoothMA5e for any future uses.

CHAIN OF CUSTODY FORM

Morris A. Turner, MD

C.L.I.A #21.1862

266 Line Road
Montelair, Delaware 00956
800-555-1567

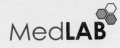 MedLAB

CHAIN OF CUSTODY FORM
SPECIMEN I.D.NO:

STEP 1—TO BE COMPLETED BY COLLECTOR OR EMPLOYER REPRESENTATIVE.

Employer Name, Address, and I.D. No.:   OR   Medical Review Officer Name and Address:

_____   _____

_____   _____

_____

Donor Social Security No. or Employee I.D. No.: _____

Donor I.D. verified: ☐ Photo I.D.   ☐ Employer Representative _____
                                                            Signature

Reason for test: (check one)   ☐ Preemployment   ☐ Random   ☐ Postaccident
                                 ☐ Periodic   ☐ Reasonable suspicion/cause
                                 ☐ Return to duty   ☐ Other (specify)

Test(s) to be performed: _____   Total tests ordered: ☐

Type of specimen obtained: ☐ Urine   ☐ Blood   ☐ Semen   ☐ Other (specify)
                    Submit only one specimen with each requisition.

STEP 2—TO BE COMPLETED BY COLLECTOR.

For urine specimens, read temperature within 4 minutes of collection.
Check here if specimen temperature is within range. ☐ Yes, 90°–100°F/32°–38°C
Or record actual temperature here: _____

STEP 3—TO BE COMPLETED BY COLLECTOR.

Collection site_____   Address _____
City _____   State _____   Zip_____   Phone _____
Collection date: _____   Time: _____   ☐ a.m.   ☐ p.m.

I certify that the specimen identified on this form is the specimen presented to me by the donor identified in step 1 above, and that it was collected, labeled, and sealed in the donor's presence.

Collector's name: _____   Signature of collector _____

STEP 4—TO BE INITIATED BY DONOR AND COMPLETED AS NECESSARY THEREAFTER.

Purpose of change	Released by Signature	Received by Signature	Date
A. Provide specimen for testing			
B. Shipment to Laboratory			
C.			

Comments:

STEP 5—TO BE COMPLETED BY THE LABORATORY:

Specimen package seal(s) intact when received in lab?   ☐ Yes   ☐ No   If no , explain.
Laboratory receiver's initials _____

Copy 1 - Original - Must accompany specimen to laboratory.

Name_____ Date_____

CHEMISTRY REQUEST FORM

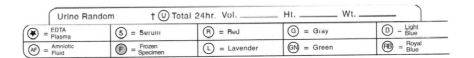

☐ ‖‖‖‖‖‖‖‖‖‖‖‖‖‖
70Y

Account No.

Specimen Date Mo Day Yr	Specimen Time Hr Min	Patient Name (Last)		(First, MI)	Sex	Date of Birth Mo Day Yr	Age Yrs Mos

50 8649 9000 4

	Patient I.D. #	Physician I.D.	Patient/Resp. Party's Phone #

* I certify that I have read the informed consent on the back and understand its content.

	Responsible Party or Insured's Name (Last, First)	Patient's SS #

_____
Patient's Signature

	Address	City	State	Zip Code

REV. 6/95

Resp. Party's Employer	Medicaid Number/HMO #	Medicare #

Physician Name	UPIN #	Physician's Signature	Provider #

Diagnosis Code (ICD-9)	Insurance Code or Company Name and Address	Insurance I.D. #	Workers Comp. Yes No

Group # or Name	Relationship to Insured (Circle One) 1-Self 2-Spouse 3-Other

(a)

Urine Random   † Ⓤ Total 24hr. Vol. _____ Ht. _____ Wt. _____

Ⓧ = EDTA Plasma	Ⓢ = Serum	Ⓡ = Red	Ⓖ = Gray	Ⓓ = Light Blue
AF = Amniotic Fluid	Ⓕ = Frozen Specimen	Ⓛ = Lavender	GN = Green	RB = Royal Blue

Apply Labels to Patient Specimens Only
Patient Control No.

‖‖‖‖‖‖‖‖‖‖
50 8649 9000 4

50 8649 9000 4
‖‖‖‖‖‖‖‖‖‖
50 8649 9000 4

50 8649 9000 4
‖‖‖‖‖‖‖‖‖‖
50 8649 9000 4

50 8649 9000 4
‖‖‖‖‖‖‖‖‖‖
50 8649 9000 4

CHEMISTRY REQUEST

58867	☐ Basic Chemistry	Ⓢ	1693	☐ Glycohemoglobin, Total	Ⓛ	4465	☐ Prolactin	Ⓢ
1396	☐ Amylase, Serum	Ⓢ	4416	☐ HCG, Beta Chain, Quant	Ⓢ	4747	☐ Prostatic Acid Phosphatase (EIA)	Ⓢ
6254	☐ Antinuclear Antibody (ANA), Qnt	Ⓢ	1453	☐ Hemoglobin A1C	Ⓛ	10322	☐ Prostate-Specific Antigen (PSA)	Ⓢ
1040	☐ BUN	Ⓢ	6510	☐ Hepatitis B Surf Antigen (HBsAg)	Ⓢ	5199	☐ Prothrombin Time	Ⓑ
7419	☐ Carbamazepine (Tegretol)	Ⓢ	6395	☐ Hepatitis B Surf Antibody (Anti HBs)	Ⓢ	6502	☐ Ra Latex Screen	Ⓢ
5009	☐ CBC With Differential	Ⓛ	58560	☐ Hepatitis Profile I (Diagnostic)	Ⓢ	5215	☐ Sedimentation Rate	Ⓛ
2139	☐ CEA-EIA Roche	△ Ⓧ	46938	☐ Hepatitis Profile II (Follow up)	Ⓢ	6072	☐ STS	Ⓢ
98012	☐ Chlamydia by DNA Probe	△	58552	☐ Hepatitis Profile VII (A and B)	Ⓢ	1149	☐ T₄ (Thyroxine)	Ⓢ
96479	☐ Chlamydia/GC, DNA Probe	△	83824	☐ HIV-1 ABS-EIA	Ⓢ	7336	☐ Theophylline (Theo-Dur)	Ⓢ
1065	☐ Cholesterol, Total	Ⓢ	7625	☐ Lead, Blood	RB	620	☐ Thyroid Profile I	Ⓢ
1370	☐ Creatinine, Serum	Ⓢ	235002	☐ Lipid Profile I (Lipoprotein Analysis)	Ⓢ	27011	☐ Thyroid Profile II	Ⓢ
7385	☐ Digoxin (Lanoxin)	Ⓢ	235028	☐ Lipid Profile III (incl Apolipoproteins)	Ⓢ	4259	☐ TSH, 3rd Generation	Ⓢ
604	☐ Electrolytes (Na, K, Cl)	Ⓢ	7708	☐ Lithium	Ⓢ	810	☐ Vitamin B-12 and Folate	Ⓢ
4598	☐ Ferritin	Ⓢ	505	☐ Liver Profile A	Ⓢ			
4309	☐ Follicle Stim. Hormone (FSH)	Ⓢ	7401	☐ Phenytoin (Dilantin)	Ⓢ	**URINE CHEMISTRY**		
1818	☐ Glucose	Ⓖ	1180	☐ Potassium	Ⓢ	3038	☐ Urinalysis (Microscopic if indicated)	Ⓤ
	☐ Glucose Tolerance	Ⓖ	4556	☐ Pregnancy, Serum, Ql.	Ⓢ	3772	☐ Urinalysis, Complete	Ⓤ
	Indicate No. Of Tubes		53520	☐ Prenatal Profile B with HBsAG	2-L Ⓡ			

ADDITIONAL TESTS

Test #	Name
☐ 1375	24 Hr Urine for Protein Ⓤ
☐ 4550	Pregnancy, Urine, Qul Ⓤ

(b)

CONSENT FORM

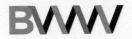

BWW Medical Associates, PC
305 Main Street, Port Snead YZ 12345-9876
Tel: 555-654-3210, Fax: 555-987-6543
Web: BWWAssociates.com

DRUG SCREEN CONSENT FORM

A urine drug test is required by _____ as part of your pre-employment screening. Please provide us with a list of all medications that you are presently taking.

_____

_____

_____

_____

_____

I understand that my prospective or continued employment is contingent on a successful screening.

Date: _____ Signature: _____

Witness: _____

Name_____ Date_____

DEA FORM 41

Sample Only

OMB Approval No. 1117-0007	U.S. Department of Justice/Drug Enforcement Administration **REGISTRANTS INVENTORY OF DRUGS SURRENDERED**	PACKAGE NO.

The following schedule is an inventory of controlled substances which is hereby surrendered to you for proper disposition.

FROM: *(Include Name, Street, City, State and ZIP Code in space provided below.)*

	Signature of applicant or authorized agent
⌐ ¬	
	Registrant's DEA Number
∟ ⌐	Registrant's Telephone Number

NOTE: CERTIFIED MAIL (Return Receipt Requested) IS REQUIRED FOR SHIPMENTS OF DRUGS VIA U.S. POSTAL SERVICE. See instructions on reverse (page 2) of form.

NAME OF DRUG OR PREPARATION Registrants will fill in Columns 1, 2, 3, and 4 ONLY.	Number of Containers	CONTENTS *(Number of grams, tablets, ounces or other units per container)*	Controlled Substance Content, *(Each Unit)*	FOR DEA USE ONLY		
				DISPOSITION	QUANTITY	
					GMS.	MGS.
1	*2*	*3*	*4*	*5*	*6*	*7*
1						
2						
3						
4						
5						
6						
23						
24						

The controlled substances surrendered in accordance with Title 21 of the Code of Federal Regulations, Section 1307.21, have been received in _____ packages purporting to contain the drugs listed on this inventory and have been: **(1) Forwarded tape-sealed without opening; (2) Destroyed as indicated and the remainder forwarded tape-sealed after verifying contents; (3) Forwarded tape-sealed after verifying contents.

DATE _____   DESTROYED BY: _____

**Strike out lines not applicable.   WITNESSED BY: _____

INSTRUCTIONS

1. List the name of the drug in column 1, the number of containers in column 2, the size of each container in column 3, and in column 4 the controlled substance content of each unit described in column 3; e.g., morphine sulfate tabs., 3 pkgs., 100 tabs., 1/4 gr. (16 mg.) or morphine sulfate tabs., 1 pkg., 83 tabs., 1/2 gr. (32 mg.), etc.

2. All packages included on a single line should be identical in name, content and controlled substance strength.

3. Prepare this form in quadruplicate. Mail two (2) copies of this form to the Special Agent in Charge, under separate cover. Enclose one additional copy in the shipment with the drugs. Retain one copy for your records. One copy will be returned to you as a receipt. No further receipt will be furnished to you unless specifically requested. Any further inquiries concerning these drugs should be addressed to the DEA District Office which serves your area.

4. There is no provision for payment for drugs surrendered. This is merely a service rendered to registrants enabling them to clear their stocks and records of unwanted items.

5. Drugs should be shipped tape-sealed via prepaid express or certified mail (**return receipt requested**) to Special Agent in Charge, Drug Enforcement Administration, of the DEA District Office which serves your area.

PRIVACY ACT INFORMATION

AUTHORITY: Section 307 of the Controlled Substances Act of 1970 (PL 91-513).
PURPOSE: To document the surrender of controlled substances which have been forwarded by registrants to DEA for disposal.
ROUTINE USES: This form is required by Federal Regulations for the surrender of unwanted Controlled Substances. Disclosures of information from this system are made to the following categories of users for the purposes stated.
  A. Other Federal law enforcement and regulatory agencies for law enforcement and regulatory purposes.
  B. State and local law enforcement and regulatory agencies for law enforcement and regulatory purposes.
EFFECT: Failure to document the surrender of unwanted Controlled Substances may result in prosecution for violation of the Controlled Substances Act.

Under the Paperwork Reduction Act, a person is not required to respond to a collection of information unless it displays a currently valid OMB control number. Public reporting burden for this collection of information is estimated to average 30 minutes per response, including the time for reviewing instructions, searching existing data sources, gathering and maintaining the data needed, and completing and reviewing the collection of information. Send comments regarding this burden estimate or any other aspect of this collection of information, including suggestions for reducing this burden, to the Drug Enforcement Administration, FOI and Records Management Section, Washington, D.C. 20537; and to the Office of Management and Budget, Paperwork Reduction Project no. 1117-0007, Washington, D.C. 20503.

DEA FORM 222

Sample Only

DEA Form-222 (Oct. 1992)	**U.S. OFFICIAL ORDER FORMS - SCHEDULES I & II** Drug Enforcement Administration **SUPPLIER'S Copy 1**	
See Reverse of PURCHASER'S Copy for Instructions	No order form may be issued for Schedule I and II substances unless a completed application form has been received. (21 CFR 1305.04).	**OMB APPROVAL No. 1117-0010**

To: (Name of Supplier)

Street Address

Address

City   State

Date (MM-DD-YYYY)   Suppliers DEA Registration No.

To Be Filled in By **PURCHASER**

Line No.	No. of Packages	Size of Package	Name of Item
1			
2			
3			
4			
5			
6			
7			
8			
9			
10			

To Be Filled in By **SUPPLIER**

National Drug Code	Packages Shipped	Date Shipped

◄ **LAST LINE COMPLETED** *(MUST BE 10 OR LESS)*

Signature of **PURCHASER** or Attorney or Agent

Date Issued

Schedules

Registered As a

No. of This Order Form

DEA Registration No.

Name and Address of Registrant

Name_____ Date_____

DEA FORM 224

Sample Only

Form-224	**APPLICATION FOR REGISTRATION** Under the Controlled Substances Act	APPROVED OMB NO 1117-0014 FORM DEA-224 (10-06) Previous editions are obsolete

INSTRUCTIONS   Save time—apply on-line at *www.deadiversion.usdoj.gov*

1. To apply by mail complete this application. Keep a copy for your records.
2. Print clearly, using black or blue ink, or use a typewriter.
3. Mail this form to the address provided in Section 7 or use enclosed envelope.
4. Include the correct payment amount. FEE IS NON-REFUNDABLE.
5. If you have any questions call 800-882-9539 prior to submitting your application.

IMPORTANT: DO NOT SEND THIS APPLICATION AND APPLY ON-LINE.

DEA OFFICIAL USE:

Do you have other DEA registration numbers?
☐ NO   ☐ YES

MAIL-TO ADDRESS   Please print mailing address changes to the right of the address in this box.

FEE FOR THREE (3) YEARS IS $551
FEE IS NON-REFUNDABLE

SECTION 1   **APPLICANT IDENTIFICATION**   ☐ **Individual Registration**   ☐ **Business Registration**

Name 1   (Last Name of individual -OR- Business or Facility Name)

Name 2   (First Name and Middle Name of individual -OR- Continuation of business name)

Street Address Line 1 (If applying for fee exemption, this must be address of the fee exempt institution)

Address Line 2

City   State   Zip Code

Business Phone Number   Point of Contact

Business Fax Number   Email Address

DEBT COLLECTION INFORMATION
Mandatory pursuant to Debt Collection Improvements Act

Social Security Number (*if registration is for individual*)

Provide **SSN** or **TIN**. See additional information note #3 on page 4.

Tax Identification Number (*if registration is for business*)

FOR Practitioner or MLP ONLY:

Professional Degree: *select from list only*

Professional School:

Year of Graduation:

National Provider Identification:

Date of Birth (*MM-DD-YYYY*):

SECTION 2
BUSINESS ACTIVITY

Check one business activity box only

☐ Central Fill Pharmacy
☐ Retail Pharmacy
☐ Nursing Home
☐ Automated Dispensing System

☐ Practitioner (DDS, DMD, DO, DPM, DVM, MD or PHD)
☐ Practitioner Military (DDS, DMD, DO, DPM, DVM, MD or PHD)
☐ Mid-level Practitioner (MLP) (DOM, HMD, MP, ND, NP, OD, PA, or RPH)
☐ Euthanasia Technician

☐ Ambulance Service
☐ Animal Shelter
☐ Hospital/Clinic
☐ Teaching Institution

FOR Automated Dispensing System (ADS) ONLY:

DEA Registration # of Retail Pharmacy for this ADS

An ADS is automatically fee-exempt. Skip Section 6 and Section 7 on page 2. You must attach a notorized affidavit.

SECTION 3
DRUG SCHEDULES

Check all that apply

☐ Schedule II Narcotic
☐ Schedule II Non-Narcotic

☐ Schedule III Narcotic
☐ Schedule III Non-Narcotic

☐ Schedule IV
☐ Schedule V

(continued)

DEA FORM 224 *(concluded)*

Sample Only

SECTION 4	You MUST be currently authorized to prescribe, distribute, dispense, conduct research, or otherwise handle the controlled substances in the schedules for which you are applying under the laws of the **state** or jurisdiction in which you are operating or propose to operate.
STATE LICENSE(S)	

Be sure to include both state license numbers if applicable

State License Number (required) ☐☐☐☐☐☐☐☐☐☐☐☐☐☐☐☐☐☐

Expiration Date (required) ___/___/___ MM - DD - YYYY

What state was this license issued in? _____

State Controlled Substance License Number (if required) ☐☐☐☐☐☐☐☐☐☐☐☐☐☐☐☐☐☐

Expiration Date ___/___/___ MM - DD - YYYY

What state was this license issued in? _____

SECTION 5

LIABILITY

IMPORTANT

All questions in this section must be answered.

1. Has the applicant ever been **convicted of a crime** in connection with controlled substance(s) under state or federal law, or is any such action pending?   YES ☐ NO ☐

   Date(s) of incident MM-DD-YYYY: ☐☐–☐☐–☐☐☐☐

2. Has the applicant ever surrendered (for cause) or had a **federal** controlled substance registration revoked, suspended, restricted, or denied, or is any such action pending?   YES ☐ NO ☐

   Date(s) of incident MM-DD-YYYY: ☐☐–☐☐–☐☐☐☐

3. Has the applicant ever surrendered (for cause) or had a **state** professional license or controlled substance registration revoked, suspended, denied, restricted, or placed on probation, or is any such action pending?   YES ☐ NO ☐

   Date(s) of incident MM-DD-YYYY: ☐☐–☐☐–☐☐☐☐

4. If the applicant is a **corporation** (other than a corporation whose stock is owned and traded by the public), association, partnership, or pharmacy, has any officer, partner, stockholder, or proprietor been **convicted of a crime** in connection with controlled substance(s) under state or federal law, or ever surrendered, for cause, or had a **federal** controlled substance registration revoked, suspended, restricted, denied, or ever had a **state** professional license or controlled substance registration revoked, suspended, denied, restricted or placed on probation, or is any such action pending?   YES ☐ NO ☐

   Date(s) of incident MM-DD-YYYY: ☐☐–☐☐–☐☐☐☐   *Note: If question 4 does not apply to you, be sure to mark 'NO'. It will slow down processing of your application if you leave it blank.*

EXPLANATION OF "YES" ANSWERS

Applicants who have answered "YES" to any of the four questions above **must provide a statement to explain each "YES" answer.**

Use this space or attach a separate sheet and return with application

Liability question # _____   Location(s) of incident: _____

Nature of incident:

Disposition of incident:

SECTION 6   EXEMPTION FROM APPLICATION FEE

☐ Check this box if the applicant is a federal, state, or local government official or institution. Does not apply to contractor-operated institutions.

Business or Facility Name of Fee Exempt Institution. **Be sure to enter the address of this exempt institution in Section 1.**

☐☐☐☐☐☐☐☐☐☐☐☐☐☐☐☐☐☐☐☐☐☐☐☐☐☐☐☐☐☐☐☐☐☐☐☐☐☐

FEE EXEMPT CERTIFIER

Provide the name and phone number of the certifying official

The undersigned hereby certifies that the applicant named hereon is a federal, state or local government official or institution, and is exempt from payment of the application fee.

Signature of certifying official (other than applicant) _____   Date _____

Print or type name and title of certifying official _____   Telephone No. (required for verification) _____

SECTION 7

METHOD OF PAYMENT

Check one form of payment only

Sign if paying by credit card

☐ Check   Make check payable to: **Drug Enforcement Administration** See page 4 of instructions for important information.

☐ American Express ☐ Discover ☐ Master Card ☐ Visa

Credit Card Number ☐☐☐☐☐☐☐☐☐☐☐☐☐☐☐☐   Expiration Date ☐☐–☐☐

Signature of Card Holder _____

Printed Name of Card Holder _____

Mail this form with payment to:

U.S. Department of Justice
Drug Enforcement Administration
P.O. Box 28083
Washington, DC 20038-8083

FEE IS NON-REFUNDABLE

SECTION 8

APPLICANTS SIGNATURE

Sign in ink

I certify that the foregoing information furnished on this application is true and correct.

Signature of applicant (sign in ink) _____   Date _____

Print or type name and title of applicant _____

WARNING: Section 843(a)(4)(A) of Title 21, United States Code states that any person who knowingly or intentionally furnishes false or fraudulent information in this application is subject to imprisonment for not more than four years, a fine of not more than $30,000.00 or both.

Name_____ Date_____

DEA FORM 224A

Sample Only
Submitted through Internet only

Form-224a	RENEWAL APPLICATION FOR REGISTRATION Under the Controlled Substances Act	APPROVED OMB NO 1117-0014 FORM DEA-224a (1-05)

INSTRUCTIONS	1 To renew by mail complete this application. Keep a copy for your records. 2 Print clearly, using black or blue ink, or use a typewriter. 3 Section 5 should be completed only if your information has changed. 4 Mail this form to the address provided in section 6 or use enclosed envelope. 5 Include the correct payment amount. FEE IS NON_REFUNDABLE. 6 If you have any questions call 800-882-9359 prior to submitting your application. 7 Save time-renew online at WWW.deadiversion.usdoj-gov. IMPORTANT: DO NOT SEND THIS APPLICATION AND RENEW ONLINE.	REGISTRATION INFORMATION: DEA# REGISTRATION EXPIRES FEE IS NON-REFUNDABLE

SECTION 1

DRUG SCHEDULES
Check all that apply.

☐ Schedule II Narcotic   ☐ Schedule III Narcotic   ☐ Schedule IV
☐ Schedule II Non-Narcotic ☐ Schedule III Non-Narcotic ☐ Schedule V

SECTION 2   ☐ Check this box if you need official order forms-for the purchase of schedule II narcotic/schedule II non-narcotic controlled substances.

SECTION 3

STATE LICENSE(S)

Be sure to Include both state license numbers if applicable

A. Are you currently authorized to prescribe, distribute, dispense, conduct research, or otherwise handle the controlled substances in the schedules for which you are applying under the laws of the state or jurisdiction in which you are operating or purpose to operate?

YES ☐   NO ☐   [   ]   State License Number

YES ☐   NO ☐   [   ]   State Controlled Substance License Number (if required)

LIABILITY:

IMPORTANT:
If you answered yes to these questions on previous application, you must continue to answer yes and provide a statement of explanation.

All questions in this section must be answered.

	YES	NO
B. Has the applicant ever been convicted of a crime in connection with controlled substances under state or federal law?	☐	☐
C. Has the applicant ever surrendered (for cause) or had a federal controlled substance registration revoked, suspended, restricted, or denied?	☐	☐
D. Has the applicant ever surrendered (for cause) or had a state professional license or controlled substance registration revoked, suspended, denied, restricted, or placed on probation? Is any such action pending?	☐	☐
E. If the applicant is a corporation(other than a corporation whose stock is owned and traded by the public), association, partnership, or pharmacy, has any officer, partner, stockholder, or proprietor been convicted of a crime in connection with controlled substances under state or federal law, or ever surrendered, for cause, or had a federal controlled substance registration revoked, suspended, restricted, denied, or ever had a state professional license or controlled substance registration revoked, suspended, denied, restricted or placed on probation?	☐	☐

SECTION 4

EXPLANATION OF "YES" ANSWERS

Applicants who have answered "YES" to questions B C D or E above must provide a statement to explain such answers

Use this space or attach a separate sheet and return with application

Date(s) of incident: _____   Location(s) of incident: _____

Nature of incident:

Result of incident:

RENEWAL- Page 1

(continued)

DEA Form 224A **915**

DEA FORM 224A *(concluded)*

Sample Only
Submitted through Internet only

SECTION 5

CHANGES TO
APPLICANT
IDENTIFICATION

Last Name (if registration is for individual)-OR-Business Name (if registration is for business)

First Name and Middle Initial

DEBT COLLECTION
INFORMATION

Mandatory pursuant
to Debt Collection
Improvements ACT.

Tax Identification Number (if registration is for business)

Social Security Number (if registration is for individual)

Provide SSN or TIN.
See note #3 on
bottom of page 2

Address Line 1 (street address)

IMPORTANT:

Leave this section
blank unless the
registration
information on
front page
is incorrect.

Address Line 2

City   State   Zip Code

Business Phone Number   Business Fax Number

SECTION 6

METHOD OF
PAYMENT

Check one form of
payment only

☐ Check   Make check payable to: Drug Enforcement Administration
See page 4 of instructions for important information.

☐ American Express   ☐ Discover   ☐ Master Card   ☐ Visa

Credit Card Number   Expiration Date

Sign if paying by
credit card

Signature of Card Holder

Printed Name of Card Holder

Mail this form with payment to:

U.S. Department of Justice
Drug Enforcement Administration
P.O. Box 105616
Atlanta, GA 30348-5616

FEE IS NON-REFUNDABLE

SECTION 7

CERTIFICATION
OF EXEMPTION
from application fee

Provide the name and
phone number of the
certifying official

☐ Check this box if the applicant is a federal, state, or local government operated hospital, institution or official.
Be sure to enter the name and address of the exempt institution on address lines 1 and 2 in Section 5, if it is not already on your
current registration certificate.

The undersigned hereby certifies that the applicant named hereon is a federal, state or local government operated hospital, institution or official,
and is exempt from payment of the application fee.

Signature of certifying official (other than applicant)

Date

Print or type name and title of certifying official

Telephone No. (required for verification)

SECTION 8

APPLICANT'S
SIGNATURE

Sign in ink

I certify that the foregoing information furnished on this application is true and correct.

Signature of applicant

Date

Print or type name and title of applicant

WARNING: Section 843(a)(4)(A) of Title 21, United States Code states that any person who knowingly or intentionally furnishes false or
fraudulent information in the application is subject to imprisonment for not more than four years, a fine of not more than $30,000, or both.

---

1. No registration will be issued unless a completed application form has been received (21 CFR 1301.13).
2. In accordance with the Paperwork Reduction Act of 1995, no person is required to respond to a collection of information unless it displays a valid OMB control number. The
valid OMB control number for this collection is 1117-0014. Public reporting burden for this collection of information is estimated to average 12 minutes per response, including
the time for reviewing instructions, searching existing data sources, gathering and maintaining the data needed, and completing and reviewing the collection of information.
3. The Debt Collection Improvements Act of 1996 (PL 104-134) requires that you furnish your Taxpayer Identifying Number and/or Social Security Number on this application
This number is required for debt collection procedures should your fee become uncollectable.
4. PRIVACY ACT INFORMATION

    AUTHORITY: Section 302 and 303 of the Controlled Substances Act of 1970 (PL 91-513) and Debt Collection Improvements Act of 1996 (PL 104-134) for
taxpayer identifying number and/or social security number).
    PURPOSE: To obtain information required to register applicants pursuant to the Controlled Substances Act of 1970.
    ROUTINE USES: The Controlled Substances Act Registration Records produces special reports as required for statistical analytical purposes. Disclosures of
information from this system are made to the following categories of users for the purposes stated:
      A. Other federal law enforcement and regulatory agencies for law enforcement and regulatory purposes.
      B. State and local law enforcement and regulatory agencies for law enforcement and regulatory purposes.
      C. Persons registered under the Controlled Substances Act (PL 91-513) for the purpose of verifying the registration of customers.
    EFFECT: Failure to complete form will preclude processing of the application.

RENEWAL-Page 2

EYEWASH SAFETY INSPECTION RECORD

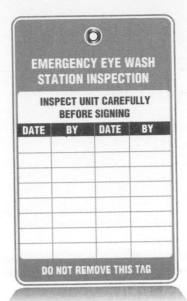

GROWTH CHART

**Birth to 36 months: Boys
Head circumference-for-age and
Weight-for-length percentiles**

NAME _____

RECORD # _____

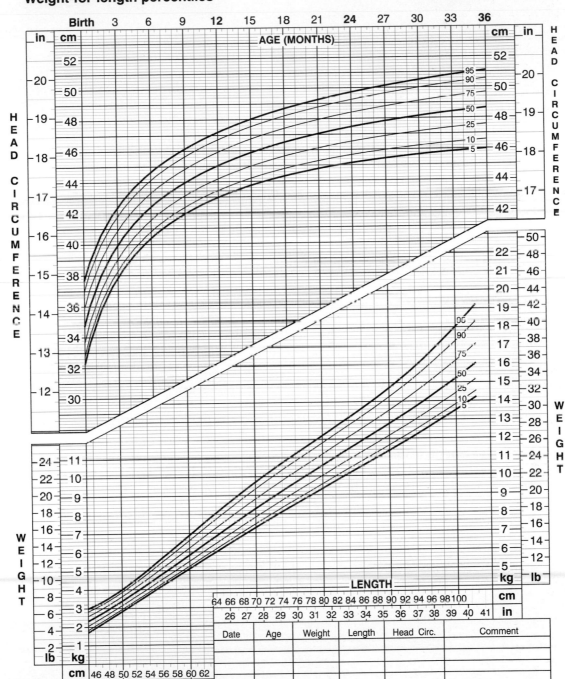

Published May 30, 2000 (modified 10/16/00).
SOURCE: Developed by the National Center for Health Statistics in collaboration with
the National Center for Chronic Disease Prevention and Health Promotion (2000).
http://www.cdc.gov/growthcharts

CDC
SAFER · HEALTHIER · PEOPLE™

This document will be used multiple times. Make photocopies before writing on this document, or download it from the
Online Learning Center at www.mhhe.com/BoothMA5e for any future uses.

Name_____ Date_____

GROWTH CHART

Birth to 36 months: Boys
Length-for-age and Weight-for-age percentiles

NAME _____

RECORD # _____

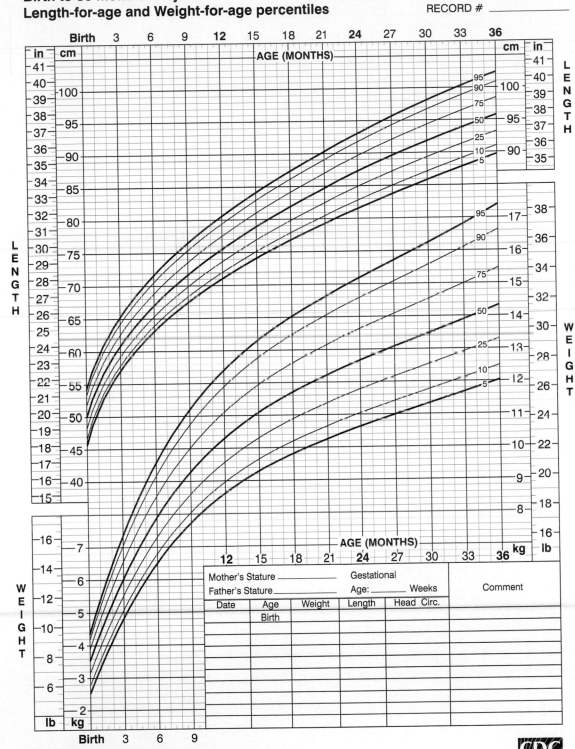

Published May 30, 2000 (modified 4/20/01).
SOURCE: Developed by the National Center for Health Statistics in collaboration with
the National Center for Chronic Disease Prevention and Health Promotion (2000).
http://www.cdc.gov/growthcharts

CDC

SAFER · HEALTHIER · PEOPLE™

This document will be used multiple times. Make photocopies before writing on this document, or download it from the Online Learning Center at www.mhhe.com/BoothMA5e for any future uses.

Name_____   Date_____

GROWTH CHART

**Birth to 36 months: Girls
Head circumference-for-age and
Weight-for-length percentiles**

NAME _____

RECORD # _____

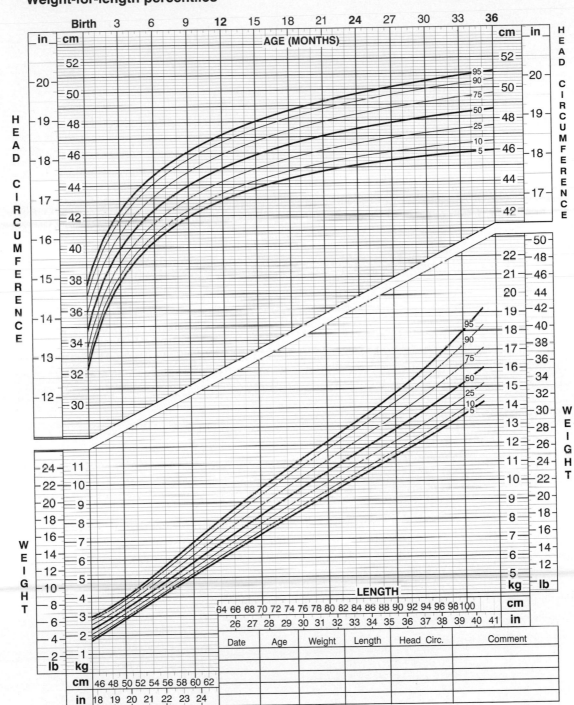

Published May 30, 2000 (modified 10/16/00).
SOURCE: Developed by the National Center for Health Statistics in collaboration with
the National Center for Chronic Disease Prevention and Health Promotion (2000).
http://www.cdc.gov/growthcharts

CDC
SAFER·HEALTHIER·PEOPLE™

Copyright © 2014 by The McGraw-Hill Companies, Inc.

This document will be used multiple times. Make photocopies before writing on this document, or download it from the
Online Learning Center at www.mhhe.com/BoothMA5e for any future uses.

Name_____ Date_____

GROWTH CHART

Birth to 36 months: Girls
Length-for-age and Weight-for-age percentiles

NAME _____

RECORD # _____

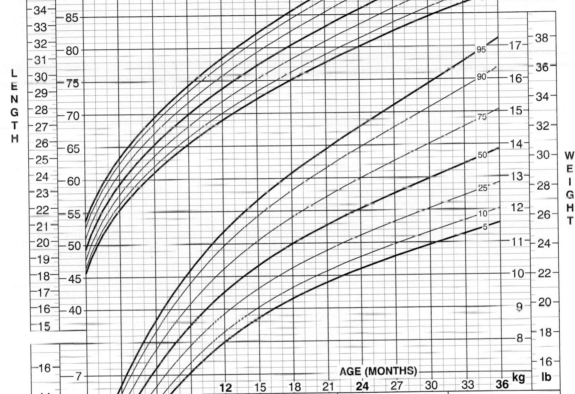

Published May 30, 2000 (modified 4/20/01).
SOURCE: Developed by the National Center for Health Statistics in collaboration with
the National Center for Chronic Disease Prevention and Health Promotion (2000).
http://www.cdc.gov/growthcharts

CDC
SAFER • HEALTHIER • PEOPLE™

This document will be used multiple times. Make photocopies before writing on this document, or download it from the
Online Learning Center at www.mhhe.com/BoothMA5e for any future uses.

GROWTH CHART

2 to 20 years: Boys
Stature-for-age and Weight-for-age percentiles

NAME _____

RECORD # _____

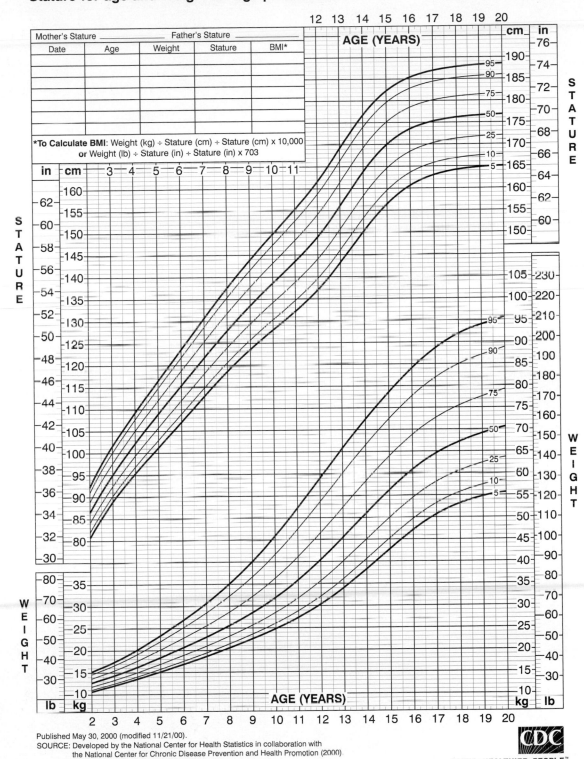

Published May 30, 2000 (modified 11/21/00).
SOURCE: Developed by the National Center for Health Statistics in collaboration with
the National Center for Chronic Disease Prevention and Health Promotion (2000).
http://www.cdc.gov/growthcharts

CDC
SAFER·HEALTHIER·PEOPLE™

This document will be used multiple times. Make photocopies before writing on this document, or download it from the Online Learning Center at www.mhhe.com/BoothMA5e for any future uses.

GROWTH CHART

2 to 20 years: Boys
Body mass index-for-age percentiles

NAME _____

RECORD # _____

Date	Age	Weight	Stature	BMI*	Comments

*To Calculate BMI: Weight (kg) ÷ Stature (cm) ÷ Stature (cm) x 10,000
or Weight (lb) ÷ Stature (in) ÷ Stature (in) x 703

BMI

BMI

95

90

85

75

50

25

10

5

35
34
33
32
31
30
29
28
27
26
25
24
23
22
21
20
19
18
17
16
15
14
13
12

27
26
25
24
23
22
21
20
19
18
17
16
15
14
13
12

kg/m²   **AGE (YEARS)**   **kg/m²**

2   3   4   5   6   7   8   9   10   11   12   13   14   15   16   17   18   19   20

Published May 30, 2000 (modified 10/16/00).

SOURCE: Developed by the National Center for Health Statistics in collaboration with
the National Center for Chronic Disease Prevention and Health Promotion (2000).
http://www.cdc.gov/growthcharts

CDC
SAFER · HEALTHIER · PEOPLE™

This document will be used multiple times. Make photocopies before writing on this document, or download it from the Online Learning Center at www.mhhe.com/BoothMA5e for any future uses.

GROWTH CHART

Weight-for-stature percentiles: Boys

NAME _____

RECORD # _____

Date	Age	Weight	Stature	Comments

STATURE

kg	lb
cm	80	85	90	95	100	105	110	115	120
in	31	32	33	34	35	36	37	38	39	40	41	42	43	44	45	46	47

Published May 30, 2000 (modified 10/16/00).
SOURCE: Developed by the National Center for Health Statistics in collaboration with
the National Center for Chronic Disease Prevention and Health Promotion (2000).
http://www.cdc.gov/growthcharts

SAFER · HEALTHIER · PEOPLE™

This document will be used multiple times. Make photocopies before writing on this document, or download it from the Online Learning Center at www.mhhe.com/BoothMA5e for any future uses.

GROWTH CHART

2 to 20 years: Girls
Stature-for-age and Weight-for-age percentiles

NAME _____

RECORD # _____

Mother's Stature _____		Father's Stature _____		
Date	Age	Weight	Stature	BMI*

*To Calculate BMI: Weight (kg) ÷ Stature (cm) ÷ Stature (cm) x 10,000
or Weight (lb) ÷ Stature (in) ÷ Stature (in) x 703

AGE (YEARS)

12 13 14 15 16 17 18 19 20

Published May 30, 2000 (modified 11/21/00).
SOURCE: Developed by the National Center for Health Statistics in collaboration with
the National Center for Chronic Disease Prevention and Health Promotion (2000).
http://www.cdc.gov/growthcharts

CDC
SAFER · HEALTHIER · PEOPLE™

This document will be used multiple times. Make photocopies before writing on this document, or download it from the Online Learning Center at www.mhhe.com/BoothMA5e for any future uses.

Name_____ Date_____

GROWTH CHART

2 to 20 years: Girls
Body mass index-for-age percentiles

NAME _____

RECORD # _____

Date	Age	Weight	Stature	BMI*	Comments

*To Calculate BMI: Weight (kg) ÷ Stature (cm) ÷ Stature (cm) x 10,000
or Weight (lb) ÷ Stature (in) ÷ Stature (in) x 703

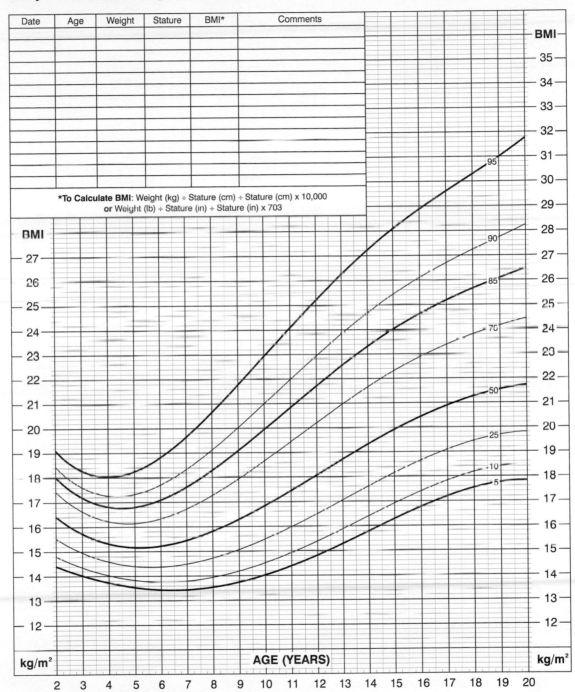

AGE (YEARS)

kg/m²

Published May 30, 2000 (modified 10/16/00).
SOURCE: Developed by the National Center for Health Statistics in collaboration with
the National Center for Chronic Disease Prevention and Health Promotion (2000).
http://www.cdc.gov/growthcharts

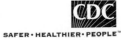

SAFER · HEALTHIER · PEOPLE™

This document will be used multiple times. Make photocopies before writing on this document, or download it from the Online Learning Center at www.mhhe.com/BoothMA5e for any future uses.

GROWTH CHART

NAME _____

Weight-for-stature percentiles: Girls

RECORD # _____

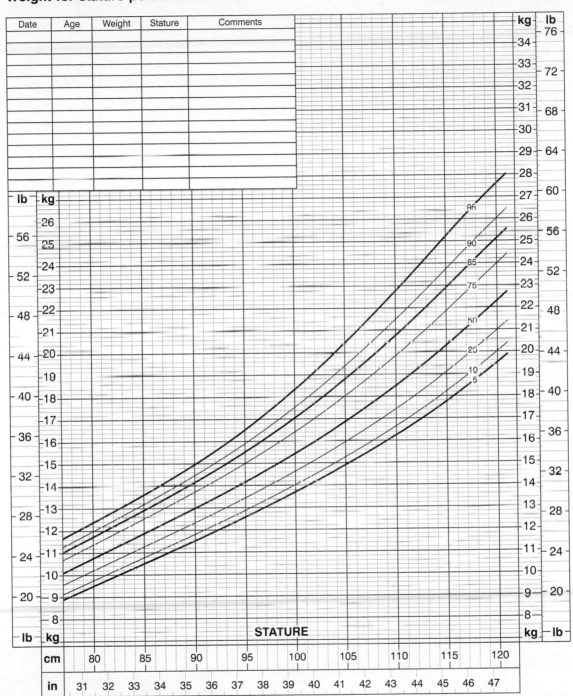

Date	Age	Weight	Stature	Comments

Published May 30, 2000 (modified 10/10/00).
SOURCE: Developed by the National Center for Health Statistics in collaboration with
the National Center for Chronic Disease Prevention and Health Promotion (2000).
http://www.cdc.gov/growthcharts

CDC
SAFER · HEALTHIER · PEOPLE™

This document will be used multiple times. Make photocopies before writing on this document, or download it from the Online Learning Center at www.mhhe.com/BoothMA5e for any future uses.

LABORATORY REPORT FORM

BWW

BWW Medical Associates, PC
305 Main Street, Port Snead YZ 12345-9876
Tel: 555-654-3210, Fax: 555-987-6543
Web: BWWAssociates.com

Paul F. Buckwalter, MD
Alexis N. Whalen, MD
Elizabeth H. Williams, MD

Patient Name_____ Medical Record#_____ Age_____ Sex_____

Address_____ Phone_____

Referring Physician_____

Laboratory Findings:

DATE	BLOOD TEST	PATIENT RESULT	NORMAL VALUE/RANGE

DATE	URINALYSIS	PATIENT RESULT	NORMAL VALUE/RANGE

Test completed by: _____   _____
                        (Print name)   (Signature)

This document will be used multiple times. Make photocopies before writing on this document, or download it from the Online Learning Center at www.mhhe.com/BoothMA5e for any future uses.

LABORATORY REQUISITION FORM

LAB USE ONLY		Laboratory Name & Address		Requesting Physician Information
Acct #				
DATE				Address
TIME				

Patient Information Patient Name (Last)	(First)	(MI)	Date of Birth / /	Phone Number
Address	City, State	Zip	Phone Number	
Patient I.D. Number	Responsible Party (Last) (First) (Phone)	Male		
		Female		
Social Security Number	Physician	Specimen Collection	Date Time	

Bill: Check One			
Our account Medicare Insurance Co./Patient			
Complete the Following Information for Billing a Patient and/or a Third Party Agency			
Policy Holder Name	Policy Holder Address:	Relation	
	Policy Holder Phone Number:	Self Spouse Child Other	
Insurance Co. Name	Address Insurance Co.	City , State, Zip	
Employer			
Policy	Group #		
	PATIENT or GUARDIAN SIGNATURE:	DATE:	

CHECK DESIRED TESTS   PLEASE PROVIDE ICD=9-CM#

√	ORGAN DISEASE PANELS, BLOOD	ICD-9	√	TEST, BLOOD	ICD-9	√	TEST, BLOOD	ICD-9	√	TEST, URINE	ICD-9
	ACUTE HEP. A,B,C			ESR			WBC with diff			U/A Routine	
	BASIC METABOLIC			EBV			PT				
	THYROID			FBS			PTT				
	ELECTROLYTES			Grp A β-hem strep			Bleeding time				
	HEPATIC FUNCTION			Hgb			PCO_2				
	LIPID PROFILE			Hct			PO_2				
	RENAL FUNCTION			HgbA1c			CO_2				
	TEST, BLOOD			HIV antibodies			HCO_3			**MICROBIOLOGY**	
	ACE			Insulin			Ca^{++}			AFB culture	
	ADH			Iron			Cl^-			C & S	
	ALT			Ketone bodies						Chlamydia screen	
	AFP			LD						Endocervical culture	
	Amylase			pH						GC screen	
	Acetone			Phenylalanine						Gram stain	
	AST			K^+ and Na^+			**TEST, URINE**			O & P	
	Bilirubin			Proteins, Albumin			Cys			Strep A culture	
	BUN			Proteins, Fibrinogen			CrCl			Throat culture	
	CEA			PSA			Glucose			Urine culture	
	Calcium, total			RBC			HCG			Viral culture	
	Carbon dioxide, total			Sickle cells			UBG			Wound culture	
	Cholesterol, total			TSH			UFC				
	Cholesterol, HDLs			T3			UK				
	Cholesterol, LDLs			T4			UNA				
	CK			Uric Acid			Uosm				
	CMV			WBC			UUN				

This document will be used multiple times. Make photocopies before writing on this document, or download it from the Online Learning Center at www.mhhe.com/BoothMA5e for any future uses.

Name_____ Date_____

MEDICAL VISIT FORM

Name _____ DOB _____ Date _____

ALLERGIES _____

Review of Systems

Systems	NL	Note	Systems	NL	Note
Constitutional			Musculoskeletal		
Eyes			Skin/breasts		
ENT/mouth			Neurologic		
Cardiovascular			Psychiatric		
Respiratory			Endocrine		
GI			Hem/lymph		
GU			Allergy/immun		

Current Medicines	Date	Current Diagnosis

Note

H: _____ W: _____ T: _____ P: _____ R: _____

B/P Sitting _____ or Standing _____ Supine _____

Last Tetantus _____

L.M.P. _____

O2 Sat: _____

Pain Scale: _____

Social Habits	Yes	No
Tobacco	__	__
Alcohol	__	__
Rec. Drugs	__	__

CC:

HPI:

MEDICATION FLOW SHEET

BWW

BWW Medical Associates, PC
305 Main Street, Port Snead YZ 12345-9876
Tel: 555-654-3210, Fax: 555-987-6543
Web: BWWAssociates.com

Paul F. Buckwalter, MD
Alexis N. Whalen, MD
Elizabeth H. Williams, MD

MEDICATION FLOW SHEET

Patient Name		Allergies		
DATE	**MEDICATION**	**REFILLS**		
Start — Stop	Dosage/Direction/Amount	Date/Amount/Initials		

NOMOGRAM

Weight

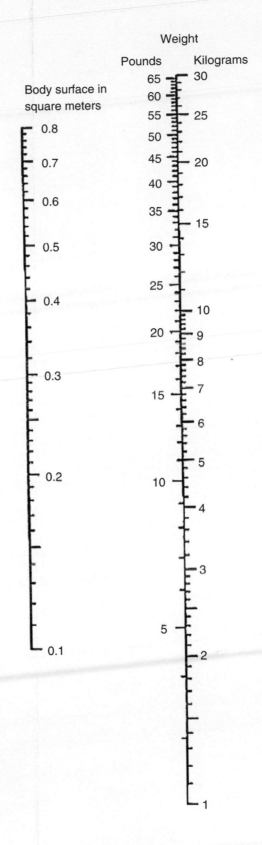

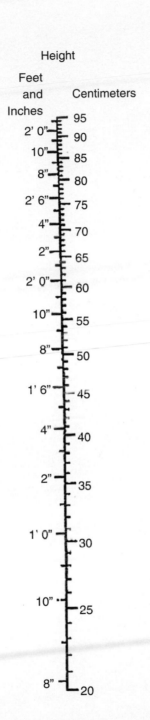

Name_____ Date_____

PATIENT MEDICAL HISTORY FORM

HEALTH HISTORY
(Confidential)

Name_____ Today's Date_____

Age_____ Birthdate_____ Date of last physical examination_____

What is your reason for visit?_____

SYMPTOMS Check (✓) symptoms you currently have or have had in the past year.

GENERAL	GASTROINTESTINAL	EYE, EAR, NOSE, THROAT	MEN only
☐ Chills	☐ Appetite poor	☐ Bleeding gums	☐ Breast lump
☐ Depression	☐ Bloating	☐ Blurred vision	☐ Erection difficulties
☐ Dizziness	☐ Bowel changes	☐ Crossed eyes	☐ Lump in testicles
☐ Fainting	☐ Constipation	☐ Difficulty swallowing	☐ Penis discharge
☐ Fever	☐ Diarrhea	☐ Double vision	☐ Sore on penis
☐ Forgetfulness	☐ Excessive hunger	☐ Earache	☐ Other
☐ Headache	☐ Excessive thirst	☐ Ear discharge	**WOMEN only**
☐ Loss of sleep	☐ Gas	☐ Hay fever	☐ Abnormal Pap smear
☐ Loss of weight	☐ Hemorrhoids	☐ Hoarseness	☐ Bleeding between periods
☐ Nervousness	☐ Indigestion	☐ Loss of hearing	☐ Breast lump
☐ Numbness	☐ Nausea	☐ Nosebleeds	☐ Extreme menstrual pain
☐ Sweats	☐ Rectal bleeding	☐ Persistent cough	☐ Hot flashes
MUSCLE/JOINT/BONE	☐ Stomach pain	☐ Ringing in ears	☐ Nipple discharge
Pain, weakness, numbness in:	☐ Vomiting	☐ Sinus problems	☐ Painful intercourse
☐ Arms ☐ Hips	☐ Vomiting blood	☐ Vision – Flashes	☐ Vaginal discharge
☐ Back ☐ Legs	**CARDIOVASCULAR**	☐ Vision – Halos	☐ Other
☐ Feet ☐ Neck	☐ Chest pain	**SKIN**	Date of last
☐ Hands ☐ Shoulders	☐ High blood pressure	☐ Bruise easily	menstrual period_____
GENITO-URINARY	☐ Irregular heart beat	☐ Hives	Date of last
☐ Blood in urine	☐ Low blood pressure	☐ Itching	Pap smear_____
☐ Frequent urination	☐ Poor circulation	☐ Change in moles	Have you had
☐ Lack of bladder control	☐ Rapid heart beat	☐ Rash	a mammogram?_____
☐ Painful urination	☐ Swelling of ankles	☐ Scars	Are you pregnant?_____
	☐ Varicose veins	☐ Sore that won't heal	Number of children_____

CONDITIONS Check (✓) conditions you have or have had in the past.

☐ AIDS	☐ Chemical Dependency	☐ High Cholesterol	☐ Prostate Problem
☐ Alcoholism	☐ Chicken Pox	☐ HIV Positive	☐ Psychiatric Care
☐ Anemia	☐ Diabetes	☐ Kidney Disease	☐ Rheumatic Fever
☐ Anorexia	☐ Emphysema	☐ Liver Disease	☐ Scarlet Fever
☐ Appendicitis	☐ Epilepsy	☐ Measles	☐ Stroke
☐ Arthritis	☐ Glaucoma	☐ Migraine Headaches	☐ Suicide Attempt
☐ Asthma	☐ Goiter	☐ Miscarriage	☐ Thyroid Problems
☐ Bleeding Disorders	☐ Gonorrhea	☐ Mononucleosis	☐ Tonsillitis
☐ Breast Lump	☐ Gout	☐ Multiple Sclerosis	☐ Tuberculosis
☐ Bronchitis	☐ Heart Disease	☐ Mumps	☐ Typhoid Fever
☐ Bulimia	☐ Hepatitis	☐ Pacemaker	☐ Ulcers
☐ Cancer	☐ Hernia	☐ Pneumonia	☐ Vaginal Infections
☐ Cataracts	☐ Herpes	☐ Polio	☐ Venereal Disease

MEDICATIONS List medications you are currently taking	**ALLERGIES** To medications or substances
Pharmacy Name_____ Phone_____	

(continued)

This document will be used multiple times. Make photocopies before writing on this document, or download it from the Online Learning Center at www.mhhe.com/BoothMA5e for any future uses.

Name_____ Date_____

PATIENT MEDICAL HISTORY FORM *(concluded)*

(All information is strictly confidential)

FAMILY HISTORY Fill in health information about your family.

Relation	Age	State of Health	Age at Death	Cause of Death	Check (✓) if your blood relatives had any of the following: Disease	Relationship to you
Father					Arthritis, Gout	
Mother					Asthma, Hay Fever	
Brothers					Cancer	
					Chemical Dependency	
					Diabetes	
					Heart Disease, Strokes	
Sisters					High Blood Pressure	
					Kidney Disease	
					Tuberculosis	
					Other	

HOSPITALIZATIONS

Year	Hospital	Reason for Hospitalization and Outcome

PREGNANCY HISTORY

Year of Birth	Sex of Birth	Complications if any

HEALTH HABITS Check (✓) which substances you use and describe how much you use.

Caffeine	
Tobacco	
Drugs	
Other	

Have you ever had a blood transfusion? ☐ Yes ☐ No
If yes, please give approximate dates._____

SERIOUS ILLNESS/INJURIES	DATE	OUTCOME

OCCUPATIONAL CONCERNS
Check (✓) if your work exposes you to the following:

Stress	
Hazardous Substances	
Heavy Lifting	
Other	

Your occupation:

I certify that the above information is correct to the best of my knowledge. I will not hold my doctor or any members of his/her staff responsible for any errors or omissions that I may have made in the completion of this form.

_____   _____
Signature   Date

_____   _____
Reviewed By   Date

Copyright © 2014 by The McGraw-Hill Companies, Inc.

This document will be used multiple times. Make photocopies before writing on this document, or download it from the Online Learning Center at www.mhhe.com/BoothMA5e for any future uses.

PATIENT PHYSICAL EXAMINATION FORM

BWW

BWW Medical Associates, PC
305 Main Street, Port Snead YZ 12345-9876
Tel: 555-654-3210, Fax: 555-987-6543
Web: BWWAssociates.com

Paul F. Buckwalter, MD
Alexis N. Whalen, MD
Elizabeth H. Williams, MD

Review of Systems and Physical Examination
ROS

HEENT:_____

CV_____

Resp_____

GI_____

GU_____

MS_____

Integ_____

Neuro_____

Psych_____

Endo_____

Allergic/Immuno_____

Physical Examination

T_____ P_____ BP_____ R_____ HT_____ WT_____

Appearance_____ Skin_____ Mucus membrane_____

Eyes_____ Vision_____ Pupils_____ Fundus_____

Ears_____ Nose_____ Throat_____

Chest_____ Breasts_____

Heart_____

Lungs_____

Abdomen_____

Genitalia_____

Rectum_____

Pelvic_____

Extremities_____ Pulses_____

Lymph nodes_____ Neck_____ Axilla_____ Inguinal_____ Abd_____

Neuro_____

This document will be used multiple times. Make photocopies before writing on this document, or download it from the Online Learning Center at www.mhhe.com/BoothMA5e for any future uses.

PRESCRIPTION

BWW

Medical Associates, PC
305 Main Street, Port Snead YZ 12345-9876
Tel: 555-654-3210, Fax: 555-987-6543
Web: BWWAssociates.com

Paul F. Buckwalter, MD
Lic: J87877 DEA AJ3434343

Pt: Valarie Ramirez
198 Elm St
Sherman, TX 77521

11/27/XX

DOB: 08/04/19XX

R_X Allegra 180 mg
    disp: 30 thirty
  sig: i po q am
  Refill: 6

Paul F. Buckwalter, MD
*****Electronic Signature Verified*****

Paul F. Buckwalter, MD

A generically equivalent drug product may be dispensed unless the
practitioner hand writes the words 'BRAND NECESSARY' or 'BRAND
MEDICALLY NECESSARY' on the prescription face

PRIVACY VIOLATION COMPLAINT FORM

BWW

BWW Medical Associates, PC
305 Main Street, Port Snead YZ 12345-9876
Tel: 555-654-3210, Fax: 555-987-6543
Web: BWWAssociates.com

Paul F. Buckwalter, MD
Alexis N. Whalen, MD
Elizabeth H. Williams, MD

Privacy Violation Complaint

As per our Privacy Policies and Procedures, we are providing this form for individuals who feel they have a complaint regarding how their protected health information was handled by our office. You have the right to make a complaint and we may take no retaliatory actions against you because of it. We will respond to this complaint within 30 days of its receipt.

Patient Name: _____

Address: _____

DOB: _____ Date of Complaint: _____

Phone: Home _____ Cell _____ Work _____

Best time to reach you: _____

Reason for the complaint (Please be as specific as possible, attaching additional documentation as necessary): _____

_____

_____

_____

_____

_____

_____   _____
Signature   Date

Office Use Only

Received by: _____ Date _____

Follow-up Started on (date): _____

PROGRESS NOTE

BWW

BWW Medical Associates, PC
305 Main Street, Port Snead YZ 12345-9876
Tel: 555-654-3210, Fax: 555-987-6543
Web: BWWAssociates.com

Paul F. Buckwalter, MD
Alexis N. Whalen, MD
Elizabeth H. Williams, MD

PROGRESS NOTES

Name _____ Chart #_____

DATE	

This document will be used multiple times. Make photocopies before writing on this document, or download it from the Online Learning Center at www.mhhe.com/BoothMA5e for any future uses.

Name_____ Date_____

QUALITY CONTROL LOG

Quality Control Daily Log								
Name of Unit	Glucose Control Solution	Strip Lot No./ Exp. Date	Low Control Value 35–65 mg/dL	High Control Value 175–235 mg/dL	Analyzed By	Date	Remedial Action Taken If Control Values Abnormal	Retest After Remedial Action Taken

This document will be used multiple times. Make photocopies before writing on this document, or download it from the Online Learning Center at www.mhhe.com/BoothMA5e for any future uses.

Name_____ Date_____

RECEIPT OF PRIVACY PRACTICES

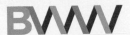

BWW Medical Associates, PC
305 Main Street, Port Snead YZ 12345-9876
Tel: 555-654-3210, Fax: 555-987-6543
Web: BWWAssociates.com

Paul F. Buckwalter, MD
Alexis N. Whalen, MD
Elizabeth H. Williams, MD

Notice of Privacy Practices

I understand that BWW Medical Associates, PC creates and maintains medical records describing my health history, symptoms, examinations, test results, diagnoses, treatments, and plans for my future care and/or treatment. I further understand that this information may be used for any of the following:

1. Plan and document my care and treatment
2. Communicate with health professionals involved in my care and treatment
3. Verify insurance coverage for planned procedures and/or treatments for the applicable diagnoses
4. Application of any medical or surgical procedures and diagnoses (codes) to my medical insurance claim forms as application for payment of services rendered
5. Assessment of quality of care and utilization review of the health care professionals providing my care

Additionally, it has been explained to me that:

1. A complete description of the use and disclosure of this information is included in the *Notice of Information of Privacy Practices* which has been provided to me
2. I have had a right to review this information prior to signing this consent
3. BWW Medical Associates, PC has the right to change this notice and their practices
4. Any revision of this notice will be mailed to me at the address I provided to them prior to its implementation
5. I may object to the use of my health information for specific purposes
6. I may request restrictions as to the manner my information may be used or disclosed in order to carry out treatment, payment, or health information
7. I understand that it is not required that my requested restrictions be honored
8. I may revoke this consent in writing, except for those disclosures which may have taken place prior to the receipt of my revocation

At the time of the document signing, I request the following restrictions to disclosure or use of my health information: _____

_____

_____   _____
Printed Name of Patient or Legal Guardian   Signature of Parent or Legal Guardian

_____   _____
Printed Name of Witness/Title   Signature of Witness/Title

Date: _____

REPORTABLE DISEASE REPORTING FORM

DEPARTMENT OF PUBLIC HEALTH
Division of Disease Surveillance

ENTERIC ILLNESS CASE INVESTIGATION
(Please check appropriate illness)

_____Shigellosis   _____Giardiasis
_____Non-typhoid Salmonellosis   _____Amebiasis
_____Campylobacter enteritis

CASE INFORMATION

Name: _____ Age or Birthdate: _____ Sex: _____ Race: _____

Address: _____ Phone: _____
              (Street)   (City)   (County)   (Zip)

Occupation:_____ *High Risk: Y   N
              (What)   (Where)
          (If infant or student list school, nursery or day care center)

Attending   Address or   Was the patient
Physician: _____   Phone:_____   hospitalized: Y   N

Hospital: _____ Dates: _____
                                                   (Admission)   (Discharge)

Onset: _____ Date recovered: _____ Symptom Summary: _____

_____

Suspected Causative Agent: _____
(include species or serotype if known)

HOUSEHOLD CONTACTS INFORMATION

Name	Age	Family Relationship	Occupation	*High Risk Y N	Provide date of onset for all household members with concurrent similar illness
1)					
2)					
3)					
4)					
5)					
6)					
7)					
8)					
9)					
10)					

*"High Risk" = occupation as food handler, direct patient care worker, day care center worker or person attending day care or who is institutionalized. Stool specimens should be obtained on "high risk" cases and "high risk" household contacts as appropriate for the illness. Results may be recorded in Laboratory Information Section of this form (see over).

Name of the person who completed this form:_____ County:_____

Information obtained from: _____ Date:_____

Telephone Interview: _____ Home Visit: _____ Outbreak Investigation: _____

C-30 Rev. 10/83   AUTH: Act 368, P.A. 1978

(continued)

REPORTABLE DISEASE REPORTING FORM (concluded)

NON-HOUSEHOLD CONTACTS WITH A CONCURRENT SIMILAR ILLNESS

Name	Approximate date of onset of symptoms	Address and/or Phone	Relationship to case (Nature of contact)
1)			
2)			
3)			
4)			
5)			

ADDITIONAL EXPOSURES OR COMMENTS

Home Sewage System: Municipal   Septic Tank   Other_____

Home drinking Water Type: Municipal   Private Well   Other_____

As appropriate for the illness, ask about meals eaten away from home, stores where groceries bought, brand of poultry, meat, dairy products consumed, overnight travel, recent foreign travel, group functions, exposure to raw milk, untreated water, animals, etc. within one incubation period before onset.

(shigellosis to 7 days, salmonellosis - up to 3 days, Campylobacter enteritis - up to 10 days)

Be specific, provide place name(s) and date(s).

FOLLOW-UP FECAL CULTURE RESULTS FOR "HIGH RISK" CASE AND/OR CONTACTS.

Name or Initials	Date(s) Obtained and Findings
1)	
2)	
3)	
4)	
5)	

ARIZONA DEPARTMENT OF HEALTH SERVICES COMMUNICABLE DISEASE REPORT Important Instructions on Reverse Side PLEASE PRINT OR TYPE	County/IHS ID Number/Chapter	State ID Number	
PATIENT'S NAME (Last) (First)	DATE OF BIRTH	SEX ☐ Male ☐ Female	ETHNICITY ☐ Hispanic ☐ Non-Hispanic
STREET ADDRESS	CENSUS TRACT	CITY	RACE ☐ White ☐ Am. Indian ☐ Asian ☐ Black ☐ Other ☐ Unknown
COUNTY STATE	ZIP CODE	PHONE NO.	
DIAGNOSIS OR SUSPECT REPORTABLE CONDITION			COUNTY USE ONLY:
DATE ONSET DATE OF DIAGNOSIS	LAB RESULTS		LAB CONFIRMATION DATE:_____ ☐ Negative ☐ Positive ☐ Not Done
PATIENT OCCUPATION OR SCHOOL			☐ Unknown
PHYSICIAN OR OTHER REPORTING SOURCE PHONE NUMBER			COUNTY USE ONLY: ☐ Confirmed case ☐ Probable case
STREET ADDRESS	CITY	STATE ZIP CODE	☐ Outbreak Associated ☐ Ruled Out

Original and 1st copy to County Health Department   ☐ CHECK IF ADDITIONAL FORMS ARE NEEDED (Quantity)_____

SELF-EVALUATION OF PROFESSIONAL BEHAVIORS

Behavior	Example(s)	Rate Yourself (5 = Best)					Improvements Needed
		1	2	3	4	5	
Integrity	Consistently honest; able to be trusted with the property of others; can be trusted with confidential information; completes tasks accurately.						
Appearance	Clothing and uniform appropriate for circumstance; neat, clean, and well-kept appearance; good personal hygiene and grooming.						
Teamwork	Places the success of the team above self-interest; does not undermine the team; helps and supports other team members; shows respect to all team members; remains flexible and open to change; communicates with others to help resolve problems.						
Self-confidence	Demonstrates the ability to trust personal judgment; demonstrates an awareness of strengths and limitations; exercises good personal judgment.						
Communication	Speaks clearly; writes legibly, listens actively; adjusts communication strategies to various situations.						
Commitment to diversity	Consistently demonstrates respect for varied cultural backgrounds, ethnicities, religions, sexual orientations, social classes, abilities, political beliefs, and disabilities.						
Punctuality and attendance	Arrives at class and work on the appointed day and time.						
Acceptance of criticism	Listens when constructive criticism is given; does not become defensive with criticism; appreciates constructive criticism and incorporates suggestions into behavior as appropriate.						
Organization	Coordinates more than one task at a time; keeps work area neat and orderly; anticipates future work; works efficiently and systematically.						
Knowledge and comprehension	Learns new things easily; retains new information; associates theory with practice.						

SURGICAL GUIDELINES (SAMPLE)

BWW

BWW Medical Associates, PC
305 Main Street, Port Snead YZ 12345-9876
Tel: 555-654-3210, Fax: 555-987-6543
Web: BWWAssociates.com

Paul F. Buckwalter, MD
Alexis N. Whalen, MD
Elizabeth H. Williams, MD

Pre-Operative Instructions for Surgery
Use the following guidelines to prepare for your upcoming surgery.

Medications:
1. If you take anticoagulants such as aspirin, warfarin, Coumadin, Plavix, Heparin, Ticlid, or Lovenox, you may need to stop taking the medication before the surgery.
2. STOP all herbal medications, vitamin E, diet pills, multivitamins, and NSAIDS such as ibuprofen, Advil, Nuprin, Aleve, Naprosyn, or Naproxen 7 to 10 days prior to surgery.
3. STOP all cholesterol lowering medications, such as Lipitor, Zocor, or Pravachol, 48 HOURS PRIOR to surgery.
4. DO NOT TAKE ANY diuretics or water pills the morning of surgery.
5. DO NOT TAKE these medications the morning of surgery: BENAZEPRIL, CAPTOPRIL, ALAPRIL, QUINAPRIL.
6. DO TAKE any HEART MEDICATIONS or BLOOD PRESSURE MEDICATIONS the morning of surgery with a sip of water, unless otherwise indicated.
7. You MAY USE PRESCRIBED INHALERS AND you MUST BRING THEM WITH YOU the day of surgery.
8. If you are a diabetic, DO NOT TAKE ANY DIABETIC PILLS OR INSULIN the morning of surgery. Your blood sugar will be checked at the hospital prior to surgery and will be taken care of as needed.

Skin Preparation:
BEFORE surgery, your body must be thoroughly cleaned with a special soap to decrease the amount of germs on the skin. Dial antibacterial soap may be used for this purpose. Using this soap will help reduce the chance of getting a wound infection after surgery.

Follow these instructions for proper skin preparation:
DO NOT shave the day of surgery. Shaving can cause small abrasions or nicks in the skin, which allow germs to enter. If you want to shave, it must be done the night before surgery.

DO NOT use any creams, lotions, powders, or underarm deodorant in the area where your surgery will take place. These items interfere with the solution used to prepare your skin in the operating room.

The evening before surgery:
Take a shower and wash your entire body with antibacterial soap. Work the soap up into lather. Wash your body, especially the surgical area, with a clean, fresh washcloth. Rinse thoroughly because soap can leave a film, which may interfere with the antiseptics used to clean the skin in the operating room. Dry your body with a clean, fresh towel. Wear clean, fresh pajamas to bed.

(continued)

SURGICAL GUIDELINES (SAMPLE) *(concluded)*

BWW

BWW Medical Associates, PC
305 Main Street, Port Snead YZ 12345-9876
Tel: 555-654-3210, Fax: 555-987-6543
Web: BWWAssociates.com

Paul F. Buckwalter, MD
Alexis N. Whalen, MD
Elizabeth H. Williams, MD

The morning of surgery:

Take a shower or wash the surgical area again with antibacterial soap. Work into lather and clean your body or the surgical site with a clean, fresh washcloth. Again, rinse thoroughly. Dry your body with a clean, fresh towel, and put on clean, fresh clothes.

Additional Instructions:

1. DO NOT eat or drink anything after midnight the day before surgery, or the morning of surgery (except for certain morning medications). This includes candy, mints, coffee, water, gum, and cigarettes.

2. DO NOT wear any jewelry, makeup, nail polish, hair clips, or contact lenses the day of surgery. Bring your contact lens case and cleaning solution to the hospital if you wear contacts.

3. DO NOT bring any valuables with you to the hospital or they will have to be placed with security or left with the accompanying person.

4. It is recommended that you wear loose, comfortable clothing to the hospital the day of surgery. Wear something that is loose enough to fit over the operated site, which may have a bandage over it, especially if you are going home the same day.

5. Plan to arrive at the hospital 2 hours prior to your surgery time as told by your doctor's office.

6. If you are having OUTPATIENT SURGERY, it is REQUIRED that you have a responsible person provide you with transportation after surgery, and someone must be able to stay with you 24 hours following surgery. You cannot take the bus or a taxicab home alone.

7. If you are staying overnight after your surgery, you will be transported to your room after a short stay in the recovery room.

8. ALL patients for ALL surgeries REQUIRE pre-testing unless otherwise told by your surgeon. Additional pre-testing information will be given to you.

9. Please call our office if you have any further questions or concerns.

X-RAY EXAMINATIONS RECORD

X-RAY EXAMINATIONS RECORD

Patient	Date	Type X-Ray	No. Taken	Referring Doctor	Comments